Practical Transfusion Medicine

Practical Transfusion Medicine

FIFTH EDITION

Edited By

Michael F. Murphy, MD, FRCP, FRCPath, FFPath
Professor of Blood Transfusion Medicine
University of Oxford
Consultant Haematologist
NHS Blood and Transplant and Department of Haematology, Oxford University Hospitals
Oxford, UK

David J. Roberts, MB, ChB, D.Phil, FRCPath
Professor of Haematology
University of Oxford
Consultant Haematologist
NHS Blood and Transplant and Department of Haematology, Oxford University Hospitals
Oxford, UK

Mark H. Yazer, MD
Professor of Pathology
University of Pittsburgh
Adjunct Professor of Clinical Immunology
University of Southern Denmark
Odense, Denmark
Medical Director
RBC Serology Reference Laboratory, ITXM Centralized Transfusion Service
Associate Medical Director
ITXM Centralized Transfusion Service
Pittsburgh, USA

WILEY Blackwell

Registered Offices
John Wiley & Sons, Inc., 111 River Street, Hoboken, NJ 07030, USA
John Wiley & Sons Ltd, The Atrium, Southern Gate, Chichester, West Sussex, PO19 8SQ, UK

Editorial Office
9600 Garsington Road, Oxford, OX4 2DQ, UK
For details of our global editorial offices, customer services, and more information about Wiley products visit us at www.wiley.com.

Wiley also publishes its books in a variety of electronic formats and by print-on-demand. Some content that appears in standard print versions of this book may not be available in other formats.

Library of Congress Cataloging-in-Publication Data

Names: Murphy, Michael F. (Michael Furber), editor. | Roberts, David J. (David John)
    (Consultant hematologist), editor. | Yazer, Mark H., editor.
Title: Practical transfusion medicine / edited by Michael F. Murphy, David J. Roberts, Mark H. Yazer.
Description: Fifth edition. | Hoboken, NJ : John Wiley & Sons Inc., 2017. |
    Preceded by Practical transfusion medicine / edited by Michael F. Murphy,
    Derwood H. Pamphilon, Nancy M. Heddle. 4th ed. 2013. |
    Includes bibliographical references and index.
Identifiers: LCCN 2016053360 | ISBN 9781119129417 (cloth) | ISBN 9781119129448 (Adobe pdf) |
    ISBN 9781119129424 (epub)
Subjects: | MESH: Blood Transfusion | Blood Grouping and Crossmatching |
    Hematopoietic Stem Cell Transplantation | Blood Preservation |
    Cross Infection–prevention & control
Classification: LCC RM171 | NLM WB 356 | DDC 615.3/9–dc23
LC record available at https://lccn.loc.gov/2016053360

Set in 10/12pt Warnock by SPi Global, Pondicherry, India

Printed in Singapore by C.O.S. Printers Pte Ltd

10 9 8 7 6 5 4 3 2 1

Contents

List of Contributors

Louis H. Alarcon
Professor of Departments
of Surgery and Critical
Care Medicine, University
of Pittsburgh School of
Medicine, Pittsburgh, USA

Jean Pierre Allain
NHS Blood and Transplant
and Division of Transfusion
Medicine,
Department of Hematology,
University of Cambridge,
Cambridge, UK

Imelda Bates
Professor of Clinical
Tropical Haematology,
Liverpool School of
Tropical Medicine,
Liverpool, UK

Ravishankar Rao Baikady
Consultant in Anaesthesia,
The Royal Marsden,
NHS Foundation Trust,
London, UK

Neil Blumberg
Department of Pathology
and Laboratory Medicine,
University of Rochester;
Blood Bank/Transfusion
Service of Strong Memorial
Hospital, Rochester, USA

Franklin Bontempo
University of Pittsburgh
Medical Center, Pittsburgh,
USA;
Institute for Transfusion
Medicine, Pittsburgh, USA

Colin J. Brown
NHS Blood and Transplant,
Histocompatibility and
Immunogenetics Services,
Colindale Centre, London,
UK

Susan J. Brunskill
NHS Blood and Transplant,
Systematic Review Initiative,
Oxford, UK

Rebecca Cardigan
NHS Blood and Transplant,
Cambridge, UK

Akila Chandrasekar
NHS Blood and Transplant,
Tissue and Eye Services,
Liverpool, UK

Irina Chibisov
University of Pittsburgh
Medical Center, Pittsburgh,
USA;
Institute for Transfusion
Medicine, Pittsburgh,
USA

Nicola Curry
Oxford Haemophilia &
Thrombosis Centre, Churchill
Hospital, Oxford, UK

Brian R. Curtis
Platelet and Neutrophil
Immunology Laboratory and
Blood Research Institute,
Blood Center of Wisconsin,
Milwaukee, USA

Robert D. Danby
Churchill Hospital, Oxford
University Hospitals NHS
Foundation Trust, Oxford,
UK

Geoff Daniels
International Blood Group
Reference Laboratory, NHS
Blood and Transplant,
Bristol, UK

Robertson D. Davenport
University of Michigan Health
System, Ann Arbor,
USA

Meghan Delaney
Bloodworks Northwest and
Department of Laboratory
Medicine and Paediatrics,
University of Washington,
Seattle, USA

Roger Y. Dodd
American Red Cross, Jerome
H. Holland Laboratory for
the Biomedical Sciences,
Rockville, USA

Carolyn Dorée
NHS Blood and Transplant,
Systematic Review Initiative,
Oxford, UK

Katharine A. Downes
Medical Director of
Transfusion Medicine,
University Hospitals,
Cleveland Medical Center;
Associate Professor of
Pathology, Case Western
Reserve University,
Cleveland, OH

Walter H. "Sunny" Dzik
Department of Pathology
and Medicine, Massachusetts
General Hospital,
Harvard Medical School,
Boston, USA

Khaled El-Ghariani
NHS Blood and Transplant
and Sheffield Teaching
Hospitals NHS Trust and
University of Sheffield,
Sheffield, UK

Lise J. Estcourt
NHS Blood and Transplant,
John Radcliffe Hospital,
Oxford, UK; Radcliffe
Department of Medicine,
University of Oxford,
Oxford, UK

Dean Fergusson
Senior Scientist, University
of Ottawa Center for
Transfusion Research,

Clinical Epidemiology
Program, Ottawa, Canada;
Health Research Institute,
Ottawa, Canada

Stephen P. Field
Welsh Blood Service,
Pontyclun, Wales, UK

Peter Flanagan
New Zealand Blood Service,
Auckland, New Zealand

Ronan Foley
Department of Pathology
and Molecular Medicine,
McMaster University,
Hamilton, Canada

Richard O. Francis
Assistant Professor,
Department of Pathology
and Cell Biology, Columbia
University College of
Physicians and Surgeons,
New York, USA;
Director, Special Hematology
and Coagulation Laboratory
New York Presbyterian
Hospital – Columbia
University Medical Center,
New York,
USA

Steven M. Frank
Department of
Anesthesiology/Critical Care
Medicine, Johns Hopkins
Medical Institutions,
Baltimore, USA

Mark K. Fung
Department of Pathology
and Laboratory Medicine,
University of Vermont
Medical Center,
Burlington, USA

Marc Germain
Héma-Québec, Quebec City,
Canada

Mindy Goldman
Medical Director,
Donor and Clinical Services,
Canadian Blood Services,
Medical Services and
Innovation, Ottawa,
Canada

Lawrence Tim Goodnough
Departments of Pathology
and Medicine, Stanford
University, Stanford,
USA

Andreas Greinacher
Department of Immunology
and Transfusion Medicine,
Universitätsmedizin
Greifswald, Greifswald,
Germany

Joanna M. Heal
Department of Pathology
and Laboratory Medicine,
University of Rochester;
Blood Bank/Transfusion
Service of Strong
Memorial Hospital,
Rochester, USA

Paul C. Hébert
Professor, Department of
Medicine, Centre Hospitalier
de L'Université de Montreal;
Centre Recherche de le
Centre Hospitalier de
Montreal, Montreal, Canada

Nancy M. Heddle
Department of Medicine,
McMaster University and
Canadian Blood Services,
Hamilton, Ontario, Canada

John R. Hess
Professor of Laboratory
Medicine and Hematology,
University of Washington
School of Medicine,
Seattle, USA; Director,
Harborview Transfusion
Service, Seattle, USA

Christopher D. Hillyer
Chief Executive Officer,
New York Blood Center,
New York, USA;
Weill Cornell Medical
College, New York, USA

Daniel Hollyman
Diagnostics Development and
Reference Services, NHS Blood
and Transplant, Bristol,
UK

Sally Hopewell
Oxford Clinical Trials
Research Unit, University of
Oxford, Oxford, UK

Rachael Hough
University College London
Hospital's NHS Foundation
Trust, London, UK

Seema Kacker
Medical Student, The Johns
Hopkins University School
of Medicine and Bloomberg
School of Public Health,
Baltimore, USA

Louis M. Katz
Chief Medical Officer,
America's Blood Centers,
Washington, DC, USA;
Adjunct Clinical Professor,
Infectious Diseases, Carver
College of Medicine,
University of Iowa Healthcare,
Iowa City, USA

Richard M. Kaufman
Brigham and Women's
Hospital, Boston,
USA

John N. Kearney
NHS Blood and Transplant,
Tissue and Eye Services,
Liverpool, UK

Alan D. Kitchen
National Transfusion
Microbiology Laboratory
and NHS Blood and
Transplant, Colindale,
London, UK

Steven H. Kleinman
University of British
Columbia, Victoria,
Canada

Daryl J. Kor
Mayo Clinic, Rochester,
USA

Marissa Li
United Blood Services,
Ventura, USA

Mark W. Lowdell
Professor of Cell and
Tissue Therapy, University
College London; Director of
Cellular Therapy, Honorary
Consultant Scientist, Royal
Free London NHS Foundation
Trust, London, UK

Edwin J. Massey
NHS Blood and Transplant,
Bristol, UK

Ellen McSweeney
Irish Blood Transfusion
Service, National Blood Centre,
Dublin, Republic of Ireland

Jay E. Menitove
Director and CEO, Greater
Kansas City Blood Center,
Kansas City, USA (Retired)

Hira Mian
Department of Oncology,
McMaster University,
Hamilton, Ontario

Siraj A. Misbah
Oxford University Hospitals,
University of Oxford, Oxford,
UK

Emma Morris
Professor of Clinical Cell
& Gene Therapy, UCL
Institute of Immunity
and Transplantation,
London, UK

William G. Murphy
Irish Blood Transfusion
Service, and University
College Dublin, Dublin,
Republic of Ireland

Gavin J. Murphy
British Heart Foundation
Professor of Cardiac Surgery,
School of Cardiovascular
Sciences, University of
Leicester, Leicester, UK

Cristina V. Navarrete
NHS Blood and Transplant,
Histocompatibility and
Immunogenetics Services,
Colindale Centre, London, UK;
University College London,
London, UK

Matthew D. Neal
Assistant Professor of
Departments of Surgery
and Critical Care Medicine,

University of Pittsburgh School of Medicine, Pittsburgh, USA

Paul M. Ness
Director, Transfusion Medicine Division: Professor, Pathology and Medicine, Johns Hopkins Medical Institutions, Baltimore, USA

Enrico M. Novelli
Division of Hematology/ Oncology, Vascular Medicine Institute, University of Pittsburgh, Pittsburgh, USA

Pamela O'Hoski
Department of Pathology and Molecular Medicine, McMaster University, Hamilton, Canada

Nishith N. Patel
Clinical Research Fellow in Cardiac Surgery, School of Clinical Sciences, University of Bristol, Bristol, UK

Rachel Protheroe
Bristol Adult Bone Marrow Transplant Unit, University Hospitals Bristol, Bristol, UK

Lirong Qu
Department of Pathology, University of Pittsburgh, Pittsburgh, USA; Institute for Transfusion Medicine, Pittsburgh, USA

Sandra Ramírez-Arcos
Development Scientist, Canadian Blood Services, Medical Services and Innovation, Ottawa, Canada

Majed A. Refaai
Department of Pathology and Laboratory Medicine, University of Rochester; Blood Bank/Transfusion Service of Strong Memorial Hospital, Rochester, USA

Toby Richards
Professor of Surgery, University College London, London, UK

Martin Rooms
Consultant in Anaesthesia, The Royal Marsden, NHS Foundation Trust, London, UK

Paul Rooney
NHS Blood and Transplant, Tissue and Eye Services, Liverpool, UK

Amy E. Schmidt
Department of Pathology and Laboratory Medicine, University of Rochester; Blood Bank/Transfusion Service of Strong Memorial Hospital, Rochester, USA

Neil Shah
Department of Pathology, Stanford University, Stanford, USA

Beth H. Shaz
Chief Medical and Scientific Officer, New York Blood Center, New York, USA; Columbia University Medical Center, New York, USA

Andrew W. Shih
Department of Pathology and Molecular Medicine,

Transfusion Medicine Fellowship Program, McMaster University, Hamilton, Canada

Edward L. Snyder
Director, Transfusion Medicine Service, Cellular Therapy Center, Yale-New Haven Medical Center, Yale University, New Haven, Connecticut, USA

Simon J. Stanworth
NHS Blood and Transplant, Oxford University Hospitals, Oxford, UK; Department of Hematology, Oxford University Hospitals, Oxford, UK; Radcliffe Department of Medicine, University of Oxford, Oxford, UK

Susan L. Stramer
American Red Cross, Scientific Support Office, Gaithersburg, USA

Ronald G. Strauss
Professor Emeritus, Department of Pathology and Pediatrics, University of Iowa College of Medicine, Iowa City, USA; Associate Medical Director, LifeSource/ITxM, Chicago, USA

Zbigniew (Ziggy) M. Szczepiorkowski
Transfusion Medicine Service, Cellular Therapy Center, Dartmouth-Hitchcock Medical Center and Geisel School of Medicine at Dartmouth, Hanover, USA

Stephen Thomas
Assistant Director –
Manufacturing Development,
NHS Blood and Transplant,
Watford, UK

Alan T. Tinmouth
Head, Division of
Hematology, Department
of Medicine, Ottawa Hospital,
Ottawa, Canada; Scientist,
University of Ottawa Centre
for Transfusion Research,
Clinical Epidemiology
Program, Ottawa Health
Research Institute, Ottawa,
Canada

Aaron A. R. Tobian
Associate Professor of
Pathology, Medicine and
Epidemiology,
The Johns Hopkins University
School of Medicine and
Bloomberg School of Public
Health, The Johns Hopkins
University, Baltimore, USA

Darrell J. Triulzi
Department of Pathology,
University of Pittsburgh,
Pittsburgh, USA; Institute
for Transfusion Medicine,
Pittsburgh, USA

S. Marieke van Ham
Head, Department of
Immunopathology,
Sanquin Research,
Landsteiner Laboratory,
Academic Medical Center,
and SILS, Faculty of
Science, University of
Amsterdam, Amsterdam,
The Netherlands

Ralph Vassallo
Adjunct Associate Professor
of Medicine, Perelman School
of Medicine at the University
of Pennsylvania, Philadelphia

Timothy S. Walsh
Professor of Critical Care,
Clinical and Surgical Sciences,
Edinburgh University,
Edinburgh, Scotland, UK;
Anaesthetics and Intensive
Care, Edinburgh Royal
Infirmary, Edinburgh,
Scotland, UK

Theodore E. Warkentin
Department of Pathology
and Molecular Medicine
and Department of
Medicine, Michael G.
DeGroote School of
Medicine, McMaster
University, Hamilton,
Canada; Transfusion
Medicine, Hamilton
Regional Laboratory
Medicine Program
and Service of Clinical
Hematology, Hamilton
Health Sciences, Hamilton,
Ontario, Canada

Jack O. Wasey
Department of
Anesthesiology/Critical Care
Medicine, Johns Hopkins
Medical Institutions,
Baltimore, USA

Jonathan H. Waters
Department of Anesthesiology,
Magee Womens Hospital
of UPMC, Pittsburgh,
USA; Departments of

Anesthesiology and
Bioengineering, University of
Pittsburgh, Pittsburgh, USA;
Patient Blood Management
program of UPMC;
Acute Interventional Pain
Program of UPMC

Barbee I. Whitaker
Senior Director, Research
and American Association
of Blood Banks Center
for Patient Safety,
Bethesda, USA

Kathryn E. Webert
Canadian Blood Services,
and Department of Medicine
and Department of Pathology
and Molecular Medicine,
McMaster University,
Hamilton, Ontario, Canada

Erica M. Wood
Transfusion Research Unit,
Department of Epidemiology
and Preventive Medicine,
Monash University,
Melbourne, Australia;
Department of Clinical
Hematology, Monash Health,
Melbourne, Australia

Jaap Jan Zwaginga
Jon J. van Rood Center
for Clinical Transfusion
Research, Sanquin, Leiden
and the Department of
Immunohematology and
Blood Transfusion, Leiden
University Medical Center,
Leiden, The Netherlands

Preface

The pace of change in transfusion medicine is relentless, with new scientific and technological developments and continuing efforts to improve clinical transfusion practice through patient blood management (PBM), which implores us to use the best available evidence when optimising pre-, peri- and post-operative management to reduce anaemia, prevent blood loss and reduce the need for transfusions. This fifth edition has become necessary because of rapid changes in transfusion medicine since the fourth edition was published in 2013.

The primary purpose of the fifth edition remains the same as the first: to provide a comprehensive guide to transfusion medicine. This book aims to include information in more depth than contained within handbooks of transfusion medicine and yet to present that information in a more concise and approachable manner than seen in more formal standard reference texts. The feedback we have received from reviews and colleagues is that these objectives continue to be achieved and that this book has a consistent style and format. We have again striven to maintain this in the fifth edition to provide a text that will be useful to the many clinical and scientific staff, both established practitioners and trainees, who are involved in some aspect of transfusion medicine and require an accessible text.

We considered that this book had become big enough for its purpose, and the number of chapters has only been increased by one from 48 to 49. It is divided into seven sections that systematically take the reader through the principles of transfusion medicine, complications of transfusion, practice in blood centres and hospitals, clinical transfusion practice, PBM, cellular and tissue therapy and organ transplantation and development of the evidence base for transfusion. The final chapter on *Scanning the Future of Transfusion Medicine* has generated much interest, and it has been updated for this edition by three new authors.

We wish to continue to develop the content and to refresh the style of this book and are very pleased to welcome Professors David Roberts and Mark Yazer as co-editors. The authorship likewise has become more international with each successive edition to provide a broad perspective. We are very grateful to the colleagues who have contributed to this book at a time of continuing challenges and change. Once again, we acknowledge the enormous support we have received from our publishers, particularly James Schultz and Claire Bonnett.

1 Introduction: Two Centuries of Progress in Transfusion Medicine

Walter H. (Sunny) Dzik[1] and Michael F. Murphy[2]

[1] Department of Pathology and Medicine, Massachusetts General Hospital, Harvard Medical School, Boston, USA
[2] University of Oxford; NHS Blood and Transplant and Department of Haematology, Oxford University Hospitals, Oxford, UK

'States of the body really requiring the infusion of blood into the veins are probably rare; yet we sometimes meet with cases in which the patient must die unless such operation can be performed'. So begins James Blundell's 'Observations on transfusion of blood' published in *The Lancet*, marking the origins of transfusion medicine as a clinical discipline. Blundell (Figure 1.1) was a prominent London obstetrician who witnessed peripartum haemorrhage and whose interest in transfusion had begun as early as 1817 during his medical education in Edinburgh. He established that transfusions should not be conducted across species barriers and noted that resuscitation from haemorrhage could be achieved using a volume of transfusion that was smaller than the estimated blood loss. Despite life-saving results in some patients, clinical experience with transfusion was restricted by lack of understanding of ABO blood groups – a barrier that would not be resolved for another century.

The Nobel Prize-winning work of Karl Landsteiner (Figure 1.2) established the primacy of ABO blood group compatibility and set the stage for safer transfusion practice. Twentieth-century transfusion was advanced by the leadership of many physicians, scientists and technologists and repeatedly incorporated new diagnostics (monoclonal antibodies, genomics) and new therapeutics (plasma fractionation, apheresis and recombinant proteins) to improve patient care.

Today, the field of transfusion medicine is composed of a diverse range of disciplines including the provision of a safe blood supply; the fields of haemostasis, immunology, transplantation and cellular engineering; apheresis technology; treatment using recombinant and plasma-derived plasma proteins; and the daily use of blood components in clinical medicine (Figure 1.3). Without transfusion resources, very little of modern surgery and medicine could be accomplished.

For decades, the challenge of transmitting new information in transfusion fell to Dr Patrick Mollison (Figure 1.4) whose textbook became the standard of its era. Mollison highlighted the importance of both laboratory practice (immunohaematology, haemostasis, complement biology) and clinical medicine in our field. *Practical Transfusion Medicine*, here in its fifth edition, seeks to build on that tradition and to give readers the foundation knowledge required to contribute both academically and clinically to our discipline. For readers about to enjoy the content of this book, the following provides a sampling of the topics presented within the text by leading experts in our field.

Practical Transfusion Medicine, Fifth Edition. Edited by Michael F. Murphy, David J. Roberts and Mark H. Yazer.
© 2017 John Wiley & Sons Ltd. Published 2017 by John Wiley & Sons Ltd.

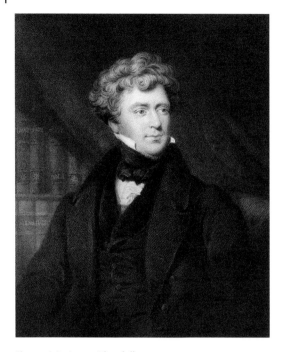

Figure 1.1 James Blundell.

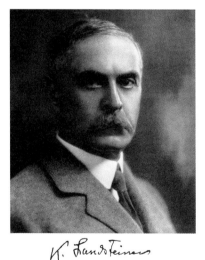

Figure 1.2 Karl Landsteiner.

Blood Donation Worldwide

Each year, approximately 100 million blood donations are made worldwide (Figure 1.5). A safe and adequate blood supply is now an

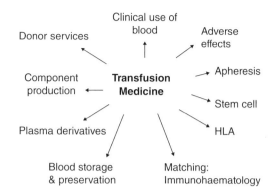

Figure 1.3 The range of transfusion medicine.

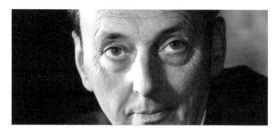

Figure 1.4 Patrick Mollison. *Source:* Garratty, Transfusion 2012;52:684–85. Reproduced with permission of John Wiley & Sons.

essential infrastructure requirement of any modern national healthcare system. The recruitment and retention of healthy blood donors is a vital activity of the field and the challenges and responsibilities faced by stewards of the blood supply are presented to readers in Chapters 18–22. Whilst the economically advantaged nations of the world have established all volunteer donor programmes with great success, data from the World Health Organization presented in Chapter 24 document that blood donation rates per capita in many low-income nations are insufficient to meet their needs. More research and investment is required so that all regions of the world can rely upon an adequate supply of safe blood.

Changing Landscape of Transfusion Risks

During the final two decades of the twentieth century, intense focus on screening blood donations for infectious diseases led to substantial

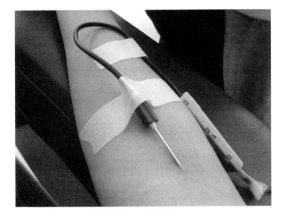

Figure 1.5 Blood donation.

progress in blood safety and a significant reduction in the risk of transfusion-transmitted diseases (Figure 1.6). Chapters 15–17 present an authoritative summary of this success. We currently enjoy a grace period when the risk of transfusion-transmitted infections is at an all-time low. However, progressive encroachment of humans upon the animal kingdom is expected to result in the emergence of new infections that cross species barriers. Haemovigilance, robust screening technologies and chemical pathogen inactivation are all being applied to address this concern and are reviewed within the text.

With the advent of the twenty-first century, the landscape of transfusion risk shifted its emphasis towards non-infectious hazards (Figure 1.7). Recent years have focused on improved understanding and prevention of transfusion-related acute lung injury, a topic covered in detail in Chapter 10. More recently, we have learned that circulatory overload from

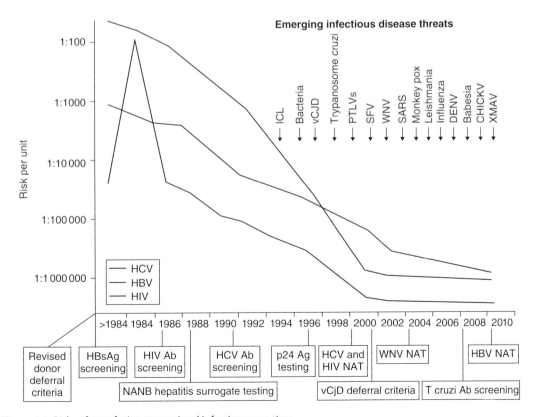

Figure 1.6 Risks of transfusion-transmitted infections over time.

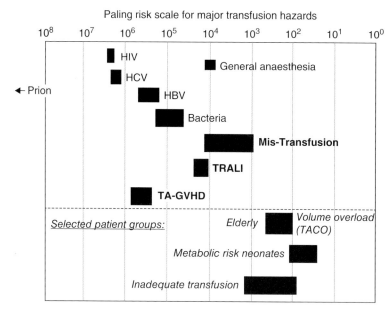

Figure 1.7 Paling scale of transfusion risk.

excessive transfusion is far more common than previously recognised. Yet Blundell himself specifically warned of it in his first description of transfusion: 'to observe with attention the countenance of the patient, and to guard ... against an overcharge of the heart' [1]. In addition, haemolytic reactions remain a serious hazard of transfusion. It is quite surprising that despite unimagined advances in internet connectivity, most nations still do not have a system for sharing patient blood group results or antibody profiles between hospitals, thereby failing to share information that would prevent acute and delayed reactions. Much can still be done to further reduce non-infectious hazards of transfusion. Readers will find that Chapters 7–17 provide state-of-the-art summaries of our current understanding regarding the full range of adverse effects and complications of transfusion.

Immunohaematology

Knowledge of the location and functional role of red cell surface proteins that display blood group epitopes has brought order out of what was once a chaotic assembly of information in blood group serology (Figure 1.8). Readers will enjoy an up-to-date treatment of this topic in Chapters 2–6.

Today, red cell genomics has become a practical clinical tool and DNA diagnostics in immunohaematology extends far beyond the reach of erythrocyte blood groups. Genotyping has always been the preferred method for defining members of the human platelet antigen system and is well established for HLA genes in the field of histocompatibility (Figure 1.9). The clinical practice of transfusion medicine is now supported by DNA diagnostics targeting a wide range of genes, including those coding for complement proteins, human neutrophil antigens, haemoglobin polymorphisms and coagulation factors.

Despite advances in defining antigens, both clinical illness and blood group incompatibilities remain dominated by antibody responses of the patient. A robust form of antibody analysis and better control of the immune response remain important frontiers of our field. The ability to downregulate specific alloimmune responses would revolutionise the approach to

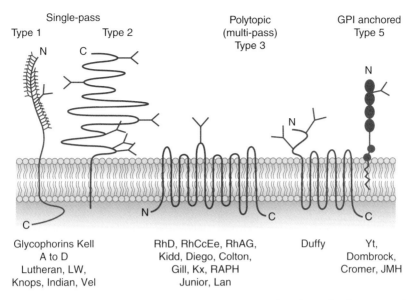

Figure 1.8 Red blood cell antigens. *Source:* Daniels G, Bromilow I. Essential Guide to Blood Groups, 3rd edn. Wiley: Chichester, 2014. Reproduced with permission of John Wiley & Sons.

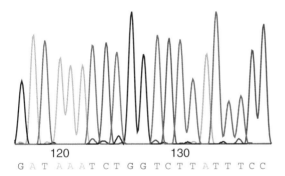

Figure 1.9 DNA sequence.

solid organ transplantation, haemophilia complicated by inhibitors, platelet refractoriness, red cell allosensitisation, haemolytic disease of the newborn and a host of other challenges that confront transfusion specialists every day.

In the meantime, we can offer patients powerful, yet nonspecific immune suppressants. And while the focus of many treatments is on reduction of pathological antibodies, it is increasingly clear that antibodies themselves do not injure tissues nearly as much as the complement proteins that antibodies attract.

Complement is at the centre of a wide variety of disorders, including drug-mediated haemolysis or thrombocytopenia, severe alloimmune or autoimmune haemolysis, cryoglobulinaemic vasculitis, HLA antibody-mediated platelet refractoriness and organ rejection, paroxysmal nocturnal haemoglobinuria, atypical haemolytic-uremic syndrome, hereditary angioedema, glomerulonephritis and age-related macular degeneration. With the development in the future of better agents to suppress complement, it can be anticipated that the focus of treatment may shift from removal of pathological antibodies to control of their effect.

Clinical Use of Blood Components: Evolution Based on Evidence

Recent years have witnessed a growing body of evidence derived from clinical research and focused on the proper use of blood components (Figure 1.10). While such research has lagged for plasma products, progress has been made for both red cells and platelets. Ever since the landmark publication of the TRICC trial by Hebert and others [2], clinical investigators have repeatedly challenged the traditional 100 g/L haemoglobin threshold for red cell transfusion. There are now at least 11 well-designed, sufficiently powered randomised controlled trials documenting that a conservative haemoglobin threshold for red cell transfusion is as beneficial

for patient outcomes as a more liberal threshold (Figure 1.11). These studies cut across a broad range of patient categories from infants to the elderly. As a result, in hospitals worldwide, red cell use is more conservative and transfusions are now withheld in nonbleeding patients until the haemoglobin concentration falls to 70 g/L. Looking ahead, we anticipate that future clinical research will seek to further refine the indication for red cells by addressing the fact that the haemoglobin concentration is but one dimension of tissue oxygenation and that the decision to transfuse red cells should include measures of both oxygen delivery and tissue oxygen consumption.

The last decade has also witnessed evidence-based refinements in the indication for platelet transfusion. The modern era of evidence begins with the work of Rebulla et al [3] who documented that a platelet threshold of $10 \times 10^9/L$ was equivalent to $20 \times 10^9/L$ for prophylactic platelet transfusions. Further advances came with the TRAP trial [4], demonstrating that reducing the number of leucocytes (and not the number of donors) was key to preventing HLA alloimmunisation, and the PLADO trial [5] which demonstrated that the traditional dose of platelets (approximately equivalent of that found in 4–6 units of whole blood) resulted in the same outcome as transfusion of three units or

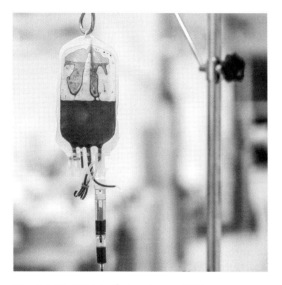

Figure 1.10 RBC transfusion. *Source:* REX by Shutterstock. © Garo.

Randomised trials of RCB transfusion threshold

Author	Name	Setting	Trigger	'n'
Hebert, 1999	TRIC	Adult ICU	7 vs 9	836
Kirpalami, 2006	PINT	Infants <1 kg	10 vs 12	457
Lacroix, 2007	---	Paediatric ICU	7 vs 9.5	637
Hajjar, 2010	TRAC	Cardiac surgery	8 vs 10	502
Cooper, 2011	CRIT	Acute MI (pilot)	8 vs 10	45
Carson, 2011	FOCUS	Hip surgery elderly	8 vs 10	2,016
Villaneuva, 2013	---	UGI bleed	7 vs 9	921
Walsh, 2013	RELIEVE	Older patients ICU	7 vs 9	100
Robertson, 2014	---	Traumatic brain	7 vs 10	200
Holst, 2014	TRISS	Septic shock	7 vs 9	998
Murphy, 2015	---	Cardiac surgery	7.5 vs 9	2,007

Figure 1.11 Trials examining the RBC transfusion threshold.

12 units as judged by the proportion of days with grade 2 or higher bleeding. Finally, the TOPPS trial [6] revealed that there was little value to prophylactic platelets among clinically stable patients undergoing autologous bone marrow transplantation. The goal now is to conduct more research on platelet transfusion outside the context of haematological malignancy. While we still have much more to do if we are to refine the clinical use of the traditional blood components, Chapters 34–37 on patient blood management and 45–46 in the section on developing the evidence base for transfusion should give readers a solid foundation upon which to improve clinical decisions regarding transfusion.

Urgent Transfusion

Care of the haemorrhaging patient has always been an essential aspect of transfusion practice. The tragedies of war and human conflict have repeatedly stimulated research focused on urgent transfusion during haemorrhage. Demand for knowledge in this area sadly continues and is amplified within violent societies by civilian trauma from firearms and in other societies by automobile injury. This is an area of changing practice patterns and readers will welcome the up-to-date focus found in Chapters 26 and 27. With the advent of increasingly complex surgery and deployment of life support systems such as extracorporeal membrane oxygenators, massive transfusion is no longer restricted to trauma. In fact, recent studies document that the majority of massive transfusion episodes are associated with surgical and medical conditions unrelated to trauma [7]. More research in these patient groups is needed.

Patients Requiring Chronic Transfusion Support

Chapters 29 and 30 address the needs of patients with haematological disorders who often require chronic transfusion support (Figure 1.12). Patients with haemoglobinopathies, thalassaemia,

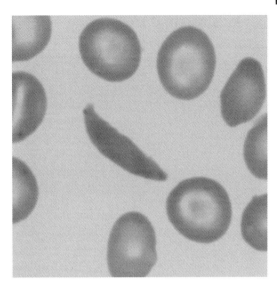

Figure 1.12 Sickle cell anaemia.

myelodysplastic syndromes, aplastic anaemia, refractory anaemia, congenital and acquired haemolytic anaemia and those with chronic bleeding disorders such as hereditary haemorrhagic telangiectasia depend upon transfusion to sustain them. Worldwide, the numbers of individuals with severe uncorrectable anaemia is enormous. For these conditions, blood transfusion is seen at its raw, primal best: the sharing of blood from those in good health to those in need.

Obstetric, Neonatal and Paediatric Transfusion Medicine

Care of the low-birthweight, premature infant remains very challenging. Anaemia and thrombocytopenia result from physiology unique to these youngest of patients, as described in Chapter 33. Neonatal and paediatric transfusion medicine is filled with customary practices often based more on tradition than evidence. We applaud those who have conducted controlled trials that are summarised within the text, and look forward to additional clinical research designed to answer fundamental questions that confront the paediatric transfusion specialist.

Haemostasis and Transfusion

No area of transfusion medicine has seen such explosive recent innovation as the field of haemostasis. A wide range of anticoagulants is now available and the balance between anticoagulation, haemostasis and thrombophilia has become more complex. Transfusion therapy continues a long evolution from plasma replacement to the targeted use of a growing number of plasma-derived or recombinant products that influence haemostasis. Tools and treatments used in the past and then put aside, such as viscoelastic testing and antifibrinolytics, have made a strong resurgence and are finding new positions in the evaluation and treatment of bleeding. Additional haemostasis agents, which we will need to clinically master, are on the way. Chapters 25, 28 and 31 address these topics and will give readers new information on the important role of transfusion in the care of patients with disorders of haemostasis and thrombosis.

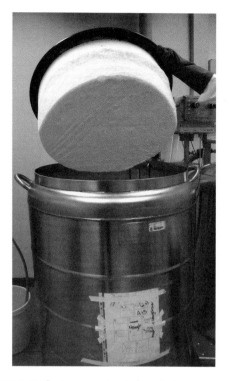

Figure 1.13 Cryopreservation in liquid nitrogen.

Cellular Therapies, Transplantation, Apheresis

Cellular therapy is a major growth area in transfusion medicine. The ability to mobilise haematopoietic progenitor cells, then harvest them safely in bulk numbers, process, freeze and successfully reinfuse them as a stem cell tissue transplant has completely revolutionised the field of bone marrow transplantation (Figure 1.13). Other therapeutic areas, such as treatment with harvested and manipulated dendritic cells, mesenchymal cells, T-cells and antigen-presenting cells, have progressed far more slowly. Nevertheless, with advances in gene engineering, the potential to treat illnesses with autologous reengineered cellular therapies is very bright. Chapters 38–44 present a detailed account of the current state of the art in cellular therapies as well as a glimpse of where this field is heading.

The Future

This fifth edition of this textbook concludes, as have previous editions, with reflections on the future of the field. While speculation on the future is never easy, our own view is that the ability to perform targeted gene editing is one of the most promising current research endeavours. CRISPR (clustered regularly interspaced short palindromic repeats) technology allows for the targeted excision of DNA at any known sequence (Figure 1.14).

Short tandem repeat DNA sequences (eventually renamed as CRISPR) were originally discovered as part of normal bacterial defence against viruses. Several genes in bacteria, called CRISPR-associated genes (cas), were found to code for nucleases specific for these repeat sequences, thereby disrupting viral genomes within bacteria. One of these cas genes, *Cas9*, was found to work efficiently within eukaryotic cells as a nuclease

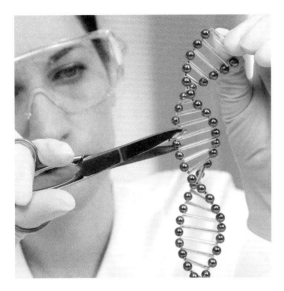

Figure 1.14 CRISPR technology allows targeted excision of DNA. *Source:* Shutterstock. © GeK.

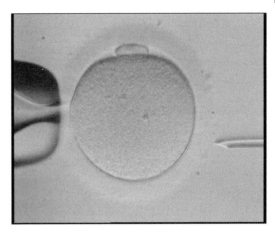

Figure 1.15 Cellular therapies of the future.

that could be guided by RNA to a specific DNA target. This RNA guide can be synthesised to match the cellular DNA area of choice. By delivering the *Cas9* nuclease and the guiding RNA into a cell, the genome of that cell can be disrupted or edited in a controlled manner.

One example of the application of CRISPR technology has focused on haemoglobin F production [8]. The *BCL11A* gene is the natural suppressor of haemoglobin F. *BCL11A* is turned on after birth, resulting in active downregulation of haemoglobin F transcription. CRISPR technology has been used to disrupt the promoter region of the *BCL11A* gene, thus removing its suppression with a resulting increase in haemoglobin F production. This approach has an obvious potential application in sickle cell disease where even a small increase in haemoglobin F expression can ameliorate

clinical symptoms. One can imagine the *ex vivo* manipulation of autologous CD34-positive cells using CRISPR technology followed by their transplantation into the sickle cell patient so as to produce a posttransplant phenotype with higher haemoglobin F expression (Figure 1.15).

Conclusion

James Blundell would immediately recognise a red cell transfusion if he saw one today. However, the great part of what we do would be incomprehensibly advanced and far beyond his understanding. In a similar way, the technologies of the future will revolutionise medical care in ways we can hardly imagine. Let us look forward to a time when we can reflect back on nonspecific immune suppression, apheresis therapy, blood group incompatibilities and one-dimensional laboratory triggers for transfusion care as practices that we needed to understand today so that we could achieve the promise of tomorrow.

References

1 Blundell J. Observations on transfusion of blood. Lancet 1828;**II**:321–4.
2 Hebert PC, Wells G, Blajchman MA et al. A multicenter, randomized, controlled clinical trial of transfusion requirements in critical care. N Engl J Med 1999;**340**:409–17.
3 Rebulla P, Finazzi G, Marangoni F et al. The threshold for prophylactic platelet transfusions

in adults with acute myeloid leukemia. N Engl J Med 1997;**337**:1870–5.

4 TRAP Trial Investigators. Leukocyte reduction and ultraviolet B irradiation of platelets to prevent alloimmunization and refractoriness to platelet transfusions. N Engl J Med 1997;**337**:1861–9.

5 Slichter SJ, Kaufman RM, Assmann SF et al. Dose of prophylactic platelet transfusions and prevention of hemorrhage. N Engl J Med 2010;**362**:600–13.

6 Stanworth SJ, Hudson CL, Estcourt LJ et al. Risk of bleeding and use of platelet transfusions in patients with hematologic malignancies: recurrent event analysis. Haematologica 2015;**100**:740–7.

7 Dzik WS, Ziman A, Cohen C et al. Survival after ultramassive transfusion: a review of 1360 cases. Transfusion 2016;**56**:558–63.

8 Canver MC, Smith EC, Sher F et al. BCL11A enhancer dissection by Cas9-mediated in situ saturating mutagenesis. Nature 2015;**527**:192–7.

2

Essential Immunology for Transfusion Medicine

Jaap Jan Zwaginga[1] and S. Marieke van Ham[2]

[1] *Jon J. van Rood Center for Clinical Transfusion Research, Sanquin, Leiden and the Department of Immunohematology and Blood Transfusion, Leiden University Medical Center, Leiden, The Netherlands*
[2] *Department of Immunopathology, Sanquin Research, Landsteiner Laboratory, Academic Medical Center, and SILS, Faculty of Science, University of Amsterdam, Amsterdam, The Netherlands*

Cellular Basis of the Immune Response

Leucocytes from the myeloid and lymphoid lineage form the different arms of the innate and adaptive immune system. Each cell type has its own unique functions.

Innate Immune Cells

Phagocytes and Antigen-Presenting Cells

Monocyte-derived macrophages, neutrophils (polymorphonuclear neutrophils, PMNs) and dendritic cells (DCs) function as phagocytes that remove dead cells and cell debris or immune complexes. In addition, these cells act as the first line of innate defence, ingesting and clearing pathogens. The first step is recognition of pathogen-derived signals (pathogen associated molecular patterns, PAMPs) or danger-derived signals from inflamed tissues (danger-associated molecular patterns, DAMPs) via pattern recognition receptors (PRR). This triggers their differentiation and expression and/or secretion of signalling proteins. Some of these proteins (such as interleukin (IL)-1, IL-6 and tumour necrosis factor (TNF)) increase acute-phase proteins that activate complement, while others (chemokines) attract circulating immune cells to the site of infection. DCs and macrophages also serve as antigen-presenting cells (APCs) that present digested proteins as antigen to specific T-cells of the lymphoid lineage. PRR ligation in this setting induces maturation of APCs with the acquisition of chemokine receptors, which allows their migration to the lymph nodes where the resting T-cells reside. Simultaneously, mature APCs acquire co-stimulatory molecules and secrete cytokines. All are needed for T-cell activation and differentiation and eventually the immune response to the specific pathogen. The type of PRR ligation determines the production of cytokines, which in turn induces the optimal pathogen class-specific immune response.

Adaptive Immune Cells

T-Lymphocytes

After migration of progenitor T-cells to the thymus epithelium, billions of T-cells are formed with billions of antigen receptor variants. Each lymphocyte expresses only one kind of heterodimeric T-cell receptor (TCR). Immature T-cells initially express a TCR receptor in complex with CD4 and CD8 molecules, which respectively interact with major histocompatibility complex (MHC) class II and class I molecules. The presentation of self-antigens within such MHC molecules on thymic stromal cells determines the fate of the immature T-cells.

First of all, these interactions induce T-cells that express only CD4 or CD8. Most important, however, is that these interactions are responsible for the removal of T-cells that have a TCR with high binding affinity for a self-antigen MHC complex. The cells that survive this so-called 'negative selection' process migrate to the secondary lymphoid organs. There, TCR-specific binding to complexes of MHC can activate them with non-self (e.g. pathogen-derived) antigens on matured APCs. Interactions between the co-stimulatory molecules CD80 and CD86 on the APC with CD28 on the T-cell subsequently drive the activated T-cells into proliferation. Without this co-stimulation (e.g. by not fully differentiated APCs or by insufficient or absent PRR ligation), T-cells become nonfunctional (anergised). The requirement of PRR-induced danger signals thus forms a second checkpoint of T-cell activation to prevent reactivity to self-antigens. Hence, the normal removal of autologous apoptotic or dead cells and cell debris by fagocytes will not lead to alloimmunization.

While immunoglobulins bind to amino acids in the context of the tertiary structure of the antigen, the TCR recognises amino acids on small digested antigen fragments in the context of an MHC molecule. MHC characteristics ensure near endless protein/antigen binding capacities and thus adaptation of the immune response to new/rapidly evolving pathogens. MHC class I is expressed on all nucleated cells and presents so-called 'endogenous' antigen-constituting self-antigens, but also antigens from viruses and other pathogens that use the replication machinery of eukaryotic cells for their propagation. Viruses and parasites (like *Plasmodium falciparum*) can hide in red blood cells because the latter lack MHC but fortunately red cells also lack the DNA replication machinery for such pathogens.

MHC class II molecules of APCs present antigenic proteins that are ingested or endocytosed from the extracellular milieu. The described antigen expression routes, however, are not absolute. Specialised DCs in this respect can also express pathogen-derived proteins that have been taken up by the DCs via the endocytic route and other extracellular-derived proteins on MHC class I to CD8+ cytotoxic T-lymphocytes (CTLs). Conversely, cytosolic proteins can become localised in the endocytic system via the process of autophagy and become expressed in MHC class II.

Paradoxically, the fact that T-cells become activated only when the specific TCR recognises alloantigens in the context of its own MHC (termed MHC restriction) seems to refute the condition whereby MHC/HLA mismatched tissue transplants are rejected. Many acceptor T-cells, however, can be activated only by a donor-specific MHC; an additional alloantigen is not needed for this. A large circulating pool of T-cells reacting with non-self MHC is usually present and explains the acute CD8-dependent rejection of non-self MHC in transplant rejection that occurs without previous immunisation.

T Helper (Th) Cells

Differentiation into Th cells is dependent on cytokines and/or plasma membrane molecules derived from the APC. Different Th subsets can be characterised by their cytokine release and their action in infected tissues. Th1 cells that release interferon (IFN)-gamma and IL-2 aid macrophages to kill intracellular pathogens upon cognate (i.e. antigen-specific) recognition of the macrophage. In addition, Th1 cells support CTL function and are required for optimal CTL memory formation. Th17 cells releasing IL-17 and IL-6 probably enhance the early innate response by activating granulocytes and seem most needed for antifungal immunity. Both Th1 and Th17 cells are drivers of strong pro-inflammatory immune responses that also induce (partly) collateral tissue damage, which might explain their association with autoimmunity. Classically, Th2 cells support B-cell differentiation and the formation of antibodies. These IL-4, -5 and -13 releasing Th2 cells, furthermore, help to kill parasites by inducing IgE production, which activates mast cells, basophils and eosinophils.

The recently defined follicular T helper cells (Tfh) have now been recognised as the main CD4 T-cell subset that supports induction and regulation of humoral immunity (antibody responses). They are required to induce IgG and IgE antibody formation and to generate long-lived immunity via induction of long-lived plasma cells and memory B-cells upon primary immunisation and upon reactivation of memory B-cells in the case of antigen re-encounter.

B-Lymphocytes

In the bone marrow, progenitor B cells divide upon local cues from stromal cells, and are directed towards acquisition of their antigen-specific B-cell receptor (BCR). With initially millions of different binding affinities of this surface-expressed immunoglobulin, immature B-cell clones that show self-antigen binding affinity are eliminated by premature stimulation. B-cells mature in the peripheral lymphoid tissues where they respond to foreign antigens via activation of the BCR. Upon receipt of additional survival signals, they proliferate and differentiate into short-lived or long-lived plasma cells that in their turn secrete immunoglobulins with identical binding specificities as the activated B-cells they are derived from. Depending on their differentiation pathway, plasma cells secrete specific classes of effector antibodies (i.e. IgM, IgD, IgG, IgA and IgE). In addition to plasma cells, memory B-cells are formed during the first antigen encounter, awaiting reactivation in a following infection.

B-Cell Activation and T-Cell-Dependent Antibody Formation

The APC function of B-cells is primarily designed to recruit specific Th cells that have previously become activated by DCs that have presented the same antigen. This process ensures that Th cells only support B-cell differentiation of those B-cells that have become activated by the same pathogen, thus minimising the risk of activation of autoreactive B-cells. Activated Th cells express CD40L, which provides co-stimulation to the B-cells. Ligation of the B-cell via the CD40 co-stimulatory molecule, together with cytokines secreted by the Th cells, modulate the direction of B-cell differentiation. The main Th subset helping B-cell differentiation are the follicular T helper cells (Tfh). In addition, they support the generation of class switched B-cells, that no longer express IgM but secrete immunoglobulins of the IgG (sub)class or IgE (see below). Some pathogens that have a repetitive structure (called thymus-independent antigens) can activate B-cells to produce IgM antibodies against mostly extracellular pathogens without T-cell help. This offers a fast response mechanism but of low affinity. Higher affinity antibody formation requires T-cell helper interactions.

Humoral Immune Response

Immunoglobulins (Igs) are in fact the secreted form of the B-cell receptor. This specific effector molecule is secreted by plasma cells. The Ig's basic structure is a roughly Y-shaped molecule made up of two identical heavy chains with four or five domains and two identical (kappa or lambda) light chains of 23 kd with two domains. Two identical highly specific antigen-binding sites (the arms of the Y) are formed by the amino terminus domains of the heavy and light chains and form the variable (Fab) domain. The specificity and variability of these antigen-binding sites are a result of two extra beta strands in these variable domains. Connected to the normal seven beta strands found in the 'constant' domains, these additional amino acid sequences form tertiary protein structures with an almost unending repertoire of different three-dimensional 'binding locks' for antigens (Figure 2.1). Both heavy chains combine with the so-called constant (Fc) region (the trunk of the Y) of the Ig, which is more or less flexibly attached to the antigen-binding part by a so-called hinge area in the heavy chains. The Fc region determines the Ig class and consequently the Ig effector function, which is different for each Ig class. Some effector Igs form higher order structures, with secreted IgA being a dimer and IgM a pentamer.

Basis of Antibody Variability

The BCR/antibody variability originates from random DNA recombination of two or three of many variable region gene segments (see Figure 2.1) resulting in an enormous B-cell

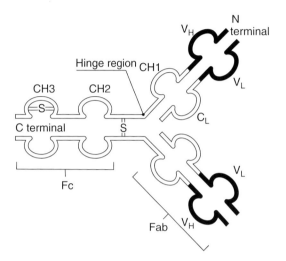

Figure 2.1 Basic structure of an immunoglobulin molecule. Domains are held in shape by disulfide bonds, though only one is shown. CH1–3, constant domains of an H chain; C_L, constant domain of a light chain; V_H, variable domain of an H chain; V_L, variable domain of a light chain.

repertoire in the bone marrow. Again, self-reactive BCRs will be deleted after which a secondary diversification of the remaining cells takes place in extrafollicular tissues or in the germinal centres of the lymphoid organs with the help of CD4 T-cell-derived signals. This consists of several sequential enzyme-driven steps leading to point mutations or so-called somatic hypermutations (SHM) of the variable regions of both the heavy and light chains. This results in B-cells with an increased affinity for the specific antigen, while others will express a BCR with a reduced affinity.

A process called affinity maturation leads to selection and survival of those B-cells with a BCR type that has the highest affinity for the antigen. Immunoglobulin (sub)class switching by helper T-cell-released cytokines induces transcription of so-called switch regions. This process enables the first produced IgM by naive B-cells to evolve into, for instance, IgG or IgE class antibodies with subclasses that determine their effector functions as well as their serum half-life and their ability for placental transfer (Table 2.1). The simultaneous regulation of SHM, affinity maturation and class switching explains why, during immune responses, the

Table 2.1 Immunoglobulin classes and their functions.

Structure				Function		
Isotype	Heavy chain	Light chain	Configuration	Complement activation*	Cells reacting with FcR	Placental passage
IgM	μ	κ, λ	Pentamer	+++	L	–
IgG1	γ1	κ, λ	Monomer	++	M, N, P, L, E	+++
IgG2	γ2	κ, λ	Monomer	+	P, L	+
IgG3	γ3	κ, λ	Monomer	+++	M, N, P, L, E	++
IgG4	γ4	κ, λ	Monomer	–	N, L, P	++
IgA1	α1	κ, λ	Monomer	+	–	–
IgA2	α2	κ, λ	Dimer in secretion	–	–	–
IgD	δ	κ, λ	Monomer	–	–	–
IgE	ε	κ, λ	Monomer	–	B, E, L	–

*Classical pathway.

B, basophils/mast cells; E, eosinophils; L, lymphocytes; M, macrophages; N, neutrophils; P, platelets.

initial IgM Igs generally show low binding affinity to the antigen, while those that are formed later on show enhanced antigen binding.

Antibody Effector Functions

While IgM only functions in circulation, IgA in this respect is mostly localised in epithelial tissues like the gut and exocrine (e.g. milk, saliva and tear producing) glands. It acts there as an early defence to pathogen invasion of these tissues and of the newborn via the mother's milk. Apart from the class, Ig functionality can also be modulated by glycosylation. Particular for the IgG heavy chain (the Fc tail) but also of the Fab binding region, glycosylation can accommodate different extensions of N-acetylglucosamine and mannose residues by galactose, sialic acid, etc. The extent and composition of these are influenced by many factors including cytokines, age, pregnancy, hormones and bacterial DNA and determine the stability and binding characteristics of the IgG. The knowledge in this area will be of major importance for engineering monoclonal antibodies and immunoglobulin preparations [1]. Finally, increasing antibody specificities and subclass changes also depend on the molecular structure of the V domains (like the predominant use of IGHV3 superspecies genes). This selective use of V genes in antibody production against a certain antigen was found in pregnancy-induced RhD immunised females who volunteered for further immunisation with RhD [2]. The latter is needed for the production of therapeutic quantities of anti-D antibodies.

Although antibodies can neutralise toxins and pathogens, the clearing of these pathogens from the body is achieved by the following processes.

- For pathogens, an IgG-mediated process is responsible for the clearance of antigen–Ig complexes from circulation by spleen and liver phagocytes.
- For parasites, by exocytosis of stored mediators, e.g. from mast cells that are triggered by their Fc epsilon receptor recognising the Fc region of IgE.

- Activation of the complement cascade. This system is part of innate immunity but is also vital to the effector functions of complement-fixing immunoglobulin isotypes. Central to the complement's function is the activation of C3 by three routes, as outlined in Figure 2.2: the classical, alternative and lectin pathways.

The fate of antibody-coated cells and thus also for red blood cells in auto- or alloimmune haemolysis is dependent on whether there is partial or total activation of the cascade downstream from C3. Total activation in this respect generates the membrane attack complex with the formation of the trimolecular complex of C4b2a3b or C5 convertase. This complex cleaves C5 into two fragments, C5a and C5b. C5b forms a complex with C6, C7 and C8, which facilitates the insertion of a number of C9 molecules in the membrane. This so-called membrane attack complex (MAC) creates lytic pores in the membrane that destroy the target cell. IgM mediates this process especially well. MAC can also be transferred to cells close by and leads to so-called bystander lysis.

Partially activated complement, in contrast, recruits and activates phagocytes to sites of infection but it can also mediate homing and clearance of complement-coated cells in macrophage areas of the spleen or liver, which next to Fc receptors also carry complement receptors.

Red Blood Cell Antibodies Illustrating the Above Principles

Several hundred red cell transfusion-related antigens have been identified. Alloimmunisation can happen after contact with non-self blood antigens by transfusion or transplantation or during pregnancy and delivery but can also be elicited by contact with bacterial antigens structurally similar to non-self blood-borne antigens. Where the cellular mechanisms are still largely unclear [1,3], the humoral response is easier to investigate through direct analyses of antibody levels. IgM class antibodies form first but are

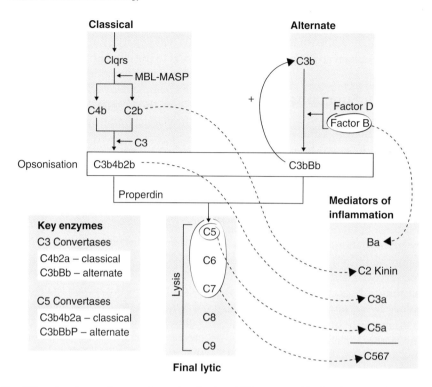

Figure 2.2 The different pathways for complement activation. MBL, mannan-binding lectin; MASP, MBL-associated serine protease.

transient as T-cell-independent B-cell activation IgM-producing plasma cells can be in part short-lived while others are long-lived. So-called naturally occurring IgM antibodies, can also be present permanently, indicating that they derived at least in part from long-lived plasma cells or that they are formed upon continuous turnover of memory B cells into antibody-secreting plasma cells. The best known of these IgM antibodies are those directed against the A or B blood group antigens, which are likely stimulated by exposure to gastrointestinal bacteria bearing A- and B-like antigens. This explains their presence as early as in the first months of life.

Although some IgM to IgG switching does occur for the antibodies against the A and B antigens, the T-cell-independent antibody formation for these carbohydrate antigens has to be discerned from the thymic or T-cell-dependent high-affinity IgG-forming mechanisms against polypeptide blood groups.

Fortunately, A and B antigens are only expressed at low levels on fetal red blood cells. Therefore, while the natural IgM cannot cross the placenta, anti-A or -B IgG transferred from the mother's blood usually do not lead to hae-molysis in the fetus.

Antibody and Complement-Mediated Blood Cell Destruction

A red cell transfusion to a recipient with circulating antibodies against antigens on these red cells can cause acute (within 24 hours) or delayed haemolytic reactions. As the acute form can be life-threatening, especially when intra-vascular haemolysis is induced, the delayed form is typically less severe [3].

Most red blood group allo- and autoanti-bodies of the IgG isotype bring about lysis via the interaction of the IgG constant domain with Fc gamma receptors on cells of the mononuclear phagocytic system.

- Fc gamma RI is the most important receptor that causes red cell destruction. This is a high-affinity receptor found predominantly on monocytes. The consequence of adherence of IgG-coated red cells to Fc gamma RI-positive cells is phagocytosis and lysis. This is usually extravascular and takes place in the spleen.
- Fc gamma RII is a lower affinity receptor found on monocytes, neutrophils, eosinophils, platelets and B-cells.
- Fc gamma RIII is also of relatively low affinity and found on macrophages, neutrophils, eosinophils and NK cells.
- There is also an FcRn (neonatal) on the placenta and other tissues of a different molecular family, which mediates the transfer of IgG into the fetus and is involved in the control of IgG concentrations.

The severity of haemolysis by IgG antibodies is determined by the concentration of antibody, its affinity for the antigen, the antigen density, the IgG subclass and their complement activating capacity. IgG2 antibodies generally do not reduce red cell survival, while IgG1 and IgG3 do.

The complement system, either working alone or in concert with an antibody, plays an important part in immune red cell destruction. In contrast to extravascular Fc gamma R-mediated destruction, complement-mediated lysis occurs in the intravascular compartment. The ensuing release of anaphylatoxins such as C3a and C5a contributes to acute systemic effects. IgM anti-A and -B can cause such potentially lethal effects should an error in patient identification or ABO typing occur, leading to a mistransfusion.

Red cells coated with C3b undergo extravascular haemolysis mainly in liver cells carrying receptors for C3b (CR1 or CD35). If, however, the bound C3b degrades to its inactive components iC3b and C3dg then the cell is effectively protected from lysis. Membrane-bound molecules such as decay accelerating factor (DAF) and membrane inhibitor of reactive lysis (MIRL) also protect red cells from lysis in this way.

Clinical Aspects Related to Alloimmunisation Against Blood Cell Antigens

The incidence of red cell alloimmunisation has been reported to vary between 2% and 21% in nonsickle cell disease patients. This reported variation is certainly influenced by the type and number of transfusions [4]. On the other hand, medication-suppressed immunity [5] or an activated immune system by the presence of autoimmune disorders, infection [6] or preexisting haemolysis priming APCs with danger signals are all likely to influence immunisation efficacy. Finally, alloimmunisation efficacy is influenced by the genetic or ethnic differences between donor and patient. The latter is not only the case for red cell blood groups themselves but also for HLA differences between donor and recipient. Certain HLA types are associated with a higher red blood cell alloimmunisation risk, suggesting specific HLA restriction for the presentation of some red cell antigens [7,8]. The fact that a first alloimmunisation increases the risk of further antibody formation might indicate the existence of a subgroup of so-called *responder* patients who have an intrinsic higher risk for alloimmunisation [9]. Better identification of clinical or genetic patient factors for red cell antigen alloimmunisation will be of great importance; this might enable a cost-effective matching in specific high-risk conditions.

The immediate documentation of newly detected antibodies, and perhaps screening for antibodies after transfusion, is essential because antibodies can become undetectable over time. New antigen exposure, for example via a new transfusion, will immediately boost their production and can cause delayed and potentially serious haemolysis. The rate of antibody evanescence is inversely proportionate to the primary immunisation strength (e.g. antibody titres reached), i.e. the higher the initial antibody titre, the slower the rate of evanescence. The rate is also dependent on the nature of antigen exposure, such as the difference between intrauterine transfusion and fetal blood immunisation [10].

Although alloimmunisation against red cell antigens is important enough, (co-)transfused platelets and leucocytes, respectively expressing MHC class I and both class I and II, are more effective in inducing alloimmunisation [11]. HLA and HPA antibodies are associated with various subsequent effects. First, these antibodies can cause refractoriness to platelet transfusions because donor platelets express varying amounts of incompatible HLA class I molecules. HPA antibodies can cause neonatal alloimmune thrombocytopenia. HLA antibodies in this respect do not seem able to cross the placental barrier, they are at least partly instrumental in causing transfusion-related acute lung injury. Finally, HLA antibodies in the recipient itself can cause cytokine-induced febrile nonhaemolytic transfusion reactions when reacting with and destroying donor leucocytes in transfusion products. Mechanistically less clear, posttransfusion purpura and hyperhaemolysis [12] are also associated with antibodies against transfused blood components [13].

KEY POINTS

1) Allogeneic blood are intrinsically non-self and capable of eliciting an immune response; additional danger signals (as in inflammatory conditions) are needed to prime and activate the immune cells that are most important for alloantibody formation.
2) The ability of antibodies to bring about erythrocyte or platelet destruction varies according to their isotype and their antigenic, Fc receptor and complement binding and activating capacities. Glycosylation determining antibody functionality is a new term in these equations.
3) Many clinical problems encountered in transfusion medicine are antibody based; in many cases, the causal mechanisms still need more elucidation [14].
4) Better identification of high-risk patients (responders) who are more likely to become alloimmunised, together with the increasing availability of donor red cell and platelet genotyping, will enable selective preventive and cost-effective donor–recipient matching [14].
5) High alloimmunisation risk patients and conditions might additionally benefit from immunomodulatory therapies shown to be preventing alloimmunization.

References

1 Vidarsson G, Dekkers G, Rispens T. IgG subclases and allotypes: from structure to effector functions. Front Immunol 2014;**5**:520.
2 Dohmen SE, Verhagen OJHM, Muit J, Ligthart PC, van der Schoot CE. The restricted use of IGHV3 super-species genes in anti-Rh is not limited to hyperimmunized anti-D donors. Transfusion 2006;**46**: 2162–8.
3 Vamvakas EC, Pineda AA, Reisner R, Santrach PJ, Moore SB. The differentiation of delayed hemolytic and delayed serologic transfusion reactions: incidence and predictors of hemolysis. Transfusion 1995;**35**:26–32.
4 Zalpuri S, Zwaginga JJ, Le Cessie S, Elshuis J, Schonewille H, van der Bom JG. Red-blood-cell alloimmunisation and number of red-blood-cell transfusions. Vox Sang 2012;**102**:144–9.
5 Zalpuri S, Evers D, Zwaginga JJ et al. Immunosuppressants and alloimmunization against red blood cell transfusions. Transfusion 2014;**54**(8):1981–7.
6 Evers D, van der Bom JG, Tijmensen J et al. Red cell alloimmunisation in patients with different types of infections. Br J Haematol 2016 Aug 18. doi: 10.1111/bjh.14307 (epub ahead of print).

7 Hoppe C, Klitz W, Vichinsky E, Styles L. HLA type and risk of alloimmunisation in sickle cell disease. Am J Hematol 2009;**84**:462–4.

8 Noizat-Pirenne F, Tournamille C, Bierling P et al. Relative immunogenicity of Fya and K antigens in a Caucasian population, based on HLA class II restriction analysis. Transfusion 2006;**46**: 1328–33.

9 Higgins JM, Sloan SR. Stochastic modelling of human RBC alloimmunisation: evidence for a distinct population of immunologic responders. Blood 2008;**112**: 2546–53.

10 Verduin EP, Brand A, van de Watering LM et al. Factors associated with persistence of red blood cell antibodies in woman after pregnancies complicated by fetal alloimmune haemolytic disease treated with intrauterine transfusions. Br J Haematol 2015;**168**:443–51.

11 Buetens O, Shirey RS, Goble-Lee M et al. Prevalence of HLA antibodies in transfused patients with, without red cell antibodies. Transfusion 2006;**46**:754–6.

12 Win N. Hyperhemolysis syndrome in sickle cell disease. Expert Rev Hematol 2009;**2**:111–15.

13 Hebert PC, Fergusson D, Blajchman MA et al., for the Leukoreduction Study Investigators. Clinical outcomes following institution of the Canadian universal leukoreduction program for red blood cell transfusions. JAMA 2003;**289**:1941–9.

14 Zimring JC, Welniak L, Semple JW et al, for the NHLBI Alloimmunisation Working Group. Current problems and future directions of transfusion-induced alloimmunisation: summary of an NHLBI working group. Transfusion 2011;**51**:435–41.

Further Reading

Murphy K. Janeway's Immunobiology, 8th edn. London: Garland Science, 2011.

3

Human Blood Group Systems

Geoff Daniels

International Blood Group Reference Laboratory, NHS Blood and Transplant, Bristol, UK

Introduction

A blood group may be defined as an inherited character of the red cell surface detected by a specific alloantibody. This definition would not receive universal acceptance as cell surface antigens on platelets and leucocytes might also be considered blood groups, as might uninherited characters on red cells defined by autoantibodies or xenoantibodies. The definition is suitable, however, for the purposes of this chapter.

Most blood groups are organised into blood group systems. Each system represents a single gene or a cluster of two or more closely linked homologous genes. Of the 347 blood group specificities recognised by the International Society for Blood Transfusion, 303 belong to one of 36 systems (Table 3.1). All these systems represent a single gene, apart from Rh, Xg and Chido/Rodgers, which have two closely linked homologous genes, and MNS with three genes [1,2].

Most blood group antigens are proteins or glycoproteins, with the blood group specificity determined primarily by the amino acid sequence, and most of the blood group polymorphisms result from single amino acid substitutions, though there are many exceptions. Some of these proteins cross the membrane once, with either the N-terminal or C-terminal outside the membrane, some cross the membrane several times and some are outside the membrane to which they are attached by a glycosylphosphatidylinositol anchor.

Some blood group antigens, including those of the ABO, P1PK, Lewis, H and I systems, are carbohydrate structures on glycoproteins and glycolipids. These antigens are not produced directly by the genes controlling their polymorphisms, but by genes encoding transferase enzymes that catalyse the final biosynthetic stage of an oligosaccharide chain.

The ABO System

ABO is often referred to as a histo-blood group system because, in addition to being expressed on red cells, ABO antigens are present on most tissues and in soluble form in secretions. At its most basic level, the ABO system consists of two antigens, A and B, indirectly encoded by two alleles, *A* and *B*, of the *ABO* gene. A third allele, *O*, produces neither A nor B. These three alleles combine to effect four phenotypes: A, B, AB and O (Table 3.2).

Clinical Significance

Two key factors make ABO the most important blood group system in transfusion medicine. First, the blood of almost all adults contains antibodies to those ABO antigens lacking from their red cells (see Table 3.2). In addition to anti-A and anti-B, group O individuals have anti-A,B, an antibody to a determinant common

Practical Transfusion Medicine, Fifth Edition. Edited by Michael F. Murphy, David J. Roberts and Mark H. Yazer.
© 2017 John Wiley & Sons Ltd. Published 2017 by John Wiley & Sons Ltd.

Table 3.1 Human blood group systems.

Number	Name	Symbol	Number of antigens	Gene symbol(s)	Chromosome
001	ABO	ABO	4	*ABO*	9
002	MNS	MNS	48	*GYPA, GYPB, GYPE*	4
003	P1PK	P1PK	3	*A4GALT*	22
004	Rh	RH	54	*RHD, RHCE*	1
005	Lutheran	LU	22	*BCAM*	19
006	Kell	KEL	35	*KEL*	7
007	Lewis	LE	6	*FUT3*	19
008	Duffy	FY	5	*DARC*	1
009	Kidd	JK	3	*SLC14A1*	18
010	Diego	DI	22	*SLC4A1*	17
011	Yt	YT	2	*ACHE*	7
012	Xg	XG	2	*XG, CD99*	X/Y
013	Scianna	SC	7	*ERMAP*	1
014	Dombrock	DO	10	*ART4*	12
015	Colton	CO	4	*AQP1*	7
016	Landsteiner–Wiener	LW	3	*ICAM4*	19
017	Chido/Rodgers	CH/RG	9	*C4A, C4B*	6
018	H	H	1	*FUT1*	19
019	Kx	XK	1	*XK*	X
020	Gerbich	GE	11	*GYPC*	2
021	Cromer	CROM	18	*CD55*	1
022	Knops	KN	9	*CR1*	1
023	Indian	IN	4	*CD44*	11
024	Ok	OK	3	*BSG*	19
025	Raph	RAPH	1	*CD151*	11
026	John Milton Hagen	JMH	6	*SEMA7A*	15
027	I	I	1	*GCNT2*	6
028	Globoside	GLOB	2	*B3GALT3*	3
029	Gill	GIL	1	*AQP3*	9
030	RHAG	RHAG	4	*RHAG*	6
031	Forssman	FORS	1	*GBGT1*	9
032	JR	JR	1	*ABCG2*	4
033	Lan	LAN	1	*ABCB6*	2
034	Vel	VEL	1	*SMIM1*	1
035	CD59	CD59	1	*ABCG2*	11
036	Augustine	AUG	2	*SLC29A1*	6

Table 3.2 The ABO system.

Phenotype	Genotypes	Frequency			Antibodies present
		Europeans*	Africans[†]	Indians[§]	
O	*O/O*	43%	51%	31%	Anti-A, -B, -A,B
A_1	$A^1/A^1, A^1/O, A^1/A^2$	35%	18%	26%	Anti-B
A_2	$A^2/A^2, A^2/O$	10%	5%	3%	Sometimes anti-A_1
B	*B/B, B/O*	9%	21%	30%	Anti-A
A_1B	A^1/B	3%	2%	9%	None
A_2B	A^2/B	1%	1%	1%	Sometimes anti-A_1

* English donors.
[†] Donors from Kinshasa, Congo.
[§] Makar from Mumbai.

to A and B. Second, ABO antibodies are IgM, though they may also have an IgG component, have thermal activity at 37 °C, activate complement and cause immediate intravascular red cell destruction, which can give rise to severe and often fatal haemolytic transfusion reactions (HTRs) (see Chapter 8). Major ABO incompatibility (i.e. donor red cells with an ABO antigen not possessed by the recipient) must be avoided in transfusion and, ideally, ABO-matched blood (i.e. of the same ABO group) would be provided.

ABO antibodies seldom cause haemolytic disease of the fetus and newborn (HDFN) and when they do, it is usually mild.

Biosynthesis and Molecular Genetics

Red cell A and B antigens are expressed predominantly on oligosaccharide structures on integral membrane glycoproteins, but are also on glycosphingolipids embedded in the membrane. The tetrasaccharides that represent the predominant form of A and B antigens on red cells are shown in Figure 3.1, together with their biosynthetic precursor, the H antigen, which is abundant on group O red cells. The product of the *A* allele is a glycosyltransferase that catalyses the transfer of *N*-acetylgalactosamine (GalNAc)

from a nucleotide donor substrate, UDP-GalNAc, to the fucosylated galactose (Gal) residue of the H antigen, the acceptor substrate. The product of the *B* allele catalyses the transfer of Gal from UDP-Gal to the fucosylated Gal residue of the H antigen. GalNAc and Gal are the immunodominant sugars of A and B antigens, respectively. The *O* allele produces no transferase, so the H antigen remains unmodified.

The *ABO* gene on chromosome 9 consists of seven exons. The *A* and *B* alleles differ by four nucleotides in exon 7 encoding amino acid substitutions. These determine whether the gene product is a GalNAc-transferase (A) or Gal-transferase (B) [3]. The most common *O* allele (O^1) has an identical sequence to *A*, apart from a single nucleotide deletion in exon 6, which shifts the reading frame and introduces a translation stop codon before the region of the catalytic site, so that any protein produced would be truncated and have no enzyme activity.

H, the Biochemical Precursor of A and B

H antigen is the biochemical precursor of A and B (see Figure 3.1). It is synthesised by an α1,2-fucosyltransferase, which catalyses the transfer of fucose from its donor substrate to the terminal

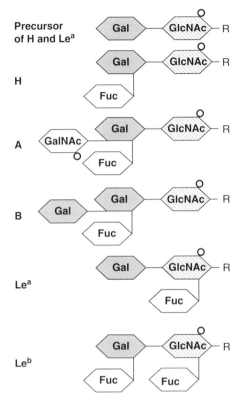

Figure 3.1 Diagram of the oligosaccharides representing H, A, B, Le^a and Le^b antigens and the biosynthetic precursor of Hand Le^a. R, remainder of molecule.

Gal residue of its acceptor substrate. Without this fucosylation, neither A nor B antigens can be made. Two genes, active in different tissues, produce α1,2-fucosyltransferases: *FUT1* responsible for H on red cells; *FUT2* for H in many other tissues and in secretions. Homozygosity for inactivating mutations in *FUT1* leads to an absence of H from red cells and, therefore, an absence of red cell A or B, regardless of *ABO* genotype. Such mutations are rare, as are red cell H-deficient phenotypes. In contrast, inactivating mutations in *FUT2* are relatively common and about 20% of white Europeans (non-secretors) lack H, A and B from body secretions, despite expressing those antigens on their red cells. Very rare individuals who have H-deficient red cells and are also H nonsecretors (Bombay

phenotype) produce anti-H together with anti-A and -B and can cause a severe transfusion problem.

The Rh System

Rh is the most complex of the blood group systems, with 54 specificities. The most important of these is D (RH1).

Rh Genes and Proteins

The antigens of the Rh system are encoded by two genes, *RHD* and *RHCE*, which produce D and CcEe antigens, respectively. The genes are highly homologous, each consisting of 10 exons. They are closely linked, but in opposite orientations, on chromosome 1 [4] (Figure 3.2). Each gene encodes a 417 amino acid polypeptide that differs by only 31–35 amino acids, according to Rh genotype. The Rh proteins are not glycosylated and span the red cell membrane 12 times, with both termini inside the cytosol and with six external loops, the potential sites of antigenic activity (see Figure 3.2).

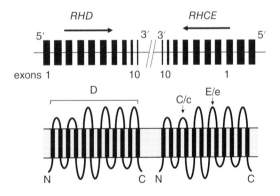

Figure 3.2 Diagrammatic representation of the Rh genes, *RHD* and *RHCE*, shown in opposite orientations as they appear on the chromosome, and of the two Rh proteins in their probable membrane conformation, with 12 membrane-spanning domains and six extracellular loops expressing D, C/c and E/e antigens.

D Antigen

The most significant Rh antigen clinically is D. About 85% of white people are D+ (Rh-positive) and 15% are D– (Rh-negative). In Africans, only about 3–5% are D– and in the East Asia D– is rare.

The D– phenotype is usually associated with the absence of the whole D protein from the red cell membrane. This explains why D is so immunogenic, as the D antigen comprises numerous epitopes on the external domains of the D protein. In white people, the D– phenotype almost always results from homozygosity for a complete deletion of *RHD*. D-positives are either homozygous or heterozygous for the presence of *RHD*. In Africans, in addition to the deletion of *RHD*, D– often results from an inactive *RHD* (called *RHD*ψ) containing translation stop codons within the reading frame.

Numerous variants of D are known, though most are rare [5,6]. They are often split into two types, partial D and weak D, though this dichotomy is not adequately defined and of little value for making clinical decisions. Partial D antigens lack some or most of the D epitopes. If an individual with a partial D phenotype is immunised by red cells with a complete D antigen, they might make antibodies to those epitopes they lack. The D epitopes comprising partial D may be expressed weakly or may be of normal or even enhanced strength. Weak D antigens appear to express all epitopes of D, but at a lower site density than normal D. D variants result from amino acid substitutions in the D protein occurring either as a result of one or more missense mutations in *RHD* or from one or more exons of *RHD* being exchanged for the equivalent exons of *RHCE* in a process called gene conversion.

Anti-D

Anti-D is almost never produced in D– individuals without exposure to by D+ red cells. D is highly immunogenic and approximately 20% of D– recipients of transfused D+ red cells make anti-D. Anti-D can cause severe immediate or delayed HTRs and D+ blood must never be transfused to a patient with anti-D.

Anti-D is one of the most common causes of severe HDFN.

Prediction of Fetal Rh Phenotype by Molecular Methods

Knowledge of the molecular bases for D– phenotypes has made it possible to devise tests for predicting fetal D type from fetal DNA. This is a valuable tool in assessing whether the fetus of a woman with anti-D is at risk from HDFN [7]. Most methods involve PCR tests that detect the presence or absence of *RHD*. The usual source of fetal DNA is the small quantity of free fetal DNA present in maternal plasma. This noninvasive form of fetal D typing is now provided as a service in many countries for alloimmunised D– women. In addition, in a few European countries noninvasive fetal *RHD* genotyping is offered to all D– pregnant women, so that only those with a D+ fetus receive routine antenatal anti-D prophylaxis (see Chapter 33).

C and c, E and e

C/c and E/e are two pairs of antigens representing alleles of *RHCE*. The fundamental difference between C and c is a serine–proline substitution at position 103 in the second external loop of the CcEe protein (see Figure 3.2), and E and e represent a proline–alanine substitution at position 226 in the fourth external loop [8].

Anti-c is clinically the most important Rh antibody after anti-D and may cause severe HDFN. On the other hand, anti-C, -E and -e rarely cause HDFN and when they do, the disease is generally mild, though all have the potential to cause severe disease.

Other Rh Antigens

Of the 54 Rh antigens, 20 are polymorphic, i.e. have a frequency between 1% and 99% in at least one major ethnic group, 22 are rare antigens and 12 are very common antigens. Antibodies to many of these antigens have proved to be clinically important and it is prudent to treat all Rh antibodies as being potentially clinically significant [9].

Other Blood Group Systems

Of the remaining blood group systems (see Table 3.1), the most important clinically are Kell, Duffy, Kidd and MNS.

Kell System

The original Kell antigen, K (KEL1), has a frequency of about 9% in Caucasians, but is rare in other ethnic groups. Its antithetical (allelic) antigen, k (KEL2), is common in all populations. The remainder of the Kell system consists of one triplet and five pairs of allelic antigens – Kp^a, Kp^b and Kp^c; Js^a and Js^b; K11 and K17; K14 and K24; VLAN and VONG; KYO and KYOR – plus 17 high-frequency and three low-frequency antigens. Almost all represent single amino acid substitutions in the Kell glycoprotein.

Anti-K can cause severe HTRs and HDFN. About 10% of K– patients who are given one unit of K+ blood produce anti-K, making K the next most immunogenic antigen after D. In most cases of HDFN caused by anti-K, the mother will have had previous blood transfusions. HDFN caused by anti-K differs from Rh HDFN in that anti-K appears to cause fetal anaemia by suppression of erythropoiesis, rather than immune destruction of mature fetal erythrocytes [9]. Most other Kell system antibodies are rare and best detected by an antiglobulin test.

The Kell antigens are located on a large glycoprotein, which belongs to a family of endopeptidases that process biologically important peptides, and is able to cleave the biologically inactive peptide big endothelin-3 to produce endothelin-3, an active vasoconstrictor.

Duffy System

Fy^a and Fy^b represent a single amino acid substitution in the extracellular N-terminal domain of the Duffy glycoprotein. Their incidence in Caucasians is Fy^a 68%, Fy^b 80%. But about 70% of African Americans and close to 100% of West Africans are Fy(a–b–) (Table 3.3). Fy(a–b–)

Table 3.3 The Duffy system: phenotypes and genotypes.

Phenotype	Genotype	Frequency (%)	
		Europeans	Africans
Fy(a + b–)	*FY*A/A* or *FY*A/Null*[†]	20	10
Fy(a + b+)	*FY*A/B*	48	3
Fy(a–b+)	*FY*B/B* or *FY*B/Null*	32	20
Fy(a–b–)	*FY*Null/Null*	0	67

[†] *Null* represents the allele that produces no Duffy antigens on red cells.

Table 3.4 Nucleotide polymorphisms in the promoter region and in exon 2 of the three common alleles of the Duffy gene.

Allele	GATA box sequence –64 to –69 (promoter)	Codon 42 (exon 2)	Antigen
FY*A	TTATCT	GGT (Gly)	Fy^a
FY*B	TTATCT	GAT (Asp)	Fy^b
FY*Null	TTACCT	GAT (Asp)	Red cells – none
			Other tissues – probably Fy^b

Africans are homozygous for an *FY*B* allele containing a mutation in a binding site for the erythroid-specific GATA-1 transcription factor, which means that Duffy glycoprotein is not expressed in red cells, though it is present in other tissues [10] (Table 3.4). The Duffy glycoprotein is the receptor exploited by *Plasmodium vivax* merozoites for penetration of erythroid cells. Consequently, the Fy(a–b–) phenotype confers resistance to *P. vivax* malaria. The Duffy glycoprotein (also called Duffy antigen chemokine receptor, DARC) is a red cell receptor for a variety of chemokines, including interleukin-8.

Anti-Fy^a is not infrequent and is found in previously transfused patients who have usually made other antibodies. Anti-Fy^b is very rare.

Both may cause acute or delayed HTRs and HDFN varying from mild to severe [9].

Kidd System

Kidd has two common alleles, *JK*A* and *JK*B*, which represent a single amino acid change in the Kidd glycoprotein. Both Jk^a and Jk^b antigens have frequencies of about 75% in Caucasian populations. A Kidd-null phenotype, Jk(a–b–), results from homozygosity for inactivating mutations in the Kidd gene, *SLC14A1*. It is very rare in most populations, but reaches an incidence of greater than 1% in Polynesians. The Kidd glycoprotein is a urea transporter in red cells and in renal endothelial cells.

Anti-Jk^a is uncommon and anti-Jk^b is very rare, but both cause severe transfusion reactions and, to a lesser extent, HDFN [9]. Kidd antibodies have often been implicated in delayed HTRs. They are often difficult to detect serologically and tend to disappear rapidly after stimulation.

MNS System

MNS, with a total of 48 antigens, is second only to Rh in complexity. MNS antigens are present on one or both of two red cell membrane glycoproteins, glycophorin A (GPA) and glycophorin B (GPB). They are encoded by homologous genes, *GYPA* and *GYPB*, on chromosome 4.

The M and N antigens, both with frequencies of about 75%, differ by amino acids at positions 1 and 5 of the external N-terminus of GPA. S and s have frequencies of about 55% and 90%, respectively, in a Caucasian population and represent an amino acid substitution in GPB. About 2% of black West Africans and 1.5% of African Americans are S– s–, a phenotype virtually unknown in other ethnic groups, and most of these lack the U antigen, which is present when either S or s is expressed. The numerous MNS variants mostly result from amino acid substitutions in GPA or GPB and from hybrid GPA–GPB molecules, formed by intergenic recombination between *GYPA* and *GYPB*. The phenotypes resulting from these hybrid proteins are rare in Europeans and Africans, but the GP.Mur (previously Mi.III) variant phenotype occurs in up to 10% of East Asians. GPA and GPB are exploited as receptors by the malaria parasite *Plasmodium falciparum*.

Anti-M and -N are not generally clinically significant, though anti-M is occasionally haemolytic [9]. Anti-S, the rarer anti-s, and anti-U can cause HDFN and have been implicated in HTRs. Although rare elsewhere, anti-Mur, which detects red cells of the GP.Mur phenotype, is common in East Asia and Oceanic regions and causes severe HTRs and HDFN.

Biological Significance of Blood Group Antigens

The functions of several red cell membrane protein structures bearing blood group antigenic determinants are known, or can be deduced from their structure. Some are membrane transporters, facilitating the transport of biologically important molecules through the lipid bilayer: band 3 membrane glycoprotein, the Diego antigen, provides an anion exchange channel for HCO_3^- and Cl^- ions; the Kidd glycoprotein is a urea transporter; the Colton glycoprotein is aquaporin 1, a water channel; the GIL antigen is aquaporin 3, a glycerol transporter; JR and Lan glycoproteins are probably porphyrin transporters; Augustine glycoprotein is a nucleoside transporter; and RhAG may form a carbon dioxide and, possibly, oxygen channel, and could function as an ammonia/ammonium transporter [11–13]. The Lutheran, LW and Indian (CD44) glycoproteins are adhesion molecules, possibly serving their primary functions during erythropoiesis. The MER2 antigen is located on the tetraspanin CD151, which associates with integrins within basement membranes, but its function on red cells is not known. The Duffy glycoprotein is a chemokine receptor and could function as a 'sink' or scavenger for unwanted chemokines. The Cromer (CD55), Knops (CD35) and CD59 antigens are markers for complement regulatory proteins that protect the cells from destruction by autologous complement. Some blood group glycoproteins appear to be enzymes, though their functions on red cells are not known: the Yt antigen is acetylcholinesterase, the Kell antigen is an endopeptidase and the sequence of the Dombrock glycoprotein suggests that it belongs to a family of adenosine diphosphate (ADP)-ribosyltransferases. The C-terminal domains of the Gerbich antigens, GPC and GPD and the N-terminal domain of the Diego glycoprotein, band 3, are attached to components of the cytoskeleton and function to anchor it to the external membrane. The carbohydrate moieties of the membrane glycoproteins and glycolipids, especially those of the most abundant glycoproteins, band 3 and GPA, constitute the glycocalyx, an extracellular coat that protects the cell from mechanical damage and microbial attack.

The Rh proteins are associated as heterotrimers with the glycoprotein RhAG in the red cell membrane, and these trimers are part of a macrocomplex of red cell surface proteins that include tetramers of band 3 plus LW, GPA, GPB and CD47, and are linked to the red cell cytoskeleton through protein 4.2 and ankyrin. There is probably another protein complex containing Rh proteins and dimers of band 3, plus Kell, Kx and Duffy blood group proteins, and is linked to the cytoskeleton through glycophorin C (Gerbich blood group), MMP1 and protein 4.1R.

The structural differences between antithetical red cell antigens (e.g. A and B, K and k, Fy^a and Fy^b) are small, often being just one monosaccharide or one amino acid. The biological importance of these differences is unknown and there is little evidence to suggest that the product of one allele confers any significant advantage over the other. Some blood group antigens are exploited by pathological microorganisms as receptors for attaching and entering cells, so in some cases absence or changes in these antigens could be beneficial. It is likely that interaction between cell surface molecules and pathological microorganisms has been a major factor in the evolution of blood group polymorphism.

KEY POINTS

1) The International Society of Blood Transfusion recognises 347 blood group specificities, 303 of which belong to one of 36 blood group systems.
2) The most important blood group systems clinically are ABO, Rh, Kell, Duffy, Kidd and MNS.
3) ABO antibodies are almost always present in adults lacking the corresponding antigens and can cause fatal intravascular HTRs.
4) ABO antigens are carbohydrate structures on glycoproteins and glycosphingolipids.
5) Anti-RhD is the most common cause of HDFN.
6) Red cell surface proteins serve a variety of functions, though many of their functions are still not known.

References

1 Red Cell Immunogenetics and Blood Group Terminology Working Party of the International Society of Blood Transfusion. Available at: www.isbtweb.org/workingparties/red-cell-immunogenetics-and-blood-groupterminology

2 Storry JR, Castilho L, Daniels G et al. International Society of Blood Transfusion Working Party on red cell immunogenetics and blood group terminology: Cancun report (2012). *Vox Sang* 2014;**107**:90–6.

3 Yamamoto F, Clausen H, White T, Marken J, Hakomori S. Molecular genetic basis of the

histo-blood group ABO system. Nature 1990;**345**:229–33.

4 Wagner FF, Flegel WA. *RHD* gene deletion occurred in the *Rhesus box*. Blood 2000;**95**:3662–8.

5 Daniels G. Variants of RhD – current testing and clinical consequences. Br J Haematol 2013;**161**:461–70.

6 Rhesus base website: www.rhesusbase.info.

7 Daniels G, Finning K, Martin P, Massey E. Noninvasive prenatal diagnosis of fetal blood group phenotypes: current practice and future prospects. Prenat Diagn 2009;**29**:101–7.

8 Mouro I, Colin Y, Chérif-Zahar B, Cartron J-P, Le Van Kim C. Molecular genetic basis of the human Rhesus blood group system. Nature Genet 1993;**5**:62–5.

9 Poole J, Daniels G. Blood group antibodies and their significance in transfusion medicine. Transfus Med Rev 2007;**21**:58–71.

10 Tournamille C, Colin Y, Cartron JP, Le Van Kim C. Disruption of a GATA motif in the *Duffy* gene promoter abolishes erythroid gene expression in Duffy-negative individuals. Nature Genet 1995;**10**:224–8.

11 Daniels G. Functions of red cell surface proteins. Vox Sang 2007;**93**:331–40.

12 Anstee DJ. The functional importance of blood group active molecules in human red blood cells. Vox Sang 2011;**100**:140–9.

13 Mohandas N, Gallagher PG. Red cell membrane: past, present, and future. Blood 2008;**112**:3939–48.

Further Reading

Anstee DJ. Red cell genotyping and the future of pretransfusion testing. Blood 2009;**114**:248–56.

Anstee DJ. The relationship between blood groups and disease. Blood 2010;**115**:4635–43.

Avent ND, Reid ME. The Rh blood group system: a review. Blood 2000;**95**:375–87.

Daniels G. Human Blood Groups, 3rd edn. Oxford: Wiley-Blackwell, 2013.

Daniels G. The molecular genetics of blood group polymorphism. Hum Genet 2009;**126**:729–42.

Daniels G, Bromilow I. Essential Guide to Blood Groups, 3rd edn. Oxford: Blackwell Publishing, 2013.

Daniels G, Reid ME. Blood groups: the past 50 years. Transfusion 2010;**50**:3–11.

Fung MK, Grossman BJ, Hillyer C, Westhoff CM. AABB Technical Manual, 18th edn. Bethesda: AABB, 2014.

Reid ME, Lomas-Francis C. The Blood Group Antigen Facts Book, 3rd edn. New York: Academic Press, 2012.

Watkins WM (ed.) Commemoration of the centenary of the discovery of the ABO blood group system. Transfus Med 2001;**11**:239–351.

4 Human Leucocyte Antigens

Cristina V. Navarrete[1,2] and Colin J. Brown[1]

[1] *NHS Blood and Transplant, Histocompatibility and Immunogenetics Services, Colindale Centre, London, UK*
[2] *University College London, London, UK*

Introduction

The genes coding for the human leucocyte antigens (HLAs) are located on the short arm of chromosome 6, spanning a distance of approximately 4 Mb. This genomic region is divided into three subregions [1,2].

- Class I subregion contains genes coding for the heavy (α) chain of the classical (HLA-A, -B and -C) and nonclassical (HLA-E, -F and -G) class I molecules. The nonclassical major histocompatibility complex class I chain-related gene *A* and gene *B* (MICA and MICB) have also been mapped to this subregion, centromeric to the *HLA-B* gene (Figure 4.1).
- Class II subregion contains the classical HLA-DR, -DQ and -DP genes and the nonclassical HLA-DMA, -DMB, -DOA and -DOB genes. The low molecular polypeptide genes LMP2 and LMP7, TAP1 and TAP2 transporters and the Tapasin (*Tpn*) genes involved in the processing, transport and loading of HLA class I antigenic peptides are also located in this subregion (see Figure 4.1).
- Class III subregion lies between the other two subregions and contains genes coding for a diverse group of proteins, including complement components (C4Bf), tumour necrosis factor (TNF) and heat-shock proteins (HSPs).

The nonclassical class I-like gene HFE has been mapped to a locus located 4 Mb telomeric to HLA-F. Single point mutations in this gene are associated with the development of hereditary haemochromatosis (HH).

HLA Class I Genes

HLA class I genes are defined, according to their structure, expression and function, as classical (HLA-A, -B and -C) and nonclassical (HLA-E, -F and -G). Both classical and nonclassical HLA class I genes code for a heavy (α) chain, of approximately 43 kd, non-covalently linked to a nonpolymorphic light chain, the β_2-microglobulin of 12 kd, which is coded for by a gene on chromosome 15. The extracellular portion of the heavy chain has three domains (α1, α2 and α3) of approximately 90 amino acids long. These domains are encoded by exons 2, 3 and 4 of the class I gene, respectively. The α1 and α2 are the most polymorphic domains of the molecule and they form a peptide-binding groove that can accommodate antigenic peptides of approximately eight to nine amino acids long.

The exon/intron organisation of the nonclassical HLA class I genes (E, F and G) is very similar to the classical class I genes, but they have a more restricted polymorphism. The MICA and MICB gene products, however, do not bind β_2-microglobulin and do not present antigenic peptides.

A schematic representation of the classical HLA class I gene and molecule is shown in Figure 4.2.

Practical Transfusion Medicine, Fifth Edition. Edited by Michael F. Murphy, David J. Roberts and Mark H. Yazer.
© 2017 John Wiley & Sons Ltd. Published 2017 by John Wiley & Sons Ltd.

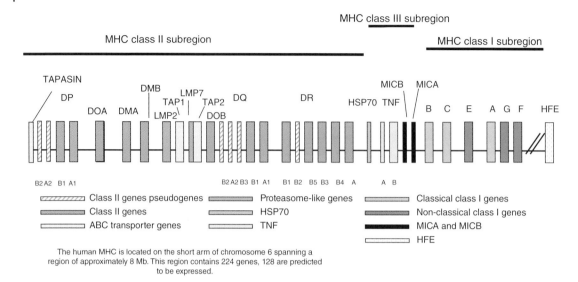

Figure 4.1 Map of the human leucocyte antigen complex. HSP, heat-shock protein; TNF, tumour necrosis factor. *Source:* Based on Trowsdale and Campbell, 1997, in Charron D (ed.) HLA Genetic Diversity of HLA: Functional and Medical Implications, Vol. 1, pp. 499–504.

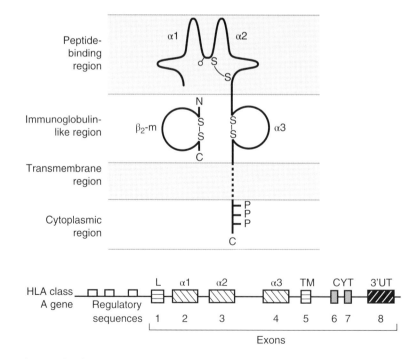

Figure 4.2 HLA class I molecule. β_2-m, β_2-microglobulin.

HLA Class II Genes

The classical HLA class II DR, DQ and DP A and B genes code for a heterodimer formed by non-covalently associated α and β chains of approximately 34 and 28 kd, respectively. The expressed α and β chains consist of two extracellular domains and a transmembrane and cytoplasmic domain. The α1/β1 and α2/β2 domains are encoded by exon 2 and exon 3 of the class II gene respectively. The majority of the polymorphism is located in the β1 domain of the DR molecules and in the α1 and β1 domains of the DQ and DP molecules. Similar to the class I molecules, these domains also form a peptide-binding groove. However, in the case of the class II molecules (DR), the groove is open at both sides and can accommodate antigenic peptides of varying size, although most of them are approximately 13–25 amino acids long.

A schematic representation of the HLA class II gene and molecule is shown in Figure 4.3.

The nonclassical HLA class II DMA, DMB, DOA and DOB genes have a similar structure to the classical class II genes, but show limited polymorphism.

Genetic Organisation and Expression of HLA Class II Genes

There is one DRA gene of limited polymorphism and nine DRB genes, of which B1, B3, B4 and B5 are highly polymorphic and B2, B6 and B9 are pseudogenes. The main serologically defined DR specificities (DR1–DR18) are determined by the polymorphic DRB1 gene. The number of DRB genes expressed in each individual varies according to the *DRB1** allele expressed

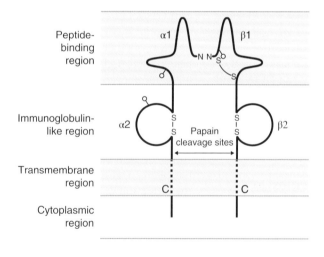

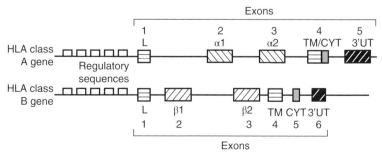

Figure 4.3 HLA class II molecule.

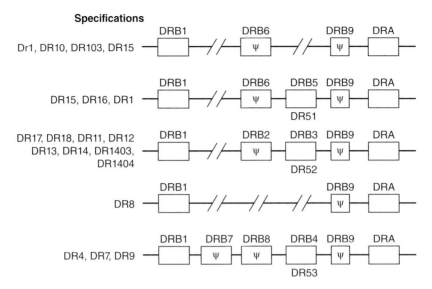

Figure 4.4 Expression of HLA-DRB genes.

(Figure 4.4). There are a few exceptions to this pattern of gene expression, for example a DRB5 gene has been found to be expressed with some *DR1* alleles. Some nonexpressed or null DRB5 and DRB4 genes have also been identified. In contrast to the *DRB* genes, there are two DQA and three DQB genes, but only the DQA1 and DQB1 are expressed and both are polymorphic. Similarly, there are two DPA and two DPB genes, but only the DPA1 and DPB1 are expressed and both are polymorphic.

Expression of HLA Molecules

The HLA class I molecules (A, B, C) are present on the majority of tissues and blood cells, including T- and B-lymphocytes, granulocytes and platelets. Low levels of expression have been detected in endocrine tissue, skeletal muscle and cells of the central nervous system. HLA-E and -F are also expressed on most tissues tested, but HLA-G shows a more restricted tissue distribution and to date, HLA-G products have only been found on extravillous cytotrophoblasts of the placenta and mononuclear phagocytes. MICA and MICB molecules are expressed on fibroblasts, endothelial, intestinal and tumour epithelial cells.

The HLA class II molecules are constitutively expressed on B-lymphocytes, monocytes and dendritic cells, but can also be detected on activated T-lymphocytes and activated granulocytes. It is not clear whether they are also present on activated platelets. HLA class II expression can be induced on a number of cells such as fibroblasts and endothelial cells as the result of activation and/or the effect of certain inflammatory cytokines, such as interferon (IFN)-γ, TNF and interleukin (IL)-10.

Both classical and nonclassical HLA molecules can also be found in soluble forms and it has been suggested that they may play a role in the induction of peripheral tolerance.

Genetics

HLA genes which are co-dominantly expressed and inherited in a mendelian fashion are highly polymorphic. Some alleles of these genes segregate in strong linkage disequilibrium (LD), i.e. the observed frequency of alleles of different loci segregating together is greater than the frequency expected by random association. Some of these alleles and the patterns of LD are present with similar frequencies in all populations but others are unique to some population groups.

For example, HLA-A*02 is expressed at a relatively high frequency in most population groups studied so far, whereas HLA-B*53 is found predominantly in black African populations.

The genetic region containing all HLA genes on each chromosome is termed the 'haplotype'. Some HLA haplotypes are also found across different ethnic groups, such as HLA-B*44-DRB1*07, whereas others are unique to a particular population, such as HLA-B*42-DRB1*03:02 in black Africans. This characteristic is particularly relevant for the selection of HLA-compatible family donors for patients requiring solid organ or haemopoietic stem cell (HSC) transplantation.

Function of HLA Molecules

The main function of HLA molecules is to present antigenic peptides to T-cells, and this requires a fine interaction between the HLA molecules, the antigenic peptide and the T-cell receptor. A number of co-stimulatory molecules (e.g. CD80 and CD86) and adhesion molecules such as ICAM-1 (CD54) and LFA-3 (CD58) also contribute to these interactions.

The HLA class I molecules are primarily, but not exclusively, involved in the presentation of endogenous antigenic peptides to CD8 cytotoxic T-cells. Both the classical and nonclassical HLA class I molecules also interact with a new family of receptors present on natural killer (NK) cells [3]. Some of these receptors, which are polymorphic and differentially expressed, have an inhibitory role, whereas others are activating. The killer-activating and killer-inhibitory receptors belong to two distinct families: the immunoglobulin superfamily called killer immunoglobulin receptors (KIRs) and the C-type lectin superfamily CD94-NKG2. The interaction between the inhibitory receptors and the relevant HLA ligand results in the prevention of NK lysis of the target cell. Thus, NK cells from any given individual will be alloreactive towards cells lacking their corresponding inhibitory KIR ligands, such as tumour or allogeneic cells. In contrast, NK cells will be tolerant to cells from individuals who

express the corresponding KIR ligands. The MICA and MICB molecules, which are induced by stress, are polymorphic but do not have a peptide-binding groove and nor do they bind β2m. These molecules also interact with the NK activatory receptor NKG2D and with γδT cells.

The *LMP2* and *LMP7* genes are thought to improve the capacity of the proteaosomes to generate peptides of the appropriate size and specificity to associate with the class I molecules whereas *TAP1* and *TAP2* are primarily involved in the transport of the proteaosome-generated peptides to the endoplasmic reticulum, where they associate with the class I molecules.

The HLA class II molecules (DR, DQ and DP) are mostly involved in the presentation of exogenous antigenic peptides to CD4 helper T-cells. Once activated, these CD4 cells can initiate and regulate a variety of processes leading to the maturation and differentiation of cellular (CD8 cytotoxic T-cells) and humoral effectors (such as antibody production by plasma cells). Activated effectors also secrete pro-inflammatory cytokines (IL-2, IFN-γ, TNF-α) and regulatory cytokines (IL-4, IL-10 and transforming growth factor (TGF)-β).

HLA-DM molecules facilitate the release of the class II-associated invariant chain (Ii) peptide from the peptide-binding groove of the HLA-DR molecules so that the groove can be loaded with the relevant antigenic peptide and this function is modulated by the DO molecules [4].

Identification of HLA Gene Polymorphism

The HLA polymorphisms were initially identified and defined using serological and cellular techniques. The development of gene cloning and DNA sequencing allowed a detailed analysis of these genes at the single nucleotide level. This analysis revealed the existence of locus-specific nucleotide sequences in both coding (exons) and non-coding (introns) regions of the genes and the existence of nucleotide sequences that are common to several alleles of the same and/or different loci.

HLA	HLA region
HLA-DR	Identifies the HLA locus
HLA-DR13	A serologically-defined antigen
HLA-DRB1*	Identifies the HLA locus and gene, the asterisk indicates the HLA allele(s) have been defined using DNA-based techniques.
HLA-DRB1*13	A group of HLA alleles with a common DRB1*13 sequence, termed **first field resolution**, that is the field before the first colon.
HLA-DRB1*13:01	A specific HLA allele, termed **second field resolution** as the numerals appear in the second field between the first and the second colon.
HLA-DRB1*13:01	A **null allele**, there is o cell surface expression of the DRB1*13 gene product.
HLA-DRB1*13:01:02	An allele that differs by a synonymous (silent or non-coding) mutation.
HLA-DRB1*13:01:01:02	An allele that contains a mutation outside the coding region.
HLA-DRB1*13:01:01:02N	A null allele which contains a mutation outside the coding region.

Figure 4.5 An example of a current HLA nomenclature. *Source:* Reproduced from Nunes et al [6].

Due to the complexity of the HLA polymorphism and to the vast number of new alleles defined each year, a revised nomenclature has been implemented [5,6] (Figure 4.5). In this revised version, optional suffixes may be added to an allele to indicate its expression status, i.e. the suffix 'N' for **n**ull alleles; these alleles are not expressed on the cell surface; 'L' for **l**ow expression; 'S' for **s**ecreted, these are soluble HLA molecules; 'C' for **c**ytoplasmic expression, 'A' for **a**berrant expression; and 'Q' for when the expression of the allele is **q**uestionable.

The number of recognised serologically defined antigens and DNA-identified HLA alleles is shown in Table 4.1 and can be accessed at http://hla.alleles.org/nomenclature/stats.html.

DNA sequencing of a number of HLA alleles of various loci also demonstrated that the majority of the variation was located in the α1 and α2 domain of the class I molecules, and in the α1 and β1 domain of the class II molecules. These are called hypervariable regions. Based on this information, a number of techniques have been developed to characterise these polymorphisms. Most of the described techniques make use of the polymerase chain reaction (PCR) to amplify

Table 4.1 Number of recognised HLA antigens/alleles.

Gene	Alleles	Protein	Antigens[*]
HLA class I			
HLA-A	3192	2245	24
HLA-B	3997	2938	50
HLA-C	2740	1941	9
HLA-E	17	6	
HLA-F	22	4	
HLA-G	50	16	
HLA class II			
HLA-DRB1	1764	1290	17
HLA-DRA1	7	2	—
HLA-DRB3	59	47	1
HLA-DRB4	16	9	1
HLA-DRB5	21	18	1
HLA-DQB1	807	539	6
HLA-DQA1	54	32	—
HLA-DPB1	550	447	6[†]
HLA-DPA1	40	20	—

Source: Adapted from Marsh et al. [5]
[*] Serologically defined.
[†] Cellular defined.

the specific genes or region to be analysed and include PCR sequence-specific priming (PCR-SSP), PCR sequence-specific oligonucleotide probing (PCR-SSOP) and DNA sequencing-based typing using the Sanger method (SBT) or by parallel or clonal sequencing, also called new-generation sequencing (NGS) [7].

PCR Sequence-Specific Priming

This technique involves the use of specific primers designed to only anneal with DNA in the area of interest initiating DNA synthesis. Amplification only takes place if the primer can bind and the product of amplification is visualised by agarose gel electrophoresis, which allows for rapid identification of the HLA types in individual samples. However, as the HLA system is very polymorphic, a large number of specific primers are required to obtain a low-resolution HLA type. PCR-SSP requires prior knowledge of the sequence to be detected and may not detect novel HLA types.

PCR Sequence-Specific Oligonucleotide Probing

In this technique, the gene of interest is amplified using primers designed to anneal with DNA sequences common to all alleles. Oligonucleotide probes are designed to bind to specific HLA sequences of interest. This may be achieved by immobilising the DNA to be typed to an inert support and hybridising with sequence-specific oligonucleotide probes (SSOP) or immobilising the probes and hybridising with the amplified DNA (reverse SSOP). Detection of hybridisation and analysis of reaction patterns is largely automated, and is more amenable to typing large numbers of samples (e.g. stem cell registry typing and disease association studies).

DNA Sequencing-Based Typing

DNA sequencing involves the denaturation of the DNA to be analysed to provide a single-strand template. Sequencing primers, exon or locus specific, are then added and the DNA extension is performed by the addition of Taq polymerase in the presence of excess nucleotides. The sequencing mixture is divided into four tubes, each of which contains specific dideoxyribonucleoside triphosphate (ddATP). When these are incorporated into the DNA synthesis, elongation is interrupted with chain-terminating inhibitors. In each reaction, there is random incorporation of the chain terminators and therefore products of all sizes are generated. The sequencing products are detected by labelling the nucleotide chain inhibitors with radioisotopes and, more recently, with fluorescent dyes. The products of the four reactions are then analysed by electrophoresis in parallel lanes of a polyacrylamide–urea gel and the sequence is read by combining the results of each lane using an automated DNA sequencer. In HLA SBT, some ambiguous results can be obtained with heterozygous samples and these may need to be retested by using PCR-SSP or reverse PCR-SSOP. SBT permits high-resolution HLA typing, which is known to be important in the selection of HLA-matched HSC unrelated donors.

A major advantage of all DNA-based techniques is that no viable cells are required to perform HLA class I and II typing. Furthermore, since all the probes and primers are synthesised to order, there is a consistency of reagents used, allowing the comparison of HLA types from different laboratories. However, although serological typing is being rapidly replaced by DNA-based typing techniques, serological reagents may still be required for antigen expression studies.

More recently, a new approach to performing high-resolution and high-throughput HLA typing involving massive parallel clonal sequencing strategies and NGS platforms has been described [8]. The availability of HR HLA typing will be particularly useful for the selection of HLA matched donors for patients in need of an HSC transplant.

The advantages and disadvantages of the various techniques described above are detailed in Table 4.2.

Formation of HLA Antibodies

HLA-specific antibodies are induced by pregnancy, transplantation, blood transfusions and planned immunisations. The affinity, avidity and class of the antibodies produced depend on various factors, including the route of

Table 4.2 Advantages and disadvantages of DNA-based techniques.

Technique	Advantages	Disadvantages
Sequence-specific oligonucleotide probing (SSOP)	Needs only one pair of genetic primers; fewer reactions to set up Larger number of samples can be processed simultaneously Requires small amount of DNA Inexpensive	Different temperatures required for each probe Probes can cross-react with different alleles Large numbers of probes required to identify specificity Difficult to interpret pattern of reactions
Sequence-specific priming (SSP)	Provides rapid typing with higher resolution than SSOP All PCR amplifications are carried out at same time, temperature and conditions Fast and simple to read and interpret	Too many sets of primers are needed to fulfil HLA type Requires a two-stage amplification to provide HR typing
Sequencing-based typing (SBT)	Does not require previous sequence data to identify new allele	Requires expensive reagents and equipment
Sequencing-based typing by NGS	Provides the highest level of resolution and unambiguous results Requires automation for high-throughput testing	Requires more training Cost-effective for high throughput only Requires expensive reagents and equipment Requires complex algorithms for the analyses and provision of results

HR, high resolution; NGS, next-generation sequencing; PCR, polymerase chain reaction.

immunisation, the persistence and type of immunological challenge and the immune status of the host. Cytotoxic HLA antibodies can be identified in approximately 20% of human pregnancies. The antibodies produced are normally multispecific, high titre, high affinity and of the IgG class. Although these HLA IgG antibodies can cross the placenta, they are not harmful to the fetus. Antibodies produced following transplantation are mostly IgG, although rarely HLA IgM antibodies have been identified. In contrast, the majority of HLA antibodies found in multitransfused patients are multispecific IgM and IgG and are mostly directed at public epitopes. The introduction of leucocyte-reduced blood components (see Chapter 22) may lead to a reduction in alloimmunisation in naive recipients, but it may not be very effective in preventing alloimmunisation in already sensitised recipients, i.e. women who have become immunised as a result of pregnancy.

The deliberate immunisation of healthy individuals to produce HLA-specific reagents is nowadays difficult to justify ethically. However, planned HLA immunisation is still carried out in some countries to treat women with a history of recurrent miscarriages. These women are immunised with leucocytes from their partners or from a third party to attempt to induce an immunomodulatory response that results in the maintenance of the pregnancy.

Detection of HLA Antibodies

A number of techniques to detect HLA antibodies have been developed. These include the complement-dependent lymphocytotoxicity (LCT) test, enzyme linked immunosorbent assay (ELISA) and flow cytometry and, more recently, a Luminex-based technique [9].

Complement-Dependent Cytotoxicity (CDC) Test

The complement-dependent cytotoxicity (CDC) test, developed by Terasaki and McClelland [10], allows the detection of complement-fixing antibodies reacting with the HLA antigen present on the cell surface, leading to the activation of complement via the classical pathway and in cell death. The CDC assay, however, does not discriminate between HLA and non-HLA cytotoxic lymphocyte-reactive antibodies such as IgM autoantibodies, although these antibodies are not thought to be of clinical significance in solid organ transplant recipients or in patients immunologically refractory to random donor platelet transfusions.

Since the CDC test only detects cytotoxic HLA-specific antibodies, other techniques such as the ELISA, flow cytometry or Luminex technology using beads coated with HLA antigens HLA-specific antibodies are currently being used.

Enzyme-Linked Immunosorbent Assay

In this technique, purified HLA antigens may be pooled for detection of HLA antibodies or derived from specific donors to allow the definition of HLA specific antibodies. The purified antigen is immobilised on a microwell plate, serum or plasma under investigation is added to the microplate and washed. Antibody binding is detected by an enzyme linked antihuman immunoglobulin for visualisation and analysis.

One of the main advantages of this ELISA technique is that it detects both complement fixing and noncomplement fixing HLA antibodies and is specific for HLA.

Flow Cytometry

In this technique, the bound antibody is detected by using an antibody against human immunoglobulin labelled with a fluorescent marker, such as fluorescein isothiocyanate or R-phycoerythrin. At the end of the incubation period, the cells are passed through the laser beam of the flow cytometer to identify the different cell populations based on their morphology/granularity and on the fluorescence. Normally, test sera with median fluorescence values greater than the mean +3 SD of the negative controls are considered positive, but each laboratory needs to establish its own positive and negative cut-off point values. By using a second antibody against cell-specific markers such as CD3 or CD19, it is possible to identify T- or B-cell reactivity.

Flow cytometric techniques are more sensitive when compared with LCT- and ELISA-based techniques, and for the detection of noncomplement-fixing antibodies produced early in the sensitisation. However, one of the disadvantages is that they also detect non-HLA lymphocyte-reactive antibodies that are of unclear clinical relevance.

The use of flow cytometric techniques was initially investigated as an alternative cross-match technique and was shown to be more sensitive than CDC, since it can detect both cytotoxic and noncytotoxic antibodies, some of which may be HLA specific.

Luminex

This technique uses fluorochrome-dyed polystyrene beads coated with specific HLA antigens. The precise ratio of these fluorochromes creates 100 distinctly coloured beads, each of which is coated with a single antigen. The beads are then incubated with the patient's serum and the reaction is detected using a PE-conjugated antihuman IgG (Fc-specific) antibody. The Luminex analyser has two lasers, the first to detect the internal fluorescence of the bead and the second to detect PE-labelled antihuman IgG indicating the presence of antibodies directed against the specific HLA antigen on that specific bead.

The CDC test and flow cytometry are the two main techniques used to perform antibody cross-matching between the patient's serum and the potential donor's cells in the solid organ transplant setting, whereas the Luminex technique is the main technique used for HLA antibody detection and definition.

Clinical Relevance of HLA Antigens and Antibodies

Although the main role of the HLA molecules is to present antigenic peptides to T-cells, HLA molecules can themselves be recognised as foreign by the host T-cells by a mechanism known as allorecognition. Two pathways of allorecognition have been identified: direct and indirect.

In the direct pathway, the host's T-cells recognise HLA molecules (primarily class II) expressed on donor tissues such as tissue dendritic cells and endothelial cells. Indirect allorecognition involves the recognition by the host T-cells of donor-derived HLA class I and II antigenic peptides presented by the host's own antigen-presenting cells. Because of this mechanism, HLA antigen incompatibility is one of the main barriers to success of solid organ or HSC transplantation and also results in the strong alloimmunisation seen in patients following transplantation or blood transfusion. Also, HLA antibodies are responsible for some of the serious immunological reactions to the transfusion of blood and blood components and play a pivotal role in the rejection of solid organ transplants [11].

HLA and Solid Organ Transplantation

Matching for HLA-A, -B and -DR antigens is an important factor influencing the outcome of solid organ transplantation and particularly renal transplants. Application of the PCR-based techniques has allowed the identification of molecular differences between otherwise serologically identical HLA types of donor and recipient pairs, particularly in the HLA-DRβ1 chain. Correlation of these results with graft survival has shown a higher kidney graft survival rate when recipients and donors are HLA-DR identical by serological and molecular techniques than when they are HLA-DR identical by serological but not molecular methods (87% versus 69%) [12].

The presence of circulating HLA-specific antibodies directed against donor antigens in renal and cardiac recipients has been associated with hyperacute rejection of the graft. It is therefore important that these antibodies are detected and identified as soon as the patient is registered on the transplant waiting list, to ensure that incompatible donors are not considered for transplantation [13]. Antibodies against HLA-C, DQ and DP also appear to influence graft outcome, and many centres test for these antibodies in patients awaiting transplantation.

Furthermore, the appearance of donor-specific antibodies after transplantation has been associated with graft rejection, indicating the importance of posttransplant antibody monitoring for some groups of patients.

HLA and Haemopoietic Stem Cell Transplantation

HLA incompatibility is one of the main factors associated with the development of acute graft-versus-host disease (aGVHD), particularly when using matched unrelated donors. Although HSC transplantation between HLA-identical siblings ensures matching for all HLA-A, -B, -C, -DRB1 and -DQB1 genes, acute GVHD still develops in about 20–30% of these patients. This is probably due to the effect of untested HLA antigens, such as DP, or minor histocompatibility antigens in the activation of donor T-cells. However, patients receiving grafts from HLA-matched unrelated donors have a higher risk of developing GVHD than those transplanted using an HLA-identical sibling [14].

The use of DNA-based methods has provided a unique opportunity to improve the HLA matching of patients and unrelated donors and to reduce the development of GVHD. However, it has been shown that the increased GVHD seen as a result of HLA mismatch is also associated with lower relapse rates, probably due to a graft-versus-leukaemia (GVL) response associated with the graft-versus-host response. The use of T-cell-depleted marrow, which has successfully decreased the incidence of GVHD, has also resulted in an increased incidence of leukaemia relapse. Thus, it appears that cells in the bone marrow, responsible for GVHD, may also be involved in the elimination of residual leukemic cells. Conversely, the rate of graft rejection is significantly higher in recipients of an HLA-mismatched transplant than in those receiving a transplant from an HLA-identical sibling (12.3% versus 2.0%) [14,15].

Haemopoietic stem cell transplantation using cord blood from HLA-matched and HLA-mismatched donors has been associated with a reduced risk and severity of GVHD and with no increase in relapse rates. It is possible that the immaturity of the immunological effectors present in cord blood may contribute to the reduced GVHD without impairment of the GVL effect.

Graft failure, which is thought to be mediated by residual recipient T- and/or NK cells reacting with major or minor histocompatibility antigens present in the donor marrow cells, has been shown to be associated also with antibodies reacting with donor's HLA antigens. Thus, rejection is particularly high in HLA-alloimmunised patients. HLA antibodies are also more relevant in the posttransplant period, where highly immunised patients can develop immunological refractoriness to random platelet transfusions due to the presence of HLA antibodies. These patients require transfusions of HLA-matched platelets (see Chapter 27).

HLA and Blood Transfusion

White cells and platelets present in transfused products express antigens that, if not identical to those expressed by the recipient, are able to activate T-cells and lead to the development of antibodies and/or effector cells responsible for some of the serious complications of blood transfusion. Also, antibodies (and T-cells) present in the transfused product may react directly with the relevant antigens in the recipient and lead to the development of a transfusion reaction. Amongst the transfusion reactions due to the presence of antibodies in the recipient are a febrile nonhaemolytic transfusion reaction (FNHTR) (Chapter 9) and immunological refractoriness to random platelet transfusions (Chapter 29) [11].

The occurrence of FNHTR is most commonly associated with the presence of HLA antibodies and to a lesser extend with human platelet antigen (HPA) or human neutrophil antigen (HNA) antibodies in the recipient reacting with white blood cells or platelets present in the transfused product. However, FNHTRs may also be triggered by the direct action of cytokines such as IL-1β, TNF-α, IL-6 and/or by chemokines such as IL-8, which are found in transfused products.

Immunological refractoriness to random platelet transfusions is primarily due to the presence of HLA and, to a lesser extent, HPA

and high-titre ABO alloantibodies in the patient reacting with the transfused incompatible platelets leading to the lack of platelet increments after the transfusion. Following the introduction of universal leucocyte reduction, the proportion of multitransfused patients with HLA antibodies seems to have decreased to approximately 10–20% and these patients are, in general, previously sensitised transplanted or transfused recipients and multiparous women.

The development of transfusion-related acute lung injury (TRALI) (Chapter 10) has been associated with the transfusion of blood components containing HLA and HNA antibodies able to recognise the relevant antigen(s) on recipient white cells and triggering an immunological reaction leading to the accumulation of neutrophils in the lungs and oedema. TRALI has sometimes been associated with the presence of HLA or HNA antibodies in recipients reacting with transfused leucocytes and/or to interdonor antigen–antibody reactions in pooled platelets.

Transfusion-associated (TA) GVHD (Chapter 13), which is a rare but often severe and fatal transfusion reaction, is the result of immunocompetent HLA-matched T-lymphocytes present in blood or blood components reacting with HLA and/or minor histocompatibility antigens present on the recipient cells. TA-GVHD occurs primarily in immunosuppressed individuals, although it can also occur in immunocompetent recipients. The diagnosis of TA-GVHD depends on finding evidence of donor-derived cells, chromosomes or DNA in the blood and/or affected tissues of the recipient.

HLA and Disease

HLA genes are known to be associated with a number of autoimmune and infectious diseases [16,17] and different mechanisms to explain these associations have been postulated, including linkage disequilibrium with the relevant disease susceptibility gene, the preferential presentation of the pathogenic peptide by certain HLA molecules and molecular mimicry between certain pathogenic peptides and host-derived peptides.

Box 4.1   HLA-associated diseases.

HLA class I genes
  Birdshot chorioretinopathy: *HLA-A*29*
  Behçet's disease: *HLA-B*51*
  Ankylosing spondylitis: *HLA-B*27*
  Psoriasis: *HLA-Cw*06*
  Malaria: *HLA-B*53*

HLA class II genes
  Rheumatoid arthritis
  HLA-DRB1*04:01
  HLA-DRB1*04:04
  HLA-DRB1*04:05
  HLA-DRB1*04:08
  HLA-DRB1*01:01/01:02
  HLA-DRB1*14:02
  HLA-DRB1*10:01
Narcolepsy: *HLA-DQB1*06:02/DQA1*01:02*
Celiac disease: *HLA-DQB1*02:01/DQA1*05:01(DQ2)* ;
HLA-DQB1*03:02/DQA1*03:01(DQ8)
HPA-1a Antibody production in neonatal allo-
immune thrombocytopenia: *HLA-DRB3*01:01*
Malaria: *HLA-DRB1*13:02/DQB1*05:01*
Insulin-dependent diabetes mellitus: *HLA-
DQB1*03: 02/DQA1*03:01*

HLA-linked diseases
  Haemochromatosis: HFE gene, *C282Y*, *H63D*
  and *S65C*
  21-OH deficiency: *(HLA-B*47) 21-OH* gene
  Abacavir hypersensitivity: *B*57:01*

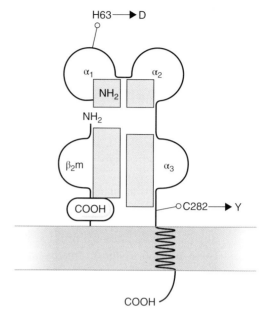

Figure 4.6 HFE molecule. β_2-m, β_2-microglobulin.

More recently, it has been shown that HLA genes are also involved in the response to certain drugs, such as the association of HLA-B*57:01 and abacavir, a drug used in the treatment of HIV [18].

A number of diseases associated with both HLA class I and II are described in Box 4.1.

Hereditary Haemochromatosis

Hereditary haemochromatosis (HH) is caused by an inherited disorder in the genes involved in the metabolism of iron. HH is a common genetic disorder in northern Europe, where between 1 in 200 and 1 in 400 individuals suffer from the disease,

with an estimated carrier frequency of between 1 in 8 and 1 in 10. Clinical manifestations of HH include cirrhosis of the liver, diabetes and cardiomyopathy. Detection of asymptomatic iron overload is important since removal of excess iron by phlebotomy can prevent organ damage [19].

Hereditary haemochromatosis, originally described associated to HLAA3, was later found to be related to mutations in the HFE gene located 3 Mb telomeric from the HLA-F gene. At least three of these mutations (C282Y, H63D and S65C) may predispose to and affect the clinical outcome of this condition. Over 90% of HH patients in the UK are homozygous for the mutation that replaces a cysteine (C) with a tyrosine (Y) at codon 282 in the HFE gene. The second and third mutations (H63D and S65C) are thought to be less important, although they may have an additive effect if inherited with the first mutation (Figure 4.6). Recent studies on blood donors have shown that approximately 1 in 280 donors is homozygous for the mutations. DNA-based techniques allow a simple, rapid and unambiguous definition of these mutations.

Neonatal Alloimmune Thrombocytopenia

This is a serious condition affecting newborns and is due to fetomaternal incompatibility for HPAs (see also Chapters 5 and 33). More than 80% of cases occur in women who are homozygous for the *HPA-1b* allele. The majority of cases are associated with the presence of HPA-1a antibodies; about 15% of cases are due to anti-HPA-5b. The production of HPA-1a antibodies is strongly associated with the *HLA-DRB3*0101* allele. However, only approximately 35% of HPA-1a-negative, DRB3*0101-positive women develop antibodies upon exposure to the antigen, suggesting that other genes or factors may be involved in the development of alloimmunisation against HPA-1a.

Other Diseases

Diseases in which the molecular mimicry mechanism has been postulated include HLA-B*27 with ankylosing spondylitis and *Klebsiella* infection although the precise pathogenic mechanisms involved remain unknown.

Recent genome-wide association studies [20] using over 1000 single nucleotide polymorphisms (SNPs) located in the MHC have identified a number of SNP in strong linkage disequilibrium with some of the HLA-associated diseases such as rheumatoid arthritis and systemic lupus erythematosus.

KEY POINTS

1) HLA molecules are crucial in the induction and regulation of immune responses and in the outcome of transplantation using allogeneic-related and -unrelated donors and are also responsible for some of the serious immunological complications of blood transfusion.
2) The main feature of HLA genes is their high degree of polymorphism and linkage disequilibrium and, depending on their molecular structure, expression and function, they are classified as classical or nonclassical.
3) The definition of HLA polymorphisms is currently performed using DNA-based techniques at various degrees of resolution depending on the clinical need and relevance.
4) The techniques currently used to screen and define the specificity of HLA antibodies allow the discrimination of HLA and non-HLA cytotoxic and noncytotoxic antibodies.
5) HLA antibodies produced following transfusion, transplantation or pregnancy are responsible for some of the most serious complications of blood transfusion.
6) HLA matching and cold ischemia time are the two most important factors influencing the outcome of renal transplantation.
7) In the HSC transplantation setting, HLA matching for HLA class I and II genes is essential to minimise the development of GVHD.
8) HLA genes are involved in the pathogenesis of a variety of diseases either directly through the presentation of pathogenic peptides or indirectly through their linkage disequilibrium with the relevant disease susceptibility gene(s).

References

1 Campbell RD. The human major histocompatibility complex: a 4000-kb segment of the human genome replete with genes, in Genome Analysis, Vol.5: Regional Physical Mapping (eds KE Davies, SM Tilghman), Cold Spring Harbor Laboratory Press, New York, 1993, pp.1–33.

2 Horton R, Wilming L, Rand V et al. Gene map of the extended human MHC. Nat Rev 2004;**5**:889–99.

3 Parham P, McQueen KL. Alloreactive killer cells: hindrance and help for haematopoietic transplants. Nat Rev Immunol 2003;**3**:108–21.

4 Traherne JA. Human MHC architecture and evolution: implications for disease association studies. J Immunogenet 2008;**35**:179–92.

5 Marsh SG, Albert ED, Bodmer WF et al. Nomenclature for factors of the HLA system. Tissue Antigens 2010;**75**:291–455.

6 Nunes E, Heslop H, Fernandez-Vina M et al. Definitions of histocompatibility typing term. Blood 2011;**118**:e180–e183.

7 Metzker ML. Sequencing technologies – the next generation. Nature Rev Genet 2010;**11**:31–46.

8 Shiina T, Suzuki S, Ozaki Y et al. Super high resolution for single molecule – sequence-based typing of classical HLA loci at the 8-digit level using next generation sequencers. Tissue Antigens 2012;**80**:305–16.

9 Howell WM, Carter V, Clark B. The HLA system: immunobiology, HLA typing, antibody screening and crossmatching techniques. J Clin Pathol 2010;**63**:387–90.

10 Terasaki PL, McClelland JD. Microdroplet assay of human serum cytokines. Nature 2000;**204**:998–1000.

11 Brown CJ, Navarrete CV. Clinical relevance of the HLA system in blood transfusion. Vox Sang 2011;**101**:93–105.

12 Opelz G, Döhler B. Effects of human leucocyte antigen compatibility of kidney graft survival: comparative analysis of two decades. Transplantation 2007;**84**:137–43.

13 Dyer PA, Claas FHJ. A future for HLA matching in clinical transplantation. Eur J Immunogenet 1997;**24**:17–28.

14 Madrigal JA, Arguello R, Scott I, Avakian H. Molecular histocompatibility typing in unrelated donor bone marrow transplantation. Blood Rev 1997;**11**:105–17.

15 Petersdorf EW, Malkki M, Gooley TA et al. MHC haplotype matching for unrelated hematopoietic cell transplantation. PloS Med 2007;**4**:59–68.

16 Caillat-Zucman S. Molecular mechanisms of HLA association with autoimmune diseases. Tissue Antigens 2009;**73**(1):1–8.

17 Gambaro G, Anglani F, d'Angelo A. Association studies of genetic polymorphisms and complex disease. Lancet 2000;**355**:308–11.

18 Profaizer T, Eckels D. HLA alleles and drug hypersensitivity reactions. Int J Immunogenet 2011;**39**:99–105.

19 Bomford A. Genetics of haemochromatosis. Lancet 2002;**360**:1673–81.

20 Dilthey A, Cox C, Iqbal Z, Nelson M R, McVean G. Improved genome inference in the MHC using a population reference graph. Nature Genet 2015;**47**:682–8.

Further Reading

Brown C, Navarrete C. HLA antibody screening by LCT, LIFT and ELISA, in Histocompatibility Testing (eds J Bidwell, C. Navarrete), Imperial College Press, London, 2000, pp.65–98.

Brown C. Human leucocyte antigens and their clinical significance, in Transfusion & Transplantation Science (ed. R Knight), Oxford University Press, Oxford, 2012, pp.162–86.

Contreras M, Navarrete C. Immunological complications of blood transfusion, in ABC of Transfusion, 4th edn (ed. M Contreras), Wiley-Blackwell, Oxford, 2009, pp.61–8.

Harrison J, Navarrete C. Selection of platelet donors and provision of HLA matched platelets, in Histocompatibility Testing (eds J Bidwell, C. Navarrete), Imperial College Press, London, 2000, pp.379–90.

Navarrete C. Human leucocyte antigens, in Practical Transfusion Medicine, 3rd edn (eds MF Murphy, DH Pamphilon), Wiley-Blackwell, Oxford, 2009, pp.30–43.

Ouwehand H, Navarrete C. The molecular basis of blood cell alloantigens, in Molecular Hematology, 3rd edn (eds D Proven, J Gribben), Blackwell Publishing, Oxford, 2010, pp.259–75.

Parham P, Moffett A. How did variable NK-cell receptors and MHC class I ligands influence immunity, reproduction and human evolution? Nat Rev Immunol 2013;**13**(2):133–44.

5

Platelet and Neutrophil Antigens

Brian R. Curtis

Platelet and Neutrophil Immunology Laboratory and Blood Research Institute, Blood Center of Wisconsin, Milwaukee, USA

Antigens on Platelets and Granulocytes

Antigens on human platelets and granulocytes can be categorised according to their biochemical nature into:

- carbohydrate antigens on glycolipids and glycoproteins:
  - A, B and O
  - P and Le on platelets, I on granulocytes
- protein antigens:
  - human leucocyte antigen (HLA) class I (A, B and C)
  - glycoprotein (GP)IIb/IIIa, GPIa/IIa, GPIb/IX/V, etc., on platelets
  - FcγRIIIb (CD16), CD177, etc., on granulocytes
- drug-dependent antigens:
  - quinine, quinidine
  - some antibiotics, e.g. penicillins and cephalosporins, vancomycin
  - heparin.

These antigens can be targeted by some or all of the following types of antibodies:

- autoantibodies
- alloantibodies
- isoantibodies
- drug-dependent antibodies.

Many platelet and granulocyte antigens, for example ABO and HLA class I, are shared with other cells (Table 5.1); others, however, are restricted to single lineages.

This chapter is divided into two sections: the first focuses on proteins expressed predominantly on platelets, and in particular the human platelet alloantigens (HPAs), while the second section focuses on the equivalent proteins and alloantigens expressed predominantly on neutrophils (human neutrophil antigens, HNAs).

Human Platelet Antigens

Twenty-nine platelet polymorphisms have been described (Table 5.2); most were first discovered during investigation of cases of neonatal alloimmune thrombocytopenia (NAIT). The majority of these antigens are located on the GPIIIa subunit of the GPIIb/IIIa integrin (αIIb/β3, CD41/CD61), which is present at high density on the platelet membrane and seems to be particularly polymorphic and immunogenic. Others are located on the GPIIb subunit, on the GPIa subunit of GPIa/IIa (CD49b/CD29), GPIb/IX/V (CD42b/CD42a/CD42d) and CD109 [1].

These receptor complexes are critical to platelet function and are responsible for the stepwise process of platelet attachment to the damaged vessel wall. GPIb/IX/V is the receptor for the von Willebrand factor (vWF) and is implicated in the initial tethering of platelets to damaged

Practical Transfusion Medicine, Fifth Edition. Edited by Michael F. Murphy, David J. Roberts and Mark H. Yazer.
© 2017 John Wiley & Sons Ltd. Published 2017 by John Wiley & Sons Ltd.

Table 5.1 Antigen expression on peripheral blood cells.

Antigen	Erythrocytes	Platelets	Neutrophils	B-lymphocytes	T-lymphocytes	Monocytes
A, B, H	+++	+/+++*	−	−	−	−
I	+++	++	++	−	−	−
Rh**	+++	−	−	−	−	−
K	+++	−	−	−	−	−
HLA class I	−/(+)	+++	++	+++	+++	+++
HLA class II	−	−	−/+ ++†	+++	−/+++†	+++
GPIIb/IIIa	−	+++	(+)‡	−	−	−
GPIa/IIa	−	++	−	−	++	−
GPIb/IX/V	−	+++	−	−	−	−
CD109	−	(+)/+†	−	−	−/++†	(+)
FcγRIIIb (CD16b)	−	−	+++	−	−	−
CD177	−	−	+++§	−	−	−
CTL-2	−	(+)	++	++	+++	?/-
CD11b/18	−	−	++	++	++	++¶
CD11a/18	−	−	++	++	++	++
CD36 (GPIV)	-/+∫	+++	-	-	-	+++

+++, ++, + Level of antigen expression in decreasing order. (+)weak expression, ? not known.
* Platelets from 4–6% of individuals have 'high expression' of A and/or B antigens.
** Nonglycosylated.
† On activated cells.
‡ GPIIIa in association with an alternative α chain (α_v).
§ Expressed on a subpopulation of neutrophils.
¶ Also expressed on natural killer cells.
∫ On nucleated erythrocytes.

endothelium. The GPIbα-bound vWF interacts with collagen, facilitating the interaction of collagen with its signalling (GPVI) and attachment receptors (GPIa/IIa). Outside-in signalling via GPVI leads to conformational changes in integrins GPIIb/IIIa and GPIa/IIa from 'locked' to 'open' configurations, exposing the high-affinity binding sites for collagen and fibrinogen, respectively. GPIIb/IIIa is the major platelet fibrinogen receptor and is critical to the final phase of platelet aggregation, but it also binds fibronectin, vitronectin and vWF. The function of CD109 has not been fully elucidated although recent studies suggest a role in regulation of transforming growth factor β (TGF-β)-mediated signalling. Glanzmann's thrombasthenia and Bernard–Soulier syndrome are rare and severe, autosomal recessive, platelet bleeding disorders caused by deletions or mutations in the genes encoding GPIIb and GPIIIa, or GPIbα, GPIbβ and GPIX, respectively [2].

Inheritance and Nomenclature

Most HPAs have been shown to be biallelic, with each allele being co-dominant, although recently the HPA-1, -5 and -7 systems have been shown to have third alleles. The nomenclature for HPAs involves consecutive numbering (HPA-1, -2, -3 and so on) (see Table 5.2) according to the date of discovery, with the major allele in each system designated 'a' and the minor allele 'b' [1,3].

Table 5.2 Human platelet antigens.

Antigens	Phenotypic frequency*	Glycoprotein	Amino acid change	Encoding gene	Nucleotide change	dbSNP number
HPA-1a	72% a/a	GPIIIa	Leu33Pro	*ITGB3*	176 T > C	rs5918
HPA-1b	26% a/b					
	2% b/b					
HPA-2a	85% a/a	GPIbα	Thr145Met	*GPIBA*	482C > T	rs6065
HPA-2b	14% a/b					
	1% b/b					
HPA-3a	37% a/a	GPIIb	Ile843Ser	*ITGA2B*	2621 T > G	rs5911
HPA-3b	48% a/b					
	15% b/b					
HPA-4a	>99.9% a/a	GPIIIa	Arg143Gln	*ITGB3*	506G > A	rs5917
HPA-4b	<0.1% a/b					
	<0.1% b/b					
HPA-5a	88% a/a	GPIa	Glu505Lys	*ITGA2*	1600G > A	rs10471371
HPA-5b	20% a/b					
	1% b/b					
HPA-6bw	<1% b/b	GPIIIa	Arg489Gln	*ITGB3*	1544G > A	rs13306487
HPA-7bw	<1% b/b	GPIIIa	Pro407Ala	*ITGB3*	1297C > G	
HPA-8bw	<1% b/b	GPIIIa	Arg636Cys	*ITGB3*	1984C > T	
HPA-9bw	<1% b/b	GPIIb	Val837Met	*ITGA2B*	2602G > A	
HPA-10bw	<1% b/b	GPIIIa	Arg62Gln	*ITGB3*	263G > A	
HPA-11bw	<1% b/b	GPIIIa	Arg633His	*ITGB3*	1976G > A	
HPA-12bw	<1% b/b	GPIbβ	Gly15Glu	*GPIBB*	119G > A	
HPA-13bw	<1% b/b	GPIa	Met799Thr	*ITGA2*	2483C > T	
HPA-14bw	<1% b/b	GPIIIa	Lys611del	*ITGB3*	1909_1911del^{AAG}	
HPA-15bw	35% a/a	CD109	Ser682Tyr	*CD109*	2108C > A	rs10455097
	42% a/b					
	23% b/b					
HPA-16bw	<1% b/b	GPIIIa	Thr140Ile	*ITGB3*	497C > T	
HPA-17bw	<1% b/b	GPIIIa	Thr195Met	*ITGB3*	662C > T	
HPA-18bw	<1% b/b	GPIa	Gln716His	*ITGA2*	2235G > T	
HPA-19bw	<1% b/b	GPIIIa	Lys137Gln	*ITGB3*	487A > C	ss120032848
HPA-20bw	<1% b/b	GPIIb	Thr619Met	*ITGA2B*	1949C > T	ss120032852
HPA-21bw	<1% b/b	GPIIIa	Glu628Lys	*ITGB3*	1960G > A	ss120032849
HPA-22bw	<1% b/b	GPIIb	Lys164Thr	*ITGA2B*	584A > C	rs142811900
HPA-23bw	<1% b/b	GPIIIa	Arg622Trp	*ITGB3*	1942C > T	rs139166528
HPA-24bw	<1% b/b	GPIIb	Ser472Asn	*ITGA2B*	1508G > A	
HPA-25bw	<1% b/b	GPIa	Thr187Met	*ITGA2*	3347C > T	
HPA-26bw	<1% b/b	GPIIIa	Lys580Asn	*ITGB3*	1818G > T	
HPA-27bw	<1% b/b	GPIIb	Leu841Met	*ITGA2B*	2614C > A	rs149468422
HPA-28bw	<1% b/b	GPIIb	Val740Leu	*ITGA2B*	2311G > T	ss550827881
HPA-29bw	<1% b/b	GPIIIa	Thr7Met	*ITGB3*	98C > T	ss1221285311

* Based on studies of Caucasians.
rs, international SNP reference number in dbSNP database; SNP, single nucleotide polymorphism.

Antigens are only included in a system if antibodies against the alloantigen encoded by both the major and minor alleles have been reported; if an antibody against only one antigen has been reported, a 'w' (for workshop) is added after the antigen name, e.g. HPA-10bw.

For all but one of the 29 HPAs, the difference between the two alleles is a single nucleotide polymorphism (SNP), which changes the amino acid in the corresponding protein (Figure 5.1). Six HPAs are grouped into biallelic HPA systems (HPA-1–5 and HPA-15) and for all of these, except HPA-3 and HPA-15, the minor allele frequency is ≤0.2 in Caucasian populations. Homozygosity for the minor allele is therefore relatively rare so providing compatible blood components for patients with antibodies against high-frequency HPA antigens can be difficult. Some SNPs are population specific, for example SNP rs5918 (HPA-1 system) is absent in populations of the Far East; conversely, SNP rs5917 (HPA-4) is not present in Caucasians but is present in Far Eastern and Hispanic and Latino populations. It is therefore important to take ethnicity into account when investigating clinical cases of suspected HPA alloimmunisation.

Typing for HPAs

Many DNA-based typing techniques have been developed to determine HPA genotypes [4]. One such assay is the polymerase chain reaction using sequence-specific primers (PCR-SSP). This is a fast and reliable technique and has become a cornerstone in platelet immunology laboratories. High-throughput HPA SNP typing techniques with automated readout, such as Taqman assays, are now also in routine use and allow rapid, high-throughput genotyping that is especially useful for routine donor typing in blood centres.

Genotyping of fetal DNA from amniocytes or chorionic villus biopsy samples is of clinical value in cases of HPA alloimmunisation in pregnancies where there is a history of severe NAIT and the father is heterozygous for the implicated HPA SNP. Noninvasive HPA genotyping assays based on the presence of trace amounts of fetal DNA in maternal plasma have been recently described and reduce the risk to the fetus from invasive sampling procedures [5].

Platelet Isoantigens, Autoantigens and Drug-Dependent Antigens

GPIV/CD36 is absent from the platelets of 2–8% of individuals of black African descent and 3–10% of Japanese and other Eastern Asian populations. If these individuals are exposed to GPIV-positive blood through pregnancy or transfusion, they may produce GPIV isoantibodies. These antibodies can cause NAIT, posttransfusion purpura or platelet refractoriness and may be responsible for febrile nonhaemolytic transfusion reactions (FNHTRs). Similarly, formation of isoantibodies can complicate both the pregnancies and transfusion support of patients with Glanzmann's thrombasthenia and Bernard–Soulier syndrome. Interestingly, GPIV-negative platelet transfusions are effective in raising platelet levels in GPIV-immunised patients.

The GPs carrying the HPAs are the targets of autoantibodies in autoimmune thrombocytopenia (AITP); these autoantibodies bind to the platelets of all individuals, regardless of their HPA type. Platelet autoimmunity is frequently associated with B-cell malignancies and during immune cell reengraftment following haemopoietic stem cell transplantation. In both situations, the presence of autoantibodies may contribute to the refractoriness to donor platelets.

Numerous drugs, and even some foods and herbal remedies, can associate with platelet GPs or preformed antibodies to form antigens that elicit the formation of drug-dependent antibodies (DDAbs) in certain patients [6]. DDAbs only bind to the GP in the presence of drug; a classic example is quinine. Typically, quinine-dependent antibodies bind to GPIIb/IIIa and/or GPIb/IX/V although other GPs are sometimes the target. Other drugs frequently associated with drug-induced thrombocytopenia (DITP) include vancomycin, sulfamethoxazole-trimethoprim,

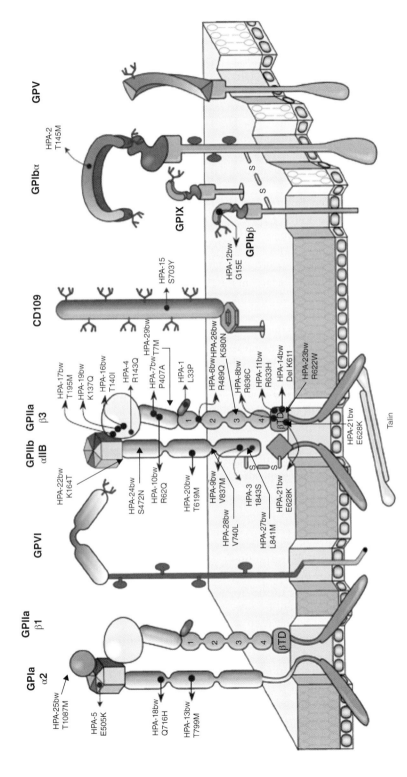

Figure 5.1 Representation of the platelet membrane and the glycoproteins (GP) on which the human platelet antigens (HPA) are localised. From left to right are depicted GPIa/IIa, GPIIb/IIIa, CD109 and GPIb/IX/V. The molecular basis of the HPAs is indicated by black dots, with the amino acid change in single-letter code and by residue number in the mature protein.

piperacillin, carbamazepine, rifampin and oxaliplatin. In haematooncology patients, who often receive a spectrum of drugs, unravelling the causes of persistent thrombocytopenia or poor responses to platelet transfusions can be complex because of the many possible causes of thrombocytopenia. Testing the patient's serum for the presence of DDAbs can help in determining if thrombocytopenia is drug induced. If the thrombocytopenia is drug mediated, withdrawal of the drug will result in recovery of the platelet count once the drug is eliminated from the circulation.

Another form of drug-dependent thrombocytopenia may be observed in coronary artery disease patients treated with ReoPro (abciximab). This function-blocking chimeric human–mouse F(ab) fragment against GPIIb/IIIa causes precipitous thrombocytopenia in approximately 1% of patients due to the presence of preexisting antibodies against ReoPro-induced neoepitopes.

The interaction of heparin with platelet factor 4 induces epitope formation that can cause antibody production and lead to heparin-induced thrombocytopenia (HIT) (see Chapter 31), but the reduction in platelet count is less profound than in classic examples of drug-mediated immune thrombocytopenia. The risk of thrombotic complications is the main concern in patients with HIT who show a mild but significant reduction in their platelet count after heparin administration.

Detection of HPA Alloantibodies

Optimal testing for platelet antibodies requires use of multiple methods. The platelet immunofluorescence test (PIFT) by flow cytometry is a highly sensitive assay, but is unable to distinguish between HPA and HLA class I antibodies. Despite this limitation, it remains widely used as a whole-cell assay capable of detecting a wide range of antibody specificities and is especially useful in detecting both autoantibodies and alloantibodies. The principles of the PIFT are shown in Plate 5.1 (see the plate section). Assays that use purified or captured GPs, such as the MAIPA assay, were developed for the detection and identification of HPA antibodies.

The widely used MAIPA assay captures specific GPs using monoclonal antibodies and can be used to analyse complex mixtures of platelet antibodies in patient sera [7]. The principle of this assay is shown in Figure 5.2. The MAIPA assay requires considerable operator expertise in order to ensure maximum sensitivity and specificity, and selection of appropriate screening cells is critical. Use of monoclonal antibodies that block binding of the patient's HPA antibodies, platelets heterozygous for the relevant HPA or from donors who have a low expression of particular antigens, e.g. HPA-15, may result in failure to detect clinically significant alloantibodies. Furthermore, recent evidence suggests that integrin conformation is an important factor in assay sensitivity. Recently, monoclonal antigen capture assays similar to MAIPA that use individual beads coated with GP-specific monoclonal antibodies have been developed. These assays are highly sensitive and allow for multiplexing for simultaneous detection of antibodies against multiple HPAs.

Clinical Significance of HPA Alloantibodies

Human platelet alloantigen alloantibodies are responsible for the following clinical conditions:

- NAIT: this condition is described in detail below (but also see Chapter 33)
- refractoriness to platelet transfusions (described in detail in Chapter 29)
- posttransfusion purpura (described in detail in Chapter 14).

Neonatal Alloimmune Thrombocytopenia
History
Neonatal alloimmune thrombocytopenia is a well-recognised clinical entity and the platelet counterpart of haemolytic disease of the newborn (HDFN), with an estimated incidence of severe thrombocytopenia due to maternal HPA antibodies of 1 per 1000–1200 live births [8]. Unlike HDFN, about 30% of cases of NAIT occur in first pregnancies.

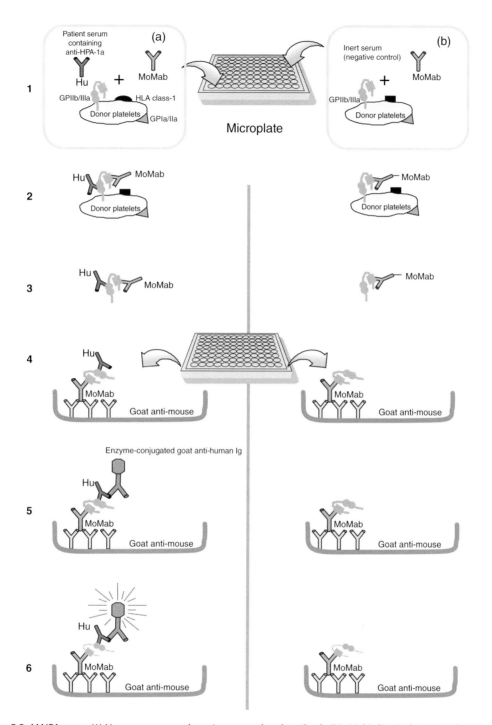

Figure 5.2 MAIPA assay. (1) Human serum and murine monoclonal antibody (MoMab) directed against glycoprotein being studied, e.g. GPIIb/IIIa are sequentially incubated with target platelets: in (a) the test serum contains anti-HPA-1a and in (b) no platelet antibodies are present. (2) After incubation, a trimeric (a) or dimeric (b) complex is formed. Excess serum antibody and MoMab are removed by washing. (3) The platelet membrane is solubilised in nonionic detergent, releasing the complexes into the fluid phase; particulate matter is removed by centrifugation. (4) The lysates containing the glycoprotein/antibody complexes are added to wells of a microtitre plate previously coated with goat anti-mouse antibody. (5) Unbound lysate is removed by washing and enzyme-conjugated goat antihuman antibody is added. (6) Excess conjugate is removed by washing and substrate solution is added. Cleavage of substrate, i.e. a colour reaction, indicates binding of human antibody to target platelets.

Definition and Pathophysiology

Neonatal alloimmune thrombocytopenia is due to maternal HPA alloimmunisation caused by fetomaternal incompatibility for a fetal HPA inherited from the father that is absent in the mother. Maternal IgG alloantibodies against the fetal HPA cross the placenta, bind to fetal platelets and, depending on a number of factors, may reduce platelet survival. Severe thrombocytopenia in the term neonate, accompanied by haemorrhage, is generally caused by HPA-1a antibodies if the mother is Caucasian. Antibodies against HPA-2 and HPA-4 antigens are more often implicated in cases of Far Eastern ethnicity. In the latter and in black Africans, GPIV deficiency should also be considered. Antibodies against HPA-5b and -5a tend to cause much less severe NAIT than anti-HPA-1a, probably due to the low copy number of the GPIa/IIa complex (3000/platelet versus 80 000/platelet for GPIIb/IIIa).

Neonatal alloimmune thrombocytopenia due to alloantibodies against other HPAs is infrequent and HLA class I antibodies, present in 15–25% of multiparous women, are rarely, if ever, the cause of NAIT. Clearance of IgG-coated fetal platelets takes place predominantly in the spleen through interaction with mononuclear cells bearing Fcγ receptors for the constant domain of IgG.

HPA-1a is known to be expressed on fetal platelets from 16 weeks' gestation and placental transfer of IgG antibodies can occur as early as 14 weeks, so thrombocytopenia can occur early in pregnancy and intracranial haemorrhage (ICH) has been reported as early as 16 weeks' gestation.

Incidence

Prospective screening of pregnant Caucasian women has shown that about 1 in 1200 neonates has severe thrombocytopenia ($<50 \times 10^9/L$) because of alloimmunisation against HPA-1a. However, the authors' experience and other studies, where prospective screening was not carried out [9], indicate that the number of samples referred for investigation of suspected NAIT is considerably less, which suggests that many cases are undiagnosed.

Clinical Features

A typical case of NAIT presents with skin bleeding (purpura, petechiae and/or ecchymoses) or more serious haemorrhage, such as ICH, in a full-term and otherwise healthy newborn with a normal coagulation screen and isolated thrombocytopenia. There are less common presentations *in utero*, including ventriculomegaly, cerebral cysts and hydrocephalus, which may be discovered by routine ultrasound. Although rare, hydrops fetalis has been reported in association with NAIT and this diagnosis should be considered if there are no other obvious reasons for the hydrops.

The precise incidence of ICH due to NAIT is unknown, but conservative estimates suggest that it is as low as 1 in 20 000 live births. Nearly 50% of severe ICHs occur *in utero*, usually between 30 and 35 weeks' gestation, but sometimes before 20 weeks. At the other end of the clinical spectrum, and more commonly, NAIT is discovered incidentally when a blood count is performed for other reasons.

Differential Diagnosis

Other causes of neonatal thrombocytopenia are infection, prematurity, intrauterine growth retardation, inherited chromosomal abnormalities (particularly trisomy 21), maternal autoimmune thrombocytopenic purpura (AITP) and, very rarely, inherited forms of inadequate megakaryopoiesis. Maternal platelet autoimmunity is rarely associated with severe thrombocytopenia in the neonate, but should be considered in women with a history of AITP.

Laboratory Investigations

Only antibodies against HPAs or isoantibodies against GPIIb/IIIa, GPIb/IX, CD109 and GPIV are thought to cause alloimmune thrombocytopenia in the fetus and neonate, although there are reports of platelet autoantibodies from patients with AITP crossing the placenta and causing neonatal thrombocytopenia.

For appropriate clinical management, the cause of severe thrombocytopenia in an otherwise healthy neonate should be urgently investigated. Screening for maternal HPA antibodies must be carried out, preferably by an experienced reference lab using techniques with appropriate sensitivity and specificity. HPA antibodies are detected in approximately 30% of referrals of suspected NAIT referred to the Platelet and Neutrophil Immunology Reference Laboratory, Milwaukee, USA. The most frequently detected antibody specificities are HPA-1a and HPA-5b, which are implicated in about 85% and 10% of clinically diagnosed cases of NAIT, respectively. The ability of an HPA-1a-negative mother to form anti-HPA-1a is significantly controlled by the class II HLA *DRB3*01:01* allele. This allele is present in approximately 30% of Caucasoid women, and the chance of HPA-1a antibody formation is greatly enhanced in HPA-1a-negative women who are HLA *DRB3*01:01*-positive compared to *DRB3*01:01*-negative women (odds ratio of 140). The absence of HLA *DRB3*01:01* has a negative predictive value of as high as 99% for HPA-1a alloimmunisation but its positive predictive value is only 35%, limiting its potential usefulness as part of an antenatal screening programme. However, it remains of clinical use when counselling female siblings from index cases who have formed HPA-1a antibodies in pregnancy. About 10% of HPA-1a-negative women develop anti-HPA-1a in pregnancy, and of these, about 30% will deliver a neonate with a platelet count $<50 \times 10^9$/L.

Molecular typing of the parents and neonate for HPA-1, -2, -3, -5 and HPA-15 should be performed because the results will be informative when interpreting antibody investigation results. For patients from the Far East, HPA-4 must also be included and the platelets should be investigated for GPIV expression status.

Alloimmunisation against low-frequency HPAs, e.g. HPA-9bw, explain some NAIT referrals that have a negative antibody screen for the common HPA antibody specificities. A practical approach to detecting antibodies against low-frequency antigens that are absent from cells used in antibody screening panels is to perform a cross-match of maternal serum against paternal platelets, and genotype paternal or affected infants' DNA samples for low-frequency HPA SNPs when GP-specific antibodies are detected against paternal platelets only. It is also necessary to exclude positive findings due to ABO or HLA class I antibodies.

Neonatal Management

A cord platelet count of $<100 \times 10^9$/L should be repeated using a venous sample and a blood film examined. The neonate should be examined for skin or mucosal bleeding if a low platelet count is confirmed. If the platelet count is $<30 \times 10^9$/L or if there are signs of bleeding with a low count, it is strongly recommended that the neonate is transfused with donor platelets that are HPA-1a and -5b negative, as these will be compatible with the maternal HPA alloantibody in ≥95% of NAIT cases, but if HPA-compatible platelets are not immediately available and there is an urgent clinical need for transfusion then random, ABO and RhD-compatible, donor platelets should be used [10]. In a typical case, the platelet count should recover to normal within a week, although a more protracted recovery can occur. Intravenous immunoglobulin (IvIgG) is not recommended as a first-line treatment as it is only effective in about 75% of cases and there is a delay of 24–48 hours before a satisfactory count is achieved; this is in contrast to the immediate effect of transfusion of HPA-compatible donor platelets. A cerebral ultrasound scan of the baby within the first week of life should be considered if the platelet count is $<50 \times 10^9$/L and is recommended when the platelet count is 30×10^9/L.

Antenatal Management

In a subsequent pregnancy of a mother with serologically confirmed NAIT, the clinical management needs to be planned by a team experienced in the management of the risks of this condition. Treatment during the subsequent pregnancy is based on the history of haemorrhage and fetal/neonatal thrombocytopenia in previous pregnancies.

Infusions of high-dose IvIgG to the mother is the safest and most effective intervention to reduce the risk of ICH in the at-risk fetus [11]. The dose is 1 g/kg bodyweight at weekly intervals, usually from 20 weeks' gestation onwards; some fetal medicine specialists will use a higher dose (2 g/kg/week) and/or between 12 and 20 weeks' gestation, depending on the history of NAIT in previous pregnancies. Early commencement of treatment is indicated where there is a history of antenatal ICH in previous pregnancies, because the earliest reports of ICH are at 16 weeks. A beneficial effect of IvIgG on the fetal platelet count occurs in approximately 70% of cases.

The delivery needs careful planning between obstetric, paediatric and haematology teams to ensure an appropriate mode of delivery, and close liaison with blood transfusion services for timely provision of HPA-compatible platelets for the neonate. For neonates who have been transfused *in utero*, irradiation of cellular blood components is recommended.

Counselling

Counselling of couples with an index case about the risks of severe fetal/neonatal thrombocytopenia in a subsequent pregnancy needs to be based on disease severity in the infant(s) and outcome of immunological investigations. The following should be taken into account:

- thrombocytopenia in subsequent cases is as severe or, generally, more severe
- the best predictors of severe fetal thrombocytopenia in a future pregnancy are antenatal ICH and severe thrombocytopenia (platelet count $<30 \times 10^9$/L) in a previous pregnancy
- antibody specificity
- antibody titre and bioactivity have been investigated to determine if these parameters have a predictive role in determining the severity

of NAIT – contradictory data have been obtained and currently are probably of no value in informing clinical management
- HPA zygosity of the partner. If the father is heterozygous, there is a 50% chance a future fetus will inherit the implicated HPA and be at significant risk of developing NAIT.

Human Neutrophil Antigens

Neutrophils, like platelets, express their own unique cell surface antigens. There are common antigens that have a wider distribution on other blood cells and tissues, e.g. I and P blood group systems and HLA class I. Unlike erythrocytes and platelets, neutrophils do not express ABO antigens. There are 'shared' antigens that have a limited distribution among other cell types, such as HNA-4 and HNA-5 polymorphisms associated with CD11/18. There are also a limited number of truly neutrophil-specific antigens, such as HNA-1a, HNA-1b, HNA-1c polymorphisms on FcγRIIIb/CD16b. The current nomenclature for HNA includes polymorphisms that are both cell specific and 'shared' (Table 5.3) [12].

HNA-1

The three antigens that comprise the HNA-1 antigens are localised on neutrophil FcγRIIIb (CD16), one of two low-affinity receptors (R) for the constant domain (Fc) of human IgG(γ) that are found on neutrophils. There are normally 100 000–200 000 copies of FcγRIIIb per neutrophil. Four amino acid differences in FcγRIIIb define the difference between HNA-1a and -1b, while a single amino acid substitution (alanine 78 > asparagine) defines the HNA-1c polymorphism. The expression of HNA-1c is frequently associated with the presence of an additional FcγRIIIb gene and increased expression of FcγRIIIb. The expression of HNA-1 antigens varies with ethnicity, with HNA-1a being more common in Chinese and Japanese populations and HPA-1b more common in Caucasians.

The FcγRIIIb 'Null' phenotype is rare and is based on a double deletion or mutation of the

Table 5.3 Human neutrophil antigens.

Antigen	Genotype frequency (%)*	Glycoprotein	Amino acid change	Encoding gene
1a	54	FcγRIIIb/CD16b	<u>36 38 65 78 82 106</u>	*FCGR3B*
1b	88		Arg Leu Asn Ala Asp Val	
1c	5		Ser Leu Ser Ala Asn Ile[†]	
			Ser Leu Ser Asp Asn Ile[†]	
2	97	CD177	nk	*CD177*
3a	94	CTL2	Arg152Gln	*SLC44A2*
3b	40	CTL2		
4a	99	CD11b	Arg61His	*ITGAM*
4b	1			
5a	85	CD11a	Arg766Thr	*ITGAL*
5bw	54			

* Frequencies based on studies of Caucasians.
[†] HNA-1b also carries the HNA-1d epitope, and HNA-1c also carries the HNA-1b epitope.
nk, not known.

FcγRIIIb gene and is, in some cases, associated with a deletion of the *FcγRIIc* gene. A maternal deficiency of FcγRIIIb can cause immune neutropenia in the newborn due to maternal FcγRIIIb isoantibodies. The FcγRIIIb molecule can also be the antigenic target in autoimmune neutropenias. Of note, as many as 23% of autoantibodies in autoimmune neutropenia of infancy have 'relative/stronger' reactivity for HNA-1a.

HNA-2

HNA-2, formerly known as HNA-2a or NB1, is localised on CD177 and expressed as a glycosylphosphatidylinositol-anchored membrane GP found both on the neutrophil surface membrane and on secondary granules. The term HNA-2a should no longer be used since it is now known that there is no antithetical antigen; rather, the HNA-2-negative phenotype is associated with particular sequence haplotypes from which nonproductive HNA-2 transcripts are generated, thereby causing a failure of CD177/HNA-2 expression, and such individuals are capable of producing CD177/HNA-2 antibodies when exposed to the protein.

The percentage of neutrophils expressing HNA-2 varies between individuals and HNA-2 alloantibodies typically give a bimodal fluorescence profile with granulocytes from HNA-2-positive donors in immunofluorescence tests with a flow cytometric endpoint. HNA-2 antigen status can be determined by phenotyping with polyclonal or monoclonal antibodies. A SNP (829A>T) was recently reported that introduces a stop codon in CD177 resulting in lack of CD177 expression on neutrophils. If confirmed, genotyping for this SNP will allow for a molecular screen of individuals at risk of CD177 isoimmunisation.

HNA-3

HNA-3a and HNA-3b antigens are expressed on choline transporter-like protein 2 (CTL2), and in addition to neutrophils are also expressed on T- and B-lymphocytes and weakly on platelets. The polymorphism is determined by a SNP in the *SLC44A2* gene that results in a A152G amino change in CTL2 that determines HNA-3a and HNA-3b, respectively. HNA-3b/b individuals can make HNA-3a antibodies, and 5–6% of Caucasians and 16% of Han Chinese have the HNA-3b/b type. HNA-3a antibodies have been implicated in neonatal alloimmune neutropenia (NAIN) and cause particularly severe cases of TRALI.

HNA-4 and HNA-5

The genes encoding the α_M and α_L subunits of the β_2 integrins CD11b/18 and CD11a/18 are polymorphic and are associated with HNA-4a/4b and HNA-5a/5bw, respectively. Alloantibody formation against these two polymorphisms has been observed in transfusion recipients, and recently cases of NAIN due to HNA-4a, HNA-4b and HNA-5a antibodies have been described. The low incidence of neonatal neutropenia associated with these antibodies is probably explained by the wide distribution of these proteins on granulocytes, monocytes and lymphocytes.

Detection of Neutrophil Antibodies

Reliable detection and identification of neutrophil antibodies are technically difficult due to the daily requirement for fresh, typed donor neutrophils since neutrophils cannot be stored. The incidence of antibody-mediated neutropenias is comparatively rare and, therefore, the best strategy for investigation of clinical cases is a national reference laboratory where adequate technical expertise and reagents are available.

The granulocyte immunofluorescence test by flow cytometry (GIFT-FC) and the granulocyte chemiluminescence tests have the advantage of good sensitivity but are not specific, i.e. they cannot readily distinguish between granulocyte-specific and HLA class I antibodies without further investigations. For some HNA systems, such as antigens expressed on CD16, CD177 and CD11/18, the monoclonal antibody immobilisation of granulocyte antigens (MAIGA) assay can be applied to determine HNA specificity. The principles of the granulocyte immunofluorescence test and the MAIGA assays are analogous to the equivalent platelet tests (see Plate 5.1 and Figure 5.2, respectively). Increased understanding of the molecular nature of HNAs has opened up the potential to develop recombinant HNAs and both cell lines expressing recombinant proteins (rHNA) and soluble rHNA coupled to a solid phase have been described. These new assays have shown promise but, currently, generally lack the sensitivity and specificity of established techniques.

Like for HPA, HNA typing is performed by PCR-SSP or sequence-based typing techniques with the exception of HNA-2, which currently requires typing fresh neutrophils with CD177 monoclonal antibodies by GIFT-FC.

Clinical Significance of HNA Antibodies

Neutrophil-specific antibodies are implicated in:

- neonatal alloimmune neutropenia (NAIN)
- febrile nonhaemolytic transfusion reactions
- transfusion-related acute lung injury (TRALI) (see Chapter 10)
- autoimmune neutropenia
- persistent postbone marrow transplant neutropenia.

Neonatal Alloimmune Neutropenia
Maternal alloimmunisation against neutrophil-specific alloantigens on fetal/neonatal neutrophils is a condition analogous to NAIT in terms of pathophysiology but, with an estimated incidence of 0.1–0.2% of live births, is comparatively rare as a clinically significant entity although there are no reliable figures. Clinical presentation is mainly one of bacterial infections with isolated neutropenia being the only haematological abnormality. The neutropenia may be severe but is reversible and newborn infants may require treatment with antibiotics and/or G-CSF to control bacterial infections and hasten recovery to a normal neutrophil count. The neutropenia in some cases has been reported to extend for up to 32 weeks. HNA-1a and -2 are the most commonly implicated antibody specificities.

FNHTR and TRALI (see Chapter 10)
Febrile nonhaemolytic transfusion reactions have a number of different causes. They can occasionally be associated with the presence of leucocyte (HLA and HNA) alloantibodies in the recipient. Serological investigations for platelet, HLA and granulocyte antibodies are of limited

clinical value as the diagnostic specificity of these tests for FNHTRs is low. Nonetheless, testing for HNA antibodies may be required in rare cases in which a severe FNHTR cannot be otherwise explained and washed components have proved ineffective.

Transfusion-related acute lung injury is a severe and sometimes life-threatening transfusion reaction [13]. The majority of cases are caused by donor leucocyte alloantibodies against alloantigens present on the patient's leucocytes, although patient alloantibodies may be involved. HLA class I- and II-specific antibodies and HNA antibodies have been implicated as causal agents, with HNA-1a and HNA-3a antibody specificities being found most commonly [14]. TRALI investigations are logistically complex because of the need to contact all the implicated donors to obtain fresh blood samples. The donor samples are screened for both HLA and HNA alloantibodies. If antibodies are found, it is necessary to type the patient to determine whether they have the cognate antigen and to type the donor to establish that they lack the antigen. In some cases, it may be necessary to screen a recipient's serum for antibodies or to perform a cross-match between donor sera and the patient's granulocytes and lymphocytes.

Many blood transfusion services have taken steps to reduce the incidence of TRALI, for example by reducing the proportion of female donors for plasma and platelet components, and more recently by screening female donors for HLA and HNA antibodies. The success of these strategies has been demonstrated by the reduced incidence of TRALI in haemovigilance schemes [15].

Autoimmune Neutropenia

Autoimmune neutropenia is a rare condition that can occur as a transient, self-limiting autoimmunity in young children [16] or a chronic form in adults [17]. The autoantibodies tend to target the FcγRIIIb (CD16), CD177 or CD11/18 molecules but can also be HNA specific, for example antibodies with 'relative' HNA-1a

specificity are found in as many as 23% of childhood cases of autoimmune neutropenia.

The most sensitive method for the detection of autoantibodies is to test the patient's neutrophils using the direct immunofluorescence test. However, the combination of severe neutropenia, high blood sample volume requirements to recover sufficient granulocytes and the need for a fresh sample limits the applicability of this test, especially in children. Screening of a patient's serum with a panel of typed neutrophils in the indirect granulocyte immunofluorescence and granulocyte chemiluminescence or granulocyte agglutination tests provides a suitable alternative and, in some studies, this approach has been found to be only slightly less sensitive than performing a direct test.

Persistent Postbone Marrow Transplant Neutropenia

Antibody-mediated neutropenia may be a serious complication of bone marrow transplantation [18]. In this context, as the neutrophil antibodies may be autoimmune and/or alloimmune in nature, laboratory investigation requires serological and typing studies to elucidate the nature of the antibodies involved.

Drug-Induced Neutropenia

Drug-induced immune neutropenia (DIIN) occurs when drug-dependent antibodies form against neutrophil membrane glycoproteins and cause neutrophil destruction. Affected patients have fever, chills and infections; severe infections left untreated can result in death. Severe neutropenia or agranulocytosis associated with exposure to nonchemotherapy drugs ranges from approximately 1.6 to 15.4 cases per million population per year. Unlike for drug-induced immune thrombocytopenia and anaemia, studies of DIIN are limited so knowledge of possible mechanisms and utility of laboratory testing for antibodies is not well understood [19]. However, in cases of severe neutropenia, in which other causes have been ruled out, discontinuation of the suspected drug(s) should be considered.

KEY POINTS

1) Allo-, auto-, iso- and drug-dependent antigens may be found on platelets and neutrophils and are implicated in a range of immune cytopenias.
2) Alloantigens on platelets are known as HPAs; alloantigens on neutrophils are known as HNAs.
3) Reliable detection and identification of HPA- and HNA-specific antibodies require the use of both whole-cell type assays such as the PIFT/GIFT and antigen-capture type assays such as the MAIPA/MAIGA assays.
4) HPA and HNA types can mostly be determined using PCR-based methodologies.
5) NAIT is a common disorder and HPA-1a or HPA-5b antibodies are responsible for approximately 95% of cases.
6) Optimal postnatal treatment of NAIT is the transfusion of donor platelets lacking the HPA targeted by maternal antibodies.
7) Optimal antenatal treatment of NAIT is IvIgG with or without addition of steroids.
8) HNA antibodies can be associated with both alloimmune and autoimmune neutropenia.
9) TRALI can be a life-threatening condition, especially if HNA-3a antibodies are involved.
10) The incidence of antibody-mediated TRALI has been significantly reduced by implementation of a number of different strategies to reduce transfusion of leucocyte antibodies.

References

1 Curtis BR, McFarland JG. Human platelet antigens – 2013. Vox Sang 2014;**106**(2):93–102.
2 Nurden P, Nurden AT. Congenital disorders associated with platelet dysfunctions. Thromb Haemost 2008;**99**(2):253–63.
3 Metcalfe P, Watkins NA, Ouwehand WH et al. Nomenclature of human platelet antigens. Vox Sang 2003;**85**(3):240–5.
4 Curtis BR. Genotyping for human platelet alloantigen polymorphisms: applications in the diagnosis of alloimmune platelet disorders. Semin Thromb Hemost 2008;**34**(6):539–48.
5 Le Toriellec E, Chenet C, Kaplan C. Safe fetal platelet genotyping: new developments. Transfusion 2012;**53**(8):1755–62.
6 Curtis BR. Drug-induced immune thrombocytopenia: incidence, clinical features, laboratory testing, and pathogenic mechanisms. Immunohematology 2014;**30**(2):55–65.
7 Curtis BR, McFarland JG. Detection and identification of platelet antibodies and antigens in the clinical laboratory. Immunohematology 2009;**25**(3):125–35.
8 Bussel JB, Primiani A. Fetal and neonatal alloimmune thrombocytopenia: progress and ongoing debates. Blood Rev 2008;**22**(1):33–52.
9 Tiller H, Killie M, Skogen B, Oian P, Husebekk A. Neonatal alloimmune thrombocytopenia in Norway: poor detection rate with nonscreening versus a general screening programme. Br J Obstet Gynaecol 2009;**116**(4):594–8.
10 Kiefel V, Bassler D, Kroll H et al. Antigen-positive platelet transfusion in neonatal alloimmune thrombocytopenia (NAIT). Blood 2006;**107**(9):3761–3.
11 Pacheco LD, Berkowitz RL, Moise KJ Jr, Bussel JB, McFarland JG, Saade GR. Fetal and neonatal alloimmune thrombocytopenia: a management algorithm based on risk stratification. Obstet Gynecol 2011;**118**(5):1157–63.
12 Bux J. Human neutrophil alloantigens. Vox Sang 2008;**94**(4):277–85.
13 Bux J, Sachs UJ. The pathogenesis of transfusion-related acute lung injury (TRALI). Br J Haematol 2007;**136**(6):788–99.

14 Reil A, Keller-Stanislawski B, Gunay S, Bux J. Specificities of leucocyte alloantibodies in transfusion-related acute lung injury and results of leucocyte antibody screening of blood donors. Vox Sang 2008;**95**(4):313–17.

15 Lucas G, Win N, Calvert A et al. Reducing the incidence of TRALI in the UK: the results of screening for donor leucocyte antibodies and the development of national guidelines. Vox Sang 2012;**103**(1):10–17.

16 Bruin M, Dassen A, Pajkrt D, Buddelmeyer L, Kuijpers T, de Haas M. Primary autoimmune neutropenia in children: a study of neutrophil antibodies and clinical course. Vox Sang 2005;**88**(1):52–9.

17 Autrel-Moignet A, Lamy T. Autoimmune neutropenia. Presse Med 2014;**43**(4):e105–e118.

18 Stroncek DF, Shapiro RS, Filipovich AH, Plachta LB, Clay ME. Prolonged neutropenia resulting from antibodies to neutrophil-specific antigen NB1 following marrow transplantation. Transfusion 1993;**33**(2):168–3.

19 Curtis BR. Drug-induced immune neutropenia/agranulocytosis. Immunohematology 2014;**30**(2):95–101.

Further Reading

Bassler D, Greinacher A, Okascharoen C et al. A systematic review and survey of the management of unexpected neonatal alloimmune thrombocytopenia. Transfusion 2008;**48**:92–8.

Capsoni F, Sarzi-Puttini P, Zanella A. Primary and secondary autoimmune neutropenia. Arthritis Res Ther 2005;**7**:208–14.

Fung YL, Minchinton RM, Fraser JF. Neutrophil antibody diagnostics and screening: review of the classical versus the emerging. Vox Sang 2011;**101**:282–90.

Kjeldsen-Kragh J, Ni H, Skogen B. Towards a prophylactic treatment of HPA-related foetal and neonatal alloimmune thrombocytopenia. Curr Opin Hematol 2012;**19**(6):469–74.

Lucas GF, Metcalfe P. Platelet and granulocyte glycoprotein polymorphisms. Transfus Med 2000;**10**:157–74.

Murphy MF, Bussel JB. Advances in the management of alloimmune thrombocytopenia. Br J Haematol 2007;**136**:366–78.

Stroncek DF, Fadeyi E Adams S. Leukocyte antigen and antibody detection assays: tools for assessing and preventing pulmonary transfusion reactions. Transfus Med Rev 2007;**21**(4):273–86.

6 Pretransfusion Testing and the Selection of Red Cell Products for Transfusion

Mark H. Yazer[1] and Meghan Delaney[2]

[1] *Department of Pathology, University of Pittsburgh, Pittsburgh, USA; Department of Clinical Immunology, University of Southern Denmark, Odense, Denmark; ITXM Centralized Transfusion Service, Pittsburgh, USA*
[2] *Bloodworks Northwest and Department of Laboratory Medicine and Paediatrics, University of Washington, Seattle, USA*

Introduction

The goal of pretransfusion compatibility testing is to ensure that serologically safe blood products are issued to the recipient. It is therefore crucial to accurately determine the recipient's blood type (ABO group, D type) and whether they have any unexpected red cell antibodies. To this end, a 'type and screen' is often ordered together, although as detailed below, they are actually two separate tests.

Determining the Recipient's ABO Group and Screening for Unexpected Antibodies

Clerical Check and Verification of Recipient's Identity

The first step in ensuring the recipient's serological safety that the blood bank performs is a check of the recipient's name and unique identifiers that are supplied on the tube of blood and the requisition that specifies the nature of the testing to be performed. The name and unique identifiers on the tube of blood and the requisition must match exactly, as it has been demonstrated

that even a seemingly innocuous discrepancy can lead to an unacceptably high risk for a wrong blood in tube (WBIT) error [1]. WBIT errors, or miscollections, occur when the blood in the tube does not come from the recipient whose name is on the tube. These are serious errors that can lead to ABO-incompatible mistransfusions and possibly the death of the recipient. Any samples in which an identification discrepancy has been identified must be rejected, and a new, properly labelled sample obtained for testing. In some countries, it is mandatory for a recipient's ABO group to be tested twice on the same sample if the recipient does not have an ABO group on record at that hospital. This process merely validates the precision of the typing – it does not help to prevent WBIT errors.

To improve the accuracy of the typing, many hospitals have a requirement for a recipient without a historical type to have, at a minimum, their ABO group performed on two separately collected samples before ABO-identical components are issued [2]. If the ABO group of both samples match each other, confidence that the intended recipient's blood was actually drawn increases. Thus the historical type that is maintained on file functions as an important means of detecting miscollections, and the more recipients who are covered by a database of historical ABO groups, the further their serological safety is enhanced [3–5].

Determining the Recipient's ABO Group

To determine the recipient's ABO group, two complementary tests are used. The forward type (also known as front or cell typing) is used to detect the antigens on the recipient's red cells using monoclonal IgM anti-A and anti-B reagent blends and observing for agglutination. Pentameric IgM antibodies can cross-link antigens on adjacent cells, causing direct agglutination of red cells without requiring additional reagents. The reverse type (also known as back or plasma typing) makes use of the fact that virtually everyone older than a few months of age will have naturally occurring IgM antibodies to the A or B (or both) antigens lacking on their own red cells. This test is performed by separately mixing the recipient's serum or plasma with commercially available A_1 and B red cells and observing for agglutination. A reverse type is not performed on neonates whose serum is not typically tested until they are older than four months of age as any anti-A or anti-B detected in their serum is presumed to be of maternal origin. Expected patterns of agglutination are demonstrated in Table 6.1.

Occasionally discrepancies between the forward and reverse typings occur. Some common causes of ABO discrepancies include being immunosuppressed, receipt of IvIg and converting to the donor blood group after a stem cell transplant. Furthermore, genetic subtypes of A and B can also cause weak or absent agglutination on the forward type that can lead to discrepant results [6,7]. In very unusual cases, naturally occurring chimeras or individuals with mosaic phenotypes can produce very confusing and apparently discrepant results [8]. In all situations when an ABO discrepancy is detected, a thorough investigation into its cause should be performed, starting by ensuring that a WBIT error or accidental mistyping in the blood bank did not occur, before group-specific blood products can be issued.

Determining the Recipient's D Type

To determine the recipient's D type, a procedure similar to the forward type is performed. The recipient's red cells are exposed to an IgM monoclonal anti-D reagent which does not detect the DVI variant (because individuals with this phenotype can become alloimmunised if transfused with D-positive red cells; thus as recipients they should be typed as D negative and transfused with D-negative red cells). As with the forward type, agglutination is the positive endpoint of this test. D typing can be complicated when the recipient has weak or partial D alleles [9].

Difficulties in D Typing: Weak and Partial D

A weak D allele is one that typically encodes a protein with mutations in its intramembrane or intracellular regions such that it is unstable in the red cell membrane and fewer than normal numbers of the protein are expressed on the red cell surface (Figure 6.1). The RhD protein is thought to be fully intact with all its epitopes present; there are simply fewer proteins on the surface resulting in weaker than normal agglutination with some D typing reagents.

- Some recipients with rare weak D alleles have been demonstrated to be susceptible to alloimmunisation if transfused with D-positive red cells, some authors have suggested that

Table 6.1 Expected ABO grouping patterns.

	Forward type		Reverse type	
Group	Anti-A	Anti-B	A1 cells	B cells
A	+++	–	–	+++
B	–	+++	+++	–
O	–	–	+++	+++
AB	+++	+++	–	–

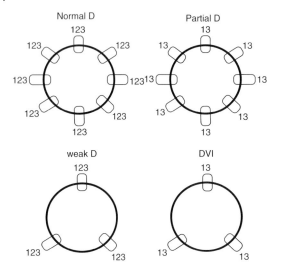

Figure 6.1 Comparison of weak D and partial D with a normal D-positive RBC. The circles represent the RBC membrane, the rectangles represent an RhD protein and the numbers above each RhD protein are a stylised representation of different D epitopes on the protein. The D epitopes are arbitrarily numbered 1, 2 and 3. The number of antigens and epitopes, as well as the size of the RhD protein, is not to scale. In this example, eight D antigens on the RBC surface are schematically shown as normal, and each D antigen has three D epitopes. In reality, the number of D antigens ranges from 10 000 to 25 000 and more than 30 D epitopes are expressed on the D antigen. The weak D RBC features D antigens with the full complement of D epitopes but the number of D antigens is reduced compared to normal. The partial D RBC demonstrates the normal number of D epitopes but each protein is lacking at least one D epitope. The partial D type DVI demonstrates both weak D and partial D features. *Source:* This figure originally appeared in Flegel WA, Denomme GA, Yazer MH. On the complexity of D antigen typing: a handy decision tree in the age of molecular blood group diagnostics. J Obstet Gynaecol Can 2007;**29**:746–52, and is reprinted here with the kind permission of Elsevier.

recipients with the more common weak D alleles (types 1, 2 or 3) are not vulnerable to alloimmunisation [10].

Partial D recipients, on the other hand, usually type very strongly with anti-D reagents and are usually indistinguishable from those with normal D proteins because they have a normal copy number of RhD proteins embedded in their red cell membrane (see Figure 6.1). However, partial D proteins are lacking at least one D epitope often due to genetic cross-over events with the structurally similar *RHCE* gene.

- When partial D recipients are exposed to D-positive red cells, they can become D alloimmunised.
- Detecting partial D recipients before they are mistaken for normal D-positive recipients can usually only be done using sophisticated *RHD* genotyping methods.
- The usual presentation of a partial D recipient in the blood bank is the conundrum they create when they present following transfusion of D-positive red cells with an allo anti-D.

Both weak and partial D recipients are uncommon. The further reading list at the end of the chapter provides some additional sources for more detailed information on the genetics, frequency and management of donors and recipients with these alleles.

Antibody Screening and Identification

Overall, fewer than 5% of transfused recipients will develop an antibody to foreign red cell antigens other than A or B. This percentage is often much higher in sickle cell disease patients, where the alloimmunisation rate can approach 50% [5,11]. Hence, these antibodies are collectively referred to as 'unexpected antibodies' due to their relative rarity. However, it is important to detect red cell antibodies when they are present because transfusing a recipient who has an unexpected antibody with antigen-positive red cells can result in a variety of outcomes, ranging from shortening the lifespan of the transfused red cell without significant untoward consequences for the recipient to an outright immediate haemolytic reaction with severe clinical consequences. Although most red cell antibodies are allogeneic (following exposure to foreign red cell antigens via transfusion or pregnancy), some are autoantibodies that do not require exposure to foreign red cells for development.

To detect the presence of unexpected red cell antibodies, the recipient's serum/plasma should be tested against two or more screening cells (hence the meaning of the second part of the phrase 'type and screen'). The reagent screening cells are always group O and should between them express all the clinically significant antigens; ideally the Rh phenotypes R_1R_1, rr and R_2R_2 should be represented in the screening cell set. Different national standards and guidelines exist but in many countries, it is recommended that the screening cells express the Jk^a, Jk^b, S, s, Fy^a and Fy^b antigens, and incorporate the following phenotypes: $Jk(a+b-)$, $Jk(a-b+)$, $S+s-$, $S-s+$, $Fy(a+b-)$, $Fy(a-b+)$, since stronger reactions may be obtained with cells expressing double dose antigen expression.

If an unexpected red cell antibody is detected in the antibody detection (screening) test, the blood bank must identify its specificity and, when clinically significant, select antigen-negative units for crossmatching (see below). The antibody's specificity is determined by testing the recipient's serum/plasma against a large panel of reagent group O red cells of known phenotypes (i.e. the antigens on the surface of the red cells). The reagent red cells in the panel used to determine the specificity of an antibody are similar to those used in the screen, but because typically 10–11 reagent red cells are used in the panel (compared to only 2–3 in the screen), the antibody's specificity can be determined. Antibody specificity can be assigned when the serum/plasma is reactive with at least two examples of red cells bearing the antigen, and non-reactive with at least two examples of red cells lacking the antigen.

Antibody Detection Methods

Test methods have been developed to detect antibodies of different isotypes. Antibodies with specificities for red cell antigens are usually IgG or IgM. As stated above, pentameric IgM antibodies can cross-link antigens on adjacent cells, causing direct agglutination of red cells. Conversely, IgG antibodies are monomeric and, although divalent, the distance between the Fab

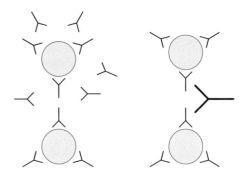

Red cells incubated with serum containing IgG antibody. Unbound antibody washed away. Anti-human globulin added to precipitate cells

Figure 6.2 Indirect immunoglobulin test.

regions on a single IgG molecule is generally insufficient to allow for direct agglutination. That is, the antigen density on the red cells is usually insufficient to permit the Fab regions of IgG molecules to span the distance between two adjacent red cell and cause direct agglutination. Methods such as the antiglobulin test (sometimes referred to as the Coombs' test) that use a secondary antiisotype antibody (Figure 6.2) or the enzyme method (which uses proteolytic enzymes such as papain or ficin to cleave negatively charged, hydrophilic residues from red cell membranes) must therefore be used to detect most IgG red cell antibodies.

Test systems for detection of serological reactions can be classified into three broad categories.

Liquid-Phase ('Tube') Systems
Liquid-phase systems rely on visualisation of haemagglutination reactions in individual glass/plastic test tubes or microplates. The presence or absence of agglutinated red cells distinguishes positive and negative reactions, allowing grading of reaction avidity according to strength of haemagglutination. While not the most sensitive methods available today, implicit association test (IAT) methods using red cells suspended in low ionic strength solution (LISS) remain the gold standard for the detection of clinically significant red cell alloantibodies. Using polyethylene glycol is another enhancement technique.

Column-Agglutination Systems

Introduction of column-agglutination systems (commonly referred to as 'gel') has resulted in very significant changes to routine laboratory practice. Synthetic gel mixtures or glass microbeads configured into vertical columns on small cards form density barriers, retaining agglutinated red cells and allowing passage of the nonagglutinated cells. Positive reactions (antibody/antigen interactions) are distinguished by agglutinates at or near the top of the gel column and negative reactions appear as buttons of red cells at the bottom (Figure 6.3).

Reagent (IgM) antibody can be incorporated into the columns, allowing phenotyping simply by addition of test cells to the top of the column. Similarly, the IAT can be performed in columns containing antiglobulin reagent to which plasma and reagent red cells are added. Manual and automated methods for performing and interpreting these tests are now widely available.

Solid-Phase Systems

These systems use microplates for testing. The positive reaction endpoint is characterised by a red cell monolayer in the wells, while discrete buttons of red cells at the bottom of the well indicate negative reactions (Figure 6.4). Solid-phase systems require carefully standard-ised centrifugation and washing steps, but fully automated equipment is also widely available.

Autoantibodies

Autoantibodies may be suspected when the recipient's serum/plasma reacts with the A_1 and B cells used in the reverse ABO group (cold autoantibodies) or with all cells in the antibody screen and antibody identification panel, including the patient's own red cells. Autoantibodies are common, but not all autoantibodies give rise to clinically significant haemolysis. Serological investigations should focus on determining the patient's ABO and D group and excluding

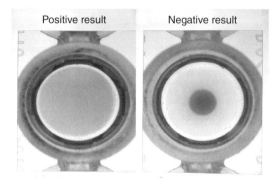

Positive result   Negative result

Figure 6.4 Solid-phase blood grouping technology.

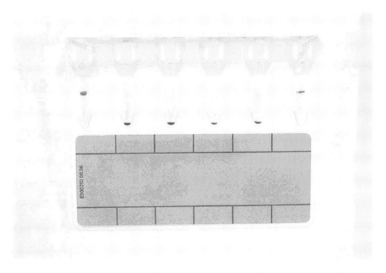

Figure 6.3 Column-agglutination technology for blood grouping and antibody screening. Samples may consist of patient cells and reagent antisera or reagent red cells and patient serum/plasma. Positive results are seen in the first and last columns, the other columns show negative reactions.

the presence of underlying alloantibodies. Cold type autoantibodies tend not to confound alloantibody identification unless they react at 37 °C. Warm type autoantibodies will usually cause the red cells to have a positive direct antiglobulin test (DAT) due to coating with IgG with or without complement, and an eluate prepared from these cells typically reacts with all the panel cells. Chapter 29 has more information on the clinical management of patients with immune-mediated haemolysis.

Crossmatching Techniques

The crossmatch ensures that an ABO-compatible red cell has been selected for transfusion, and that the unit is antigen negative in the case of a recipient with an unexpected antibody.

Crossmatch Techniques for Patients Without Current or Historical Antibodies

If a recipient has a negative antibody screen and no record of historical red cell antibodies, an immediate spin (IS) crossmatch can be used to issue red cells. The recipient's plasma is mixed and centrifuged with the potential donor's red cells. As anti-A and anti-B are IgM antibodies (often called isohaemagglutinins) that can directly agglutinate red cell, this IS crossmatch provides a final confirmation of ABO compatibility between the recipient and the blood donor. There is negligible risk in omitting the IAT crossmatch in recipients with a negative screen [12]. Antibodies directed against low-frequency antigens may be missed, but the majority of these are clinically insignificant. False-positive IS results arising from rouleaux or cold agglutinins can occur and can also cause ABO discrepancies.

Many centres now perform electronic crossmatching (also known as the computer crossmatch) to confirm donor/recipient ABO compatibility before release of ABO type specific RBCs. There are several essential prerequisites for using this technique.

- The computer system contains logic to prevent assignment and release of ABO-incom-

patible blood, including 'hard stops' to prevent release of ABO-incompatible blood.
- No clinically significant antibodies are detected in the recipient's current antibody screen and there is no record of previously having detected such antibodies.
- There are concordant results of at least two determinations of the recipient's ABO and D groups on file, at least one of which is from a current sample.
- Critical system elements (application software, readers and interfaces) have been validated on site, and there are mechanisms to verify the correct entry of data prior to the release of red cell units, such as barcode identifiers to enter information when it cannot be automatically transferred.

Electronic red cell issue has been widely used for over a decade, and is now routine practice in many countries. It has several advantages over serological crossmatching.

- Reduced technical workload.
- Rapid availability of blood. The electronic crossmatch can be performed in under five minutes whereas even the fastest serological crossmatch technique requires at least 20 minutes.
- Improved blood stock management through reduced numbers of crossmatched red cells and reduced wastage.
- Less handling of biohazardous material.
- Elimination of insignificant false-positive results in the IS.
- Ability to issue blood electronically at remote sites, using trained nonlaboratory staff.

This last characteristic has allowed development of systems for electronic remote blood issue. When patient details are entered, the system checks that criteria for electronic issue are fulfilled and either allows access to ABO- and D-compatible units in the remote blood refrigerator or dispenses compatible units. A compatibility label is printed and attached to the unit and rescanned to ensure it is the correct one for the unit. Such systems reduce the time taken for the issue of blood, particularly in small hospitals without transfusion laboratories [13].

Crossmatch Techniques for Patients With Current or Historical Antibodies

For patients with current or historical antibodies, a full IAT crossmatch is required. This means that the recipient's plasma is mixed with the potential donor's red cells, and the antihuman globulin reagent is added. The absence of agglutination or haemolysis indicates compatibility between recipient and donor. This type of crossmatch takes approximately 45 minutes to perform and thus extra time is required to provide red cells to recipients with antibodies.

Selection of Red Cells for Transfusion

Selecting ABO-Compatible Red Cells

Table 6.2 shows the donor ABO groups that are compatible with the recipient's ABO group. For patients without antibodies, ABO compatibility is the only necessary compatibility consideration.

Selecting D compatible red cells

Typically D negative recipients should receive D negative RBCs. However, in circumstances when the D negative RBC inventory is unusually low or in an emergency situation when the recipient's D status is unknown, some transfusion services will issue D positive RBCs to selected D negative recipients who meet certain criteria. These criteria usually consider the age and gender of the recipient, as well as if the recipient has a history of having formed anti-D. These switching strate-

gies are designed to preserve the D negative RBC inventory for D negative females of childbearing age and children. Sometimes a lower age threshold for switching a D negative male compared to a D negative female to D positive RBCs is employed as alloimmunization in the former does not carry the risk of causing hemolytic disease of the fetus and newborn (HDFN). The rate of D alloimmunization of hospitalized D negative recipients of at least one unit of D positive RBCs has been shown to be approximately 22%.

Clinical Significance of Unexpected Antibodies

Table 6.3 lists some of the more common unexpected antibodies and suggests how to select and crossmatch red cells for recipients with these antibodies. Most clinically significant antibodies are of the IgG isotype.

Use of Uncrossmatched Red Cells

As group O red cells are the 'universal donor' type, they can be safely administered to recipients of any ABO blood group. Group O red cells may be issued in life-threatening situations where even the short time required to perform pretransfusion testing would jeopardise a bleeding recipient's life. In these emergency situations, if the patient is a premenopausal female, group O-negative uncrossmatched red cells should be used. Otherwise, if the patient is an older female or a male, O-positive units can be selected. Group-specific units can be provided as soon as the patient's group is known.

Concerns about the potential for haemolysis to occur when uncrossmatched units are used sometimes arise because often these units are transfused before the antibody screen is complete. Thus there is a potential for recipients with antibodies to receive uncrossmatched units that bear the antigen to which they have become sensitised. Fortunately, even in these cases when an incompatible uncrossmatched unit has been transfused, the risk of overt haemolysis is quite low.

- In a study of seven recipients of uncrossmatched red cells who received at least one unit that was incompatible with their antibody, only

Table 6.2 ABO compatibilities between donor and recipient for red cell and plasma-containing products.

Donor ABO group	Compatible red cell donor	Compatible plasma-containing product donor
A	A, O	A, AB
B	B, O	B, AB
O	O only	All ABO groups
AB	All ABO groups	AB only

Table 6.3 Recommendations for selection of blood for patients with red cell alloantibodies.

	Typical examples	Procedure
Antibodies considered clinically significant	Anti-RhD, -C, -c, -E, -e Anti-K, -k Anti-Jk^a, -Jk^b Anti-S, -s, -U Anti-Fy^a, -Fy^b	Select ABO-compatible, antigen-negative blood for serological crossmatching
Antibodies directed against antigens with an incidence of <5%, and where the antibody is often not clinically significant	Anti-C^w Anti-Kp^a Anti-Lu^a Anti-Wr^a (anti-Di3)	Select ABO-compatible blood for serological crossmatching
Antibodies primarily reactive below 37 °C, and never or only very rarely clinically significant	Anti-A$_1$ Anti-N Anti-P$_1$ Anti-Le^a, -Le^b, -Le^{a+b} Anti-HI (in A$_1$ and A$_1$B patients)	Select ABO-compatible blood for serological crossmatching, performed strictly at 37 °C
Antibodies sometimes reactive at 37 °C and clinically significant	Anti-M	If reactive at 37 °C, select ABO-compatible, antigen-negative blood for serological crossmatching If unreactive at 37 °C, select ABO-compatible blood for serological crossmatching performed strictly at 37 °C
Other antibodies active by IAT at 37 °C	Many specificities	Seek advice from blood centre

IAT, implicit association test.

one recipient actually demonstrated biochemical evidence of haemolysis, although it was unclear if the patient haemolysed the uncrossmatched unit or one of the earlier units that he had received to treat his gastrointestinal bleed (a condition that could also confound the interpretation of the biochemical markers) [14].

- Overall, of the 265 emergency issued red cells in that study, this was the only reported haemolytic event representing only 0.4% of all of the uncrossmatched units.
- A low rate of haemolysis following uncrossmatched red cell transfusion was also found in several other studies (Table 6.4).
- Thus, if a patient is exsanguinating and requires urgent red cell transfusion before the type and screen is finished, uncrossmatched red cells can be a safe and life-saving intervention [15].

Selection of Platelets and Plasma Components

ABO- and D-compatible platelets are preferable but when these are not available, ABO- and D-incompatible platelets may be used in adults. The D alloimmunisation rate following D-positive platelet transfusion to a D-negative recipient is low [16].

Plasma must be ABO compatible with the recipient, but AB plasma is the universal plasma donor group (see Table 6.2). In some countries, plasma can only be maintained in the thawed state for up to 24 hours at refrigerator temperatures (1–6 °C), while in others the plasma can be kept in the refrigerator for an additional four days after thawing. Thawed plasma has the advantages of being readily available for issue and reducing waste, hence

Table 6.4 Summary of clinical studies on the rate of haemolysis following the transfusion of uncrossmatched red cells. Please see original text for complete reference citations.

Study	Number of recipients	Number of uncrossmatched red cell units issued	Rate of haemolysis	Rate of new antibody formation
Mulay, 2012	1407	4144	1/1407 (0.02%)	7/232* (3%)
Radkay, 2012	218	1065	1/218 (0.5%)	4/218 (1.8%)
Miraflor, 2011	132	1570	1/132 (0.8%)	1/132
Goodell, 2010	262	1002	1/262 (0.4%)	Not reported
Ball, 2009	153	511	0	Not reported
Dutton, 2005	161	581	0	1/161 (0.6%)
Unkle, 1991	135	Not reported	0	3/135 (2.2%)
Lefebre, 1987	133	537	0	Not reported
Schwab, 1986	99	410	0	Not reported
Gervin, 1984	160	875	0	Not reported
Blumberg, 1978	46	221	0	Not reported
Total	2906	10916	4/2906 (0.1%)	16/878 (1.8%)

Source: Reprinted with kind permission of Wolters Kluwer Health Inc, originally published in Boisen M, Collins RA, Yazer MH, Waters JH. Pretransfusion testing and transfusion of uncrossmatched erythrocytes. Anesthesiology 2015;**122**:191–5.

its growing popularity in the USA [17]. Other preparations, such as pooled, solvent-detergent plasma or plasma that has been virally inactivated using other techniques, are also available in some regions.

Cryoprecipitate is prepared from whole-blood donations. It should ideally be of the same ABO group as the recipient, but in adults this is not essential due to its very small volume. Cryoprecipitate is mainly used as a source of fibrinogen, where a virally inactivated fibrinogen concentrate is not available.

Frozen products must always be thawed using an approved device and method.

KEY POINTS

1) Pretransfusion testing establishes the recipient's ABO group and also detects unexpected antibodies. This process can take several hours or longer, depending on the number and nature of the antibodies present, so it is always best ordered far in advance of the patient's surgery or procedure to avoid delays in obtaining crossmatched red cells.
2) Distinguishing between weak and partial D phenotypes is not always possible with serological methods and a genotype should be obtained in patients with unusual D phenotypes.
3) Electronic red cell crossmatching is a time-saving technique and can be used in the vast majority of recipients.
4) Uncrossmatched red cells, when used in emergency life-threatening situations, pose a low risk of haemolysis to the recipient and can be life-saving.

References

1 Linden JV, Paul B, Dressler KP. A report of 104 transfusion errors in New York State. Transfusion 1992;**32**(7):601–6.

2 Goodnough LT, Viele M, Fontaine MJ et al. Implementation of a two-specimen requirement for verification of ABO/Rh for blood transfusion. Transfusion 2009;**49**(7):1321–8.

3 MacIvor D, Triulzi DJ, Yazer MH. Enhanced detection of blood bank sample collection errors with a centralized patient database. Transfusion 2009;**49**(1):40–3.

4 Delaney M, Dinwiddie S, Nester TN, Aubuchon JA. The immunohematologic and patient safety benefits of a centralized transfusion database. Transfusion 2013;**53**(4):771–6.

5 Harm SK, Yazer MH, Monis GF, Triulzi DJ, Aubuchon JP, Delaney M. A centralized recipient database enhances the serologic safety of RBC transfusions for patients with sickle cell disease. Am J Clin Pathol 2014;**141**(2):256–61.

6 Hult AK, Olsson ML. Many genetically defined ABO subgroups exhibit characteristic flow cytometric patterns. Transfusion 2010;**50**(2):308–23.

7 Hult AK, Yazer MH, Jorgensen R et al. Weak A phenotypes associated with novel ABO alleles carrying the A(2)-related 1061C deletion and various missense substitutions. Transfusion 2010;**50**(7):1471–86.

8 Cho D, Lee JS, Yazer MH et al. Chimerism and mosaicism are important causes of ABO phenotype and genotype discrepancies. Immunohematology 2006;**22**(4):183–7.

9 Flegel WA, Denomme GA, Yazer MH. On the complexity of D antigen typing: a handy decision tree in the age of molecular blood group diagnostics. J Obstet Gynaecol Can 2007;**29**(9): 746–52.

10 Sandler SG, Flegel WA, Westhoff CM et al. It's time to phase in RHD genotyping for patients with a serologic weak D phenotype. Transfusion 2015;**55**(3):680–9.

11 Chou ST, Jackson T, Vege S, Smith-Whitley K, Friedman DF, Westhoff CM. High prevalence of red blood cell alloimmunization in sickle cell disease despite transfusion from Rh-matched minority donors. Blood 2013;**122**(6):1062–71.

12 Mintz PD, Haines AL, Sullivan MF. Incompatible crossmatch following nonreactive antibody detection test. Frequency and cause. Transfusion 1982;**22**(2):107–10.

13 Staves J, Davies A, Kay J, Pearson O, Johnson T, Murphy MF. Electronic remote blood issue: a combination of remote blood issue with a system for end-to-end electronic control of transfusion to provide a "total solution" for a safe and timely hospital blood transfusion service. Transfusion 2008;**48**(3):415–24.

14 Goodell PP, Uhl L, Mohammed M, Powers AA. Risk of hemolytic transfusion reactions following emergency-release RBC transfusion. Am J Clin Pathol 2010;**134**(2):202–6.

15 Radkay L, Triulzi DJ, Yazer MH. Low risk of hemolysis after transfusion of uncrossmatched red blood cells. Immunohematology 2012;**28**(2):39–44.

16 Cid J, Lozano M, Ziman A et al. Low frequency of anti-D alloimmunization following D+ platelet transfusion: the Anti-D Alloimmunization after D-incompatible Platelet Transfusions (ADAPT) study. Br J Haematol 2015;**168**(4):598–603.

17 US Department of Health and Human Services. The 2011 National Blood Collection and Utilization Survey Report. Available at: www.aabb.org/research/hemovigilance/ bloodsurvey/Documents/11-nbcus-report.pdf (accessed 9 November 2016).

Further Reading

Boisen ML, Collins RA, Yazer MH, Waters JH. Pretransfusion testing and transfusion of uncrossmatched erythrocytes. Anesthesiology 2015;**122**(1):191–5.

Cho D, Lee JS, Yazer MH et al. Chimerism and mosaicism are important causes of ABO phenotype and genotype discrepancies. Immunohematology 2006;**22**:183–7.

Chou ST, Jackson T, Vege S, Smith-Whitley K, Friedman DF, Westhoff CM. High prevalence of red blood cell alloimmunization in sickle cell disease despite transfusion from Rh-matched minority donors. Blood 2013;**122**: 1062–71.

Cottrell S, Watson D, Eyre TA, Brunskill SJ, Dorée C, Murphy MF. Interventions to reduce wrong blood in tube errors in transfusion: a systematic review. Transfus Med Rev 2013;**27**:197–205.

Flegel WA, Denomme GA, Yazer MH. On the complexity of D antigen typing: a handy decision tree in the age of molecular blood group diagnostics. J Obstet Gynaecol Can 2007;**29**:746–52.

Judd WJ. Requirements for the electronic crossmatch. Vox Sang 1998;**74** (Suppl. 2):409–17.

Sandler SG, Flegel WA, Westhoff CM et al. It's time to phase in RHD genotyping for patients with a serologic weak D phenotype. Transfusion 2014;**55**:680–9.

Zarandona JM, Yazer MH. The role of the Coombs test in the evaluation of hemolysis in adults. Can Med Assoc J 2006;**174**:305–7.

7 Investigation of Acute Transfusion Reactions

Kathryn E. Webert[1] and Nancy M. Heddle[2]

[1] Canadian Blood Services, and Department of Medicine and Department of Pathology and Molecular Medicine, McMaster University, Hamilton, Ontario, Canada
[2] Department of Medicine, McMaster University and Canadian Blood Services, Hamilton, Ontario, Canada

Introduction

The investigation of suspected acute reactions to blood components and plasma derivatives cannot be summarised in a single simple algorithm for several reasons:

- signs and symptoms are not specific for one type of reaction
- the frequency and type of reactions vary with different blood components, e.g. leucocyte-reduced or not
- risks are variable with different patient populations
- the severity and risk of reactions must be taken into account to ensure a balance between the safety, availability and costs due to wastage.

In this chapter, an algorithmic approach is provided for the clinical management and laboratory investigation of transfusion reactions.

Understanding the Clinical Presentation and Differential Diagnosis

Acute reactions are defined as adverse events occurring during or within 4–6 hours of transfusion. They can usually be placed into the following categories [1,2]:

- acute haemolysis (AHTR)
- allergic
- anaphylactic
- transfusion-related acute lung injury (TRALI)
- febrile nonhaemolytic reactions (FNHTR)
- bacterial sepsis
- hypotension
- transfusion-associated circulatory overload (TACO)
- acute pain reaction
- metabolic complications (hyperkalaemia, hypokalaemia, hypocalcaemia, hypothermia).

There are other types of reactions that can occur following the acute period, including delayed haemolytic reactions, transfusion-associated graft-versus-host disease, posttransfusion purpura, alloimmune thrombocytopenia and alloimmune neutropenia. These reactions are discussed in other chapters.

The diagnosis of an acute transfusion reaction can be challenging as signs and symptoms are not specific for each type of reaction, all possible signs and symptoms do not present with every reaction and different types of reactions can occur simultaneously. In Table 7.1, signs and symptoms have been grouped into nine categories. The information summarised in this table illustrates how similar signs and symptoms can occur in different reactions (e.g. bacterial sepsis, allergic and anaphylactic reactions can all present with cutaneous symptoms).

Practical Transfusion Medicine, Fifth Edition. Edited by Michael F. Murphy, David J. Roberts and Mark H. Yazer.

Table 7.1 Summary of the signs/symptoms typically observed with different types of acute transfusion reactions.

Reaction type	Cutaneous	Pain	Inflammatory	Respiratory	Hypotension	Hypertension	Other cardiovascular	GI	Neuromuscular	CNS	DIC	Haemoglobinuria	Renal failure
AHTR		√		√	√						√	√	√
Allergic	√			√									
Anaphylactic	√		√*	√	√	√	√						
TRALI			√	√	√		√						
FNHTR		√	√					√					
Bacterial sepsis	√	√	√	√	√	√	√	√			√	√	
Hypotensive		√	√	√	√								
TACO		√		√		√	√	√					
Acute pain		√	√	√		√	√		√				
Hyperkalaemia							√	√	√				
Hypokalaemia		√					√		√	√			
Hypocalcaemia		√	√				√	√	√				
Hypothermia				√			√						
Hypotensive		√	√	√	√								

*Flushing only.

AHTR, acute haemolytic transfusion reaction; CNS, central nervous system; DIC, disseminated intravascular coagulation; FNHTR, febrile nonhaemolytic transfusion reaction; GI, gastrointestinal; TACO, transfusion-associated circulatory overload; TRALI, transfusion-related acute lung injury.

To ensure management strategies and investigations that minimise risks to patients, healthcare professionals need to understand the aetiology and pathophysiology of each type of acute reaction (Table 7.2). It is also essential to understand the typical clinical presentation for each type of reaction so that a differential diagnosis can be formulated as part of the investigative process. Some considerations to assist in the decision-making process and investigation are summarised below [3,4].

Patient History

- The reason for the patient's admission and current diagnosis may give some indication as to the type of reaction. For example, if the patient is being transfused because of anaemia but is also in congestive heart failure, TACO could be the cause of the reaction.
- Consider whether the patient has been previously transfused or pregnant as this can lead to alloimmunisation to red cell and leucocyte antigens, which are known to be associated with certain types of reactions (acute haemolytic, FNHTR).
- What blood components have been transfused and what is the transfusion timeline? If plasma-containing products have recently been transfused, consider whether the reaction could be caused by passive infusion of antibody or soluble allergens that may now be reacting with the product being transfused.
- Has the patient had a history of reactions when blood components are transfused? Some patients are prone to developing recurrent FNHTR and/or allergic reactions when transfused.
- Is the patient known to be IgA deficient? Some patients with IgA deficiency develop anti-IgA antibodies, which may cause anaphylactic transfusion reactions when an IgA-containing blood component is transfused.

Medications

- Determine what medications the patient is receiving or has received in the time period leading up to the transfusion. Considerations should include:
  - the use of premedications given to prevent acute reactions such as allergic (antihistamines) or FNHTR (antipyretics)
  - antimicrobial medication
  - pyrogenic agents that are known to cause fever such as amphotericin or monoclonal antibodies
  - ACE inhibitors, which have been associated with hypotensive reactions
  - pruritogenic agents such as vancomycin, narcotics, etc.

Type of Blood Component Being Transfused

- Does the component contain significant volumes of plasma? Infusion of plasma is associated with a variety of reactions, including allergic, anaphylactic, TRALI and acute haemolysis caused by passive antibody incompatibility with the patient's red cells [3,4].
- Does the component contain a significant number of red cells? If greater than 50 mL of red cells are present in the component, acute haemolysis needs to be considered as a possible cause of the adverse reaction.
- Was the component stored at room temperature or in a refrigerator? Platelets have a higher risk of bacterial contamination if they are stored at room temperature. However, products stored at colder temperatures can also be contaminated with bacteria, especially those strains that are known to grow at cold temperatures [3].
- Is the component leucocyte reduced and if so, was leucocyte reduction performed before or after storage? Nonleucocyte-reduced blood components (especially platelets) are associated with a higher frequency of FNHTR. Post-storage leucocyte reduction also has limited effectiveness in preventing FNHTR to platelets whereas prestorage leucocyte reduction is highly effective. In contrast, both post- and prestorage leucocyte reduction are effective in preventing most FNHTR to red cells [5].

Table 7.2 Summary of acute transfusion reactions. Data from Callum et al [3] and Popovsky [4].

Reaction	Frequency	Mechanism	Clinical presentation	Differential diagnosis	Laboratory investigations	Management
AHTR	1:25 000 (fatal 1:600 000)	Result from the destruction of donor red cells by preformed recipient antibodies	Fever, flank pain and red/brown urine	FNHTR bacterial contamination TRALI Non-immune causes of haemolysis	Positive DAT free haemoglobin in plasma and urine Positive cross-match	Stop the transfusion immediately Begin infusion of normal saline
		Antibodies fix complement and cause rapid intravascular haemolysis	Hypotension, shock, death			Alert the blood transfusion laboratory, check for clerical error, send entire transfusion set-up to blood transfusion laboratory for testing
		Usually due to ABO incompatibility which is most often the result of clerical error				Obtain bloodwork: DAT, plasma for free haemoglobin, antibody screen Obtain urine sample: haemoglobinuria
Allergic transfusion reaction	1:100–300 transfusions	Soluble allergenic substances in the plasma of the donated blood product react with preexisting IgE antibodies in the recipient	Hives Urticaria Flushing	Anaphylactic transfusion reaction TRALI TACO	Rule out anaphylactic reaction	Stop the transfusion until a more serious reaction is ruled out Antihistamine may improve symptoms
		Causes mast cells and basophils to release histamine, leading to hives or urticaria				If no evidence of dyspnoea or anaphylaxis, the transfusion may be continued with close observation
Anaphylactic transfusion reaction	1:20 000–50 000 transfusions	Usually due to the presence of anti-IgA antibodies in recipients who are IgA deficient	Rapid onset of shock, hypotension, angioedema and respiratory distress (2° to bronchospasm and laryngeal oedema)	Allergic transfusion reaction TRALI TACO	IgA level Testing for anti-IgA (if IgA deficient)	Stop the transfusion Adrenaline Airway maintenance, oxygenation Maintain haemodynamic status (IV fluids, vasopressor medications)

TRALI	2–8 cases per 10000 allogeneic transfusion (0.014–0.08%) 0.5–2 cases per 1000 patients transfused (0.04–0.16%)	Antibodies or neutrophil-priming agents in the infused blood product likely interact with the recipient's leucocyte antigens Activation of the WBC results in the production of inflammatory mediators that increase vascular permeability Leads to capillary leak and pulmonary tissue damage	Shortness of breath Fever Hypotension or hypertension Acute noncardiogenic pulmonary oedema (elevated JVP, bilateral lung crackles)	Bacterial contamination TACO Anaphylactic transfusion reaction Cardiogenic pulmonary oedema ARDS Pneumonia	Antigranulocyte or anti-HLA antibodies in the donor CXR (bilateral pulmonary infiltrates) BNP (possibly useful)	Stop the transfusion Respiratory support as required (supplemental oxygen, mechanical ventilation) Maintain haemodynamic status (IV fluids, vasopressor medications)
FNHTR	Commonly occurs during transfusions of red cells, platelets or plasma 1:100 red cell transfusions; 1:5 platelet transfusions	Likely caused by cytokines that are generated and accumulate during the storage of blood components Less frequently caused by leucocyte antigen/antibody interactions between recipient and blood product	Fever, rigours, chills Other: nausea, vomiting, dyspnoea, hypotension Typically occurs during or within 2 hours of transfusion but may present up to 6 hours after transfusion	AHTR Bacterial contamination TRALI Co-morbid conditions causing fever (i.e. infection, haematological malignancies, solid tumour) Drugs causing fever	No specific tests Rule out other transfusion reactions	Stop the transfusion until a more serious reaction is ruled out Antipyretics to decrease fever and meperidine may help patients with severe chills and rigours
Bacterial contamination	Previously estimated as 1:10000 for symptomatic reactions (platelets), 1:>1 million (RBC) Likely lower if pretransfusion bacterial detection is in place	Bacteria in the blood product from: donor skin (venipuncture site); donor with bacteraemia; contamination during collection/storage	High fever, rigours Hypotension	AHTR FNHTR Allergic transfusion reaction	Gram stain and culture of remaining blood component Gram stain and culture of patient's blood	Stop the transfusion IV fluids Broad-spectrum antibiotics
Hypotensive transfusion reaction	Unknown but thought to be rare	Unknown	AHTR Bacterial contamination			Stop the transfusion

(Continued)

Table 7.2 (Continued)

Reaction	Frequency	Mechanism	Clinical presentation	Differential diagnosis	Laboratory investigations	Management
	May be related to generation of bradykinin and/or its active metabolite Majority of reactions occur within minutes of the beginning of the transfusion and resolve rapidly with cessation of the transfusion and supportive care administered through a negatively charged filter or to patients receiving an angiotensin-converting enzyme (ACE) inhibitor	Hypotension Dyspnoea, urticaria, flushing, pruritus, GI symptoms Most reactions occur within minutes of the beginning of the transfusion and resolve rapidly with cessation of the transfusion and supportive care	TRALI Anaphylactic transfusion reaction Unrelated to blood transfusion (i.e. due to blood loss)	No specific tests Rule out other transfusion reactions		Maintain haemodynamic status (IV fluids, vasopressor medications)
TACO	May be as high as 1:100 transfusions	Increase in central venous pressure, increase in pulmonary blood volume and decrease in pulmonary compliance with resultant secondary congestive heart failure and pulmonary oedema	Elevated JVP Bilateral crackles on auscultation Hypertension Dry cough Orthopnoea Pedal oedema	TRALI Anaphylactic transfusion reaction	Chest x-ray Clinical examination BNP (possibly useful)	Stop the transfusion Supplemental oxygen Diuretics
Acute pain reaction	Unknown Data suggest it may occur with 0.02% of blood products transfused	Unknown	Acute pain during transfusion (chest, abdominal, back or flank) Other symptoms include: dyspnoea, hypertension, chills, tachycardia, restlessness, flushing, headache	AHTR TRALI TACO Allergic	No specific tests	Temporarily stop transfusion Rule out other causes of reaction Pain management

Hyperkalaemia	Unknown Likely more common in infants and children and individuals receiving massive transfusion	During storage of red blood cells, increasing potassium concentration of the supernatant occurs	Muscle weakness Cardiac effects: ECG changes (e.g. peaked T waves, loss of P wave amplitude, prolonged PR interval and QRS duration), arrhythmias, cardiac arrest Death		Electrolytes ECG	May possibly be prevented by such modalities as: slow rate of infusion, the use of fresher blood, washing of red cells, use of in-line potassium filters (in development)
Hypokalaemia	Rare May occur in association with massive transfusion (especially large amounts of FFP)	Unknown Possibly caused by metabolic alkalosis secondary to citrate metabolism, release of catecholamines, aldosterone and/or antidiuretic hormone	ECG changes (flattened or inverted T waves, U wave, ST depression, wide PR interval) Muscle weakness Cardiac arrthythmias	Rapid infusion of other solutions low in potassium	Electrolytes ECG	Consider replacement of potassium
Hypocalcaemia	Rare May occur in association with massive transfusion	May occur in massive transfusion recipients with liver failure Liver normally rapidly metabolises transfused citrate. If rate of citrate delivery exceeds liver's ability to clear citrate, citrate may be able to bind to calcium, resulting in hypocalcaemia	ECG changes (prolongation of QT interval), depressed left ventricular function, increased neuromuscular excitability, hypotension		Calcium level Magnesium level (also bound by citrate)	Consider calcium replacement when ionised calcium concentration is less than 50% of normal value with symptoms of hypocalcaemia
Hypothermia	Unknown Most commonly seen with rapid massive transfusion of red cells (stored between 1° and 6°C)	Occurs with rapid transfusion of large volumes of cold blood (red cells)	Decreased core body temperature Hypothermia may be associated with metabolic derangements (hyperkalaemia, increased lactate, increased oxygen affinity of haemoglobin), abnormalities in haemostasis and cardiac disturbances	Other causes associated with massive transfusion and trauma include infusion of cold fluids, opening of body cavities due to injuries, impaired thermoregulatory control		May be prevented by use of blood warmers when rapid massive transfusion is required

AHTR, acute haemolytic transfusion reaction; ARDS, adult respiratory distress syndrome; BNP, brain natriuretic peptide; CXR, chest x-ray; DAT, direct antiglobulin test; ECG, electrocardiogram; FFP, fresh frozen plasma; FNHTR, febrile nonhaemolytic transfusion reaction; GI, gastrointestinal; HLA, human leucocyte antigen; IV, intravenous; JVP, jugular venous pressure; RBC, red blood cell; TACO, transfusion-associated circulatory overload; TRALI, transfusion-related acute lung injury; WBC, white blood cell.

Was Fever Present?

- Fever is a common finding in most types of reactions. However, it does not occur in allergic transfusion reactions or with anaphylaxis. Therefore, fever can be useful to help differentiate between severe hypotension caused by bacterial contamination, acute haemolysis or TRALI (fever may be present) versus hypotension caused by anaphylactic shock (fever is absent).

- Was the rise in temperature ≥2 °C? Significant temperature increases are typically seen with bacterial contamination, especially if the patient has not been premedicated with an antipyretic or is not receiving antibiotic therapy. Increases in temperature greater than 2 °C are not usually seen with other types of reactions [6].

Volume of Component Transfused

The volume of the component transfused can also be an important consideration for a differential diagnosis.

- Some types of reactions are dose dependent; hence, they tend to occur towards the end of the transfusion after most of the component has been given. Such reactions include allergic reactions, FNHTR and TRALI. This observation becomes less useful when symptoms occur during the transfusion of multiple blood components. In this situation, it is difficult to determine if the reaction is caused by the first unit transfused or the current unit that is being administered.

- Anaphylactic reactions can present after a small amount of component is transfused (1–10 mL) [7].

- Acute haemolytic reactions usually require at least 50–100 mL of red cells to be transfused before symptoms appear.

Other Considerations

- Always remember that the patient's clinical co-morbidities and therapies could also be causing many of the symptoms typical of acute transfusion reactions. Hence, these always need to be considered as part of the differential diagnosis.

- Although most reactions are relatively infrequent, it is possible for a patient to have more than one type of reaction concurrently. This possibility should always be considered when the patient presents with atypical findings.

- For many reaction types, there is a spectrum of severity, ranging from mild to severe, depending on such factors as characteristics of the patient and blood component, and amount of blood transfused. For example, bacterial contamination of a blood component may result in an acute septic reaction with high fever and hypotension. Alternatively, such a component may cause no or only mild symptoms.

- Consider how well you know the patient and their previous response to blood component transfusions. Less concern may be appropriate for a patient who develops hives every time they are transfused, whereas action would be appropriate for the sudden development of moderate respiratory symptoms in the multitransfused patient who has previously had no adverse events.

General Approach for Investigation and Treatment of Acute Transfusion Reactions

Using all the information noted above, the clinician must make a decision whether to stop the administration of the blood component temporarily or discontinue the transfusion and must decide the extent of the investigations to be performed. Stopping and investigating every transfusion reaction is often assumed to provide the highest level of safety for the patient, but in reality may contribute to other morbidities such as bleeding or respiratory/cardiovascular morbidity if an essential transfusion is delayed. Hence, some clinical judgement is required to ensure a balance between risk and benefit. The following approach should be used if there is any concern about patient safety and an investigation is required.

Action to Be Taken on the Clinical Unit

- Stop the transfusion immediately. The severity of some reactions is dose dependent. For example, the risk of severe morbidity and mortality with acute haemolysis is generally proportional to the volume of component transfused.

- Keep the IV line open with saline (or other appropriate IV solution) in case a decision is made to continue the transfusion or the patient requires other IV therapy.

- Support the patient's clinical symptoms with appropriate medical therapy.
- Perform a bedside clerical check to ensure that the name on the blood component and requisition matches the patient's armband/identifier.
- Look carefully at the remaining blood component to determine if there is any evidence of haemolysis or particulate matter. A contaminated unit of red cells may have discolouration either in the primary bag or in the first few segments closest to the blood bag.
- Complete a transfusion reaction form and notify the blood transfusion laboratory that a reaction has occurred. The transfusion laboratory will perform relevant investigations, notify the blood supplier if applicable so appropriate actions can be taken and ensure that relevant reactions are reported to the country's haemovigilance system (see Chapter 18). This reporting provides cumulative statistics about reactions that may be the first clue of a new emerging threat to the blood supply or a problem with component manufacturing.
- If a decision is made to perform a more extensive investigation to rule out problems with a donor unit (e.g. serological incompatibility causing haemolysis, bacterial contamination, TRALI), the remainder of the blood bag should be returned to the blood transfusion laboratory and/or blood service for further testing. Local policies should be followed for additional patient samples to be collected for specialised testing.

Action to Be Taken in the Laboratory

When a reaction is reported to the blood transfusion laboratory, a clerical check should always be performed to verify that the paperwork is accurate and that the correct component was issued for transfusion. To rule out haemolysis from the differential diagnosis, the following screening tests should be performed:

- clerical check as mentioned above
- centrifuge a posttransfusion sample of the patient's blood and observe the plasma for visual evidence of haemolysis

- a direct antiglobulin test on a posttransfusion EDTA sample taken from the patient.

If the clerical check does not indicate any problems and the two screening tests are negative, acute haemolysis as the cause of the reaction can usually be eliminated. However, if the patient's symptoms are severe and consistent with a haemolytic reaction, a complete serological work-up may be indicated, including repeating the compatibility test on both the pre- and posttransfusion patient samples and specific tests for haemolysis (i.e. lactate dehydrogenase, haptoglobin, methemalbumin, etc.).

All blood transfusion laboratories should have specific protocols for the investigation of other types of reactions. The Public Health Agency of Canada has developed guidelines for the investigation of suspected reactions caused by bacterial contamination, which can be accessed from the website (www.phac-aspc.gc.ca) [8]. Similar documents may be available in other countries. Investigation of TRALI, anaphylaxis and TACO requires specialised testing, which may be available only from a reference centre or specialised laboratory [9–11]. However, each facility should have policies and procedures in place to direct and facilitate these investigations. Results from these specialised tests are not usually available in a timely manner. Hence, treatment and prevention strategies must be made based on clinical findings and test results available on site.

Algorithm

As mentioned previously, some clinical judgement is required when deciding which reactions to investigate more fully and the management strategies required. Aggressive investigation of mild reactions can burden resources within the healthcare setting and may cause unnecessary delays in transfusion therapy for a patient in critical need of blood components. In contrast, patient safety should always be paramount. The algorithm in Figure 7.1 can be used as a guide to develop a safe but logical approach to managing acute transfusion reactions.

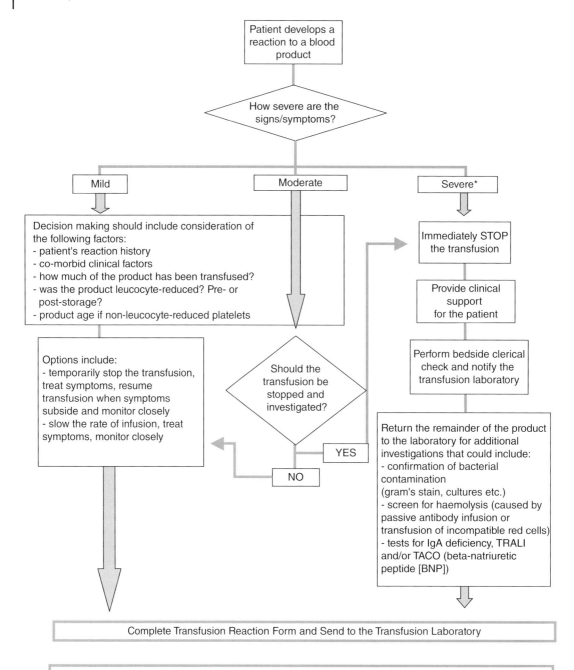

Figure 7.1 Flow diagram illustrating a possible approach for the management and investigation of an acute transfusion reaction.

KEY POINTS

1) Decisions related to the investigation of acute transfusion reactions require some clinical judgement based on the severity of the reactions.
2) Effective management decision making requires that healthcare professionals understand the types of acute transfusion reactions that can occur and their pathophysiology.
3) Patient factors to consider when formulating the differential diagnosis include the history of transfusion, pregnancy, medications, previous reactions, types of symptoms and diagnosis and clinical co-morbidities.
4) Component factors to consider when formulating the differential diagnosis include the type of component, leucocyte reduction status, volume transfused and component age.
5) Each institution must have policies and procedures for the investigation of acute reactions.

References

1 Braendstrup P, Bjerrum OW, Nielsen OJ et al. Rituximab chimeric anti-CD20 monoclonal antibody treatment for adult refractory idiopathic thrombocytopenic purpura. Am J Hematol 2005;**78**:275–80.

2 Hendrickson JE, Hillyer CD. Noninfectious serious hazards of transfusion. Anesth Analg 2009;**108**:759–69.

3 Callum J, Lin Y, Pinkerton PH et al. Bloody Easy 3, Blood Transfusions, Blood Alternatives and Transfusion Reactions: A Guide to Transfusion Medicine. Available at: http://ibta.ir/en/wp-content/uploads/111_Bloody-Easy_3rd-1.pdf (accessed 9 November 2016).

4 Popovsky M (ed.). Transfusion Reactions, 4th edn. Bethesda: AABB Press, 2012.

5 Heddle N, Webert K. Febrile nonhemolytic transfusion reactions, in Transfusion Reactions, 4th edn (ed. M Popovsky), AABB Press, Bethesda, 2012, pp.53–97.

6 Ramirez-Arcos S, Goldman M. Bacterial contamination, in Transfusion Reactions, 4th edn (ed. M Popovsky), AABB Press, Bethesda, 2012, pp.153–89.

7 Vamvakas E. Allergic and anaphylactic reactions, in Transfusion Reactions, 4th edn (ed. M Popovsky), AABB Press, Bethesda, 2012, pp. 99–147.

8 Public Health Agency of Canada. Guidelines for the Investigation of Suspected Transfusion Transmitted Bacterial Contamination. Available at: www.phac-aspc.gc.ca/publicat/ccdr-rmtc/08vol34/34s1/34s1-eng.php (accessed 9 November 2016).

9 Stroncek DF, Fadeyi E, Adams S. Leukocyte antigen and antibody detection assays: tools for assessing and preventing pulmonary transfusion reactions. Transfus Med Rev 2007;**21**:273–86.

10 Vassallo RR. Review: IgA anaphylactic transfusion reactions. Part I. Laboratory diagnosis, incidence, and supply of IgA-deficient products. Immunohematology 2004;**20**:226–33.

11 Zhou L, Giacherio D, Cooling L, Davenport RD. Use of B-natriuretic peptide as a diagnostic marker in the differential diagnosis of transfusion-associated circulatory overload. Transfusion 2005;**45**:1056–63.

Further Reading

Bakdash S, Yazer MH. What every physician should know about transfusion reactions. Can Med Assoc J 2007;**177**:141–7.

Bux J, Sachs UJH. Pulmonary transfusion reactions. Transf Med Hemother 2008;**35**:337–45.

Eder AF, Benjamin RJ. TRALI risk reduction: donor and component management strategies. J Clin Apher 2009;**24**:122–9.

Eder AF, Chambers LA. Noninfectious complications of blood transfusion. Arch Pathol Lab Med 2007;**131**:708–18.

Sandler SG. How I manage patients suspected of having had an IgA anaphylactic transfusion reaction. Transfusion 2006;**46**:10–13.

Tinegate H, Birchall J, Gray A et al. BCSH Blood Transfusion Task Force. Guideline on the investigation and management of acute transfusion reactions. Prepared by the BCSH Blood Transfusion Task Force. Br J Haematol 2012;**159**:143–53.

Vamvakas EC, Blajchman MA. Blood still kills: six strategies to further reduce allogeneic blood transfusion-related mortality. Transfus Med Rev 2010;**24**:77–124.

8

Haemolytic Transfusion Reactions

Edwin J. Massey[1], Robertson D. Davenport[2] and Richard M. Kaufman[3]

[1] *NHS Blood and Transplant, Bristol, UK*
[2] *University of Michigan Health System, Ann Arbor, USA*
[3] *Brigham and Women's Hospital, Boston, USA*

Definition of a Haemolytic Transfusion Reaction

A haemolytic transfusion reaction (HTR) is the occurrence of lysis or accelerated clearance of red cells in a recipient of a blood transfusion. With few exceptions, these reactions are caused by immunological incompatibility between the blood donor and the recipient [1].

Haemolytic transfusion reactions are usually classified with respect to the time of their occurrence following the transfusion but may also be classified on the pathophysiological basis of the site of red cell destruction, intravascular or extravascular. The classification used by the Serious Hazards of Transfusion (SHOT) haemovigilance scheme in the UK is as follows [2].

- *Acute HTRs (AHTRs)* are defined as fever and other symptoms/signs of haemolysis within 24 hours of transfusion, confirmed by one or more of the following: a fall in haemoglobin concentration (Hb), rise in lactate dehydrogenase (LDH), positive direct antiglobulin test (DAT), positive cross-match.
- *Delayed HTRs (DHTRs)* are defined as fever and other symptoms/signs of haemolysis more than 24 hours after transfusion, confirmed by one or more of the following: a fall in Hb or failure of increment, rise in bilirubin, incompatible cross-match not detectable before transfusion.

In the United States, the Centers for Disease Control and Prevention have detailed definitions for HTRs which may be classified as definitive, probable or possible. 'Definitive' HTRs fulfil the following criteria [3].

- An *AHTR* occurs during, or within, 24 hours of cessation of transfusion with new onset of **ANY** of the following signs/symptoms: back/flank pain; chills/rigours; disseminated intravascular coagulation (DIC); epistaxis; fever; haematuria (gross visual haemolysis); hypotension; oliguria/anuria; pain and/or oozing at IV site; renal failure **AND** two or more of the following: decreased fibrinogen; decreased haptoglobin; elevated bilirubin; elevated LDH; haemoglobinaemia; haemoglobinuria; plasma discolouration consistent with haemolysis; spherocytes on blood film **AND EITHER (IMMUNE-MEDIATED)** positive DAT for anti-IgG or anti-C3 **AND** positive elution test with alloantibody present on the transfused red blood cells **OR (NON-IMMUNE MEDIATED)** serological testing is negative, and physical cause (e.g. thermal, osmotic, mechanical, chemical) is confirmed.
- A *DHTR* is defined as a positive DAT for antibodies which developed between 24 hours and 28 days after cessation of transfusion **AND EITHER** a positive elution test with alloantibody present on the transfused red blood cells **OR** a newly identified red blood

Practical Transfusion Medicine, Fifth Edition. Edited by Michael F. Murphy, David J. Roberts and Mark H. Yazer.
© 2017 John Wiley & Sons Ltd. Published 2017 by John Wiley & Sons Ltd.

cell alloantibody in recipient serum **AND EITHER** an inadequate rise of posttransfusion haemoglobin level or a rapid fall in haemoglobin back to pretransfusion levels **OR** the otherwise unexplained appearance of spherocytes.

In general, with some exceptions, intravascular haemolysis is seen in AHTRs and extravascular haemolysis in DHTRs. During intravascular haemolysis, the destroyed red cells release free haemoglobin and other red cell contents directly into the intravascular space. These reactions are characterised by gross haemoglobinaemia and haemoglobinuria, which can potentially precipitate renal and other organ failure.

During extravascular haemolysis, red cells are removed from circulation primarily by the spleen. In these reactions the only feature may be a fall in Hb, but clinically significant DHTRs can occur, which may contribute to morbidity and even mortality in patients who are otherwise compromised by single or multiple organ failure prior to the reaction.

Pathophysiology of HTRs

There are three phases involved (Figure 8.1).

- Antibody binding to red cell antigens, which may involve complement activation.
- Opsonised red cells interacting with and activating phagocytes.
- Production of inflammatory mediators.

Antigen–Antibody Interactions

Where an immunological incompatibility is responsible, the course of the reaction depends upon:

- the class and subclass (in the case of IgG) of the antibody
- the blood group specificity of the antibody
- the thermal range of the antibody
- the number, density and spatial arrangement of the red cell antigen sites
- the ability of the antibody to activate complement

- the concentration of antibody in the plasma
- the amount of red cells transfused.

Characteristics of the Antibody and Antigen

The characteristics of the antibody (such as immunoglobulin class, specificity and thermal range) and those of the antigen sites against which antibody activity is directed (such as site density and spatial arrangement) are interrelated. Antibodies of a certain specificity, from different individuals, are often found only within a particular immunoglobulin class and have similar thermal characteristics; in addition, red cells of a certain blood group phenotype, from different individuals, tend to be relatively homogeneous regarding the attributes of the relevant antigen. It is for this reason that knowledge of the specificity of an antibody can be highly informative in predicting its clinical significance [4]. Three examples illustrate this concept.

- Anti-A, anti-B and anti-A,B antibodies are regularly present in moderate to high titre in the plasma of group O persons. These 'naturally occurring' antibodies are often both IgM and IgG, having a broad thermal range up to $37\,°C$, and are often strongly complement binding. The A and B antigens are often present in large numbers (e.g. up to 1.2×10^6 A_1 antigen sites per cell) and are strongly *immunogenic* (provoking an immune response in an individual lacking the antigen). If an individual who has anti-A, anti-B or anti-A,B in their plasma is transfused with donor red cells that express the cognate antigen (i.e. A and/or B), an AHTR is highly likely to occur, which may be fatal. The infusion of group O donor plasma (200–300 mL in an adult pack of platelets or plasma) can similarly cause haemolysis of the recipient's red cells if they are A, AB or B; this will be discussed later in this chapter.
- Anti-Jk^a antibodies may be produced following immunisation of a Jk(a−) person via pregnancy or transfusion. They are usually IgG (but may also have an IgM component), are

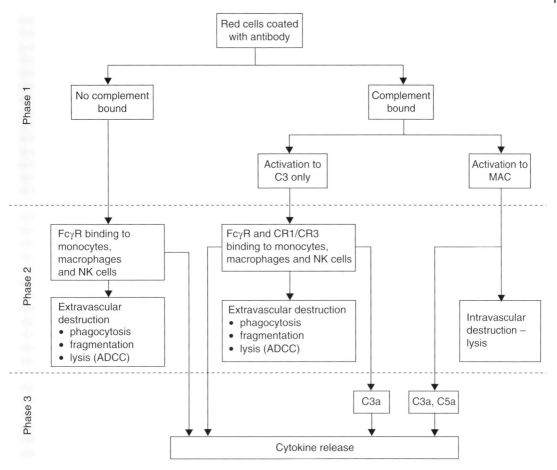

Figure 8.1 Pathophysiology of the haemolytic transfusion reaction (HTR). ADCC, antibody-dependent cell-mediated cytotoxicity; MAC, membrane attack complex; NK, natural killer.

active at 37 °C and may be complement binding. In Jk(a + b−) persons, there are about 1.4×10^4 Jkª antigen sites per cell. Jkª antigens are not particularly immunogenic but the antibody is sometimes difficult to detect in pretransfusion testing (because of the low titre of antibody); consequently, Jk(a+) blood may be inadvertently transfused to patients with preexisting anti-Jkª. These antibodies are frequently implicated in DHTRs.

- Anti-Luª antibodies may be produced following the immunisation of a Lu(a−) person, or may be 'naturally occurring'. They are usually IgM (but often have IgA and IgG components), are only sometimes reactive at 37 °C

and are not usually complement binding. The Luª antigens show variable distribution on the red cells of an individual and are poorly immunogenic. The antibody may not be detected in pretransfusion testing, because screening cells usually do not possess the Luª antigen and because antibody levels fall after immunisation. Anti-Luª antibodies have not been implicated in AHTRs and have only rarely been implicated in DHTRs, which are usually mild.

Complement Activation

Antibody-mediated intravascular haemolysis is caused by sequential binding of complement components (C1–C9) on the red cell membrane. IgM alloantibodies are more efficient activators of C1 than IgG antibodies, since the latter must be sufficiently close together on the red cell surface to be bridged by C1q in order to activate complement. Activation to the C5 stage leads to release of C5a into the plasma and assembly of the remaining components of the membrane attack complex (MAC) on the red cell surface, leading to lysis.

Extravascular haemolysis is caused by non-complement-binding IgG antibodies or those that bind sublytic amounts of complement. IgG subclasses differ in their ability to bind complement, with the following order of reactivity: IgG3 > IgG1 > IgG2 > IgG4.

Activation of C3 leads to the release of C3a into the plasma and to C3b and iC3b deposition on red cells, promoting binding of the red cell to two complement receptors, CR1 (CD35) and CR3 (CD11b), which are both expressed on macrophages and monocytes. Hence, C3b and iC3b augment macrophage-mediated clearance of IgG-coated cells, and antibodies binding sublytic amounts of complement (e.g. Duffy and Kidd antibodies) often cause more rapid red cell clearance and more marked symptoms than noncomplement-binding antibodies (e.g. Rh antibodies).

C3a and C5a are anaphylatoxins with potent pro-inflammatory effects, including oxygen radical production, granule enzyme release from mast cells and granulocytes, nitric oxide production and cytokine production [5].

Fc Receptor Interactions

IgG alloantibodies bound to red cell antigens interact with phagocytes through Fc receptors. The affinity of Fc receptors for IgG subclasses varies, with most efficient binding to IgG1 and IgG3. After attachment to phagocytes, the red cells are either engulfed or lysed through antibody-dependent cell-mediated cytotoxicity (ADCC).

Cytokines

Cytokines are generated during an HTR as a consequence of both anaphylotoxin generation (C3a, C5a) and phagocyte Fc receptor interaction with red cell-bound IgG. Some biological actions of cytokines implicated in HTRs are given in Table 8.1.

ABO incompatibility stimulates the release of high levels of tumour necrosis factor (TNF)-α into the plasma, within two hours, followed by CXCL-8 (interleukin (IL)-8) and CCL-2

Table 8.1 Cytokines implicated in haemolytic transfusion reactions.

Terminology	Biological activity
Pro-inflammatory cytokines	
TNF, IL-1	Fever
	Hypotension, shock, death
	Mobilisation of leucocytes from marrow
	Activation of T- and B-cells
	Induction of cytokines (IL-1, IL-6, CXCL-8, TNF-α, CCL-2)
	Induction of adhesion molecules
IL-6	Fever
	Acute-phase protein response
	B-cell antibody production
	T-cell activation
Chemokines	
CXCL-8	Chemotaxis of neutrophils
	Chemotaxis of lymphocytes
	Neutrophil activation
	Basophil histamine release
CCL-2	Chemotaxis of monocytes
	Induction of respiratory burst
	Induction of adhesion molecules
	Induction of IL-1
Anti-inflammatory cytokines	
IL-1ra	Competitive inhibition of IL-1 type I and II receptors

CCL, chemokine (C-C motif) ligand; CXCL, chemokine (C-X-C motif) ligand; IL, interleukin; TNF, tumour necrosis factor.

(monocyte chemotactic protein (MCP)-1). In IgG-mediated haemolysis, TNF-α is produced at a lower level together with IL-1β and IL-6. CXCL-8 production follows a similar time course to that in ABO incompatibility.

IgG-mediated haemolysis, as opposed to ABO incompatibility, also results in the production of the IL-1 receptor antagonist, IL-1ra. The relative balance of IL-1 and IL-1ra may also, at least in part, account for some of the clinical differences between intravascular and extravascular haemolysis [6].

Antibody Specificities Associated with HTRs

These are given, together with the site of red cell destruction, in Table 8.2. A helpful review paper on the clinical significance of red cell antibodies has been written by Daniels et al. [4].

Acute HTRs

Aetiology and Incidence

These reactions arise as a result of existing antibodies, in either the recipient or donor plasma, which are directed against red cell antigens of the other party. In the developed world, transfusion reactions resulting from incompatibility are more common as a cause of morbidity and mortality than transfusion-transmitted infection. This may not be the perception of patients, the public, politicians and even clinical staff. Incompatible transfusion can occur for the following reasons.

- *Clerical error*: this can occur at the point of taking and labelling the sample, laboratory compatibility testing and blood allocation, collection of the blood component from the refrigerator, freezer or agitator and bedside checking at administration.
- *Undetected antibody*: Kidd (Jk) antibodies are a typical example of antibodies that may be missed by sensitive testing systems.
- *Intentional provision of blood components* as the best available, lowest risk choice when the 'perfect' blood component is not available (e.g. ORhD negative cde/cde in an emergency to a patient who subsequently proves to have anti-c).

The majority of AHTRs have historically been due to the transfusion of ABO-incompatible red cells, but can also be due to the administration of

Table 8.2 Antibody specificities associated with haemolytic transfusion reactions.

Blood group system	Intravascular haemolysis	Extravascular haemolysis
ABO, H	A, B, H	
Rh		All
Kell	K	K, k, Kp^a, Kp^b, Js^a, Js^b
Kidd	Jk^a (Jk^b,Jk^3)	Jk^a,Jk^b,Jk^3
Duffy		Fy^a, Fy^b, Fy^3
MNS		M, S, s, U
Lutheran		Lu^b
Lewis	Le^a	
Cartwright		Yt^a
Vel	Vel	Vel
Colton		Co^a, Co^b
Dombrock		Do^a, Do^b

donor plasma containing high titres of ABO haemolysins when platelets or, less commonly, fresh frozen plasma of a different ABO blood group is transfused (classically group O donor plasma into a group A recipient). ABO-incompatible red cell transfusions are the result of the 'wrong' blood being given to the 'wrong' patient because of clerical or administrative errors, occurring at any stage during the transfusion process. ABO-incompatible platelet administration is unlikely to cause a reaction and such transfusions are 'intentional' to utilise the short shelf-life platelet stock in an efficient manner (see below).

The Serious Hazards of Transfusion (SHOT) confidential reporting scheme has shown that in cases where the patient was transfused with a blood component or plasma product that did not meet the appropriate requirements or that was intended for another patient, the sites of primary error were clinical areas in approximately 65% of cases, hospital laboratories in 34% of cases and blood establishments in 1% of cases. The reports have also highlighted that multiple errors contribute to incorrect blood component transfusion (IBCT). Examples of reported errors from several series are given in

Box 8.1. Estimates of ABO-incompatible transfusions vary and may be underestimates, since some may be unrecognised or not reported, but two surveys have found a frequency of one in approximately 30 000 transfusions [7,8].

Not all ABO-incompatible transfusions cause morbidity and mortality; mortality is dependent on the amount of incompatible red cells transfused and is reported to be 25% in recipients receiving 1–2 units of blood and reaches 44% with more than two units. However, as little as 30 mL group A cells given to a group O recipient can be fatal. Less frequently, Kell, Kidd and Duffy antibodies can be responsible and the acute reaction is due to a failure to detect, or take account of, the red cell alloantibody in either the antibody screen or cross-match.

Errors are a major cause of morbidity due to HTRs. In the UK, the number of incidents including errors and near misses reported to the SHOT haemovigilance scheme has steadily increased annually. Up to 2010, HTRs accounted for 501/8110 (6%) and IBCT 2837/8110 (35%) of errors reported. In 2014, HTRs and IBCTs accounted for 1.3% (46/3668) and 7.6% (278/3668) of incidents respectively. In both 2013 and 2014,

---

Box 8.1 Errors resulting in 'wrong blood' incidents.

Prescription, sampling and request
    Failure to identify correct recipient at sampling
    Correct patient identity at sampling but incorrectly labelled sample
    Selection of incompatible products in an emergency

Transfusion laboratory
    Took a correctly identified sample and aliquoted it into an improperly labelled test tube for testing
    Took a wrongly identified sample through testing
    Tested the correct sample but misinterpreted the results
    Tested the correct sample but recorded the results on the wrong record
    Correctly tested the sample but labelled the wrong unit of blood as compatible for the patient
    Incorrect serological reasoning, e.g. O-positive FFP to non-O-positive recipient

Collection and delivery of the wrong component to the ward
    Failure to check recipient identity with unit identity

    Bedside administration error
    Recipient identity checked through case notes or prescription chart and not wristband
    Wristband absent or incorrect

there were no reported episodes of sampling or sample labelling errors resulting in patients receiving the wrong blood component, despite a progressive increase in near misses where it was identified in a timely manner that the wrong blood was present in the sample tube (wrong blood in tube – WBIT). A 2012 recommendation that two samples from two separate venepunctures should be analysed prior to the provision of blood for a patient except in emergency situations has been widely implemented in the UK and has no doubt contributed to this improvement [2].

Nearly all deaths as a result of IBCT are due to ABO-incompatible transfusions and there were 27 deaths in which IBCT was causal or contributory between 1996 and 2010 [9]. Reports of ABO-incompatible transfusions have not increased in number despite the steady rise in all reported errors. There were 10 reported incidents of ABO incompatibility in 2014, all resulting from either an administration error or both collection and administration errors. There were no deaths and morbidity and mortality following HTR are now more commonly due to antibodies other than ABO [2].

Similar findings have been noted in other countries; details of the incompatibilities resulting in deaths reported to the Food and Drug Administration between 2010 and 2014 are provided in Table 8.3 [10].

On a positive note, the SHOT voluntary reporting scheme has demonstrated an increase in overall reporting of errors and reactions but simultaneously the number of reported errors resulting in preventable major morbidity or mortality has remained stable or fallen [2]. This suggests that increased awareness of the hazards of transfusion has led to a lower threshold to report and an improvement in patient safety. This progress is probably due to a number of initiatives to improve hospital transfusion practice, including providing better training of the large number of staff involved at some stage of the transfusion process (see Chapter 23).

Symptoms and Signs

These may become apparent when receiving as little as 20 mL of ABO-incompatible red cells. Initial clinical presentations include the following.

- Fever, chills or both.
- Pain at the infusion site or localised to the lower back/flanks, abdomen, chest or head.
- Hypotension, tachycardia or both.
- Agitation, distress and confusion, particularly in the elderly.
- Nausea or vomiting.
- Dyspnoea.
- Flushing.
- Haemoglobinuria.

In anaesthetised patients, the only signs may be uncontrollable hypotension or excessive bleeding from the operative site, as a result of DIC.

Some of these symptoms and signs can also be features of other transfusion reactions, including febrile nonhaemolytic reactions, allergic reactions, transfusion-related acute lung injury and bacterial contamination of the unit (see Chapters 9, 10 and 16).

Complications

Acute kidney injury develops in up to 36% of patients with AHTR as a result of acute tubular necrosis induced by both hypotension and DIC. Thrombus formation in renal arterioles may also cause cortical infarcts.

Disseminated intravascular coagulation develops in up to 10% of patients. TNF-α can induce tissue factor expression by endothelial cells and, together with IL-1, can reduce the endothelial expression of thrombomodulin. Thromboplastic material is also liberated from leucocytes during the course of complement activation [6].

Immediate Management of Suspected AHTR (see Chapter 7)

Actions for Nursing Staff

In the presence of a fever of more than 1 °C above the patient's pretransfusion temperature and/or any symptoms or signs mentioned above, the nursing staff should:

- stop the transfusion, leaving the infusion line ('giving set') attached to the blood pack
- use a new giving set and keep an intravenous infusion running with normal saline

Table 8.3 Fatal haemolytic transfusion reactions reported to the FDA by implicated antibody, 2010–14.

Antibody	2010 No.	2010 %	2011 No.	2011 %	2012 No.	2012 %	2013 No.	2013 %	2014 No.	2014 %	Total No.	Total %
ABO	2	29%	3	33%	3	38%	1	17%	4	50%	13	34%
Multiple antibodies*	3	43%	1	11%	2	25%	1	17%	0	0%	7	18%
Other**	0	0%	2	22%	0	0%	0	0%	2	25%	4	10%
Fy^a	0	0%	1	11%	0	0%	0	0%	0	0%	1	2%
Jk^b	1	14%	0	0%	1	13%	1	17%	0	0%	3	8%
Kell	0	0%	1	11%	1	13%	2	33%	0	0%	4	10%
Jk^a	0	0%	0	0%	0	0%	1	17%	1	12.5%	2	5%
c	0	0%	1	11%	0	0%	0	0%	0	0%	1	2%
Js^b	0	0%	0	0%	1	13%	0	0%	0	0%	1	2%
Co^a	1	14%	0	0%	0	0%	0	0%	0	0%	1	2%
C	0	0%	0	0%	0	0%	0	0%	1	12.5%	1	2%
Totals	7	100%	9	100%	8	100%	6	100%	8	100%	38	100%

* Multiple antibodies:

FY2010: antibody combinations include: D+C+K+S; Jk^b+FY^a+C+E+K+Le^a+Le^b; c+E+Jk^b+K+Le^a+panagglutinin+cold agglutinin.

FY2011: anti-Jk^a+c+E+M (warm reacting).

FY2012: antibody combinations include: S+E; C+K.

FY2013: anti-c+E.

** Other:

FY2011: includes one report of an unidentified antibody and one report of hyperhaemolysis syndrome.

FY2014: includes one report of hyperhaemolysis syndrome in which no new or additional antibody was identified.

- call a member of the medical staff
- check that the patient identity as provided on the wristband corresponds with that given on the label on the blood pack and on the compatibility form
- save any urine the patient passes for later examination for haemoglobinuria
- monitor the patient's pulse (P), blood pressure (BP) and temperature (T) at 15-minute intervals.

Actions for Medical Staff

The immediate actions depend upon the presenting symptoms and signs, and are summarised in Table 8.4.

Investigation of Suspected AHTR

Blood samples should be taken from a site other than the infusion site for the investigations listed in Table 8.5.

Other Reactions Characterised by Haemolysis

In patients with autoimmune haemolytic anaemia, transfusion may exacerbate the haemolysis and be associated with haemoglobinuria.

Donor units of red cells may also be haemolysed as a result of:

- bacterial contamination
- excessive warming
- erroneous freezing
- addition of drugs or intravenous fluids
- trauma from extracorporeal devices
- red cell enzyme deficiency.

Management of a Confirmed AHTR

The management of haemolytic transfusion reactions should be determined by the severity of the clinical manifestations.

- Maintain adequate renal perfusion while avoiding volume overload by:
  - maintenance of circulating volume with crystalloid and/or colloid infusions
  - if necessary, inotropic support.
- Transfer to a high-dependency area where continuous monitoring can take place.
- Repeat coagulation and biochemistry screens 2–4-hourly.
- If urinary output cannot be maintained at 1 mL/kg/h, seek expert renal advice.
- Haemofiltration or dialysis may be required for the acute tubular necrosis.

Table 8.4 Immediate medical management of an acute transfusion reaction.

Symptoms/signs	Likely diagnosis	Actions
Isolated fever or fever and shivering, stable observations, correct unit given	Febrile nonhaemolytic transfusion reaction (FNHTR)	Paracetamol 1 g orally/per os (PO) (in the US acetaminophen 625 mg), continue transfusion slowly observations of P, BP and T every 15 min for 1 h, then hourly. If no improvement then call haematology medical staff
Pruritus and/or urticaria	Allergic transfusion reaction	Chlorpheniramine 10 mg IV (US: diphenhydramine 25–50 mg PO or IV) and other actions as for suspected FNHTR
Any other symptoms/ signs, hypotension or incorrect unit	Assume to be an acute haemolytic transfusion reaction in first instance	Discontinue transfusion, normal saline to maintain urine output >1 mL/kg/h. Full and continuous monitoring of vital signs. Call haematology medical and transfusion laboratory staff immediately for further advice/action. Send discontinued unit of blood with attached giving set and other empty packs, after clamping securely, to the transfusion laboratory

Table 8.5 Laboratory investigation of suspected acute haemolytic transfusion reaction.

Blood test	Rationale/findings
Full blood count	Baseline parameters, red cell agglutinates on film
Plasma/urinary haemoglobin	Evidence of intravascular haemolysis
Haptoglobin, bilirubin, lactate dehydrogenase	Evidence of intravascular or extravascular haemolysis
Blood group	Comparison of posttransfusion and retested pretransfusion samples, to detect ABO error not apparent at bedside. Unexpected ABO antibodies post transfusion may result from transfused incompatible plasma. The donor ABO group should be confirmed
Direct antiglobin test (DAT)	Positive in majority, pretransfusion sample should be tested for comparison. May be negative if all incompatible cells destroyed
Compatibility testing	An indirect antiglobulin test (IAT) antibody screen and IAT cross-match using the pre- and posttransfusion sample provide evidence for the presence of alloantibody. Elution of antibody from posttransfusion red cells may aid identification of antibody or confirm specificities identified in serum in cases of non-ABO incompatibility. Red cell phenotype should also be performed on recipient pretransfusion sample and unit in cases of non-ABO incompatibility, to confirm absence in patient and presence in unit of corresponding antigen
Urea/creatinine and electrolytes	Baseline renal function
Coagulation screen	Detection of incipient disseminated intravascular coagulation
Blood cultures from the patient and implicated pack(s)	In event of septic reaction caused by bacterial contamination of unit, which may be suspected from inspection of pack for lysis, altered colour or clots

- In the event of the development of DIC, blood component therapy may be required.
- Having ascertained the nature of the incompatibility causing the AHTR, transfusion of compatible blood may be required for life-threatening anaemia.

Prevention of AHTRs

Prevention of 'Wrong Blood' Incidents

- Prevention of the multiplicity of errors that can contribute to the transfusion of ABO-incompatible red cells must depend upon the creation of an effective quality system for the entire process, which will involve:
  - adherence to national guidelines and standards
  - local procedures that are agreed, documented and validated

  - training and retraining of key staff
  - regular error analysis and review
  - reporting to local risk management/assurance committee
  - reporting to regulatory bodies such as the Medicines and Healthcare products Regulatory Agency (MHRA) in the UK, the FDA in the United States and to national haemovigilance schemes to contribute to the understanding of the extent and underlying causes.

These aspects are specifically covered in Chapter 23.

- Since the majority of errors leading to an ABO-incompatible transfusion are due to misidentification of the patient or patient's sample, due attention must be paid to the comprehensive use of unique patient identifiers throughout the hospital and automation within the laboratory [2,11,12].

- Access to previous transfusion records containing historical ABO groups should be available at all times.
- It is desirable that computerised systems are used to verify at the bedside the matches between the patient and the sample taken for compatibility testing, and at the time of transfusion between the patient and the unit of blood.

Prevention of Non-ABO AHTRs

- In the case of recurrently transfused patients, due attention should be paid to the interval between sampling and transfusion, to optimise the detection of newly developing antibodies. In the UK, for patients transfused within the previous 14 days, the pretransfusion sample should not be taken more than three days before the next transfusion [13]. In the US, the pretransfusion sample must be obtained within three days if the patient has been transfused or pregnant within the past three months. Similar requirements exist in other countries.
- In the presence of multiple red cell alloantibodies, when it is not feasible to obtain compatible red cells in an emergency, intravenous immunoglobulin (1 g/kg/day for three days) and/or steroids (hydrocortisone 100 mg six-hourly or methylprednisolone 1 g daily for three days) have been used with anecdotal reports of ameliorating a potential haemolytic or 'hyperhaemolytic' episode (see below). Similarly, other immunosuppressant/immunomodulatory drugs have been used, recently including eculizumab, a monoclonal antibody that binds to the complement component C5 and blocks its cleavage [14].

Delayed HTRs

Aetiology and Incidence

With few exceptions, DHTRs are due to secondary immune responses following reexposure to a given red cell antigen. The recipient has been primarily sensitised to the antigen in pregnancy or as a result of a previous blood transfusion and a few days after a subsequent transfusion, there is a rapid increase in the antibody concentration, resulting in the destruction of red cells.

- The antibodies most commonly implicated and reported to SHOT are those from the Kidd blood group system followed by those from the Rh, Duffy and Kell systems. One analysis showed that in approximately 10% of reported cases, more than one alloantibody was found in the serum [2,15].
- Frequently, there are no clinical signs of red cell destruction, but subsequent patient investigations reveal a positive DAT and the emergence of a red cell antibody. This situation has been termed a delayed serological transfusion reaction (DSTR) [16].
- Kidd and Duffy antibodies are more likely to cause symptoms and be associated with a DHTR rather than a DSTR.
- Estimates of the frequency of DHTR and DSTR vary, but in a series reported from the Mayo Clinic, the frequency of DHTR was one in 5405 units and of DSTR was one in 2990 units, giving a combined frequency of one in 1899 units transfused [17].
- DHTRs are in themselves rarely fatal, although in association with the underlying disease they can lead to mortality, for example in patients with poor baseline renal or hepatic function.
- Of transfusion fatalities reported to the FDA between 2010 and 2014, 21% (38) were due to HTR; 34% (13/38) were due to ABO antibodies and in 18% (7/38) more than one alloantibody was present in the serum. The most commonly implicated single specificities were Jk^a or Jk^b which constituted 13% (5/38) [10].
- In 2014, 0.76% (28/3668) of reports to SHOT were DHTRs [2]; 32% (9/28) were in patients with sickle cell disease, showing that this patient population is at particular risk as haemoglobinopathy patients receive approximately 3% of red cells in the UK.

Signs and Symptoms

These usually appear within 5–10 days following the transfusion, but intervals as short as 24 hours and as late as 41 days have been recorded. The exact onset may be difficult to define since haemolysis can be initially insidious and may only be appreciated from results of posttransfusion samples. The most common features are:

- fever
- fall in haemoglobin concentration
- jaundice and hyperbilirubinaemia.

Hypotension and kidney injury are uncommon (6% of cases). In the postoperative period in particular, the diagnosis may be overlooked and the symptoms and signs incorrectly attributed to continuing haemorrhage or sepsis. In the setting of sickle cell disease, DHTR can be particularly severe with destruction of autologous red cells (hyperhaemolysis) (see below).

Management

The majority of DHTRs require no treatment because red cell destruction occurs gradually as antibody synthesis increases. Haemolysis may, however, contribute to the development of life-threatening anaemia, particularly in patients with ongoing bleeding, and urgent investigations are required to ensure the timely provision of antigen-negative units.

Expert medical advice may be required for treatment of the hypotension and renal failure. When accompanied by circulatory instability and renal insufficiency, a red cell exchange transfusion with antigen-negative units can curtail the haemolytic process. Future transfusions of red cells should also be negative for the antigen in question.

Investigation of Suspected DHTR (see Chapter 7)

- The peripheral blood film is likely to show spherocytosis.
- Other evidence of haemolysis – namely hyperbilirubinaemia, elevated LDH, reduced serum haptoglobin, haemoglobinaemia, haemoglobinuria and haemosiderinuria – is useful to confirm the nature of the reaction and to monitor progress.
- The DAT usually becomes positive within a few days of the transfusion until the incompatible cells have been eliminated.
- Further serological testing on pre- and posttransfusion samples should be undertaken in accordance with the schedule provided for AHTR.
- The antibody may not be initially apparent in the posttransfusion serum but can be eluted from the red cells. If the red cell eluate is inconclusive, then a repeat sample should be taken after 7–10 days, to allow for an increase in antibody titre. However, additional, more sensitive techniques may have to be employed to detect the antibody and it is advisable to seek the help of a reference laboratory.
- Since a significant proportion of cases have more than one alloantibody in the serum, it is important that the panels used for antibody identification have sufficient cells of appropriate phenotypes to exclude additional specificities.

Prevention

Access to previous transfusion records may disclose the presence of antibodies undetectable at the time of cross-matching, and all patients should be questioned regarding previous transfusions and pregnancies. Patients found to have developed a clinically significant red cell alloantibody should be provided with an antibody card. When the care of patients requiring transfusion support is shared between hospitals, there must be adequate communication between laboratories and clinical teams. In England, the potential availability of patient blood groups and compatibility testing information performed in NHS Blood and Transplant via a software package to all hospitals enables the cross-checking of historical blood group and antibody information to minimise the risk of error.

Laboratories should ensure that their antibody screen is effective in detecting weak red cell alloantibodies and that screening cells are taken from homozygotes where the corresponding antibodies show a dosage effect (i.e. they are less easy to detect when red cells with heterozygous expression of the relevant antigen are used rather than cells with homozygous expression). Pretransfusion testing is covered in detail in Chapter 23.

Haemolysis Resulting from Haemopoietic Stem Cell Transplantation (see Chapter 41)

Major ABO-Incompatible Transplants

Infusion of bone marrow during major ABO-incompatible transplants can result in an AHTR (the recipient has antibodies against the donor's red cells, e.g. group A donor, group O recipient). The risk is dependent on the antibody titre of the recipient and the volume of red cells in the marrow harvest. Peripheral blood stem cell products rarely have enough red cells to result in clinical AHTR even if there is ABO incompatibility.

Minor ABO-Incompatible Transplants

Most patients transplanted with minor ABO-incompatible marrow (the donor has antibodies against the recipient's red cells, e.g. O donor, A recipient) develop a positive DAT, but only 10–15% of patients develop clinically significant haemolysis. Haemolysis in minor ABO incompatibility is short-lived and exchange transfusion is rarely required. Red cells and plasma-containing components (platelets, FFP and cryoprecipitate) should be compatible with both recipient and donor.

It has been suggested that the use of peripheral blood stem cells may increase the risk of significant haemolysis since the number of lymphocytes infused with the graft is increased, and three deaths due to an AHTR were reported between 1997 and 1999 in minor ABO-incompatible transplants. Several cases due to anti-D have been described, and antibody production has persisted for up to one year [18].

Delayed Haemolysis Following Organ Transplantation (Passenger Lymphocyte Syndrome)

Donor-derived B lymphocytes within the transplanted organ may mount an anamnestic response against the recipient's red cell antigens. Donor-derived antibodies are usually directed against antigens within the ABO and Rh systems. If ABO-mismatched organs are transplanted, the frequency of occurrence of donor-derived antibodies and haemolysis increases with the lymphoid content of the graft, from kidney to liver to heart–lung transplants. The figures for haemolysis are 9%, 29% and 70%, respectively. The frequency of haemolysis increases with an O donor and an A recipient. Pretransplant isohaemagglutinin titres do not appear to predict the incidence or severity of haemolysis. The ABO antibodies, which appear 7–10 days after transplant, last for approximately one month. Haemolysis is usually mild, although several cases of renal failure and one death have been reported. It can be ameliorated by switching to group O cells, either at the end of surgery or postoperatively if the DAT becomes positive.

Rh antibodies have been described following kidney, liver and heart–lung transplants. They can cause haemolysis for up to six months, which can be sufficiently severe to merit therapy.

Haemolysis occurs 7–10 days after transplantation, with an unpredictable and abrupt onset [19].

Hyperhaemolytic Transfusion Reactions and Haemolytic Transfusion Reactions in Sickle Cell Disease

The frequency of alloimmunisation in sickle cell anaemia is dependent upon the nature and success of the extended red cell antigen-matching policy employed. Approximately 40% of patients who are alloimmunised have experienced or will experience a DHTR.

Although DHTRs are characteristically mild in other groups of recipients, they can be responsible for major morbidity in sickle cell disease. The term 'sickle cell haemolytic transfusion reaction (SCHTR) syndrome' has been suggested to capture some of the distinctive features that can be seen to accompany a reaction (see Chapter 30). A similar syndrome has been described in other transfusion-dependent patients, so the term 'hyperhaemolytic transfusion reaction (HHTR)' may be more appropriate. These features are as follows.

- Symptoms suggestive of a sickle cell pain crisis that develop or are intensified during the HTR.
- Marked reticulocytopenia (relative to pretransfusion levels).
- Development of a more severe anaemia after transfusion than was present before. This may be due to the suppression of erythropoiesis as a result of the transfusion but hyperhaemolysis of autologous red cells (bystander immune haemolysis) has also been suggested. There have been reports that bone marrow aspirates performed on patients suffering from this complication have shown evidence of active erythropoiesis during the reticulocytopenic phase and haemophagocytosis. Also, ferritin levels can rise drastically as seen in haemophagocytic syndromes. This has led to the suggestion that erythroid precursors and reticulocytes are removed by adhesion to monocytes via other mechanisms, in addition to IgG and Fc receptors, such as the integrins $\alpha 4\beta 1$ and VCAM-1.
- Subsequent transfusions may further exacerbate the anaemia and it may become fatal.
- Patients often have multiple red blood cell alloantibodies and may also have autoantibodies, which make it difficult or impossible to find compatible units of red blood cells.

However, in other patients the DAT may be negative, no alloantibodies are identified and serological studies may not provide an explanation for the HTR; even red cells that are phenotypically matched with multiple patient antigens may be haemolysed.

Management involves withholding further transfusion and treating with corticosteroids (methylprednisolone 1 g daily for three days), while IVIG (1 g/kg/day for two days) may have been beneficial in some cases and other immunosuppressive agents have been used anecdotally [20,21].

It is recommended that patients with sickle cell disease are phenotyped prior to transfusion and that blood is matched for Rhc, C, D, e, E and K (see Chapter 30).

Acute Haemolysis from ABO-Incompatible Platelet Transfusions

Rarely, the passive transfusion of anti-A or anti-B present in a platelet pack will cause haemolysis in the recipient. This is most commonly seen in type A recipients of type O platelets. Clinically significant reactions are rare: passive anti-A/B becomes diluted in the recipient's plasma and it will also bind to A or B antigen, both soluble in the recipient's plasma and on endothelial cells. The typical anti-A/B titre in a platelet donor is of the order of 1:128, but occasionally donors will have very high titres exceeding 10 000. Severe and even fatal AHTRs have been reported, particularly in cases where a large amount of incompatible ABO antibody is transfused into a recipient with a small plasma volume (e.g. a child). In the UK, all platelet units must be screened for anti-A/B using a cut-off titre of 1:100. Packs from donors who have titres below this level are marked 'HT negative' or high titre negative. Approximately 10% of platelet units will have titres above 1:100 and will not be marked HT negative; these are restricted to ABO-identical recipients. In the US, no preventive strategy is currently mandated and local practices vary. AABB-accredited transfusion services are simply required to have a policy concerning the transfusion of products having significant amounts of incompatible ABO antibodies.

KEY POINTS

1) HTRs are the second most common cause of immediate morbidity and mortality following a transfusion in the UK and the US. The most common cause was transfusion-related acute lung injury (TRALI), but more recently transfusion-associated circulatory overload (TACO) has overtaken TRALI.

2) The clinical presentations are diverse and they can be unrecognised or misdiagnosed.

3) Most fatal AHTRs have historically been due to the transfusion of ABO-incompatible red cells but there is evidence that increased transfusion safety awareness has reduced the frequency of this. Other causes of AHTR are overtaking ABO in countries where haemovigilance schemes have been successful.

4) The transfusion of ABO-incompatible red cells is the result of an error occurring at any stage in the transfusion process. Patient identification errors are the most frequent culprit.

5) Devising and successfully implementing measures to overcome these preventable and fatal errors is a challenge but should be a priority for those involved in transfusion practice.

References

1 Beauregard P, Blajchman MA. Haemolytic and pseudohaemolytic transfusion reactions: an overview of the haemolytic transfusion reactions and the clinical conditions that mimic them. Transfus Med Rev 1994;**8**:184–99.

2 Serious Hazards of Transfusion. Annual Report 2014. Available at: www.shotuk.org (accessed 9 November 2016).

3 Centers for Disease Control and Prevention. National Healthcare Safety Network Biovigilance Component Hemovigilance Module Surveillance Protocol v2.1.3. Available at: www.cdc.gov/nhsn/pdfs/biovigilance/bv-hv-protocol-current.pdf (accessed 9 November 2016).

4 Daniels G, Poole J, de Silva M, Callaghan T, MacLennan S, Smith N. The clinical significance of blood group antibodies. Transfus Med 2002;**12**(5):287–95.

5 Davenport RD. Hemolytic transfusion reactions, in Transfusion Reactions, 2nd edn (ed. M Popovsky), AABB Press, Bethesda, 2001, pp.2–36.

6 Davenport RD. Pathophysiology of hemolytic transfusion reactions. Semin Hematol 2005;**42**(3):165–8.

7 Linden JV, Wagner K, Voytovich AE, Sheehan J. Transfusion errors in New York State: an analysis of 10 years experience. Transfusion 2000;**40**(10):1207–13.

8 Stainsby D. ABO incompatible transfusions – experience from the UK Serious Hazards of Transfusion (SHOT) scheme. Transfus Clin Biol 2005;**12**(5):385–8.

9 Serious Hazards of Transfusion. Annual Report 2010. Available at: www.shotuk.org (accessed 9 November 2016).

10 Food and Drug Administration. Fatalities Reported to FDA Following Blood Collection and Transfusion. Annual Summary for Fiscal Year 2014. Available at: www.fda.gov/downloads/BiologicsBloodVaccines/SafetyAvailability/ReportaProblem/TransfusionDonationFatalities/UCM459461.pdf (accessed 9 November 2016).

11 National Patient Safety Agency. Right Patient, Right Blood. Safer Practice Notice No. 14. Available at: www.nrls.npsa.nhs.uk/resources/collections/right-patient-right-blood/(accessed 9 November 2016).

12 National Patient Safety Agency. Standardising Patient Wristbands Improves Patient Safety. Safer Practice Notice No. 24. Available at: www.

nrls.npsa.nhs.uk/resources/?entryid45=59824 (accessed 9 November 2016).

13 British Committee for Standards in Haematology. Guidelines for Pre-Transfusion Compatibility Procedures in Blood Transfusion Laboratories. Available at: www. bcshguidelines.com/documents/Compat_ Guideline_for_submission_to_TTF_011012. pdf (accessed 9 November 2016).

14 Weinstock C, Möhle R, Dorn C et al. Successful use of eculizumab for treatment of an acute hemolytic reaction after ABO-incompatible red blood cell transfusion. Transfusion 2015;**55**(3):605–10.

15 Stainsby D, Jones H, Asher D et al. Serious hazards of transfusion: a decade of haemovigilance in the UK. Transfus Med Rev 2006;**20**(4):273–82.

16 Vamvakas EC, Pineda AA, Reisner R, Santrach PJ, Moore SB. The differentiation of delayed haemolytic and delayed serologic transfusion reactions: incidence and predictors of haemolysis. Transfusion 1995;**35**:26–32.

17 Pineda AA, Vamvakas EC, Gorden LD, Winters JL, Moore SB. Trends in the incidence of delayed hemolytic and delayed serologic transfusion reactions. Transfusion 1999;**39**(10):1097–103.

18 Daniel-Johnson J, Schwartz J. How do I approach ABO-incompatible hematopoietic progenitor cell transplantation? Transfusion 2011;**51**(6):1143–9.

19 Petz LD. Immune hemolysis associated with transplantation. Semin Hematol 2005;**42**:145–55.

20 Win N, Sinha S, Lee E, Mills W. Treatment with intravenous immunoglobulin and steroids may correct severe anemia in hyperhemolytic transfusion reactions: case report and literature review. Transfus Med Rev 2010;**24**(1):64–7.

21 Boonyasampant M, Weitz IC, Kay B, Boonchalermvichian C, Liebman HA, Shulman IA. Life-threatening delayed hyperhemolytic transfusion reaction in a patient with sickle cell disease: effective treatment with eculizumab followed by rituximab. Transfusion 2015;**55**(10):2398–403.

Further Reading

Daniels G. Human Blood Groups, 3rd edn. Wiley-Blackwell, Chichester, 2013.

Food and Drug Administration. Fatalities Reported to FDA Following Blood Collection and Transfusion. Annual Summary for Fiscal Year 2014. Available at: www.fda.gov/ downloads/BiologicsBloodVaccines/ SafetyAvailability/ReportaProblem/ TransfusionDonationFatalities/UCM459461. pdf (accessed 9 November 2016).

Klein H, Anstee D. Haemolytic transfusion reactions, in Mollison's Blood Transfusion in Clinical Medicine, 12th edn (eds HG Klein, D Anstee), Wiley-Blackwell, Chichester, 2014.

Popovsky MA. Transfusion Reactions, 4th edn. AABB Press, Bethesda, 2012.

Serious Hazards of Transfusion (SHOT) resources and reports. Available at: www. shotuk.org

Win N. The Clinical Significance of Blood Group Alloantibodies and the Supply of Blood for Transfusion. Version 3; 2015. Available at: http://hospital.blood.co.uk/media/27446/ spn2143-the-clinical-significance-of-blood-group-alloantibodies-and-the-supply-of-blood-for-transfusion.pdf (accessed 9 November 2016).

9

Febrile and Allergic Transfusion Reactions

Mark K. Fung[1] and Nancy M. Heddle[2]

[1] Department of Pathology and Laboratory Medicine, University of Vermont Medical Center, Burlington, USA
[2] Department of Medicine, McMaster University and Canadian Blood Services, Hamilton, Ontario, Canada

Introduction

Allergic reactions are most commonly due to reactions against plasma proteins. Symptomatic relief of mild urticarial reactions can usually be achieved with the use of antihistamines, but pre-medication does not appear to reduce the incidence of allergic reactions. Although anaphylactic reactions are uncommon, close monitoring of patients during transfusions permits prompt termination of the transfusion and treatment to minimise further morbidity or mortality.

Signs and symptoms typical of these reactions can also be associated with other types of transfusion reactions and/or caused by treatments and medications that the patient may be receiving as well as comorbidities. Hence, establishing causation and an appropriate management strategy can be challenging. In this chapter, febrile non-haemolytic transfusion reactions (FNHTRs) and both mild and severe forms of allergic reactions will be discussed.

Febrile Non-haemolytic Transfusion Reactions

Clinical Presentation

The classical definition of a FNHTR includes fever (usually defined as ≥1 °C rise in temperature) during or within two hours of completing the transfusion along with other symptoms that can include a cold feeling, chills and a generalised feeling of discomfort or malaise. Less frequently, headache, nausea and vomiting may also occur and, in severe reactions, rigours can be present. Although fever is a component of the classical definition, in practice only a minority of patients develop a fever, with chills, cold and discomfort being the primary findings [1]. Therefore, the use of the International Society for Blood Transfusion (ISBT) or Centers for Disease Control and Prevention (CDC) haemovigilance definitions of a FNHTR, that include having either a ≥1 °C rise in temperature to 38 °C or greater or chills and/or rigours, may be more appropriate [2,3]. Furthermore, recent analyses of the changes in vital signs during transfusions suggest that a 1 °C or greater temperature rise is a convenient number to remember; however, relevant temperature changes may occur at smaller increments for products such as plasma, where temperature rises as small as 0.6 °C represent a greater than two standard deviation increase in temperature. This observation may merit further investigation [4]. Thus, a FNHTR can actually occur in the absence of a fever.

Differential Diagnosis

Unfortunately, the signs and symptoms that are commonly associated with a FNHTR are not

Practical Transfusion Medicine, Fifth Edition. Edited by Michael F. Murphy, David J. Roberts and Mark H. Yazer.
© 2017 John Wiley & Sons Ltd. Published 2017 by John Wiley & Sons Ltd.

specific for a FNHTR. The challenge for the transfusing physician is to consider the other possibilities as part of the differential diagnosis and to develop a systematic approach for establishing a definitive diagnosis. When a transfused patient develops fever or chills, the differential diagnosis should include:

- FNHTR
- acute haemolytic reactions
- delayed haemolytic reactions
- bacterial contamination
- transfusion-related acute lung injury (TRALI)
- transfusion-associated circulatory overload (TACO)
- acute pain reactions
- co-morbid conditions
- medications.

Although all of these reactions can be associated with fever, it is especially important to rule out acute haemolysis, bacterial contamination and hypoxia (caused by TRALI or TACO) as these conditions can frequently be associated with morbidity and mortality unless rapidly recognised and treated. More recently, TACO has been associated with inflammatory signs and symptoms in a subset of these reactions, and in two-thirds of these TACO-FNHTR cases, an inflammatory sign or symptom was the initial presentation [5]. Bacterial contamination and TRALI also have implications for donor management and handling of other components prepared from the implicated donation, emphasising the importance of considering these types of reactions in the differential diagnosis (see Chapters 10 and 16). In contrast, FNHTRs cause discomfort and distress, although not long-term morbidity, for the patient and consume additional healthcare resources for their treatment and investigation. Preliminary data suggest that patients who experience FNHTR may be more likely to develop red cell alloimmunisation. The hypothesis to explain this observation is that cytokines involved in causing FNHTR may alter the immune system towards a Th2 response to foreign red cell antigens, resulting in an increased risk of alloimmunisation [6].

Whether or not preventing an inflammatory reaction would mitigate this subsequent complication remains unknown, but it highlights the potential importance of preventing an otherwise relatively minor transfusion reaction.

To further complicate the investigative process in patient populations where transfusion-associated fever or chills occur frequently (for example, in haematology/oncology patients), clinical judgement should be incorporated into the decision-making process.

Frequency

The frequency of FNHTRs varies with the:

- patient population
- type of blood components being transfused
- age of the blood component.

Reactions to platelets occur more frequently than reactions to red cells. However, precise estimates of FNHTR associated with platelet transfusions are difficult as milder reactions are likely to be underreported. In a general hospital population, FNHTRs to red cells occur with 0.04–0.44% of transfusions, whilst the frequency of reactions to platelets is higher, ranging from 0.06% to 2.2%. The degree of variation in temperatures for red cell transfusions is much smaller than that for platelets; hence, the use of a single temperature threshold of 1 °C or higher may account for some of the differences in the frequency of reactions with different types of blood components [4]. This observation may explain the higher frequency of chills or rigour reactions observed with platelet transfusions. In specific patient populations, such as adult haematology/oncology patients, reactions to platelets are even more common, occurring in up to 37% of transfusions if non-leucocyte-reduced platelets are used [7]. When prestorage leucocyte-reduced platelets are transfused, the frequency of acute reactions decreases dramatically (<2% of transfusions) [8]. In paediatric ICU patients, 1.6% of blood components transfused (40/2509) were associated with acute reactions, with FNHTR accounting for 60% (24/40) of these events [9]. Overall, paediatric patients are approximately four times more likely to have a FNHTR than adult patients [10]. FNHTRs to blood components other than red cells and platelets are rare and there are limited data to estimate their frequency.

Pathogenesis

The pathogenesis of FNHTRs is multifactorial and varies for red cells and platelets. The current understanding of the mechanisms causing these reactions with red cells and platelets is summarised below.

Factors Associated with the Blood
Component

- *Antibody mechanism*: patients' plasma contains a leucocyte antibody that reacts with leucocytes present in the blood product. An antigen–antibody reaction occurs, resulting in the release of endogenous pyrogens/cytokines by the donor leucocytes. These biological response modifiers act on the hypothalamus to cause fever. This antigen–antibody hypothesis is believed to be the primary mechanism causing FNHTRs to red cells, but probably accounts for less than 10% of FNHTRs to platelets [7]. Interestingly, the use of platelets that contain trace amounts of ABO-incompatible red blood cells (e.g. blood group O patient receiving group A platelets), whilst predicted to generate a slight and transient inflammatory reaction associated with the destruction of these small numbers of ABO-incompatible red cells, is not associated with an increased incidence of FNHTRs [11].
- *Leucocyte/platelet-derived biological response modifiers*: during storage of the blood product, pro-inflammatory cytokines (interleukin (IL)-1, IL-6, and tumour necrosis factor (TNF)-α) are released from leucocytes present in the blood component. This typically happens when the component is stored at room temperature. Cytokines accumulate to high levels by the end of the product storage period and, when infused, cause fever by stimulation of the hypothalamus. This is the

primary mechanism responsible for FNHTRs to platelets. Platelets are stored at room temperature for a maximum of 5–7 days, depending on local regulations, and have high cytokine concentrations at the end of the storage period if leucocytes are present [12]. Platelet-derived cytokines such as CD40 ligand (sCD40L) and RANTES also accumulate in stored platelets and may play a role in some reactions. When the receptor for CD40L is engaged, pro-inflammatory cytokines are synthesised (IL-6, IL-8, monocyte chemotactic protein (MCP)-1). One study suggested an incremental effect where reactions were more frequent when high levels of multiple biological response mediators were present [13]. There are over 15 different cytokines that have been shown to accumulate in platelet products during storage.
- *Other biological response modifiers (BRMs)*: other BRMs such as complement and neutrophil priming lipids have been detected in some stored blood products and it is hypothetically possible that they may cause or contribute to FNHTRs in some patients. However, there are no clinical data linking these substances to an increased risk of an adverse event [7].

Factors Associated with Patient
Susceptibility

Patient factors may also play a role in susceptibility to FNHTRs. Reactions caused by leucocyte antibodies may be more common in females due to leucocyte antibody formation during pregnancy. Patients whose disease or treatments result in an inflammatory response may also be more likely to have reactions as the additive effect of transfusion-related cytokines may be sufficient to cause the symptoms and signs of FNHTRs. Data also suggest that certain gene polymorphisms may cause an increase in inflammatory cytokine gene expression, resulting in an increased susceptibility to FNHTR. One genotype that has been shown to increase susceptibility for FNHTRs is *IL1RN*2.2* [14].

Management of FNHTRs

The management of FNHTRs includes the exclusion of other causes of fever, which can be difficult or impossible to do in patients who are both predisposed to having a fever due to their underlying disease state and who require transfusion. For example, a patient with neutropenic fevers from chemotherapy might also require transfusion – does a sudden increase in temperature during the transfusion reflect a reaction or the patient's underlying disease state? Thus, the management strategy for FNHTRs requires clinical judgement and must balance the benefits and risks of their investigation and treatment. The following questions should be considered.

- *Is the blood component leucocyte-reduced?* The risk of an FNHTR in a setting where all red cell and platelet components are prestorage leucocyte reduced is low (see above). In this situation, stopping the transfusion and investigating every reaction not only consumes significant healthcare resources, but may put patients at risk as they may not receive the required components in a timely manner.
- *Does the patient have a history of FNHTRs?* Some patients are susceptible to repeated FNHTRs when blood products are transfused, for example because of the presence of leucocyte antibodies; hence the patient's history of reaction should be considered.
- *If a temperature increase occurred, was it greater than or equal to 2 °C?* It is uncommon for the temperature to rise more than 2 °C with a FNHTR. In this situation, bacterial contamination should be suspected, the transfusion should be stopped immediately, and appropriate investigations initiated.
- *Would you describe the patient's signs and symptoms as mild, moderate or severe?* If the symptoms are mild, a less aggressive management approach may be initiated but careful observation of the patient is essential. If the symptoms are severe, the transfusion should be stopped immediately and supportive care given to the patient. Investigations to rule out other possible causes of the reaction should be initiated. If the clinical findings are categorised as moderate, the questions above need to be considered and clinical judgement is required as to how patient management should proceed.

Finally, the management strategy for FNHTRs associated with red cell transfusions should include an approach to rule out an acute haemolytic transfusion reaction. Haemolysis following platelet transfusion is rare but can occur when the plasma of the platelet product contains a high-titre ABO antibody that reacts with the patient's red cells.

The management approach should also aim to alleviate the signs and symptoms associated with an FNHTR. This may involve temporary discontinuation of the transfusion whilst antipyretic medication is administered to the patient. Medications should never be injected into the blood component. In most cases, the transfusion can be resumed once the signs and symptoms subside. There is some evidence that pethidine (or meperidine in North America) is an effective treatment for alleviating rigours associated with transfusions, although care should be taken when administering this medication to people with compromised respiratory status and to avoid possible drug–drug interactions with pethidine or meperidine.

A conservative strategy for minimising the risk to patients whilst investigating reactions would include the following steps.

- Temporarily stop the transfusion but keep the line open with saline.
- Perform a bedside clerical check between the blood and the patient to ensure that the right blood has been transfused.
- Observe the blood product to determine whether there is discolouration or particulate matter present.
- Notify the blood transfusion laboratory and send appropriate samples if laboratory investigations are deemed necessary to rule out other causes of acute reactions with fever.

Prevention of FNHTRs

As the pathogenesis of FNHTRs is different for red cells and platelet transfusions, the strategy for their prevention also depends on the blood component being transfused.

Red Cells

Since most reactions are caused by the leucocyte antigen–antibody mechanism, the primary way to prevent these reactions is to reduce the number of leucocytes in the red cell component. Prevention can be accomplished for most patients by removing approximately one log of leucocytes to a level of less than or equal to 10^8 leucocytes/unit of red cells. This is readily achieved with the use of red cell products that are collected by apheresis or filtered (before or after storage) using current leucocyte reduction filters to generate products with less than 10^6 leucocytes, which is well below the threshold needed to prevent most FNHTRs. If a patient still reacts to a leucocyte-reduced red cell product, other options for preventing future reactions include washing and/or selecting fresher blood for transfusion [7]. Premedication with antipyretics can also be considered, but will only be effective against the febrile component of the reaction with no effect on chills or rigours (see below for further discussion).

Platelets

Most platelet reactions (90%) are caused by leucocyte-derived cytokine accumulation during storage. Hence, poststorage leucocyte reduction is not an effective strategy for preventing these reactions. FNHTRs to platelets can be prevented by prestorage leucocyte reduction by either filtration or centrifugation (buffy coat method of platelet preparation). If prestorage leucocyte-reduced platelets are not available, the plasma supernatant of the stored platelets can be removed and replaced with a suitable platelet additive solution or saline. Alternatively, washing to remove the cytokine-rich plasma can be performed, or fresher platelets (≤3 days of storage) can be transfused [7].

Premedication

Premedication of the patient with an antipyretic drug, paracetamol in the UK and acetaminophen in North America, has become standard practice to prevent FNHTRs. Aspirin should not be used as a premedication in any patient requiring platelet transfusions as it affects platelet function. In some centres, it is routine practice to premedicate all patients prior to transfusion. However, there are no clinical data to justify this universal approach, with the exception of patients with recurrent FNHTRs who can be treated with an antipyretic approximately 30 minutes prior to starting the transfusion to alleviate or prevent symptoms [15,16].

Allergic Transfusion Reactions

Clinical Presentation

Allergic transfusion reactions can be either non-systemic/localised or systemic/generalised and are classified as mild, moderate or severe.

- Non-systemic reactions are usually mild, consisting of urticaria and occasionally focal angio-oedema. These are benign and self-limiting, though they can still cause symptoms that are distressing to the patient. However, such mild reactions may progress to generalised urticaria followed by more severe and systemic reactions with repeated transfusions.
- Systemic reactions range from moderate to severe and life-threatening. Although urticaria is considered a pathognomonic finding for an allergic reaction, cutaneous signs or symptoms may not always be present in severe allergic reactions. Severe reactions usually present with a combination of skin, respiratory or circulatory changes and less commonly with gastrointestinal symptoms. However, approximately 14% of severe reactions present only with respiratory symptoms or only with hypotension [17].
- Anaphylactic and anaphylactoid reactions behave identically clinically and are managed the same way. These reactions should be

considered a medical emergency as failure to initiate prompt treatment can have fatal consequences. Anaphylaxis usually begins 1–45 minutes after starting the transfusion but can occur any time during the transfusion and, in addition to an urticarial rash, presents with hypotension/shock, upper or lower airway obstruction (hoarseness, wheezing, chest pain, stridor, dyspnoea, anxiety, feeling of impending doom), gastrointestinal symptoms and, rarely, death.

Differential Diagnosis

To ensure that appropriate treatment is administered in a timely fashion, patients presenting with systemic symptoms should also be promptly evaluated for the following.

- Other causes of respiratory distress, including circulatory overload, TRALI or any other co-morbid condition such as pulmonary embolism and exacerbations of chronic lung disease.
- Other causes of shock such as acute haemolytic transfusion reactions, sepsis and other co-morbid clinical conditions that can be associated with shock.
- Hypotension with or without cutaneous flushing due to bradykinin (BK) or des-Arg9-BK generation with the use of negatively charged bedside leucocyte reduction filters, or its transient accumulation in platelets during storage. Such hypotensive reactions may occur in a subset of patients being treated with an angiotensin-converting enzyme (ACE) inhibitor or who have inherited decreased ability to metabolise BK or des-Arg9-BK [18]. These reactions have largely disappeared as bedside leucocyte reduction filters are no longer commonly used.

Frequency

It is estimated that about 1% of transfusions are complicated by allergic reactions and that allergic reactions comprise 13–33% of all transfusion reactions. Rates of allergic transfusion reactions vary widely between the studies, depending on product type and preparation. In a review of the studies done between 1990 and 2005 [15]:

- allergic reactions associated with packed red cell transfusions were reported to range from 0.03% to 0.61% with a median of 0.15% (one reaction per 667 transfusions)
- allergic reactions associated with platelet transfusions occurred at a higher rate, ranging from 0.09% to 21% with a median of 3.7% (one reaction per 27 transfusions)
- the frequency of allergic reactions associated with the transfusion of plasma was lower than platelets but more common than reactions to red cells.

True anaphylaxis is a systemic reaction caused by antigen-specific cross linking of IgE molecules on the surface of tissue mast cells and peripheral blood basophils, with immediate release of potent mediators. In contrast, immediate systemic reactions that mimic anaphylaxis but are not caused by an IgE-mediated immune response are termed anaphylactoid reactions. Both anaphylactic and anaphylactoid reactions are severe and life-threatening, but fortunately they are rare and comprise only about 1.3% of all transfusion reactions, affecting 1/20 000–1/47 000 transfusions.

Pathogenesis

Generally, an allergic transfusion reaction is defined as a type I hypersensitivity response mediated by IgE antibodies binding to a soluble allergen and resulting in the activation of mast cells. In these reactions, the allergen is often not known and the actual mechanism continues to remain largely speculative. In contrast, severe reactions that involve anaphylaxis which is not mediated by IgE antibodies but involve IgG anti-IgA are classified as type III reactions. These reactions result in complement activation with subsequent amplified release of anaphylotoxins C3a and C5a, leading to anaphylaxis.

When the aetiology of an allergic reaction is identified, it usually falls into one of the following categories:

- recipient preexisting antibodies to foreign plasma proteins in the blood component
- recipient antibodies against a substance in the blood product that either is lacking or has a distinctly different allelic expression in the patient (i.e. IgA, haptoglobin, C4)
- extraneous substances in the component (i.e. passively transmitted donor IgE antibodies, drugs, other allergens).

For the vast majority of patients, the underlying aetiology is believed to be a recipient preexisting antibody to plasma proteins in the blood component that cannot be specifically identified. Although it is a common approach to look for deficiencies in IgA, haptoglobin or C4, they are not commonly encountered and represent a very small minority of allergic reactions. In some instances, an allergic reaction can be traced back to donor-specific factors, which confers at most a 5% chance of causing an allergic reaction in another recipient; therefore, patient-specific factors are a predominant cause of allergic reactions [19]. Patients with hay fever and food allergies tended to have more allergic reactions, and the severity of reactions tended to be milder in older patients [20].

Management

When there is a suspicion for any transfusion reaction, a general principle of treatment is to discontinue the transfusion immediately and until the patient is clinically assessed. As the signs and symptoms of a transfusion-related allergic reaction are identical to an allergic reaction caused by other allergens, excluding other causes of the reaction, such as concomitantly administered medications, is essential.

- Mild non-systemic allergic transfusion reactions are usually treated with an antihistamine, commonly diphenhydramine 25–50 mg IM or IV in North America and chlorphenamine (Piriton) 10–20 mg IM or IV in the UK. The transfusion can be restarted at a slower rate once symptoms have settled.
- Moderate reactions can also be treated with a dose of corticosteroids and the transfusion of that unit is usually discontinued indefinitely.
- In severe reactions, the unit is never restarted. Anaphylaxis is treated as for any other anaphylactic reaction.
- In addition to discontinuation of the current transfusion, other blood components collected simultaneously from the same donor should be identified and avoided for this patient, particularly apheresis platelets, where two or three doses may have been created from a single collection. However, the likelihood of donor-specific factors triggering an allergic reaction in a different recipient is low relative to patient-specific factors, so it would be considered safe to use other associated blood components from this donor for other patients [19].

The management strategy for severe allergic reactions differs for adults and paediatric patients. For adults/adolescents, immediate administration of adrenaline (epinephrine in the US) 500 μg (0.5 mL of 1:1000 solution) IM is key. Aggressive volume expansion with IV normal saline, oxygen supplementation and antihistamines are also required. If the hypotension is intractable, adrenaline 500 μg (5 mL 1:10000 solution) IV can be given every 5–10 minutes and preparations should be made to transfer the patient to an intensive care unit where an IV drip of inotropic therapy can be maintained. Intubation may be necessary if the airway becomes compromised.

For paediatric patients, the treatment of anaphylaxis should include adrenaline 10 μg/kg 1:1000 concentration IM (e.g. under six months: 50 μg or 0.05 mL of adrenaline 1 in 1000; six months to six years: 120 μg or 0.12 mL; 6–12 years, 250 μg or 0.25 mL) that can be repeated every five minutes (maximum dose 300 μg). A μg/kg dose should be used rather than a mL/kg dose as there are different concentrations of adrenaline. Administration of chlorphenamine (250 μg/kg IV for children one month to less than one year of age; 2.5–5 mg for 1–5 years; 5–10 mg for 6–12 years; 10 mg for over 12 years) or diphenhydramine 1 mg/kg IV/IM in the US and ranitidine 1 mg/kg IV (maximum dose 50 mg) are also effective for supportive management.

Whilst the above drugs are being prepared, the focus should be on resuscitation, including oxygen therapy, suctioning and positioning of patient to open the airway, maintenance of the circulation, oxygen saturation monitoring, establishing an IV if possible and administering a fluid bolus with 20 mL/kg sodium chloride 0.9% if venous access is established. If signs and symptoms persist despite a single IM dose of adrenaline, then a paediatric intensive care specialist should be consulted to provide airway and further haemodynamic support.

Prevention

Premedication with Antipyretics and/or Antihistamines

It has been reported that 50–80% of transfusion recipients in Canada and the US are premedicated. A systematic review of the literature assessing the efficacy of premedication in FNHTRs, including the results of three small prospective randomised controlled trials, found no evidence that premedication prevented non-haemolytic transfusion reactions, including allergic or febrile reactions [21]. A retrospective review of 7900 transfusions in 385 paediatric oncology patients also found no statistically significant difference in allergic transfusion reactions between those who received premedication and those who did not [22]. This study also found that there was no difference in allergic reactions with or without premedication even in those with a previous history of two or more allergic reactions. In addition, allergic reactions were not more common in those with a history of two or more allergic transfusion reactions. It is unclear whether poor timing or underdosing of premedication also contributed to a negligible impact of premedication in these studies.

Although premedication does not appear to affect the incidence of allergic reactions, there have been no studies to date evaluating whether premedication has an effect on the severity of such reactions.

Leucocyte Reduction

Unlike FNHTRs, there is no significant reduction in allergic transfusion reactions with the use of leucocyte-reduced blood products.

Washed Components/Plasma-Reduced Components

Red cells have minimal volumes of residual plasma, and would require washing to further reduce the amount of plasma proteins transfused. Washing was associated with a decrease in allergic reaction rates from 2.7% to 0.3% for red cells [23]. However, washing of red cells may lead to other complications associated with increased red cell fragility, haemolysis and hyperkalaemia in the blood product [24,25]. For apheresis platelets collected and stored in platelet additive solution (PAS), where only 35% of the volume of the product contains plasma, its use was associated with a lowering of allergic reactions from 1.85% to 1.01% compared to conventional apheresis platelets with 100% of the volume containing plasma [26]. A slight decrease in platelet count increment immediately after transfusion was noted with platelets in additive solution, but no difference in platelet count increment was seen at 12–24 hours [26]. Where manual removal of plasma was attempted with more conventional apheresis platelets in older studies, plasma reduction was associated with a lowering of allergic reactions from 5.5% to 1.7%, and was further reduced with washing to 0.5% [23]. Platelet recovery was better with plasma reduction (80.7%) than with washing (70.5%), which was not considered a significant difference. Platelet activation was significantly higher with washing (24.2% increase) than with plasma reduction (10.3% increase). In contrast, plasma reduction only removed 51.1% of plasma proteins versus 96% with washing [27]. With the exclusion of severe or life-threatening allergic reactions which would benefit from washing of cellular products, the use of plasma reduction was sufficient to decrease the number of allergic reactions in 67.4% of patients with clinically significant or multiple urticarial reactions.

The growing availability and use of apheresis platelets suspended in PAS with a consequent reduction in plasma will likely reduce the frequency of allergic transfusion reactions.

IgA-Deficient Blood Components

IgA deficiency is the most common primary immunodeficiency in the Western world, affecting up to one in 20 people. Severe IgA deficiency, defined as IgA <0.05 mg/L, can be associated with anaphylactic reactions to blood components which almost always contain IgA [18]. Patients with anaphylactic transfusion reactions should have further testing using a pretransfusion serum sample to quantify their serum IgA level as well as anti-IgA antibody titres. However, in actual experience, the vast majority of patients with anaphylactic transfusion reactions are not IgA deficient. Furthermore, only a small proportion of those who are IgA deficient have anti-IgA antibodies, of which only a few cases have been documented to have anaphylactic reactions with non-IgA deficient products [28,29]. Despite the frequency of IgA deficiency in the population, the number of fatal or severe anaphylactic reactions that have been attributable to IgA deficiency has been rare to nonexistent in those centres that have studied this rigourously, raising even the question of whether IgA deficiency-related anaphylaxis is an evidence-based reaction category [29].

A common dilemma is whether IgA-containing blood products are safe for a patient who is suspected of having IgA deficiency or a patient who has had an anaphylactic reaction where anti-IgA has not been determined as the cause. Given the near ubiquitous presence of IgA in blood products, a patient with a recent transfusion within the past 24 hours with no reaction has essentially passed an antigen (IgA) stimulus test and therefore is unlikely to have IgA deficiency as their underlying cause of anaphylaxis if it occurs on a subsequent transfusion. If serum IgA is detectable in the patient, anaphylaxis due to IgA

deficiency is very unlikely, though not entirely excluded, with 0.7% of patients with low or normal IgA levels having detectable anti-IgA [28]. Even amongst patients with anti-IgA, only rare cases of associated anaphylaxis were noted [29].

Due to the limited sensitivity of the IgA assay in most hospital laboratories (0.20–50 mg/dL with nephelometry or turbidimetry), additional testing is usually required to identify patients with severe IgA deficiency (less than 0.05 mg/dL) and to test for anti-IgA antibodies. Such testing is performed in a limited number of reference laboratories. Because of the additional time necessary to perform these confirmatory assays, it is most likely that requests for additional transfusions are made prior to availability of results. Given the rarity of this type of transfusion reaction, even amongst patients with known IgA deficiency, withholding transfusions pending the outcome of laboratory testing or the availability of IgA-deficient or washed blood products may cause greater harm than a slower transfusion with careful monitoring, depending on the clinical urgency for transfusion support [30].

If an allergic transfusion reaction secondary to IgA antibodies due to IgA deficiency is confirmed, IgA-deficient or washed products should be given for any future transfusions. Even in such circumstances, when faced with a life-threatening need for transfusion prior to the availability of IgA-deficient products, a slow transfusion with intense monitoring and immediate access to supportive care in the event of a severe reaction may outweigh the risk of anaphylaxis, as recurrence of anaphylaxis due to IgA is not a certainty [31]. Such an approach should be taken with extreme caution and only after a discussion about the risks and benefits of administering an unwashed product to such an individual between the transfusion service and the patient's attending physician. Since anaphylactic transfusion reactions are rare and often not due to IgA deficiency, whilst transfusions are common and often urgent, it is both impractical and not cost-effective to widely screen for IgA deficiency in the pretransfused population.

<table>
<tr><td colspan="2">

KEY POINTS

</td></tr>
<tr><td>

1) Allergic and FNHTRs are the most common transfusion reactions. Anaphylaxis is rare.
2) Mild allergic reactions usually only require antihistamine treatment and the transfusion can be continued unless systemic symptoms develop.
3) Mild FNHTRs usually respond to the administration of an antipyretic.
4) If a moderate to severe transfusion reaction is suspected, the transfusion must be stopped until the patient is assessed and possible causes of the reaction are investigated.
5) Systemic symptoms warrant prompt clinical

</td><td>

assessment as treatment can vary widely between diagnoses and, in particular, failure to administer adrenaline (epinephrine) in anaphylactic reactions can be fatal.
6) As the signs and symptoms of FNHTR and allergic reactions can be mimicked by a variety of other causes, the patient's underlying disease state and any other co-administered medications should be considered in the differential diagnosis. As there is usually no definitive test to determine the aetiology of these reactions, they are generally diagnosed by exclusion.

</td></tr>
</table>

References

1 Heddle NM, Klama LN, Griffith L, Roberts R, Shukla G, Kelton JG. A prospective study to identify the risk factors associated with acute reactions to platelet and red cell transfusions. Transfusion 1993;**33**:794–7.

2 ISBT Working Party on Haemovigilance. Proposed Standard Definitions for Surveillance of Non-Infectious Adverse Transfusion Reactions. Available at: www.isbtweb.org/fileadmin/user_upload/Proposed_definitions_2011_surveillance_non_infectious_adverse_reactions_haemovigilance_incl_TRALI_correction_2013.pdf (accessed 9 November 2016).

3 National Healthcare Safety Network. Biovigilance Component: Hemovigilance Module Surveillance Protocol. Available at: www.cdc.gov/nhsn/pdfs/biovigilance/bv-hv-protocol-current.pdf (accessed 9 November 2016).

4 Gehrie EA, Hendrickson JE, Tormey CA. Variation in vital signs resulting from blood component administration in adults. Transfusion 2015;**55**:1866–71.

5 Andrzejewski C, Popovsky MA, Stec TC et al. Hemotherapy bedside biovigilance involving vital sign values and characteristics of patients with suspected transfusion reactions associated with fluid challenges: can some

cases of transfusion-associated circulatory overload have proinflammatory aspects? Transfusion 2012;**52**:2310–20.

6 Yazer MH, Triulzi DJ, Shaz B, Kraus T, Zimring JC. Does a febrile reaction to platelets predispose recipients to red blood cell alloimmunization? Transfusion 2009;**49**:1070–5.

7 Heddle NM, Weibert KE. Febrile non hemolytic transfusion reactions, in Transfusion Reactions, 4th edn (ed. M Popovsky), AABB Press, Bethesda, 2012, pp.53–97.

8 Paglino JC, Pomper GJ, Fisch GS, Champion MH, Snyder EL. Reduction of febrile but not allergic reactions to RBCs and platelets after conversion to universal prestorage leukoreduction. Transfusion 2004;**44**:16–24.

9 Gauvin F, Lacroix J, Robillard P, Lapointe H, Hume H. Acute transfusion reactions in the pediatric intensive care unit. Transfusion 2006;**46**:1899–908.

10 Oakley FD, Woods M, Arnold S, Young, PP. Transfusion reactions in pediatric compared with adult patients: a look at rate, reaction type, and associated products. Transfusion 2015;**55**:563–70.

11 Yazer MH, Raval JS, Triulzi DJ, Blumberg N. ABO-mismatched transfusions are not

over-represented in febrile non-haemolytic reactions to platelets. Vox Sang 2012;**102**:175–7.

12 Heddle NM, Klama L, Singer J, Richards C, Fedak P, Walker I, Kelton JG. The role of the plasma from platelet concentrates in transfusion reactions. N Engl J Med 1994;**331**:625–8.

13 Blumberg N, Gettings KF, Turner C, Heal JM, Phipps RP. An association of soluble CD40 ligand (CD154) with adverse reactions to platelet transfusions. Transfusion 2006;**46**:1813–21.

14 Addas-Carvalho M, Salles TS, Saad ST. The association of cytokine gene polymorphisms with febrile non-hemolytic transfusion reaction in multitransfused patients. Transfus Med 2006;**16**:184–91.

15 Geiger TL, Howard SC. Acetaminophen and diphenhydramine premedication for allergic and febrile nonhemolytic transfusion reactions: good prophylaxis or bad practice? Transfus Med Rev 2007;**21**:1–12.

16 Tobian AA, King KE, Ness PM. Transfusion premedications: a growing practice not based on evidence. Transfusion 2007;**47**:1089–96.

17 Domen RE, Hoeltge GA. Allergic transfusion reactions. An evaluation of 273 consecutive patients. Arch Pathol Lab Med 2003;**127**:316–20.

18 Eastlund T. Vasoactive mediators and hypotensive transfusion reactions. Transfusion 2007;**47**:369–72.

19 Savage WJ, Tobian AA, Fuller AK, Wood RA, King KE, Ness PM. Allergic transfusion reactions to platelets are associated more with recipient and donor factors than with product attributes. Transfusion 2011;**51**:1716–22.

20 Savage WJ, Hamilton RG, Tobian AA, Milne GL, Kaufman RM. Defining risk factors and presentations of allergic reactions to platelet transfusion. J Allergy Clin Immunol 2014;**133**:1772–5.

21 Martí-Carvajal AJ, Solà I, González LE, Leon de Gonzalez G, Rodriguez-Malagon N. Pharmacological interventions for the prevention of allergic and febrile non-haemolytic transfusion reactions. Cochrane Database Syst Rev 2010;**6**:CD007539.

22 Sanders RP, Maddirala SD, Geiger TL et al. Premedication with acetaminophen or diphenhydramine for transfusion with leukoreduced blood products in children. Br J Haematol 2005;**130**:781–7.

23 Tobian AA, Savage WJ, Tisch DJ, Thoman S, King KE, Ness PM. Prevention of allergic transfusion reactions to platelets and red blood cells through plasma reduction. Transfusion 2011;**51**:1676–83.

24 O'Leary MF, Szklarski P, Klein TM, Young PP. Hemolysis of red blood cells after cell washing with different automated technologies: clinical implications in a neonatal cardiac surgery population. Transfusion 2011;**51**:955–60.

25 Harm SK, Raval JS, Cramer J, Waters JH, Yazer MH. Haemolysis and sublethal injury of RBCs after routine blood bank manipulations. Transfus Med 2012;**22**:181–5.

26 Tobian AA, Fuller AK, Uglik K et al. The impact of platelet additive solution apheresis platelets on allergic transfusion reactions and corrected count increment. Transfusion 2014;**54**:1523–9.

27 Veeraputhiran M, Ware J, Dent J et al. A comparison of washed and volume-reduced platelets with respect to platelet activation, aggregation, and plasma protein removal. Transfusion 2011;**51**:1030–6.

28 Vassallo RR. Review: IgA anaphylactic transfusion reactions. Part I. Laboratory diagnosis, incidence, and supply of IgA-deficient products. Immunohematology 2004;**20**:226–33.

29 Sandler SG, Eder AF, Goldman M, Winters JL. The entity of immunoglobulin A-related anaphylactic transfusion reactions is not evidence based. Transfusion 2015;**55**:199–204.

30 Sandler SG, Zantek ND. Review: IgA anaphylactic transfusion reactions. Part II. Clinical diagnosis and bedside management. Immunohematology 2004;**20**:234–9.

31 Sandler SG. How I manage patients suspected of having had an IgA anaphylactic transfusion reaction. Transfusion 2006;**46**:10–13.

10 Lung Injury and Pulmonary Oedema After Transfusion

Steven H. Kleinman[1] and Daryl J. Kor[2]

[1] *University of British Columbia, Victoria, Canada*
[2] *Mayo Clinic, Rochester, USA*

Definition

The clinical syndrome of transfusion-related acute lung injury (TRALI) is characterised by the acute onset of respiratory distress during or within six hours of transfusion, associated with oxygen desaturation (hypoxaemia) and bilateral lung infiltrates, without evidence for left atrial hypertension or circulatory overload [1].

Incidence, Outcomes and Recipient Risk Factors

Because TRALI is under-recognised and under-reported, it is clear that the most accurate data on TRALI incidence rates come from research studies that use an active surveillance mechanism to detect cases [2–4]. Using this approach, an overall risk of 1:5000 transfused units in the general hospital population was reported in 1985 and this incidence number is frequently cited in the literature [2]. More recently, risk mitigation methods have resulted in a decreased incidence of TRALI. A recent case–control study, which used computer-generated automatic alerts to detect respiratory distress after transfusion, reported a TRALI incidence of 1 in 12 000 units following risk mitigation procedures for transfused plasma components [4]. TRALI incidence

in critically ill patients is higher than that in the general hospital population [5,6].

Haemovigilance (HV) data are informative with regard to the clinical significance of TRALI. In the USA, TRALI was the number one cause of transfusion-associated fatalities reported to the Food and Drug Administration (FDA) from 2010 to 2014; this has not changed in the last decade [7].

Pulmonary infiltrates are thought to resolve in the majority of TRALI patients within 96 hours. Mortality is approximately 10–15%. Those who recover generally do not have any chronic sequelae.

Most cases occur in adults, but children also acquire TRALI at similar rates [8]. Previous transfusion history is unremarkable and recurrent TRALI is extremely rare. At least one case of TRALI from an autologous transfusion has been recorded. Directed donations from mother to child can cause TRALI due to maternal leucocyte antibodies against the child's leucocyte antigens.

Risk factors related to coexisting recipient medical conditions have been identified. In a case–control study of 89 TRALI cases at UCSF and Mayo Clinic, investigators identified a number of recipient risk factors for TRALI (Table 10.1) [4]. These are similar to risk factors identified in other studies [5].

Practical Transfusion Medicine, Fifth Edition. Edited by Michael F. Murphy, David J. Roberts and Mark H. Yazer.
© 2017 John Wiley & Sons Ltd. Published 2017 by John Wiley & Sons Ltd.

Table 10.1 Recipient risk factors for transfusion-related acute lung injury.

Social history	Acute conditions	Procedural factors
Chronic alcohol abuse	Preexisting shock	Liver surgery[†]
Current cigarette use	Positive fluid balance	
	High peak airway pressures*	

*Greater than $30\,cmH_2O$ if mechanically ventilated before transfusion.
[†]Primarily liver transplantation.

Clinical Manifestations

The onset of TRALI is often quite dramatic, with symptoms starting either during the transfusion or within two hours of its completion in the majority of cases. The syndrome manifests as acute respiratory distress due to non-cardiogenic (inflammatory) pulmonary oedema, and is characterised by acute onset of dyspnoea, tachypnoea and oxygen desaturation. The patient may appear cyanotic and may develop hypotension. Oxygen desaturation is often severe, requiring mechanical ventilation in 70% of cases. Patients with TRALI may experience a low-grade fever for several hours. Symptoms and signs may be muted in patients under general anaesthesia. In such cases, the first indication of TRALI might be the appearance of copious amounts of pink frothy sputum from the endotracheal tube, although this finding is not specific for TRALI.

Auscultation of the lungs will detect the presence of bilateral rales or crackles. Hypoxaemia, defined as $PaO_2/FiO_2 < 300\,mmHg$ or oxygen saturation of <90% on room air by pulse oximetry, and the development of new bilateral lung infiltrates on chest radiography are essential in making a diagnosis of TRALI [1]. Chest radiography may show 'white-out', a radiographic finding in which both lungs show uniform white opacities throughout. More commonly, pulmonary infiltrates are located peripherally, especially in the lower lung fields (Figure 10.1). Because some patients with TRALI have acute transient leucopoenia (neutropenia) around the time of symptom onset, a complete blood count with a white cell count differential can be a useful adjunct test.

Although some investigators have reported that TRALI can rarely have a delayed onset (>6 hours post transfusion), HV systems do not currently classify such cases as TRALI.

Differential Diagnosis

The diagnosis of TRALI remains difficult because patients who experience severe respiratory distress during or after transfusion are often quite ill, have multiple other morbidities, may have preexisting cardiac or pulmonary compromise and could be suffering from conditions known to cause the acute respiratory distress syndrome (ARDS) (Table 10.2). ARDS due to other causes is common in critically ill patients independent of transfusion; however, its frequency is increased in transfused patients (up to 40–45% in some studies) and shows a dose–response relationship [9]. This highlights the difficulty in determining whether ARDS following transfusion in patients with predisposing ARDS risk factors is indeed TRALI or is instead due to other aetiologies.

It is worth noting that the term acute lung injury (ALI) is no longer used by pulmonary and critical care specialists outside the transfusion context. In 2012, a consensus conference recommended that less severe cases of ARDS with PaO_2/FiO_2 ranging from 200 to 300 mmHg, previously termed ALI, should rather be referred to as ARDS and subcategorised into a severity class of mild [10].

In light of these issues, clinical evaluation of potential TRALI cases should include an investigation of other causes of ARDS (see Table 10.2). In any given patient, the presence of one or more of these factors makes the diagnosis of TRALI quite difficult. In 2004, a consensus

(a)

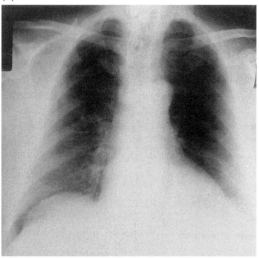

(b)

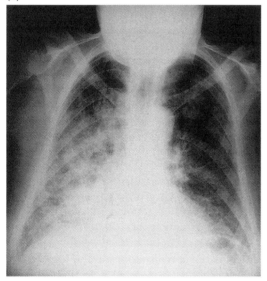

Figure 10.1 Chest x-rays of a patient with transfusion-related acute lung injury. (a) One day before a platelet transfusion and (b) shortly after transfusion showing diffuse bilateral shadowing of the lungs and a normal-sized heart. *Source:* Reproduced with permission of BMJ Publishing Group Ltd. Lesson of the week: acute non-cardiogenic lung oedema after platelet transfusion. BMJ 1997;**314**:880.

Table 10.2 Major risk factors for acute respiratory distress syndrome.

Direct lung injury	Indirect lung injury
Pneumonia	Severe sepsis
Aspiration	Shock
Lung contusion	Acute pancreatitis
Toxic inhalation	Multiple trauma
Near drowning	Severe burn
	Drug overdose
	Cardiopulmonary bypass

conference recommended that ARDS occurring within six hours of transfusion in a patient with other ARDS risk factors be designated as 'possible TRALI'. More recently, an alternative terminology of 'transfused ARDS' has been proposed [1,11]. This latter term better reflects data showing that, as a group, patients with this diagnosis have a clinical course more similar to patients with non-transfusion-related ARDS than to patients with TRALI [11]. However, in any given case, it is often extremely difficult to determine whether it was the transfusion or the alternate risk factor that caused the ARDS [11,12].

A second syndrome in the differential diagnosis of TRALI is transfusion-associated circulatory overload (TACO), which similarly results in hypoxaemic respiratory insufficiency and manifests with pulmonary oedema. However, in contrast to TRALI, the pulmonary oedema in TACO arises due to elevated pulmonary vascular pressures and is therefore hydrostatic in nature rather than inflammatory. In line with its underlying pathophysiology, TACO characteristically arises in the setting of one or more features suggestive of fluid overload or congestive heart failure. Frequently, risk factors for both TRALI and TACO are present and, to further complicate matters, there has been an increased recognition that both TRALI and TACO may coexist as contributors to posttransfusion pulmonary oedema, further challenging the specific diagnosis underlying posttransfusion hypoxaemic respiratory insufficiency [13].

There is no single finding that specifically differentiates TRALI from TACO. The lack of certain clinical findings and the presence of others may help in the differential diagnosis (Table 10.3) [4,12]. It has been reported that a 50% elevation of B-type natriuretic peptide (BNP) in a posttransfusion versus a pretransfusion sample supports a TACO diagnosis whilst a BNP level of <200 pg/mL measured immediately after the onset of acute pulmonary oedema supports the diagnosis of TRALI. In critical care patients, BNP or N-terminal-BNP levels may be higher in patients who develop TACO compared to those who develop TRALI; however, there is some concern that these analytes have limited diagnostic value due to a large overlap amongst the observed values in these patient groups [11,14].

In addition to ARDS and TACO, other conditions that can mimic TRALI include anaphylactic transfusion reactions and sepsis from transfusion of bacterially contaminated blood components. Bronchospasm, wheezing, localised or generalised skin rash and hypotension or shock favour a diagnosis of anaphylactic reaction. High fever, chills, rigour, shock, disseminated intravascular coagulation, a positive Gram stain and culture from the transfused blood component and positive blood cultures from the recipient support a diagnosis of transfusion-transmitted bacterial sepsis. Finally, a low-grade fever seen in TRALI must be differentiated from a haemolytic transfusion reaction. A clerical check of the transfusion episode showing the

Table 10.3 Conditions to be considered when attempting to differentiate TRALI from TACO.*

Feature	TRALI	TACO
Fluid overload/CHF		
Echocardiography	LVEF >40%, E/e' <15	LVEF <40%; E/e' >15
PCWP	<18 mmHg	>18 mmHg
Neck veins	Normal	Distended
Chest exam	Rales, no S3	Rales, S3
Chest radiograph	VPW <65 mm; CTR <0.55	VPW >65 mm; CTR >0.55; pleural effusion
Fluid balance	Neutral	Positive
Weight	Neutral	Increased
BNP	<200 pg/mL	>1200 pg/mL; increase in BNP >1.5 × pre-transfusion value
Diuretic response	Inconsistent	Significant improvement
Blood pressure	Hypotension	Hypertension
Inflammatory markers		
Temperature	Febrile	Unchanged
WBC	Transient leucopenia	Unchanged

*These conditions can be used to help differentiate TRALI from TACO, but none is pathognomonic for either syndrome. BNP, brain natriuretic peptide; CHF, congestive heart failure; CTR, cardiothoracic ratio; E/e', early mitral valve inflow velocity/diastolic mitral annular tissue Doppler velocity; Hg, mercury; LVEF, left ventricular ejection fraction; PCWP, pulmonary capillary wedge pressure; pg, pictogram; TACO, transfusion-associated circulatory overload; TRALI, transfusion-related acute lung injury; VPW, vascular pedicle width; WBC, white blood cell.

lack of any error, plus an absence of visual hae-molysis in the posttransfusion serum or plasma and a negative direct antiglobulin test, suggest that a haemolytic transfusion reaction is unlikely.

The term 'transfusion-associated dyspnoea' (TAD) has been endorsed for use in HV systems; it designates cases of posttransfusion dyspnoea that do not fit into any of the known pulmonary transfusion reaction categories. Such cases appear to be nonspecific and may be characterised either by less severe pulmonary compromise or by delayed onset falling outside the six-hour interval that defines TRALI or TACO; they should not be classified as mild or delayed TRALI as there are no standard definitions for these conditions.

Pathogenesis

It is generally accepted that TRALI occurs via a two-hit mechanism [15]. The first hit involves neutrophil sequestration and priming in the lung microvasculature due to recipient factors that cause endothelial injury. When neutrophils are primed, they react to a weaker signal than if unprimed. Endothelial cells are thought to be responsible for both the neutrophil sequestration (through adhesion molecules) and priming (through cytokine release). The second hit is activation of recipient neutrophils by substances in the transfused blood product. This may be due to donor antileucocyte antibodies via a mechanism that has been termed immune or antibody-mediated TRALI. The antibodies may be directed against cognate HLA or HNA (human neutrophil) antigens (i.e. a corresponding matching antigen) on recipient neutrophils, pulmonary endothelial cells or monocytes. The latter occurs with HLA class II antibodies binding to cognate antigens on monocytes, causing release of cytokines that in turn activate primed neutrophils. The second hit may also result from other soluble factors, collectively termed biological response modifiers (BRMs); potential BRMs from stored blood components include lysophosphatidylcholines, lipopolysaccharides

(neutral lipids), cytokines (interleukin (IL)-6 and IL-8), secretory phospholipase2 (sPLA2) and soluble CD40 ligand [16]. Laboratory tests to measure these bioactive substances are not widely available. TRALI resulting from these non-antibody BRMs is sometimes referred to as non-immune TRALI.

Regardless of the second hit, neutrophil activation is associated with the release from neutrophils of cytokines, reactive oxygen species, oxidases and proteases that damage the pulmonary capillary endothelium. This damage causes increased vascular permeability and results in non-hydrostatic (inflammatory) pulmonary oedema.

The two-hit theory is supported by animal experimental evidence as well as retrospective clinical studies demonstrating that most transfused blood products containing HLA antibody do not cause TRALI, even if a cognate recipient antigen is present. A modification of this theory, referred to as the threshold model, allows for the possibility that in some cases the second hit is so strong (i.e. a high-titre HLA antibody) that an initial priming event is not required and TRALI can occur even in the absence of a priming factor. This theory explains TRALI cases that have occurred in otherwise healthy individuals who have received fresh frozen plasma (FFP) as a treatment for reversing warfarin anticoagulation [8].

In older case series, 80–85% of TRALI cases were caused by the antibody mechanism and it appears that such cases are of greater clinical severity than non-immune cases and more often require mechanical ventilation [17]. The proportion of TRALI caused by antibodies versus BRMs varies by the type of component transfused, with antibody-mediated mechanisms explaining the majority of cases due to plasma and non-immune BRMs responsible for most cases from red blood cell (RBC) transfusion. Thus, in the current era of TRALI risk mitigation strategies for plasma, it is likely that the percentage of immune TRALI is lower. Implicated antibodies include HLA class I antibodies, HLA class II antibodies (directed mostly against DR antigens) and HNA antibodies. For HLA class II antibodies, the total amount of transfused antibody (a product of transfused plasma volume and antibody titre) has been demonstrated to be associated with TRALI risk [4]. Involved donors can have multiple antibody specificities against cognate antigens in the recipient and these may pose a greater risk of TRALI than does a single cognate antibody [18]. HNA-3a antibodies are important to detect as these have been associated with a substantial number of severe or fatal cases [19]. Currently, neutrophil antibody detection assays are not widely available and are just beginning to become automated. Furthermore, current automated systems have difficulty in detecting anti-HNA-3a; these antibodies may be missed unless a leucoagglutination assay or an enhanced immunofluorescence assay is used.

Lung Histology

Fatal cases of TRALI show massive alveolar oedema on histological examination (Figure 10.2) [20]. Alveolar–capillary membrane disruption is widespread with hyaline membrane formation. Interstitium and alveoli are infiltrated with inflammatory cells consisting of neutrophils and macrophages. The diffuse alveolar damage resembles findings seen in ARDS from other causes.

(a)

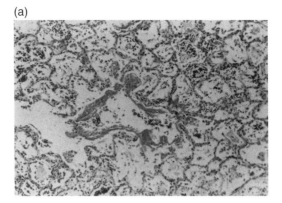

(b)

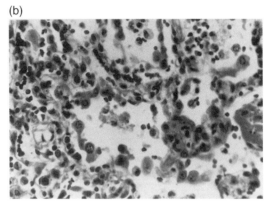

Figure 10.2 Thin sections of fixed lung from a patient with transfusion-related acute lung injury. There is acute diffuse alveolar damage with intra-alveolar oedema and haemorrhage. There was no histological evidence of infection and all postmortem cultures (bacterial, viral and fungal) were negative. Magnification: (a) ×40, (b) ×440. *Source:* Silliman et al. 1997 [20]. Reproduced with permission of John Wiley and Sons.

Types of Blood Components That Can Cause TRALI

Transfusion-related acute lung injury has been caused by many types of blood components, including red cell concentrates (even those that are leucoreduced), plasma, platelet concentrates, platelets collected by apheresis (AP) and, rarely, intravenous immunoglobulin. The length of RBC storage does not appear to influence the risk of TRALI occurrence and this is also likely the case for platelets. Plasma treated by the solvent–detergent (SD) method, manufactured

by pooling a large number of plasma units and thus diluting the leucocyte antibodies contained in donor blood, does not cause TRALI [21] and its use has been adopted as a prevention strategy in some European countries.

Plasma-rich components (e.g. plasma transfusions, AP and platelet concentrates collected by the buffy coat method, which are resuspended in a large amount of plasma from one of the platelet donors) pose a greater per unit risk than plasma-poor components (e.g. red cell concentrates). This has resulted in the implementation of policies to mitigate risk from some plasma-rich components. Due to the success of these measures, the relative percentage of TRALI cases from red cells has increased and the majority of current TRALI cases are associated with red cell transfusion.

Mitigation Strategies

When a suspected TRALI case is reported to the transfusion service, the medical director determines if the case meets the diagnostic clinical criteria for TRALI. If so, the case should be reported to the blood centre so that a donor investigation is conducted; this investigation includes testing of associated donors for HLA and possibly HNA antibodies [1]. Some laboratories in Europe also perform leucocyte crossmatching as part of the evaluation.

An 'implicated donor' is defined as one who has leucocyte antibodies that correspond to the recipient's antigen/s or a donor whose serum is reactive against the recipient's leucocytes in a crossmatch test; this is strong evidence of antibody-mediated TRALI once the clinical diagnosis of TRALI has been made. If an implicated donor is identified, that donor should be deferred, at a minimum, from future plasma apheresis or platelet apheresis donation. Furthermore, most blood transfusion laboratories will also defer an implicated donor from whole blood donation; this is particularly true if the donor has anti-HNA-3a. It remains uncertain whether the donor should be deferred if he or she has leucocyte antibodies but cognate antigens are not present in the recipient or if the crossmatch test is negative [1].

Leucocyte antibodies are much more common in ever pregnant females compared to never pregnant females or males due to maternal exposure to fetal leucocyte antigens. In 2003, this led the UK to initiate a policy of obtaining transfusable plasma units predominantly from male donors, thereby avoiding the transfusion of plasma units from female donors. With this intervention, TRALI cases from FFP transfusion reported to the UK Serious Hazards of Transfusion HV system decreased from 14 cases in 2003 to one case in 2005. Overall, 36 cases of TRALI were reported in 2003, but only 15 cases were reported in 2010 [22]. These data led to widespread international adoption of a stringent policy of not transfusing plasma from ever pregnant females. Data from multiple studies using this intervention have been aggregated in a recent meta-analysis and in a second systematic review. Both publications reported a significant reduction in TRALI risk from plasma products after the adoption of risk reduction measures (odds ratios (95% confidence interval) of 0.62 (0.42–0.92) and 0.27 (0.20–0.38) in the two analyses) [23,24].

This policy is feasible for plasma transfusion because the number of plasma units exceeds demand, except for Group AB plasma. In this latter case, plasma from nulliparous female donors is preferred to plasma from multiparous donors. However, this policy is not feasible for AP where restriction of units to male donors would seriously jeopardise the platelet supply. With regard to AP, it is becoming more common to test previously pregnant donors for HLA antibodies and then to redirect antibody-positive donors away from all high plasma volume donations, including platelet or plasma apheresis. At present, techniques for neutrophil antibody identification are cumbersome and have not been widely applied in screening. For non-antibody-mediated TRALI, no preventive steps have been recommended or undertaken.

Patient Management

If TRALI is suspected, the transfusion should be stopped and the case reported to the transfusion service. Patient management is supportive as there are no specific therapeutic interventions. TRALI is often severe and virtually all patients will require some form of oxygen supplementation to maintain acceptable oxygen saturations. Contemporary evidence suggests that assisted mechanical ventilation with or without intubation will be required in two-thirds or more of the cases [5]. When mechanical ventilation is required, lung-protective strategies with low tidal volume ventilation (<6 mL/kg of ideal bodyweight) and limited plateau airway pressures (<30 cmH$_2$O) should be ensured [25]. No definitive guidance can be provided regarding optimal positive end-expiratory pressure settings. At present, there is no convincing evidence to support the use of corticosteroids. Fluid resuscitation may be required when hypotension or shock are present. However, diuretic therapy may be indicated if hypoxaemia is severe, the blood pressure is stable, and if an element of congestive heart failure or circulatory overload cannot be

excluded. Further transfusions, if needed, do not require any other special precautions since recurrent TRALI is extremely rare.

For all suspected cases of TRALI, clinicians should obtain a chest radiograph and a blood sample that can be used for HLA phenotyping at a later time. The latter may also be used for bacterial testing if a septic transfusion reaction is under consideration. Patient testing for leucocyte antibody may be considered provided a sample has been saved, but this is not needed if only leucocyte-reduced components have been transfused. Pre- and posttransfusion BNP or NT-BNP levels are of unclear utility when attempting to specifically distinguish TRALI from TACO.

KEY POINTS

1) TRALI manifests as ARDS or non-cardiogenic pulmonary oedema during or within six hours of transfusion.
2) TRALI is a leading cause of death from transfusion.
3) Fatality occurs in 10–15% of diagnosed cases but those who recover generally show no long-term respiratory sequelae.
4) TRALI occurrence is influenced by recipient risk factors which include chronic alcohol abuse, current cigarette use, preexisting shock, positive fluid balance, peak airway pressure greater than 30 cmH$_2$O if mechanically ventilated before transfusion, liver surgery (mainly transplantation) and elevated pre-transfusion levels of interleukin-8.
5) Substances in blood components responsible for the syndrome include leucocyte antibodies (HLA and neutrophil-specific) and biological

response modifiers that act as neutrophil priming agents.
6) When TRALI is suspected, the transfusion should be stopped and the case reported to the blood transfusion laboratory.
7) Treatment is supportive and often requires mechanical ventilation.
8) TRALI is difficult to distinguish from TACO. Underlying cardiac dysfunction or evidence of fluid overload may suggest TACO.
9) Preventive measures include exclusion of blood donors implicated in TRALI cases and reducing transfusions of high plasma volume blood components from donors likely to possess leucocyte antibodies.
10) TRALI incidence has decreased due to minimising (or eliminating) transfusion of plasma manufactured from donations by ever pregnant female donors.

References

1 Kleinman S, Caufield T, Chan P et al. Toward an understanding of transfusion-related acute lung injury: statement of a consensus panel. Transfusion 2004;**44**:1774–89.

2 Popovsky MA, Moore SB. Diagnostic and pathogenetic considerations in transfusion-related acute lung injury. Transfusion 1985;**25**:573–7.

3 Clifford L, Singh A, Wilson G et al. Electronic health record surveillance algorithms facilitate the detection of transfusion-related pulmonary complications. Transfusion 2013;**53**(6):1205–16.

4 Toy P, Gajic O, Bacchetti P et al. Transfusion related acute lung injury: incidence and risk factors. Blood 2012;**119**:1757–67.

5 Vlaar APJ, Binnekade JM., Prins D et al. Risk factors and outcome of transfusion-related acute lung injury in the critically ill: a nested case–control study. Crit Care Med 2010;**38**(3):771–8.

6 Gajic O, Rana R, Winters JL et al. Transfusion-related acute lung injury in the critically ill: prospective nested case-control study. Am J Respir Crit Care Med 2007;**176**:886–91.

7 Fatalities Reported to FDA Following Blood Collection and Transfusion: Annual Summary for Fiscal Year 2014. Available at: www.fda.gov/downloads/BiologicsBloodVaccines/SafetyAvailability/ReportaProblem/TransfusionDonationFatalities/UCM459461.pdf (accessed 10 November 2016).

8 Leiberman L, Petrasko T, Yi QL et al. Transfusion-related lung injury in children: a case series and review of the literature. Transfusion 2014;**54**:57–64.

9 Silverboard H, Aisiku I, Martin G et al. The role of acute blood transfusion in the development of acute respiratory distress syndrome among the critically ill: a cohort study. J Trauma 2005;**59**:717–23.

10 Ranieri VM, Rubenfeld GD, Thompson BT et al. Acute respiratory distress syndrome: the Berlin Definition. JAMA 2012;**307**:2526–33.

11 Looney MR, Roubinian N, Gajic O et al. Prospective study in the clinical course and outcomes in transfusion-related acute lung injury. Crit Care Med 2014;**42**:1676–87.

12 Skeate RC, Eastlund T. Distinguishing between transfusion related acute lung injury and transfusion associated circulatory overload. Curr Opin Hematol 2007;**14**:682–7.

13 Wheeler AP, Bernard GR, Thompson BT. Pulmonary-artery versus central venous catheter to guide treatment of acute lung injury. N Engl J Med 2006;**354**:2213–24.

14 Li G, Daniels CE, Kojicic T et al. The accuracy of natriuretic peptides (brain natriuretic peptide and N-terminal pro-brain natriuretic) in the differentiation between transfusion-related acute lung injury and transfusion-related circulatory overload in the critically ill. Transfusion 2009;**49**:13–20.

15 Bux J, Sachs UJH. The pathogenesis of transfusion-related acute lung injury (TRALI). Br J Haematol 2007;**136**:788–99.

16 Silliman CC, Moor EE, Kehler MR et al. Identification of lipids that accumulate during routine storage of prestorage leukoreduced red blood cells and cause acute lung injury. Transfusion 2011;**51**:2549–54.

17 Middelburg RA, van Stein D, Briet E et al. The role of donor antibodies in the pathogenesis of transfusion-related acute lung injury: a systematic review. Transfusion 2008;**48**:2167–76.

18 Hashimoto S, Nakajima F, Kamada H et al. Relationship of donor HLA antibody strength to the development of transfusion-related acute lung injury. Transfusion 2010;**50**:2582–91.

19 Reil A, Keeler-Stanislawski B, Geuerney S et al. Specificities of leukocyte alloantibodies in transfusion-related acute lung injury and results of leukocyte antibody screening of blood donors. Vox Sang 2008;**95**:313–17.

20 Silliman CC, Paterson AJ, Dickey W et al. The association of biologically active lipids with the development of transfusion-related acute lung injury. Transfusion 1997;**37**:719–26.

21 Sachs UJH, Kauschat D, Bein G. White-blood cell reactive antibodies are undetectable in solvent/detergent plasma. Transfusion 2005;**45**:1628–31.

22 Knowles S, Cohen H, on behalf of the Serious Hazards of Transfusion (SHOT) Steering Group. The 2010 Annual SHOT Report (2011). Available at: www.shotuk.org/wp-content/uploads/2011/07/SHOT-2010-Report.pdf (accessed 10 November 2016).

23 Muller MCA, van Stein D, Binnekade JM et al. Low risk transfusion-related acute lung injury donor strategies and the impact on the onset of transfusion-related acute lung injury: a meta-analysis. Transfusion 2015;**55**:164–75.

24 Schnickl CN, Mastrobuoin S, Filippidis FT. Male-predominant plasma transfusion strategy for preventing transfusion-associated acute lung injury: a systematic review. Crit Care Med 2015;**43**(1):205–25.

25 Serpa Neto A, Cardoso SO, Manetta JA et al. Association between use of lung-protective ventilation with lower tidal volumes and clinical outcomes among patients without acute respiratory distress syndrome: a meta-analysis. JAMA 2012;**308**:1651–9.

Further Reading

Aubuchon JP. TRALI: reducing its risks while trying to understand its causes. Transfusion 2014;**54**:3021–5.

Bux J. Antibody-mediated (immune) transfusion-related acute lung injury. Vox Sang 2011;**100**:122–8.

Kleinman S, Caulfield T, Chan P et al. Toward an understanding of transfusion-related acute lung injury: statement of a consensus panel. Transfusion 2004;**44**:1774–89.

Muller MCA, van Stein D, Binnekade JM et al. Low risk transfusion-related acute lung injury donor strategies and the impact on the onset of transfusion-related acute lung injury: a meta-analysis. Transfusion 2015;**55**:164–75.

Popovsky MA. Transfusion-related acute lung injury: three decades of progress but miles to go before we sleep. Transfusion 2015;**55**:930–4.

Sachs UJ. Recent insights into the mechanism of transfusion-related acute lung injury. Curr Opin Hematol 2011;**18**:436.

Silliman CC, Fung YL, Ball JB, Khan SY. Transfusion-related acute lung injury (TRALI): current concepts and misconceptions. Blood Rev 2009;**23**:245.

Su L, Kamel H. How do we investigate and manage donors associated with a suspected case of transfusion-related acute lung injury. Transfusion 2007;**47**:1118.

Toy P, Gajic O, Bacchetti P et al. Transfusion-related acute lung injury: incidence and risk factors. Blood 2012;**119**:1757–67.

Vlaar APJ, Jeffermans NP. Transfusion-related acute lung injury: a clinical review. Lancet 2013;**382**:984–94.

11 Purported Adverse Effects of 'Old Blood'

Lirong Qu[1,2] and Darrell J. Triulzi[1,2]

[1] Department of Pathology, University of Pittsburgh, Pittsburgh, USA
[2] Institute for Transfusion Medicine, Pittsburgh, USA

Introduction

During red blood cell storage, well-characterised structural, biochemical and physiological changes occur over time. Although these changes have been well documented and demonstrated *in vitro*, their clinical effects on transfusion recipients remain unclear. In the United States, the mean storage duration for a unit of red cells at transfusion was 17.9 days, according to a survey conducted in part by the US Department of Health and Human Services [1]. The maximum allowable storage duration for red cells is defined by the US Food and Drug Administration (FDA) and depends on the storage media. The most common additive solutions used in the US (AS-1, AS-3, AS-5) allow for storage up to 42 days at 1–6 °C. Until recently, reports of clinical effects of red cell storage duration in the literature have been mainly from retrospective observational studies. The conclusions from these observational studies have been conflicting, possibly because of the methodological limitations. Newly published data from randomised controlled trials (RCTs) in neonates, critically ill patients and patients undergoing cardiac surgery and general hospitalized patients suggest that the duration of red cell storage is not associated with adverse clinical outcomes in these patient populations.

In Vitro Changes During Red Cell Storage

The limit of 42 days as the maximum 'shelf life' for red cell units stored in additive solution is based on the degree of haemolysis (<1%) at the end of storage and the percentage (minimum of 75%) of the red cells remaining in the circulation 24 hours after transfusion [2, 3]. During red cell storage, many changes occur in a time-dependent manner with kinetics that vary depending on the parameter [2, 3]. There is a progressive decrease in intracellular 2,3-diphosphoglycerate (DPG) and adenosine triphosphate (ATP) with concomitant accumulation of extracellular free haemoglobin and free iron. A decrease in 2,3-DPG reduces oxygen delivery to tissue although this change may be partly reversible after transfusion. Irreversible changes to the red cell membrane (including releasing of micro-vesicles) reduce deformability and may increase the likelihood of occluding the microvasculature. Extracellular haemoglobin (free or contained in micro-vesicles) may scavenge nitric oxide (NO); iron may increase circulating non-transferrin-bound iron and thus may promote inflammation [2–4]. There is a progressive accumulation of lactic acid and potassium, and a steady decrease in pH during storage. In addition, accumulation of other biological by-products,

Practical Transfusion Medicine, Fifth Edition. Edited by Michael F. Murphy, David J. Roberts and Mark H. Yazer.
© 2017 John Wiley & Sons Ltd. Published 2017 by John Wiley & Sons Ltd.

including cytokines, lipids, histamines and enzymes, may induce febrile transfusion reactions, increase oxidative membrane damage and activate or suppress the immune system [4].

Although these *in vitro* changes are clear and demonstrable (e.g. loss of 2.3-DPG by day 14 of storage), no data exist on the *in vivo* clinical significance of these changes nor a cutoff storage duration to define 'old' red cells. Therefore, defining 'old' red cells (or the age of multiple transfused units) in the clinical setting is arbitrary, which may partly explain the varied storage age definitions used in the observational studies.

Studies on Clinical Effects of 'Old' Red Cells

The study of the relationship between red cell storage duration and clinical outcomes began in 1989 with the first publication of a small randomised, single-centre trial comparing the effects of fresh whole blood (<12 hours old) with stored blood (2–5 days old) in cardiac surgery patients [5]. Until recently, with the exception of a few small RCTs, most publications on the subject were from retrospective observation studies, with the most well known being that of Koch et al [6]. In this single-centre, retrospective study of 6002 cardiac surgery patients transfused with red cells during cardiac surgery between 1998 and 2006, a total of 2872 patients received 8802 units of blood that had been stored for 14 days or less ('fresher'), and 3130 patients received 10782 units of blood that had been stored for more than 14 days ('older'). The study found that the recipients of older (median: 20 days) red cells had higher rates of hospital mortality compared with those transfused with fresher (median: 11 days) red cells (2.8% versus 1.7%, P = 0.004). Recipients of older red cells also had a higher rate of one-year mortality (7.4% versus 11.0%, P < 0.001), were more likely to have a prolonged mechanical ventilation beyond 72 hours (9.7% versus 5.6%, P < 0.001), and more likely to have renal failure (2.7% versus 1.6%, P = 0.003), sepsis or septicaemia (4.0% versus 2.8%, P = 0.01) or multisystem organ failure

(0.7% vs 0.2%, P = 0.007) compared with those transfused with fresher red cells [6]. The conclusions of this study have since been debated and challenged primarily due to the observational nature of the study and presentation of unadjusted analyses. Furthermore, other retrospective studies did not reach such conclusions [7, 8]. The largest observational study of a cohort of 854,862 adult patients who received transfusions from 2003 to 2012 found no association between the length of RBC storage and mortality [8].

One systematic review provided a detailed summary of relevant publications in adult patients over the past three decades (from 1983 to 2012) [9]. The authors identified 55 studies for detailed qualitative synthesis. Most of the 55 studies were retrospective and performed at a single institution; eight (14.5%) were small randomised studies, with three of the eight conducted in healthy volunteers. Twenty-six of the 55 studies (47%) suggested adverse effects of red cell storage on at least one clinical endpoint, where the remainder 29 (53%) showed no difference effect. The authors concluded that they could not find definitive evidence showing that fresher red cells are clinically superior to older red cells [9]. They did not perform a quantitative meta-analysis due to the considerable heterogeneity among studies and the concern with the numerous biased studies identified in their system review [9].

Two previous publications which performed a meta-analysis of studies from the mostly observational data have conflicting results [10, 11]. Wang et al performed a meta-analysis on 21 studies published between 2001 and 2011 (including six in cardiac surgery and six in trauma) totalling 409 966 patients and showed that red cell storage was associated with an increased risk of mortality (pooled odds ratio (OR) 1.16; 95% confidence interval (CI) 1.07–1.24, P = 0.0001), pneumonia (pooled OR 1.17; 95% CI 1.08–1.27, P = 0.0001) and multiple organ dysfunction syndrome (pooled OR 2.26; 95% CI 1.56–3.25, P < 0.0001) [10]. A meta-analysis by Vamvakas of only studies that included adjusted results for mortality found that the storage duration was not associated with increased risk for mortality [11].

There are several potential explanations for the conflicting conclusions from the mostly observational studies. First, a retrospective study design does not control for known or unrecognised potentially clinically important factors such as baseline patient characteristics, underlying disease, the presence of comorbidities (i.e. the need for red cell transfusion), volume transfusion, transfusion of other blood components and follow-up period. Sicker patients receive more blood transfusions and thus have a greater likelihood of receiving (at least one) older unit. An observational study cannot determine whether worse outcomes are due to the need for transfusion or transfusion itself (confounding by indication). Second, varied mortality (e.g. seven-day versus 28-day) and morbidity endpoints (outcomes) were reported among studies, making comparisons difficult. Third, various definitions of red cell storage durations were used to define 'fresher' versus 'older'. This becomes especially problematic when multiple units of various storage duration were transfused. Most importantly, there is no clinical evidence to support any of these definitions. Investigators have tried to extrapolate the *in vitro* changes to red cells as equivalent of *in vivo* effectiveness when defining age of red cell storage. This approach does not account for the fact that the kinetics of the *in vitro* changes is highly variable depending on the parameter and none have been shown to be clinically relevant. Fourth, varied red cell preparations with different storage media or modification such as leucocyte reduction were used in the studies over the years.

As a result, conclusions from these observational studies, which represent the body of literature on the subject, are conflicting. The lack of clarity on the subject prompted the design and conduct of large multicentre properly powered RCTs in an attempt to generate robust data to resolve the issue. Results from four of these studies have recently become available [12–15].

Randomised Controlled Trials

The first prospective RCT of red cell storage was carried out over 25 years ago and involved 237 patients randomised to receive units of either fresh whole blood (<12 hours) or stored blood (2–5 days) at the end of the extracorporeal circulation in primary coronary bypass operation. There were no differences in postoperative bleeding, coagulation tests or transfusion requirements between the two groups [5]. Kor et al performed a double-blind, single-centre randomised trial of 100 mechanically ventilated patients in intensive care units (ICUs) to compare the effect of fresher red cells (median age, four days) with standard red cells (median age, 26.5 days) [16]. There was no significant difference in the primary outcome of pulmonary function assessed by the partial pressure of arterial oxygen to fraction of inspired oxygen concentration ratio as well as the immunological and coagulation status between the two groups. Similar mortality was noted between the fresher group and the standard issue red cells group, but the study was not powered for this outcome [16]. Several other small, single-centre prospective randomised trials were conducted but these studies are limited by the number of patients/individuals participated in the studies (Table 11.1) [17–20].

Recently, results of four large RCTs have been published (see Table 11.1). The Age of Red Blood Cells in Premature Infants (ARIPI) study evaluated 377 premature infants with birthweight less than 1250 g in a neonatal ICU requiring at least one red cell transfusion [12]. A total of 188 patients received fresh red cells (median storage, 5.1 days; standard deviation (SD), 2.0), and 189 patients received red cells stored according to standard of care (median storage, 14.6 days; SD, 8.3). The relative risk (RR) was 1.00 (95% CI 0.82–1.21) for the primary outcome of the study, a composite measure of necrotising enterocolitis, retinopathy of prematurity, intra-ventricular haemorrhage, bronchopulmonary dysplasia and death. The rate of clinically suspected infection was 77.7% and 77.2% for the fresher red cell group and the standard red cell group, respectively (RR 1.01; 95% CI 0.90–1.12). The rate of positive cultures was 67.5 % and 64.0% for the fresher red cell

Table 11.1 Randomised controlled trials of red cell storage duration.

Author [ref], year (trial name)	Study design	Definition of storage duration	Clinical setting	No. of patients	Adverse effects with longer storage?
Heddle [15], 2016 (INFORM)	Multicentre RCT	Freshest vs oldest in the inventory	General hospital population	20,858	No difference in the rate of death
Lacroix [13], 2015 (ABLE)	Multicentre RCT	<8 days versus standard issue	ICU	2430	No for 90-day mortality No for all secondary outcomes
Steiner [14], 2015 (RECESS)	Multicentre RCT	≤10 days versus ≥21 days	Cardiac surgery	1098	No for changes in MODS No for 7-day and 28-day mortality
Fergusson [12], 2012 (ARIPI)	Multicentre RCT	<7 days versus standard of care	Premature infants	377	No for mortality No for rate of complications
Wasser [5], 1989	Single centre RCT	<12 hours vs 2–5 days	Cardiac surgery	237	No for coagulation rests, post-operative bleeding. Or transfusion requirements
Kor [16], 2012	Single centre	≤5 days versus standard issue red cells (median 21 days)	ICU	100	No difference in pulmonary function
Fernandes [17], 2001	Single centre RCT	Continuous variable	ICU (sepsis)	15 (10 transfused; 5 received albumin)	No for gastric mucosal pH
Walsh [18], 2004	Single centre RCT	≤5 days versus ≥20 days	ICU (on mechanical ventilation)	22	No for gastric mucosal pH
Yuruk [20], 2013	Single centre	<1 week versus 3–4 weeks	Haematology patients	20	Same increase in perfused vessel density in both groups
Weiskopf [19], 2012	Single centre		Healthy volunteers	35	No in pulmonary gas exchange variables

ICU, intensive care unit; MODS, multiple organ dysfunction score; RCT, randomised controlled trial.

group and the standard red cell group, respectively (RR 1.06; 95% CI 0.91–1.22) [12]. Hence, this RCT demonstrated that the use of fresher red cells compared with standard of care did not decrease or increase the rate of complications or death in this population of premature, very low-birthweight neonates [12]. This study is limited by the fact that the age of blood in the standard of care group was only 14 days old.

The Age of Blood Evaluation (ABLE) study randomised 2430 ICU patients to receive red cells that had been stored for less than eight days or standard blood transfusion laboratory issue red cells (the oldest compatible units available in the blood transfusion laboratory) [13]. A total of 1211 patients received fresh red cells (mean age, 6.1 days; SD, 4.9), and 1219 patients received standard issue red cells (mean age, 22; SD, 8.4) ($P < 0.001$). The primary endpoint of 90-day mortality occurred in 37.0% in the fresh blood group and 35.3% in the standard blood group (95% CI for the absolute difference, –2.1 to 5.5). There were no significant differences in any of the secondary outcomes (major illness; duration of respiratory, haemodynamic or renal support; infection; length of hospital stay; and transfusion reactions) between the two groups.

The Red Cell Storage Duration Study (RECESS) randomised 1096 patients to receive red cells stored for 10 days or less (shorter term storage group) or for 21 days or more (longer term storage group) [14]. The mean (±SD) durations of storage were 7.8 ± 4.8 days in the shorter term storage group (n = 538 patients) and 28.3 ± 6.7 days in the longer term storage group (n = 560 patients). No difference was seen in the median composite change in Multiple Organ Dysfunction Score (MODS) at day 7 (8.5 points for shorter term storage group and 8.7 points for longer term storage group) (95% CI for the absolute difference, -0.6 to 0.3; $P = 0.44$). The seven-day mortality was 2.8% in the shorter term storage group and 2.0% in the longer term storage group ($P = 0.43$). All-cause mortality rates at 28 days were 4.4% and 5.3%, respectively ($P = 0.57$). The study concluded that red cell storage duration was not significantly associated with seven-day changes in MODS, serious adverse events or 28-day mortality rate among patients undergoing cardiac surgery [14].

The Informing Fresh versus Old Red cell Management (INFORM) trial randomised 31,497 hospitalized adults to receive either freshest RBCs in the inventory (short-term storage group) available or the oldest available RBCs (long-term storage group) (15). Analysis was performed on 20,858 patients: 6936 patients received RBCs stored for a mean duration of 13.0 day (short-term storage group); 13,922 patients received RBCs stored for a mean of 23.6 days (long-term storage group). There was no significant difference in the rate of death between the two groups [15].

Thus, the four large RCTs provided robust data and reached consensus in showing that no differences exist between clinical outcomes and the duration of red cell storage. A meta-analysis of RCTs (1948 –May 2016) studying RBC storage from 13 clinical trials totaling 5.515 patients showed that fresher RBCs did not improve clinical outcomes [21] Although these clinical trials did not address the effects of transfusion of very fresh or 'very old' red cells, i.e. red cells stored for less than five days or more than 35 days (35–42 days old), or the effects of 'fresh' or 'old' red cells on specific patient subgroups, the results are applicable to the majority of the general medical/surgical population.

The results of two additional large RCTs are not yet available. The INFORM (Informing Fresh Versus Old Red Cell Management) trial plans to enrol hospitalised adults requiring transfusions to randomly receive either the freshest available or standard issue red cells. The TRANSFUSE (Standard Issue Transfusion Versus Fresher Red Blood Cell Use in Intensive Care) trial conducted in Australia plans to randomise adult intensive care patients to receive either the freshest available or standard issue red cells. In addition, the result from an RCT in cardiac surgery patients at the Cleveland Clinic is also awaited.

Conclusion

Observational studies of the clinical effects of the storage duration of red cells are conflicting and have methodological limitations; in addition, they are confounded by indication. These limitations prompted the design and conduction of several randomised controlled trials. Results from four of the recently published RCTs – one in paediatrics, one in critically ill patients and one in cardiac surgery patients, and one in general hospitalized patients – have provided strong evidence that the storage duration of red cells does not have measurable adverse effects on the clinical outcomes in these transfused patient populations. Additional randomised controlled trials are under way in critically ill and medical/surgical patient populations. Together, they will define whether storage duration of red cells has clinical relevance.

KEY POINTS

1) Results from retrospective observational studies of 'fresh versus old blood' are inconclusive, largely due to methodological limitations and confounding of these studies.
2) Data from recently completed RCTs have shown that duration of red cell storage is not associated with adverse clinical outcomes in premature neonates, critically ill patients and patients undergoing cardiac surgery.

References

1 Whitaker B, Henry R. The 2011 National Blood Collection and Utilization Survey Report. Available at: www.aabb.org/research/hemovigilance/bloodsurvey/Documents/11-nbcus-report.pdf (accessed 31 October 2016).

2 Hess JR. Red cell changes during storage. Transfus Apher Sci 2010;**43**(1):51–9.

3 Koch CG, Figueroa PI, Li L, Sabik JF 3rd, Mihaljevic T, Blackstone EH. Red blood cell storage: how long is too long? Ann Thorac Surg 2013;**96**(5):1894–9.

4 Spinella PC, Sparrow RL, Hess JR, Norris PJ. Properties of stored red blood cells: understanding immune and vascular reactivity. Transfusion 2011;**51**(4):894–900.

5 Wasser MN, Houbiers JG, d'Amaro J et al. The effect of fresh versus stored blood on post-operative bleeding after coronary bypass surgery: a prospective randomized study. Br J Haematol 1989;**72**(1):81–4.

6 Koch CG, Li L, Sessler DI et al. Duration of red-cell storage and complications after cardiac surgery. N Engl J Med 2008;**358**(12):1229–39.

7 Van de Watering L, Lorinser J, Versteegh M, Westendord R, Brand A. Effects of storage time of red blood cell transfusions on the prognosis of coronary artery bypass graft patients. Transfusion 2006;**46**(10):1712–18.

8 Halmin M, Rostgaard K, Lee BK, Wikman A, Norda R, Nielsen KR, et al. Length of Storage of Red Blood Cells and Patient Survival After Blood Transfusion: A Binational Cohort Study. Annals of internal medicine. 2016.

9 Lelubre C, Vincent JL. Relationship between red cell storage duration and outcomes in adults receiving red cell transfusions: a systematic review. Crit Care 2013;**17**(2):R66.

10 Wang D, Sun J, Solomon SB, Klein HG, Natanson C. Transfusion of older stored blood and risk of death: a meta-analysis. Transfusion 2012;**52**(6):1184–95.

11 Vamvakas EC. Purported deleterious effects of "old" versus "fresh" red blood cells: an updated meta-analysis. Transfusion 2011;**51**(5):1122–3.

12 Fergusson DA, Hebert P, Hogan DL et al. Effect of fresh red blood cell transfusions on clinical outcomes in premature, very low-birth-weight infants: the ARIPI randomized trial. JAMA 2012;**308**(14):1443–51.

13 Lacroix J, Hebert PC, Fergusson DA et al. Age of transfused blood in critically ill adults. N Engl J Med 2015;**372**(15):1410–18.

14 Steiner ME, Ness PM, Assmann SF et al. Effects of red-cell storage duration on patients undergoing cardiac surgery. N Engl J Med 2015;**372**(15):1419–29.

15 Heddle NM, Cook RJ, Arnold DM, Liu Y, Barty R, Crowther MA et al. Effect of Short-Term vs. Long-Term Blood Storage on Mortality after Transfusion. N Engl J Med 2016;**375**(20):1937–45.

16 Kor DJ, Kashyap R, Weiskopf RB et al. Fresh red blood cell transfusion and short-term pulmonary, immunologic, and coagulation status: a randomized clinical trial. Am J Respir Crit Care Med 2012;**185**(8):842–50.

17 Fernandes CJ Jr, Akamine N, de Marco FV, de Souza JA, Lagudis S, Knobel E. Red blood cell transfusion does not increase oxygen consumption in critically ill septic patients. Crit Care 2001;**5**(6):362–7.

18 Walsh TS, McArdle F, McLellan SA et al. Does the storage time of transfused red blood cells influence regional or global indexes of tissue oxygenation in anemic critically ill patients? Crit Care Med 2004;**32**(2):364–71.

19 Weiskopf RB, Feiner J, Toy P et al. Fresh and stored red blood cell transfusion equivalently induce subclinical pulmonary gas exchange deficit in normal humans. Anesth Analg 2012;**114**(3):511–19.

20 Yuruk K, Milstein DM, Bezemer R, Bartels SA, Biemond BJ, Ince C. Transfusion of banked red blood cells and the effects on hemorrheology and microvascular hemodynamics in anemic hematology outpatients. Transfusion 2013;**53**(6):1346–52.

21 Carson JL, Guyatt G, Heddle NM, Grossman BJ, Cohn CS, Fung MK, et al. Clinical Practice Guidelines From the AABB: Red Blood Cell Transfusion Thresholds and Storage. Jama 2016; **316**(19):2025–35.

Further Reading

Brunskill SJ, Wilkinson KL, Doree C, Trivella M, Stanworth S. Transfusion of fresher versus older red cells for all conditions. Cochrane Database of Systematic Reviews 2015;**5**:CD010801.

Qu L, Triulzi DJ. Clinical effects of red blood cell storage. Cancer Control 2015;**22**(1):26–37.

12 Transfusion-Induced Immunomodulation

Amy E. Schmidt, Majed A. Refaai, Joanna M. Heal and Neil Blumberg

Department of Pathology and Laboratory Medicine, University of Rochester; Blood Bank/Transfusion Service of Strong Memorial Hospital, Rochester, USA

Introduction

Transfusion immunomodulation refers to alterations in recipient immune function that affect clinical outcomes. In theory, this includes almost all complications of transfusion other than transmission of infectious agents. Adverse events such as alloimmunisation to blood cell or plasma protein antigens, febrile non-haemolytic transfusion reactions, anaphylaxis, transfusion-related lung injury (TRALI) and congestive heart failure following transfusion have immune effects as their primary mechanisms or as components of their pathophysiology. This chapter will focus on immune effects and clinical events thought likely to be immune in origin, which involve transfusion's effects on innate or adaptive cellular immunity. Innate immunity broadly refers to the roles of cells such as neutrophils, monocytes/macrophages and natural killer (NK) cells. Adaptive immunity includes humoral immunity (primarily B-cells and antibodies) and cellular immunity (primarily T- and dendritic cells mediating cellular cytotoxicity). Clinical outcomes potentially influenced by immunomodulation include increases in post-operative infection, cancer recurrence, metastasis or mortality, as well as facilitation of organ allograft acceptance, inflammatory changes such as systemic inflammatory response syndrome and multi-organ failure (including lung injury), necrotising enterocolitis of the newborn and enhanced success of pregnancies in patients with repetitive spontaneous abortions.

Adverse events mediated by adaptive humoral immunity (i.e. antibodies that cause red cell destruction, TRALI, anaphylaxis and allergic reactions, platelet refractoriness, post-transfusion purpura, neonatal alloimmune thrombocytopenia, organ allograft rejection, etc.) will be discussed in other chapters.

The history of transfusion immunomodulation as a comprehensive theory addressing blood transfusion's profound influence on immunity antedates our current knowledge and models of adaptive immunity (primarily T-cells) and innate immunity as distinct aspects of immune function. In the 1960s and 1970s, when lymphocytes were still considered cells of uncertain function, observational data demonstrated that renal failure patients receiving haemodialysis who required red cell transfusions had better renal allograft survival after transplantation than did patients who were not transfused [1]. This enhancing effect was reproducible, dose dependent, demonstrable in animal models and more pronounced in patients receiving whole blood or un-manipulated red cells, compared with patients receiving relatively leucocyte-reduced washed or frozen/deglycerolised red cells. Animal models demonstrated that allogeneic leucocytes, and perhaps platelets, could mediate these effects, but not allogeneic plasma. The concept that transfusion was 'immunosuppressive' grew out of these clinical observations, which have never been validated in randomised clinical trials. One lesson from this story is that important and clinically useful and actionable findings can derive from clinical cohort studies and observational data, although randomised trials are a definitive proof that is usually required.

Almost two decades later, animal model investigators Brian Shenton and colleagues in Newcastle, England, reported that allogeneic blood transfusions were associated with more rapid tumour growth in animals [2]. Paul Tartter and Lewis Burrows, surgeons in New York City, observed that colorectal cancer recurrence was more frequent in transfused patients [3]. The broad field of transfusion immunomodulation research thus began in the early 1980s. Shortly after, Tartter and colleagues noted that post-operative nosocomial infections were strikingly more frequent in transfused patients undergoing colorectal surgery [4]. Our centre later reported that this increase in post-operative nosocomial infections after surgery was not seen in patients receiving autologous transfusions. Furthermore, a role for stored supernatant plasma was proposed due to the association of whole blood with increased cancer recurrence. These findings supported an immune mechanism underlying adverse clinical outcomes [5,6].

Further animal model investigations from Cincinnati (Wesley Alexander and colleagues) [7] and San Antonio (Paul Waymack and colleagues) [8] demonstrated that promotion of infection was seen when allogeneic, as opposed to syngeneic, transfusions were given. This is key evidence that these phenomena are indeed immune mediated. More recently, randomised trials of autologous [9], leucocyte reduced [10] and restrictive red cell transfusions [11] demonstrated that each intervention is associated with clinically relevant reductions in nosocomial post-operative infections. Furthermore, observational data have shown that allogeneic platelet transfusions are associated with increases in multi-organ failure and recurrence of acute leukaemia. There are preliminary data that

removing stored supernatant from transfused red cells and platelets by washing may mitigate pro-inflammatory/immunomodulatory effects in both the surgical and haematology settings.

In this chapter, we will review the randomised trials that have definitively demonstrated that transfusion causes increases in nosocomial infection after surgery because these effects can be partially mitigated by leucocyte reduction, autologous transfusion and restrictive transfusion practices. Then, we will summarise other effects based upon observational and cohort studies, as well as animal models. The proposed immunological mechanisms underlying these findings, inferred from *in vitro* and animal model experiments, will be summarised. The question of storage age of red cells as mediators of transfusion immunomodulation will be addressed, along with future studies needed to better understand the mechanisms of transfusion immunomodulation and further mitigate the immunological toxicity of allogeneic transfusions.

Mitigation of Immunomodulation After Red Cell Transfusion

For some decades, the very existence of transfusion immunomodulation has been questioned. This raises the issue of how we establish causal associations between transfusion and altered clinical outcomes. Typical criteria supporting a causal association include reproducibility, dose dependence, mechanistic rationales and the ability to modify the association by altering the exposure to the proposed cause of the effect. Whilst it is often stated that the strongest evidence for transfusion immunomodulation is that allogeneic transfusions improve renal allograft survival, this is not the case. Whilst evidence that transfusions benefit recipients of renal allografts by enhancing graft survival is strong, it is limited to mechanistic studies, animal models, and epidemiological and cohort data. There are no modern randomised controlled trials in which patients have been selected to receive or not receive allogeneic red cells and renal allograft survival determined.

Importantly, there is conclusive evidence that the association between allogeneic red cell transfusion and post-operative infection is causal. There are mechanistic studies demonstrating that allogeneic leucocytes mediate down-regulation of host defences. Animal model studies and cohort/epidemiological data demonstrated a dose-dependent effect of red cell transfusions on post-operative infections, independent of other prognostic factors. However, the strongest and most indisputable evidence that allogeneic red cell transfusions cause increased post-operative infections, likely via an immunological mechanism, comes from randomised trials in which patients undergoing surgery have received either leucocyte-reduced or non-leucocyte-reduced red cells, autologous versus allogeneic red cell transfusions, or have been treated with restrictive versus liberal red

cell transfusion thresholds. Meta-analyses of these randomised trials confirmed that patients in the leucocyte-reduced, autologous or restricted transfusion arms experienced fewer nosocomial infections than patients in the non-leucocyte-reduced, allogeneic or liberal red cell transfusion threshold arms. Removing most allogeneic leucocytes, employing autologous red cell transfusions (which replace or minimise allogeneic red cell transfusions) or reducing the dose of allogeneic red cells through restrictive thresholds all lead to reductions in post-operative infections (Figures 12.1–12.3). These effects are likely to be clinically significant as the risk of infection is approximately 55% less in patients receiving leucocyte-reduced red cells and reductions in infection of a similar order of magnitude are seen in those received autologous transfusions compared to allogeneic transfusions or those transfused using restrictive compared to liberal transfusion thresholds.

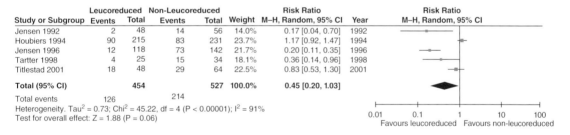

Figure 12.1 The metaanalytic summary of randomised trials of leucocyte-reduced red cell transfusions to mitigate post-operative infection in colorectal cancer surgery is shown. The risk of infection is approximately 55% less in patients receiving leucocyte-reduced red cells. Data extracted from original papers and reference [12].

Study or Subgroup	Autologous Transfusion Events	Total	Allogeneic Transfusion Events	Total	Weight	Risk Ratio M–H, Random, 95% CI	Risk Ratio M–H, Random, 95% CI
Busch 1993	65	239	59	236	28.6%	1.09 [0.80, 1.47]	
Farrer 1997	3	23	12	27	15.1%	0.29 [0.09, 0.91]	
Heiss 1993	7	62	17	58	20.3%	0.39 [0.17, 0.86]	
Newman 1997	2	35	12	35	11.7%	0.17 [0.04, 0.69]	
Wong 2002	16	74	19	71	24.2%	0.81 [0.45, 1.44]	
Total (95% CI)		**433**		**427**	**100.0%**	**0.54 [0.29, 1.00]**	
Total events	93		119				

Heterogeneity. Tau^2 = 0.33; Chi^2 = 15.05, df = 4 (P = 0.005); I^2 = 73%
Test for overall effect: Z = 1.95 (P = 0.05)

0.05 0.2 1 5 20
Favours Autologous Favours Allogeneic

Figure 12.2 Meta-analytic summary of randomised trials of autologous transfusions (either pre-deposit, haemodilution or salvage) to mitigate post-operative infection after surgery. The risk of infection is approximately 46% less in patients receiving autologous red cells [9].

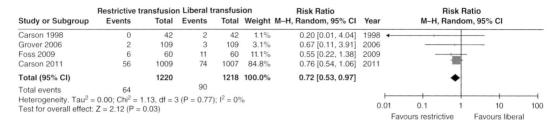

Figure 12.3 Meta-analytic summary of randomised trials of restrictive red cell transfusion thresholds (usually <70 g/L) to mitigate post-operative infection in orthopaedic surgery. The risk of infection is 28% less in patients receiving red cells according to restrictive criteria [13].

Leucocyte-Reduced Allogeneic Red Cell Transfusions Reduce Mortality In Cardiac Surgery

Although the causal effect of red cell transfusions in promoting post-operative infection might be thought of as purely immunosuppressive, it is clear that transfusion in the setting of cardiac surgery causes increased inflammatory responses. The strongest proof of this is that transfusion is associated in a dose-dependent fashion with multi-organ failure as well as subsequent mortality in cardiac surgery. One of the most important benefits of leucocyte-reduced red cell transfusions is that they reduce mortality after cardiac surgery [14]. Whilst the effect of leucocyte reduction on post-operative infection is less pronounced in the setting of cardiac surgery than in colorectal surgery, it is known that leucocyte reduction mitigates post-operative multi-organ failure in randomised trials. As multi-organ failure is believed to represent the effects of exaggerated inflammatory responses to apparent or occult infection, the mechanism of benefit may be somewhat similar to that seen in non-cardiac surgery settings.

Two groups in The Netherlands demonstrated a 50% reduction in mortality in cardiac surgery patients randomised to receive leucocyte-reduced transfusions. Thus, leucocyte reduction has been almost universally adopted for cardiac surgery worldwide, even in hospitals that do not practise universal leucocyte reduction. There is also evidence that leucocyte reduction, autologous transfusion and restrictive transfusion practices reduce recipient inflammatory responses as measured by cytokine levels *in vivo* or *in vitro*. Removal of stored supernatant from stored red cells by washing with normal saline may further reduce the inflammatory response in cardiac surgery. Thus, washing holds promise as an additional potential strategy to minimise morbidity and mortality in this heavily transfused patient population. Strategies that have been proven or proposed to mitigate transfusion immunomodulation and its adverse consequences are summarised in Box 12.1. 'Proven' is used where epidemiological/observational, mechanistic and animal model data support a cause and effect relationship, including dose response, or that randomised trials have proven the effect is, at least in part, causal.

Observational and Cohort Studies of Transfusion Immunomodulation Link Red Cell Transfusions to Both Beneficial and Adverse Outcomes

The original data supporting transfusion immunomodulation derive from cohort studies demonstrating improved renal allograft survival in transfused patients receiving red cells for anaemia caused by chronic renal failure. These patients were found to have superior renal allograft survival compared to non-transfused

---

Box 12.1 Strategies to mitigate transfusion immunomodulation effects.

- Leucocyte reduction of red cells and platelets (proven in randomised trials) – reduces postoperative infection, multi-organ failure and mortality in cardiac surgery and platelet transfusion refractoriness.
- Leucocyte reduction of transfused blood reduces inflammation, lung injury and red cell alloimmunisation in recipients by removing DNA, histones and platelets that can exacerbate innate and humoral adaptive immune responses (proposed).
- Autologous transfusion to reduce the use of allogeneic red cells in surgery – reduces postoperative infection (proven in randomised trials) and may reduce post-operative thrombosis (proposed – observational data).
- Restrictive red cell transfusion practice (proven in randomised trials) – reduces post-operative infection in some surgical settings (orthopaedic surgery) and may reduce multi-organ failure, thrombosis and mortality (proposed from both randomised trial and observational data).
- Washing of red cell and platelet transfusions – reduces treatment-related mortality and recurrence in acute myeloid leukaemia and reduces mortality in cardiac surgery (proposed from small pilot randomised trials).
- Improve red cell viability through better storage solutions and rejuvenation prior to transfusion (proposed from animal model studies, *in vitro* mechanistic studies and observational cohort studies).
- Reduced platelet activation and dysfunction during storage through improved storage solutions/conditions to reduce the likelihood of post-transfusion inflammation and organ injury (proposed from observational studies, animal models and *in vitro* mechanistic studies).

---

patients. This effect was dose dependent, and was stronger when the transfusions were red cells or whole blood rather than washed or frozen-de-glycerolysed red cells. This led Tartter and Burrows to propose that this immunosuppressive effect might be deleterious in cancer patients. A broad range of studies demonstrated a consistent dose-dependent association between red cell transfusion and earlier cancer recurrence or cancer-specific mortality. However, the effect was much greater in colorectal, gastric and head and neck cancers, and undetectable in some other cancers such as breast cancer. It was then found that, much like the observations in renal transplantation, red cells transfused as whole blood were much more potently associated with poor outcomes than relatively plasma- and leucocyte/platelet-depleted red cells [15]. This suggested a cause and effect relationship given the presence of immunomodulatory substances in greater quantities in whole blood.

Animal models demonstrated that leucocyte reduction might reduce promotion of cancer metastasis by transfusions [16], but this has not been confirmed in human trials [17]. The few randomised trials of leucocyte reduction alone have not shown a benefit in reduced cancer recurrence, suggesting that supernatant stored plasma might play a role in this association, if causal. Autologous transfusion showed promise in one randomised trial in colorectal cancer as a strategy to reduce the adverse effects of transfusion immunomodulation on cancer recurrence [18]. There have been no randomised trials of washed transfusions in cancer patients, except for a small pilot study demonstrating a 50% reduction in mortality in patients with acute leukaemia randomised to receive washed red cells and platelets.

There are also observational data that allogeneic transfusion and its attendant immunomodulatory effects have beneficial effects on the recurrence of repetitive spontaneous abortion, recurrence of regional enteritis after surgical resection and a few other inflammatory diseases. However, there are also observational data that allogeneic transfusions are associated with

> **Box 12.2 Associations between immunomodulation-mediated altered clinical outcomes and allogeneic transfusions.**
>
> - Enhancement of renal allograft acceptance (proven).
> - Increased post-operative infections (proven).
> - Increased recurrence of some solid tumours (proposed).
> - Increased inflammation (proven) leading to organ failure (proven for lung) and systemic inflammatory response syndrome/multi-organ failure in surgical patients, particularly after cardiac surgery or liver transplantation (proposed).
> - Increased thrombosis, perhaps through combined rheological and inflammatory mechanisms (proposed).
> - Reduced repetitive spontaneous abortion in some women treated with paternal or third party leucocytes (proposed).
> - Reduced recurrence of autoimmune inflammatory conditions (regional enteritis, rheumatoid arthritis) (proposed).
> - Increased reactivation of latent viral infection (proposed but the only randomised trial in HIV failed to find any evidence).
> - Increased necrotising enterocolitis in premature newborns (proposed).

with multi-organ failure, acute lung injury, acute gut injury in premature newborns and a variety of other conditions that may involve immune dysregulation or be initiated by clinically occult nosocomial infection. Box 12.2 summarises some of these studies.

Duration of Red Cell Storage and Immunomodulation

Observational data in some centres (primarily in North America) suggested that transfusion of red cells stored for a longer period of time were associated with poorer clinical outcomes, in particular nosocomial infection, multi-organ failure, thrombosis and mortality. Animal model data confirmed these results. It is clear that longer stored red cells, even when leucocyte reduced, contain more free haemoglobin, haem, iron and red cell-derived microparticles. These mediators are, hypothetically, strong candidates to cause impaired host defences, thrombosis and inflammation. Nonetheless, multiple randomised trials have demonstrated that in typical clinical practice, use of shorter storage red cells (typically 7–10 days or fewer) does not mitigate the associations between transfusion and infection, thrombosis and mortality. This may be due to the inability to compare patients receiving only very long storage red cells (i.e. >35 days) with shorter storage red cells. In addition, many of these trials included patients receiving platelet and plasma transfusions which might, in theory, obscure any benefit of shorter storage red cells.

Nonetheless, it seems likely that for most clinical settings, a few units of longer stored red cells given to an adult patient probably do not cause clinically significantly greater immune modulation and poorer outcomes than similar small quantities of shorter storage red cells. It may be that when the dose of longer storage red cells is much greater, as in infants undergoing cardiac surgery, immunomodulation is more prominent. There are observational data to suggest this may be so, particularly when red cells are exposed to stresses such as irradiation and washing, as in a study by Cholette and colleagues [19] (Figure 12.4).

Experimental Studies and Transfusion Immunomodulation

Allogeneic transfusions, as opposed to syngeneic transfusions, have been repeatedly demonstrated to alter outcomes in animal models (Box 12.3). For a phenomenon as complex as transfusion immunomodulation, exact understanding of the pleiotropic effects seen may not be possible. There is a plethora of *in vitro* and

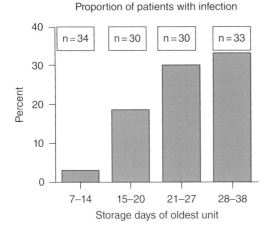

Proportion of patients with infection

Figure 12.4 The proportion of patients with infection as a function of the oldest red cell unit transfused in a randomised trial of washed, irradiated, leucocyte-reduced red cells in paediatric cardiac surgery. The almost 10-fold difference is unlikely to be totally explained by confounding, and suggests that older red cells, when transfused at doses of hundreds of millilitres per kilogram (as in infants), may be more immunomodulatory than shorter storage red cells, but these observational data require confirmation in a randomised trial [19].

Box 12.3 Effects of immunomodulation from allogeneic transfusions demonstrated in animal models.

- Enhancement of renal allograft acceptance.
- Increased post-operative infections and mortality from infection.
- Increased metastasis of solid tumours.
- Increased inflammation leading to organ failure and systemic inflammatory response syndrome/multi-organ failure.
- Increased reactivation of latent viral infection.
- Increased lung injury after infusion of DNA, histones and activated platelets in non-leucocyte-reduced donor blood.

Box 12.4 *In vitro* and *in vivo* immunological effects caused by or associated with allogeneic transfusions in model systems, animal models and/or patients.

- Reduced responses in mixed lymphocyte culture.
- Reduced cutaneous delayed type hypersensitivity reactions.
- Reduced responsiveness to mitogens and soluble antigens.
- Decreased natural killer cell number and function.
- Increased CD8 T-cell number and suppressor function.
- Decreased CD4 T-cell number.
- Decreased monocyte-macrophage function.
- Decreased cell-mediated cytotoxicity.
- Increased humoral alloimmunisation to cell-associated and soluble antigens.
- Decreased type 1 (Th1) and increased type 2 (Th2) cytokine secretion.
- Increased Treg numbers and function.
- Neutrophil priming, B-cell, endothelial cell and platelet activation by sCD40L.
- Priming of neutrophil and platelet activation by lipid mediators.
- Generation of free radicals and vascular dysfunction by cell free haemoglobin, haem and iron.
- Vascular dysfunction, platelet activation and a pro-thrombotic state due to nitric oxide scavenging and attendant inflammation.
- Activation of endothelial cells, platelets and innate immunity by microparticles.
- Monocyte and neutrophil recruitment/activation by supernatant cytokines such as IL-6, IL-8, etc.

---

animal model data demonstrating a vast range of immunological changes after allogeneic transfusions or mixing experiments (Box 12.4).

All these findings are generally consonant with up-regulation of humoral immunity, down-regulation of cellular immunity and aberrations of innate immunity (both suppressive and inappropriately activating). These findings provide logical but largely speculative explanations for the associations of allogeneic transfusion with antibody formation, inflammation, nosocomial infection, thrombosis, cancer recurrence, organ injury, reduced spontaneous abortions, necrotising enterocolitis in newborns, etc. It is reasonable to suggest that induction of type 2 immune deviation (towards interleukin (IL)-10, IL-4 and other cytokines that down-regulate cytotoxic T-cell function), promotion of Tregs (and down-regulation of T-cell cytotoxic function) and similar mechanisms make a plausible and comprehensive hypothesis about how transfusion immunomodulation mediates its effects.

Likewise, the effects of non-transferrin-bound iron, free haem and haemoglobin, as documented by the work of Hod, Spitalnik, Gladwin, Triulzi and colleagues (amongst others), make a coherent and mechanistically credible story as to why red cell transfusions down-regulate innate immunity against infection. These transfusion-derived mediators may simultaneously promote thrombosis, inflammation and organ injury, as seen in haemolytic diseases such as sickle cell anaemia and paroxysmal nocturnal haemoglobinuria. The nitric oxide scavenging effects of stored red cells may contribute to the thromboses, leucocyte, vascular and platelet dysfunction observed in transfused patients. Finally, the plasma-containing supernatant of, in particular, non-leucocyte-reduced red cells, and even of leucocyte-reduced platelets, is rich in many mediators, such as VEGF and CD40L. Speculatively, these and other mediators may immunomodulate the recipient, contributing to poorer antitumour immunity, angiogenesis and inflammation.

These hypothesised mechanisms likely operating in concert, and may partially explain the associations with transfusion that are proven (renal allograft enhancement and nosocomial infection) and those that may be causal but as yet are not proven (cancer recurrence). It is likely that mechanism will be the last thing that will be clear about transfusion immunomodulation, because not only the administered product(s) but also the clinical settings are variable and complex. Transfusion and its immune effects occur in clinical settings with multiple co-existing diseases, the added effects of anaesthesia, drugs and parenteral fluids. Whilst mechanism may remain elusive, simple modifications of transfusions, such as leucocyte reduction or washing, may mitigate devastating clinical outcomes. This is supported by the benefits of leucocyte reduction in surgical patients requiring red cell transfusions, and by the promising results seen with washing in acute leukaemia (Figure 12.5).

Conclusion

Transfusions alter cellular and innate immunity in recipients. The data are most extensive for red cell transfusions. Favourable effects, such as improved renal allograft survival, are in contrast to adverse effects, such as increased nosocomial

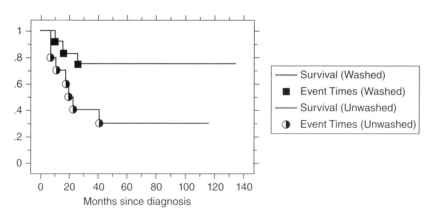

Figure 12.5 Proportion of patients surviving after diagnosis is shown for younger patients (<50 years of age) with acute leukaemia randomised to washed, leucocyte-reduced, ABO-identical, irradiated red cells and platelets versus unwashed, leucocyte-reduced, ABO-identical irradiated transfusions (n=12 for washed versus 10 for unwashed). P=0.03. Data *source:* Blumberg et al. [20].

infections. Many other associations have been proposed based upon observational and animal model data. Strategies for mitigating these unfavourable effects that have been demonstrated in randomised trials include leucocyte reduction, use of autologous transfusion, restrictive transfusion criteria and, preliminarily, removal of stored supernatant by washing. Improved techniques of red cell and platelet storage that prevent cellular damage, thus minimising exposure of the recipient to potentially toxic cellular contents such as haemoglobin, microparticles and cytokines, hold promise for further improving the benefit and reducing the risk of blood transfusions.

KEY POINTS

1) The existence of both adverse and beneficial transfusion immunomodulation effects has been convincingly demonstrated for increased post-operative infections and renal allograft enhancement.
2) In cardiac surgery, transfusion of leucocyte-reduced (compared with non-leucocyte-reduced) allogeneic red cells reduces all-cause mortality, likely due to reductions in multi-organ failure.
3) A wide range of adverse and beneficial effects has been demonstrated in transfused patients and animal models that are most likely due to immune effects of allogeneic transfusion, but most of these have not been proven to be causal.
4) A broad range of mechanisms is likely involved, including immune deviation lead-ing to up-regulation of humoral immunity and down-regulation of cytotoxic cellular immunity, and induction of Tregs.
5) Dysregulation of innate immunity (NK cells, macrophages, neutrophils and monocytes) is a prominent component of transfusion immunomodulation. Leucocyte reduction prevents accumulation of leucocytes, platelets, DNA and histones in stored blood components. These mediators may play a role in the effects seen in animal models and patients.
6) Additional manipulations such as washing, improved storage solutions or rejuvenation, re-nitrosylation, etc., may further reduce the toxicity of blood transfusions by minimising transfusion immunomodulation.

References

1 Opelz G, Sengar DPS, Mickey MR, Terasaki PI. Effect of blood transfusions on subsequent kidney transplants. Transplant Proc 1973;**5**:253–9.

2 Francis DM, Shenton BK. Blood transfusion and tumour growth: evidence from laboratory animals. Lancet 1981;**2**:871.

3 Burrows L, Tartter P. Effect of blood transfusions on colonic malignancy recurrence rate (letter). Lancet 1982;**2**:662.

4 Tartter PI, Quintero S, Barron DM. Perioperative blood transfusion associated with infectious complications after colorectal cancer operations. Am J Surg 1986;**152**:479–82.

5 Murphy P, Heal JM, Blumberg N. Infection or suspected infection after hip replacement surgery with autologous or homologous blood transfusions. Transfusion 1991;**31**:212–17.

6 Triulzi DJ, Vanek K, Ryan DH, Blumberg N. A clinical and immunologic study of blood transfusion and postoperative bacterial infection in spinal surgery. Transfusion 1992;**32**:517–24.

7 Gianotti L, Pyles T, Alexander JW, Fukushima R, Babcock GF. Identification of the blood component responsible for increased susceptibility to gut-derived infection. Transfusion 1993;**33**:458–65.

8 Waymack JP. The effect of blood transfusions on resistance to bacterial infections. Transplant Proc 1988;**20**:1105–7.

9 Vanderlinde ES, Heal JM, Blumberg N. Autologous transfusion. BMJ 2002;**324**:772–5.

10 Khanna M, Fergusson DA, Hebert PC. Leukoreduced red blood cell transfusions in surgery: a meta-analysis evaluating the efficacy of leukocyte filtered blood in reducing postoperative infections. Transfusion 2002;**42**(Suppl.):5S (abstract).

11 Salpeter SR, Buckley JS, Chatterjee S. Impact of more restrictive blood transfusion strategies on clinical outcomes: a meta-analysis and systematic review. Am J Med 2014;**127**:124–31 e3.

12 Blumberg N, Zhao H, Wang H, Messing S, Heal JM, Lyman GH. The intention-to-treat principle in clinical trials and meta-analyses of leukoreduced blood transfusions in surgical patients. Transfusion 2007;**47**:573–81.

13 Rohde JM, Dimcheff DE, Blumberg N et al. Health care-associated infection after red blood cell transfusion: a systematic review and meta-analysis. JAMA 2014;**311**:1317–26.

14 Van de Watering LMG, Hermans J, Houbiers JGA et al. Beneficial effects of leukocyte depletion of transfused blood on postoperative complications in patients undergoing cardiac surgery – a randomized clinical trial. Circulation 1998;**97**:562–8.

15 Blumberg N, Heal JM, Murphy P et al. Association between transfusion of whole blood and recurrence of cancer. BMJ 1986;**293**:530–3.

16 Blajchman MA, Bardossy L, Carmen R, Sastry A, Singal DP. Allogeneic blood transfusion-induced enhancement of tumor growth: two animal models showing amelioration by leukodepletion and passive transfer using spleen cells. Blood 1993;**81**:1880–2.

17 Jensen LS, Puho E, Pedersen L, Mortensen FV, Sorensen HT. Long-term survival after colorectal surgery associated with buffy-coat-poor and leukocyte-depleted blood transfusion: a follow-up study. Lancet 2005;**365**:681–2.

18 Heiss MM, Mempel W, Delanoff C et al. Blood transfusion-modulated tumor recurrence: first results of a randomized study of autologous versus allogeneic blood transfusion in colorectal cancer surgery. J Clin Oncol 1994;**12**:1859–67.

19 Cholette JM, Pietropaoli AP, Henrichs KF et al. Longer RBC storage duration is associated with increased postoperative infections in pediatric cardiac surgery. Pediatr Crit Care Med 2015;**16**:227–35.

20 Blumberg N, Heal JM, Rowe JM. A randomized trial of washed red blood cell and platelet transfusions in adult acute leukemia [ISRCTN76536440]. BMC Blood Disord 2004;**4**:6.

Further Reading

Blumberg N. Deleterious clinical effects of transfusion immunomodulation: proven beyond a reasonable doubt. Transfusion 2005;**45**:33S–9S; discussion 9S–40S.

Cholette JM, Henrichs KF, Alfieris GM et al. Washing red blood cells and platelets transfused in cardiac surgery reduces postoperative inflammation and number of transfusions: results of a prospective, randomized, controlled clinical trial. Pediatr Crit Care Med 2012;**13**:290–9.

Hart S, Cserti-Gazdewich CM, McCluskey SA. Red cell transfusion and the immune system. Anaesthesia 2015;**70**(Suppl. 1):38–45, e13–16.

Lannan K, Sahler J, Spinelli SL, Phipps RP, Blumberg N. Transfusion immunomodulation – the case for leukoreduced and (perhaps) washed transfusions. Blood Cells Mol Dis 2013;**50**:61–8.

Muszynski JA, Frazier E, Nofziger R et al. Red blood cell transfusion and immune function in critically ill children: a prospective observational study. Transfusion 2015;**55**(4):766–74.

Refaai MA, Blumberg N. The transfusion dilemma – weighing the known and newly proposed risks of blood transfusions against the uncertain benefits. Best Pract Res Clin Anaesthesiol 2013;**27**:17–35.

Solomon SB, Wang D, Sun J et al. Mortality increases after massive exchange transfusion with older stored blood in canines with experimental pneumonia. Blood 2013;**121**:1663–72.

Stolla M, Refaai MA, Heal JM et al. Platelet transfusion – the new immunology of an old therapy. Front Immunol 2015;**6**:28.

Teng Z, Zhu Y, Liu Y et al. Restrictive blood transfusion strategies and associated infection in orthopaedic patients: a meta-analysis of 8 randomized controlled trials. Sci Rep 2015;**5**:13421.

Torrance HD, Brohi K, Pearse RM et al. Association between gene expression biomarkers of immunosuppression and blood transfusion in severely injured polytrauma patients. Ann Surg 2015;**261**:751–9.

13 Transfusion-Associated Graft-Versus-Host Disease and Microchimerism

Beth H. Shaz[1,2], Richard O. Francis[2] and Christopher D. Hillyer[1,3]

[1] New York Blood Center, New York, USA
[2] Columbia University College of Physicians and Surgeons; Special Hematology and Coagulation Laboratory
New York Presbyterian Hospital – Columbia University Medical Center, New York, USA
[3] Weill Cornell Medical College, New York, USA

Transfusion-Associated Graft-Versus-Host Disease

Transfusion-associated graft-versus-host disease (TA-GVHD) is an uncommon yet highly fatal complication of cellular blood component transfusion; cellular components are defined as red blood cell, platelet and granulocyte components (not frozen plasma). TA-GVHD is defined by the UK Serious Hazards of Transfusion (SHOT) haemovigilance system as fever, rash, liver dysfunction, diarrhoea, pancytopenia and bone marrow hypoplasia occurring less than 30 days after transfusion, without other apparent cause. Similarly, the US National Healthcare Safety Network Biovigilance system definition for definitive diagnosis is fever, rash, hepatomegaly, diarrhoea between two days and six weeks after transfusion with laboratory evidence of liver dysfunction, pancytopenia, marrow aplasia, leucocyte chimerism and findings of TA-GVHD on skin or liver biopsy.

Development of TA-GVHD requires the product to contain immunologically competent lymphocytes and the recipient must express tissue antigens absent in the donor and not mount an effective immune response to destroy the foreign lymphocytes. Cellular blood products contain viable lymphocytes that can proliferate and result in TA-GVHD. Inactivation of these lymphocytes, usually through irradiation, prevents TA-GVHD. The identification of individuals at high risk for TA-GVHD, such as immune-impaired patients or those receiving products from blood relatives, and the subsequent requirement that these individuals receive irradiated products, reduces the incidence of TA-GVHD, but its elimination may require universal irradiation or lymphocyte inactivation of all cellular blood components.

Pathogenesis

Transfusion-associated graft-versus-host disease results from the engraftment of transfused donor T-lymphocytes in a recipient whose immune system does not reject them. The mechanism of TA-GVHD is similar to that of acute GVHD after haemopoietic stem cell (HSC) transplantation. Donor T-lymphocytes recognise recipient HLA antigens as foreign, resulting in activation and proliferation of the lymphocytes, which leads to host cell death and tissue destruction.

Clinical Features

Transfusion-associated graft-versus-host disease is an acute illness characterised by fever, rash, pancytopenia, diarrhoea and liver dysfunction which begins 4–30 days (median 8–10 days) after transfusion and results in death within three weeks from symptom onset in over 90% of the cases [1]. In neonates the clinical manifestations are similar, yet the interval between transfusion and onset is longer; the median time of onset of fever is 28 days, rash 30 days and death 51 days [2]. In the typical scenario, fever is the presenting symptom followed by an erythematous maculopapular rash, which begins on the face and trunk and spreads to the extremities. Liver dysfunction manifests as an obstructive jaundice or an acute hepatitis. Gastrointestinal complications include nausea, anorexia or diarrhoea. Leucopenia and pancytopenia, the primary reasons for death due to sepsis, candidiasis and multiorgan failure, develop later and progressively become more severe.

Diagnosis

The diagnosis of TA-GVHD is based on the characteristic clinical manifestations, pathological findings on tissue biopsy and, if possible, evidence of donor-derived lymphocytes in the recipient's blood or affected tissues. Laboratory data demonstrate pancytopenia and abnormal liver function tests. Skin biopsy changes include epidermal basal cell vacuolisation and mononuclear cell infiltration. Liver biopsy findings include degeneration of the small bile ducts, periportal mononuclear infiltrates and cholestasis. The bone marrow is usually hypocellular or aplastic, which is the primary differentiating feature between TA-GVHD and GVHD occurring after HSC transplantation. The discovery of donor lymphocytes or DNA in the patient's peripheral blood or tissue biopsy with the appropriate clinical scenario confirms the diagnosis. Donor-derived DNA is usually detected using polymerase chain reaction (PCR)-based HLA typing; other methods include the use of amplified fragment length polymorphisms, variable–number tandem repeat analysis, short tandem repeat analysis, microsatellite markers and cytogenetics.

Treatment

Most treatments of TA-GVHD are largely ineffective, including aggressive use of corticosteroids, antithymocyte globulin, ciclosporin and growth factors. However, spontaneous resolution and successful treatment with a combination of ciclosporin, steroids and OKT3 (anti-CD3 monoclonal antibody) or antithymocyte globulin have been reported. Transient improvement has been seen with nafamostat mesilate, a serine protease inhibitor that inhibits cytotoxic T-lymphocytes. There are case reports of successful treatment with autologous or allogeneic HSC transplantation.

Prevention

Since treatment options for TA-GVHD are mostly unsuccessful, patients at increased risk must be identified and transfused with lymphocyte-inactivated products, usually by γ-irradiation or pathogen inactivation technologies. Properly installed and maintained radioisotope instruments are safe, but their use requires appropriate security, radiation safety protocols and training (in the USA, blood irradiators are regulated by the Nuclear Regulatory Commission). Some pathogen reduction technologies have been shown in human clinical trials, mouse models and other lymphocyte proliferation assays to inactivate T-lymphocytes (Table 13.1). γ-Irradiation is the most common method used for irradiation to prevent TA-GVHD; in Europe the use of pathogen inactivation for platelets is growing, and irradiation by x-ray generated by linear acceleration is increasing in the USA and other locations as a nonradionuclide source.

Source and Dose of Ionising Radiation

Both γ-rays and x-rays inactivate T-lymphocytes and can be used to irradiate blood components. Usually γ–rays originate from caesium-137 or cobalt-60 while x-rays are generated from linear accelerators. Quality assurance measures should be performed, including dose mapping, adjustment of irradiation time to correct for isotopic

Table 13.1 Potential methods for leucocyte inactivation.

Method	Leucocyte inactivation
Ultraviolet B	Inhibits TA-GVHD in dog transfusion model
8-Methoxypsoralen with UV	Inhibits activation and proliferation
Aminomethyl trimethylpsoralen with UVA	Inhibits activation and proliferation
Amotosalen (S-59) with UVA	Inhibits activation and proliferation
	Inhibits TA-GVHD in murine transfusion model
Methylene blue with light	Does not inactivate leucocytes
Dimethylmethylene blue with light	No data on leucocyte inactivation
Riboflavin with UV	Inhibits proliferation
Inactine (PEN 110)	Inhibits TA-GVHD in murine transfusion model
	Inhibits activation and proliferation
Thionine with UVB Ultraviolet C	Inhibits proliferation Inhibits activation and proliferation [3]

Source: Corash and Lin 2004. Adapted with permission from Nature Publishing Group. Novel processes for inactivation of leukocytes to prevent transfusion-associated graft-versus-host disease. Bone Marrow Transplant 2004;**33**:1–7.

decay, assurance of no radiation leakage, timer accuracy, turntable operation, preventive maintenance and a qualitative indicator label to confirm that blood products have been properly irradiated.

The dose of irradiation must be sufficient to inhibit lymphocyte proliferation but not significantly damage red cells, platelets and granulocytes or their functions. Assays to assess the effect of irradiation on T-lymphocyte proliferation include mixed lymphocyte culture (MLC) assay and limiting dilution analysis (LDA). The recommended dose varies between 15 and 50 Gy (Table 13.2). Of note, there have been three patients transfused with irradiated blood products, two at doses of 20 Gy [4,5] and one at 15 Gy [6], who developed TA-GVHD, but it is unknown if there was a process or dose failure.

Adverse Effects of Irradiation

At recommended doses, radiation causes some oxidation and damage to lipid components of membranes, which continues during storage. Products irradiated immediately prior to transfusion appear to be unaffected and have virtually normal function. In stored products, radiation modestly harms red cells, but does not appear to affect platelet and granulocyte function significantly in the clinically utilised doses. The effects on red cells include an increase in extracellular potassium and a decrease in posttransfusion red cell survival [7]. The increase in extracellular potassium is usually not of clinical significance because of posttransfusion dilution of the potassium. However, there may be certain patients who are sensitive to the increased potassium resulting in transfusion-associated hyperkalaemia, such as fetuses receiving intrauterine transfusions (IUT), premature infants, infants receiving large red cell volumes and neonates undergoing exchange transfusions or intracardiac transfusions via central line catheters. Irradiating the red cell product within 24 hours of infusion can prevent the potassium increase. Also red cell products stored in additive solutions have lower extracellular potassium than CPDA-1 units of a similar age. As a consequence, red cell product outdate is variably shortened to 14–28 days after irradiation (see Table 13.2).

Blood Component Factors

Age of Blood

Use of fresh blood increases the risk of TA-GVHD. A Japanese series of cases of TA-GVHD in immunocompetent patients found that 62% of patients had received blood less than 72 hours old [1] and a US series found about 90% of cases received blood less than four days old [11]. The increased risk of fresh blood is possibly due to

Table 13.2 Comparison of irradiation guidelines, including dose and indications.

	UK [8]	USA [9]	Japan [10]
Techniques	γ-Irradiation or x-rays	γ-Irradiation or x-rays	γ-Irradiation
Dose	Minimum 2500 cGy	2500 cGy at centre of product	Between 1500 and 5000 cGy
	No part >5000 cGy	Minimum 1500 cGy at any point	
		Maximum 5000 cGy	
Type of product	All cellular products: Whole blood Red cells Platelets Granulocytes	All cellular products: Whole blood Red cells Platelets Granulocytes	All cellular products: Whole blood Red cells Platelets Granulocytes Fresh plasma
Age of product	Red cells <14 days after collection For hyperkalaemia risk, e.g. exchange or intrauterine transfusion: <24 h before transfusion Platelets – any time during 5 day storage	Red cells – any time Platelets – any time	Red cells – ≤3 days – regardless of recipient ≤14 days – if clinically indicated At any time – if patient immunocompromised
Expiry	Red cells stored for 14 days after irradiation	Red cells stored for up to 28 days after irradiation or original outdate, whichever is sooner	Irradiated red cells – up to 3 weeks after collection
General	All blood from relatives All HLA-selected products All granulocytes	All blood from relatives All HLA-selected products	All blood from relatives All HLA-selected products
Neonates	Intrauterine transfusions Exchange transfusions in IUT babies	IUT	All
Congenital immunodeficiency	All	All	All
Allogeneic HSC transplantation	All – at least 6 months post BMT; longer in selected patients	All	All
Autologous HSC transplantation	All – at least 3 months post BMT; 6 months if TBI used		
Leukaemia	No	*	To be considered
Hodgkin's disease	All stages	*	To be considered
Purine analogues	All	*	Not discussed
Non-Hodgkin's lymphoma	Not discussed	*	To be considered
Solid tumours	No	*	To be considered
Solid organ transplants	No	*	To be considered
Cardiovascular surgery	No	No	Yes
AIDS	No	No	No

* According to policies and procedures developed by the blood transfusion laboratory or blood supplier.
AIDS, acquired immune deficiency syndrome; BMT, bone marrow transplant; HLA, human leucocyte antigen; HSC, haemopoietic stem cell; IUT, intrauterine transfusion; TBI, total body irradiation.

the function and viability of lymphocytes as during storage these cells undergo apoptosis and fail to stimulate an MLC response.

Leucocyte Dose

Leucocyte reduction of blood components may decrease the risk of TA-GVHD, but it does not eliminate it. SHOT data reported a decrease in the number of TA-GVHD cases following universal leucocyte reduction of blood components in the UK in 1999 [12].

Blood Components

All cellular blood components, including red cells, platelets, granulocytes, whole blood and fresh plasma (not frozen plasma), contain viable T-lymphocytes that are capable of causing TA-GVHD (see Table 13.2). Granulocyte transfusions are the highest risk product because they have a high lymphocyte count and are administered fresh to neutropenic and immunosuppressed patients. Therefore, it is recommended that all granulocyte products undergo irradiation prior to transfusion and the remaining cellular blood components be irradiated for patients at increased risk.

Patients at Increased Risk

Patient populations have varying risk factors for developing TA-GVHD (Box 13.1). It is difficult to quantify any of these risks because the number of these patients, the number who are transfused and the number of transfusions or type of products received are unknown. The risk is therefore derived from case reports or haemovigilance data, which are biased by underrecognition, misdiagnosis and under- and passive reporting.

Congenital Immunodeficiency Patients

The first reported cases of TA-GVHD occurred in the 1960s in children with T-lymphocyte congenital immunodeficiency syndromes. Children with severe congenital immunodeficiency syndromes (SCID) and with variable immunodeficiency syndromes, such as Wiskott–Aldrich and DiGeorge syndromes, have developed TA-GVHD. These

---

Box 13.1 Indications for irradiated cellular blood components to prevent TA-GVHD.

Clear indications

Congenital immunodeficiency syndromes (suspected or known)
Allogeneic and autologous haemopoietic progenitor cell transplantation
Transfusions from blood relatives
HLA-matched or partially HLA-matched products (platelet transfusions)
Granulocyte transfusions
Hodgkin's disease
Treatment with purine analogue drugs (fludarabine, cladribine and deoxycoformycin)
Treatment with Campath (anti-CD52) and other drugs/antibodies that affect T-lymphocyte number or function
Intrauterine transfusions

Indications deemed appropriate by most authorities

Neonatal exchange transfusions
Preterm/low-birthweight infants
Infant/child with congenital heart disease (secondary to possible DiGeorge syndrome)
Acute leukaemia
Non-Hodgkin's lymphoma and other haematological malignancies
Aplastic anaemia
Solid tumours receiving intensive chemotherapy and/or radiotherapy
Recipient and donor pair from a genetically homogeneous population

Indications unsupported by most authorities

Solid organ transplantation
Healthy newborns/term infants
HIV/AIDS

---

children may be transfused prior to the recognition of these immunodeficiency syndromes. Because of the possibility of the patient not being known to be immunodeficient, it may be prudent to irradiate all blood components for children under a certain age. This is particularly true with infants undergoing cardiac surgery who may have unrecognised DiGeorge syndrome. It is recommended that all patients with suspected or confirmed congenital immunodeficiency receive irradiated products.

Allogeneic and Autologous HSC Recipients

Both allogeneic and autologous HSC transplant recipients are at increased risk of TA-GVHD. Patients who undergo allogeneic HSC transplantation have received irradiated blood products routinely for over 40 years. Many organisations in Europe and the United States recommend irradiated blood products for allogeneic and autologous HSC recipients, but it is unclear for how long before and after transplantation these patients require irradiated blood products.

Leukaemia and Lymphoma Patients

Patients with haematological malignancies are at increased risk for TA-GVHD, especially patients with Hodgkin's disease (HD). Twenty cases were reported in patients with malignant lymphoma, 13 in association with HD and seven with non-Hodgkin's lymphoma (NHL), and all undergoing therapy for active disease at the time. Five of 13 cases reported to SHOT were associated with haematological malignancies (Table 13.3). In the 1970s and 1980s, cases of TA-GVHD occurred in patients with acute leukaemia undergoing chemotherapy; the majority of these patients had received granulocyte transfusions. It is recommended that patients with haematological malignancies receive irradiated products; however, it is less clear if this requirement should be only during active treatment.

Recipients of Fludarabine and Other Purine Analogues as well as Other Drugs/Antibodies That Affect T-Lymphocyte Number or Function

Transfusion-associated graft-versus-host disease was initially reported in patients with chronic lymphocytic leukaemia (CLL) receiving fludarabine, a purine analogue that results in profound lymphopenia. There are nine cases of TA-GVHD in CLL, acute myeloid leukaemia (AML) and NHL patients who received fludarabine up to 11 months prior to transfusion. Other purine analogues, including deoxycoformycin (pentostatin) and chlorodeoxyadenosine (cladribine), have been associated with the development of TA-GVHD. Thus, it is recommended that all patients who have received fludarabine or other purine analogues as well as Campath (anti-CD52) or other drugs/antibodies that affect T-lymphocyte function or number be transfused with irradiated products; however, it is unclear if this requirement should only be for at least one year and until recovery from the resulting lymphopenia following the administration of these drugs.

Fetus and Neonate

Fetuses and neonates have immature immune systems and may be at increased risk of TA-GVHD. In neonates, most cases of TA-GVHD reported are in those with congenital immunodeficiency or who received products from related donors. At least 10 cases have been reported after neonatal exchange transfusions; four occurred in infants who had previously received IUT. Seven cases were in preterm infants (excluding those who received a product from a relative). The use of irradiated products for fetal and neonatal transfusions is recommended for exchange transfusions and IUT, preterm infants, infants with congenital immunodeficiency and those receiving products from relatives; its need is less clear for other neonatal transfusions.

Patients with Aplastic Anaemia

Since patients with aplastic anaemia are usually treated with intensive chemotherapy regimens and possible HSC transplantation, some authorities recommend they receive irradiated products, especially during myelosuppressive therapy or treatment with antithymocyte globulin.

Patients Receiving Chemotherapy and Immunotherapy

Transfusion-associated graft-versus-host disease has occurred in patients with solid tumours, including neuroblastoma, rhabdomyosarcoma

Table 13.3 Cases of TA-GVHD reported to SHOT 1996–2014.*

Year	Number of cases	Case	Diagnosis and/or possible risk factor	Red cells and/or platelets leucodepletion	Donor–recipient HLA haplotype share
1996–1997	4	1	Immunodeficient neonate, not diagnosed at time of transfusion	No	Reported as haplotype share; no other details provided
		2	Epistaxis, age 88	No	NK
		3	B-cell NHL	No	NK
		4	B-cell NHL	No	NK
1997–1998	4	5	Waldenstrom's macroglobulinaemia	No	Donor reported as homozygous; no other details provided; patient's HLA type not determined
		6	B-cell NHL	No	Yes; donor homozygous: A1; B8; DR17 Patient: A1, A31; B7, B8, Bw6; Cw7; DR17; DQ2
		7	CABG, red cells less than 3 days old	No	Yes; donor homozygous: A*01; B*0801; DRB1*0301
		8	ITP, treated with prednisolone	No	NK
1998–1999	4	9	Myeloma, 6 units of red cells, all less than 7 days old	Yes	NK
		10	Male, age 53; uncharacterised immunodeficiency; HIV negative	No	NK; 100% XX cells in marrow
		11	CABG, also received platelets	No	NK (32 donors)
		12	CABG	No	Donor homozygous: A*01; B*0801; Cw*0701/06/07; DRB1*0301; DQB1*0201/02 Patient: A*01, A 3301/03; B*0801, B*14202/03; Cw 0701/06/07; Cw 0802; DRB1 0301; DRB1 0701/03; DQB1 03032/06; DQB1 0201/02
1999–2000	0				
2000–2001	1	13	Relapsed ALL on UKALL R2. Died despite 'rescue' HSC allograft	Yes	NK; chimerism shown by variable number tandem repeat analysis but no donor HLA typing performed
2012–	1	14	Infant receiving IUT with nonirradiated maternal blood	No	NK
Total	**14**				

* No cases were reported from 2002 through 2011 and 2013–14.

ALL, acute lymphocytic leukaemia; CABG, coronary artery bypass grafting; HLA, human leucocyte antigen; HSC, haemopoietic stem cell; ITP, immune thrombocytopenia; IUT, intrauterine transfusion; NHL, non-Hodgkin's lymphoma; NK, not known.

Source: Reprinted with permission from Williamson et al. [12]. Reproduced with permission of John Wiley and Sons.

and bladder and small cell lung cancer, during intensive myeloablative therapy. Therefore, it is recommended that patients with solid tumours receive irradiated products during myelosuppressive therapy.

Solid Organ Transplantation Recipients

Graft-versus-host disease is a rare complication of solid organ transplantation, which usually results from the passenger lymphocytes contained within the solid organ and not from transfusion, even though these individuals are highly immunosuppressed and transfused. There have been five cases of TA-GVHD in recipients of solid organs, including liver, heart and inconclusive cases in kidney transplant recipients. The risk of TA-GVHD in solid organ transplant recipients appears low and the use of irradiated products is generally considered to be unwarranted.

Human Immunodeficiency Virus (HIV) and Acquired Immunodeficiency Syndrome (AIDS) Patients

HIV/AIDS is not considered a risk factor for TA-GVHD as there is only a single case report of a child with AIDS developing transient TA-GVHD. The use of irradiated blood products in HIV/AIDS patients is not warranted.

Immunocompetent Patients

Transfusion-associated graft-versus-host disease has been reported in immunocompetent patients, especially those who received transfusions of blood products donated by close relatives [13], most likely leading to a one-way haplotype match in which the donor was homozygous for a haplotype for which the recipient was heterozygous, allowing donor lymphocytes to evade immune detection yet still respond to donor tissue. The risk of receiving a blood product from a homozygous donor is greatest in populations with limited HLA haplotype polymorphisms, such as Japan [14] (Table 13.4). A recent systematic review of 348 TA-GVHD cases found that the majority of the cases involved transfusions in immunocompetent patients, with cellular blood components stored for ≤10 days, and a donor HLA profile lacking identifiably foreign antigen types compared to the recipient [15], demonstrating the importance of viable lymphocytes that are able to evade immune detection in causing TA-GVHD. Irradiation of products from close relatives and HLA-matched products is recommended, but the risk is minimal for other immunocompetent patients.

Guidelines and Requirements for Irradiated Products

The American Society for Clinical Pathology and the British Committee for Standards in

Table 13.4 Frequency of transfusion from homozygous donors to potential heterozygous recipients.

Population	Parent/child	Sibling	Unrelated
Japan	1:102	1:193	1:874
Canada Whites	1:154	1:294	1:1664
Germany	1:220	1:424	1:3144
Korea	1:183	1:356	1:3220
Spain	1:226	1:438	1:3552
South African Blacks	1:286	1:558	1:5519
US Whites	1:475	1:920	1:7174
Italy	1:434	1:854	1:12 870
France	1:762	1:2685	1:16 835

Haematology [8] published guidelines for the use of irradiation to prevent TA-GVHD. Japan has elected to irradiate all blood products [10]. In 2014, College of American Pathologists (CAP) members were surveyed about their blood product irradiation practices [16]. The most frequent indications for blood product irradiation were transfusion from blood relatives (78.6%), HLA-matched or partially matched products (68.9%), neonatal exchange transfusions (66.3%), IUT (63.3%), HSC transplant (62.7%) and preterm/low-birthweight infants (61.8%). While these patients are generally considered at risk for TA-GVHD, it was noted that several patient populations not considered at risk, including patients with HIV/AIDS (19.5%) and autoimmune disorders (17.5%), are included in organisations' irradiation policies. These results suggest that irradiation practices remain heterogeneous and that continued efforts to standardise irradiation practices are warranted.

Universal Irradiation

As case reports cited above indicate, TA-GVHD can occur in immunocompetent patients and individuals where the degree of immunocompromise was not known or properly identified prior to transfusion. Given that TA-GVHD is fatal in almost all cases and the risk of radiation of a product includes only minimal cost and effect on product potency, many authorities are in favour of universal irradiation. Consideration of universal irradiation should be undertaken on a local, regional or national basis, as appropriate.

Haemovigilance

Some countries have begun comprehensive tracking systems for adverse events of blood transfusion (Chapter 19). The continued occurrence of TA-GVHD is likely to arise from lack of agreement on the level of immunodeficiency that results in increased risk and patients with

immunocompromised conditions who receive nonirradiated products either because they are not being identified prior to transfusion or the product is not being irradiated by error. On the other hand, the low incidence reported may be secondary to underreporting and/or under-recognition, the fact that lymphocytes are no longer capable of proliferating because the blood is older by the time of transfusion, or decreasing risk due to leucocyte reduction of blood products and the genetic heterogeneity of many populations.

Transfusion-Associated Microchimerism

Chimerism is defined as the presence of two genetically distinct cell lines in a single organism. Haemopoietic chimerism refers to the persistence of allogeneic donor lymphocytes in a recipient. Microchimerism (MC) occurs when these donor cells represent a small population (less than 5%) and can be a consequence of pregnancy, organ transplantation or transfusion.

Clinical Data

Transfusion-associated MC has been reported mostly in trauma patients [17], but has also been reported in sickle cell disease and thalassaemia patients. Irradiation of products prevents TA-MC. Leucocyte reduction of blood products alone does not decrease the incidence of TA-MC among trauma patients [18]. In addition, TA-MC can be sustained for decades after transfusion [19]. When patients were evaluated for symptoms suggestive of chronic GVHD several months after transfusion, TA-MC did not correlate with these symptoms. One study reported a decrease in donor-specific lymphocyte response in TA-MC trauma patients versus non-TA-MC patients [20]. To date, no clear relationship of TA-MC to clinical outcomes has been elucidated.

KEY POINTS

1) TA-GVHD is a rare yet highly fatal complication of cellular blood component transfusion.
2) TA-GVHD can be prevented by using irradiated or leucocyte-inactivated blood components.
3) Patients at increased risk for TA-GVHD include those who are immune impaired and those receiving blood components donated from blood relatives.
4) Leucocyte dose and age of the blood component, HLA matching between the donor and the recipient and immune state of the recipi-

ent contribute to the likelihood of developing TA-GVHD.

5) While there are strong data for providing irradiated blood components to prevent TA-GVHD in some patient populations, the need for irradiation in other disease states is less clear (refer to Box 13.1).
6) Microchimerism can be detected after transfusion, but the conditions that facilitate it and its clinical consequences are unknown.

References

1 Ohto H, Anderson KC. Survey of transfusion associated graft-versus-host disease in immunocompetent recipients. Transfus Med Rev 1996;**10**:31–43.

2 Ohto H, Anderson KC. Posttransfusion graft-versus-host disease in Japanese newborns. Transfusion 1996;**36**:117–23.

3 Pohler P, Muller M, Winkler C et al. Pathogen reduction by ultraviolet C light effectively inactivates human white blood cells in platelet products. Transfusion 2015;**55**:337–47.

4 Drobyski S, Thibodeau S, Truitt RL et al. Third-party mediated graft rejection and graft-versus-host disease after T-cell-depleted bone marrow transplantation, as demonstrated by hypervariable DNA probes and HLA-DR polymorphism. Blood 1989;**74**:2285–94.

5 Sproul AM, Chalmers EA, Mills KI et al. Third party mediated graft rejection despite irradiation of blood products. Br J Haematol 1992;**80**:251–2.

6 Lowenthal RM, Challis DR, Griffiths AE et al. Transfusion-associated graft-versus-host disease: report of an occurrence following the administration of irradiated blood. Transfusion 1993;**33**:524–9.

7 Davey RJ, McCoy NC, Yu M et al. The effect of prestorage irradiation on posttransfusion red cell survival. Transfusion 1992;**32**:525–8.

8 Treleaven J, Gennery A, Marsh J et al. Guidelines on the use of irradiated blood components prepared by the British committee for standards in haematology blood transfusion task force. Br J Haematol 2011;**152**:35–51.

9 Fung MK (ed.). Technical Manual, 18th edn. AABB, Press, Bethesda, 2014, pp.687–89.

10 Asai T, Inaba S, Ohto H et al. Guidelines for irradiation of blood and blood components to prevent posttransfusion graft-vs-host disease in Japan. Transfus Med 2000;**10**:315–20.

11 Petz LD, Calhoun L, Yam P et al. Transfusion-associated graft-versus-host disease in immunocompetent patients: report of a fatal case associated with transfusion of blood from a second-degree relative, and a survey of predisposing factors. Transfusion 1993;**33**:742–50.

12 Williamson LM, Stainsby D, Jones H et al. The impact of universal leukodepletion of the blood supply on hemovigilance reports of posttransfusion purpura and transfusion-associated graft-versus-host disease. Transfusion 2007;**47**:1455–67.

13 Agbaht K, Altintas ND, Topeli A et al. Transfusion associated graft-versus-host disease in immunocompetent patients: case series and review of the literature. Transfusion 2007;**47**:1405–11.

14 Ohto H, Yasuda H, Noguchi M et al. Risk of transfusion associated graft-versus-host disease as a result of directed donations from relatives. Transfusion 1992;**32**:691–3.

15 Kopolovic I, Ostro J, Tsubota H et al. A systematic review of transfusion-associated graft-versus-host disease. Blood 2015;**126**:406–14.

16 Pritchard AE, Shaz BH. Survey of irradiation practice for the prevention of transfusion-associated graft-versus-host disease. Arch Pathol Lab Med 2016;**140**:1092–7.

17 Utter GH, Owings JT, Lee TH et al. Blood transfusion is associated with donor leukocyte microchimerism in trauma patients. J Trauma 2004;**57**:702–8.

18 Utter GH, Nathens AB, Lee TH et al. Leukoreduction of blood transfusions does not diminish transfusionassociated microchimerism in trauma patients. Transfusion 2006;**46**:1863–9.

19 Utter GH, Lee TZ, Rivers RM et al. Microchimerism decades after transfusion among combat-injured US veterans from the Vietnam, Korean, World War II conflicts. Transfusion 2008;**48**:1609–15.

20 Utter GH, Owings JT, Lee TZ et al. Microchimerism in transfused trauma patients is associated with diminished donor-specific lymphocyte response. J Trauma 2005;**58**:925–32.

Further Reading

Bloch EM, Jackman RP, Lee TH, Busch MP. Transfusion-associated microchimerism: the hybrid within. Transfus Med Rev 2013;**27**:10–20.

Corash L, Lin L. Novel processes for inactivation of leukocytes to prevent transfusion-associated graft-versus-host disease. Bone Marrow Transplant 2004;**33**:1–7.

Hume HA, Preiksaitis JB. Transfusion associated graft-versus-host disease, cytomegalovirus infection and HLA alloimmunization in neonatal and pediatric patients. Transfus Sci 1999;**21**:73–95.

Marschner S, Fast LD, Baldwin WM et al. White blood cell inactivation after treatment with riboflavin and ultraviolet light. Transfusion 2010;**50**:2489–98.

Mintz PD, Wehrli G. Irradiation eradication and pathogen reduction. Ceasing cesium irradiation of blood products. Bone Marrow Transplant 2009;**44**:205–11.

Moroff G, Luban NLC. The irradiation of blood and blood components to prevent graft-versus-host disease: technical issues and guidelines. Transfus Med Rev 1997;**11**:15–26.

Ruhl H, Bein G, Sachs UJH. Transfusion-associated graft-versus-host disease. Transfus Med Rev 2009;**23**:62–71.

Triulzi DJ, Nalesnik MA. Microchimerism, GVHD, and tolerance in solid organ transplantation. Transfusion 2001;**41**:419–26.

14 Posttransfusion Purpura

Michael F. Murphy

University of Oxford, NHS Blood and Transplant and Department of Haematology, Oxford University Hospitals, Oxford, UK

Introduction

In 1959, van Loghem and colleagues described a 51-year-old woman who developed severe thrombocytopenia seven days after elective surgery [1]. The thrombocytopenia did not respond to transfusion of fresh blood, but there was a spontaneous recovery after three weeks. The patient's serum contained a strong platelet alloantibody, which enabled the description of the first human platelet antigen (HPA) (Zw, see Chapter 5). However, the relationship of platelet alloimmunisation to posttransfusion thrombocytopenia was not recognised until two years later when Shulman and colleagues studied a similar case, naming the antibody anti-Pl^{A1} (later shown to be the same as anti-Zw), and coined the term posttransfusion purpura (PTP) [2].

Definition

Posttransfusion purpura is an acute episode of severe thrombocytopenia occurring about a week after a blood transfusion. It usually affects HPA-1a-negative women who have previously been alloimmunised by pregnancy. The transfusion precipitating PTP causes a secondary immune response, boosting the HPA-1a antibodies, although the mechanism of destruction of the patient's own HPA-1a-negative platelets remains uncertain.

Incidence

Posttransfusion purpura is considered to be a rare complication of transfusion. Only around 200 cases had been reported in the literature up to 1991 [3]. However, this may not reflect the true incidence of PTP, which is not known except through reporting to haemovigilance schemes. Thirty seven cases were reported in the first four years of the Serious Hazards of Transfusion (SHOT) scheme during which approximately 13 million blood components were transfused, giving an approximate incidence of one case in 350 000 transfusions. In the following 13 years, after the introduction of universal leucocyte reduction of blood components in the UK, only 19 cases were reported to SHOT, giving an approximate incidence of one in 2 million blood components transfused [4]. A recent study of elderly patients (65 years and older) in the United States found a PTP incidence of 1.8 in 100 000 inpatient admissions [5]. Significantly higher odds of PTP were found with platelet-containing transfusion events and with greater number of units transfused.

The low incidence of PTP relative to the 2.1% of the population who are HPA-1a negative and at risk of the condition raises the question of individual susceptibility. As in neonatal alloimmune thrombocytopenia (NAIT), the antibody response to HPA-1a is strongly associated with a certain HLA class II type (HLA-DRB3*0101) (see Chapter 5).

Practical Transfusion Medicine, Fifth Edition. Edited by Michael F. Murphy, David J. Roberts and Mark H. Yazer.
© 2017 John Wiley & Sons Ltd. Published 2017 by John Wiley & Sons Ltd.

Clinical Features

Posttransfusion purpura typically occurs in middle-aged or elderly women (mean 57 years, range 21–80), although it has also been found in males [5,6]. All patients, apart from rare exceptions, have had previous exposure to platelet antigens through pregnancy and/or transfusion. The interval between pregnancy and/or transfusion and PTP is variable, the shortest being three years and the longest 52 years. The initial maternal sensitisation to platelet antigens during pregnancy in females subsequently developing PTP is rarely of sufficient degree to cause NAIT.

Blood components implicated in causing PTP are:

- whole blood
- packed red cells
- red cell concentrates
- platelet concentrates.

There are occasional case reports of PTP following the transfusion of plasma, presumably due to the presence of platelet particles expressing platelet antigens [6].

Severe thrombocytopenia and bleeding usually occur about 5–12 days after transfusion; shorter or longer intervals are rare. The onset is usually rapid, with the platelet count falling from normal to $<10 \times 10^9$/L within 12–24 hours. Haemorrhage is very common and sometimes severe. There is typically widespread purpura and bleeding from mucous membranes and the gastrointestinal and urinary tracts. In many cases, the precipitating transfusion has been associated with a febrile nonhaemolytic transfusion reaction, probably due to the presence of coexisting HLA antibodies stimulated by previous pregnancy and/or transfusion.

Megakaryocytes are present in normal or increased numbers in the bone marrow and coagulation screening tests are normal in uncomplicated PTP.

In untreated cases the thrombocytopenia usually lasts between seven and 28 days, although it occasionally persists for longer.

Differential Diagnosis

The rapid onset of severe thrombocytopenia in a middle-aged or elderly woman should arouse suspicion of PTP and a history of recent blood transfusion should be sought. The differential diagnosis includes other causes of acute immune thrombocytopenia such as:

- autoimmune thrombocytopenia
- drug-induced thrombocytopenia, such as heparin-induced thrombocytopenia (HIT) (see Chapter 31)
- nonimmune platelet consumption, for example disseminated intravascular coagulation (DIC) and thrombotic thrombocytopenic purpura (TTP)
- a less likely possibility is passively transfused platelet-specific alloantibodies from an immunised blood donor when thrombocytopenia occurs within the first 48 hours after the transfusion [7,8]
- pseudothrombocytopenia due to ethylenediamine tetra-acetic acid (EDTA)-dependent antibodies should be excluded in any patient with unexplained thrombocytopenia by examination of the blood film.

Laboratory Investigations

A preliminary diagnosis of PTP on clinical grounds needs to be confirmed by the detection of platelet-specific alloantibodies. The majority (80–90%) of cases of PTP are associated with the development of HPA-1a antibodies in HPA-1a-negative patients [6,9]. Antibodies against HPA-1b, HPA-3a, HPA-3b, HPA-4a, HPA-5a, HPA-5b, HPA-15b and Nak^a have been associated with PTP, and occasionally multiple antibodies are present, for example anti-HPA-1a, anti-HPA-2b and anti-HPA-3a were found in one case.

Human leucocyte antigen antibodies are often present in patients with PTP. There is no evidence that they are involved in causing PTP but their presence complicates the detection of platelet-specific antibodies. Modern platelet serological techniques such as the monoclonal antibody immobilisation of platelet antigens (MAIPA) assay are useful for resolving mixtures of antibodies in patients with PTP (see Chapter 5).

Pathophysiology

The time course of events in PTP is shown in Figure 14.1. A blood transfusion triggers a rapid secondary antibody response against HPA-1a, and there is acute thrombocytopenia about a week after the transfusion. It is difficult to understand why the patient's own HPA-1a-negative platelets are destroyed. There remains no generally accepted mechanism to explain this although a number of suggestions have been made.

- Transfused HPA-1a-positive platelets release HPA-1a antigen, which is adsorbed onto the patient's HPA-1a-negative platelets, making them a target for anti-HPA-1a. Support for this hypothesis comes from observations such as the elution of anti-HPA-1a from HPA-1a-negative platelets in some cases of PTP, and the demonstration of the adsorption of HPA-1a antigen on to HPA-1a-negative platelets after incubation with plasma from HPA-1a-positive stored blood [10].

- The released HPA-1a antigen forms immune complexes with anti-HPA-1a in the plasma, and the immune complexes become bound to the patient's platelets, causing their destruction.
- The transfusion stimulates the production of platelet autoantibodies as well as anti-HPA-1a. Evidence in favour of this mechanism is the detection of positive reactions of some PTP patients' sera from the acute thrombocytopenic phase with autologous platelets.
- In the early phase of the secondary antibody response, anti-HPA-1a may be produced which has the ability to cross-react with autologous as well as allogeneic platelets.

Management

Immediate treatment is essential as the risk of fatal haemorrhage is greatest early in the course of PTP. In a review of 71 cases of PTP, five died within the first 10 days because of intracranial haemorrhage [6]. The main aim of treatment is to prevent severe haemorrhage by shortening the duration of severe thrombocytopenia.

No randomised controlled trials of treatment for PTP have been carried out. Comparison of various therapeutic measures is complicated

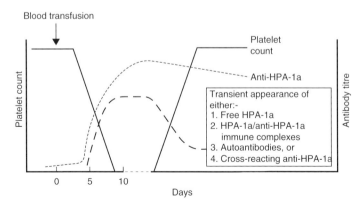

Figure 14.1 A typical time course of PTP. Purpura and severe thrombocytopenia occurred 5–10 days after a blood transfusion. The figure indicates the secondary antibody response of anti-HPA-1a, and the postulated transient appearance of either free HPA-1a antigen in the plasma, which binds to HPA-1a negative platelets, HPA-1a/anti-HPA-1a immune complexes, platelet autoantibodies or cross-reacting HPA-1a antibodies.

because it may be difficult to differentiate a response to treatment from a spontaneous remission in individual cases.

High-dose intravenous immunoglobulin (IVIgG) (2 g/kg given over two or five days) is the current treatment of choice, with responses in about 80% of cases [11]; there is often a rapid increase in the platelet count within 48–72 hours [12] (Figure 14.2). Steroids and plasma exchange were the preferred treatments before the availability of IVIgG, and plasma exchange in particular appeared to be effective in some but not all cases [6].

Platelet transfusions are usually ineffective in raising the platelet count, but may be needed in large doses to control severe bleeding in the acute phase, particularly in patients who have recently undergone surgery before there has been a response to high-dose IVIgG. There is no evidence that platelet concentrates from HPA-1a-negative platelets are more effective than those from random donors in the acute thrombocytopenic phase. There is no evidence to suggest that further transfusions in the acute phase prolong the duration or severity of thrombocytopenia.

Platelet transfusions have been reported to cause severe febrile and occasionally pulmonary reactions in patients with PTP; these were probably due to HLA antibodies reacting

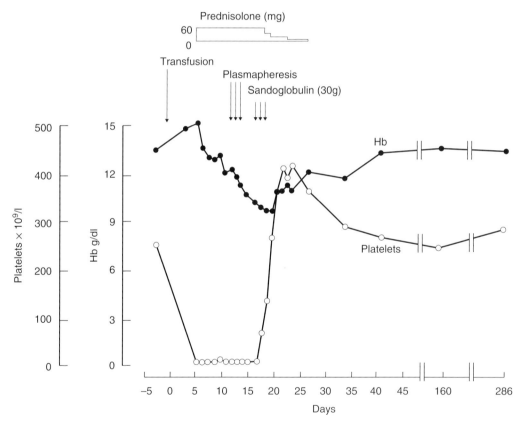

Figure 14.2 Haematological course of a patient with posttransfusion purpura showing the onset of profound thrombocytopenia six days after a blood transfusion. Initial treatment with random platelet concentrates caused rigors and bronchospasm, and there was no platelet increment. There was no response to prednisolone (60 mg/day) or plasma exchange (2.5 L/day for three days), but there was a prompt remission following high-dose IVIgG (30 g/day) for three days. *Source:* Adapted from Berney et al. [12] with permission from John Wiley & Sons.

against leucocyte in nonleucocyte-reduced platelet concentrates.

Prevention of Recurrence of PTP

Recurrence of PTP has been reported. However, it is unpredictable and has usually occurred following a delay of three years or more after the first episode. The patient should be issued with a card to indicate that he/she has previously had PTP and 'special' blood is required for future transfusions.

Future transfusion policy should be to use red cell and platelet concentrates from HPA-compatible donors or autologous transfusion. If these are not available, leucocyte-reduced blood components are considered to be safe. There have been occasional reports of recurrence of PTP with leucocyte-reduced red cell concentrates, but the implicated components would not have complied with current standards for leucocyte reduction.

KEY POINTS

1) Posttransfusion purpura is characterised by an acute episode of severe thrombocytopenia occurring about a week after a transfusion.
2) The pathophysiology remains uncertain.
3) Posttransfusion purpura typically occurs in HPA-1a-negative women who have been alloimmunised by pregnancy.
4) Haemorrhage is common and sometimes severe, although the thrombocytopenia resolves spontaneously within a few weeks.
5) High-dose intravenous immunoglobulin (2 g/kg given over two or five days) is the current treatment of choice to shorten the duration of thrombocytopenia, with responses in about 80% of cases.
6) Universal leucocyte reduction of blood components in the UK has resulted in a marked reduction in the number of reported cases.

References

1 Van Loghem JJ, Dorfmeijer H, van der Hart M, Schreuder F. Serological and genetical studies on a platelet antigen (Zw). Vox Sang 1959;**4**:161–9.

2 Shulman NR, Aster RH, Leitner A, Hiller MC. Immunoreactions involving platelets. V. Post-transfusion purpura due to a complement-fixing antibody against a genetically controlled platelet antigen. A proposed mechanism for thrombocytopenia and its relevance in 'autoimmunity'. J Clin Invest 1961;**40**:1597–620.

3 Shulman NR. Post-transfusion purpura: clinical features and the mechanism of platelet destruction, in Clinical and Basic Science Aspects of Immunohaematology (ed. SJ Nance), American Association of Blood Banks, Arlington, 1991, pp.137–54.

4 Serious Hazards of Transfusion (SHOT) Steering Group. The 2013 Annual SHOT Report. Available at: http://www.shotuk.org/wp-content/uploads/Annual-SHOT-Report-2013-Bookmarked.pdf (accessed 11 November 2016).

5 Menis M, Forshee RA, Anderson SA et al. Posttransfusion purpura occurrence and potential risk factors among the inpatient US elderly, as recorded in large Medicare databases during 2011 through 2012. Transfusion 2015;**55**:284–95.

6 Mueller-Eckhardt C. Post-transfusion purpura. Br J Haematol 1986;**64**:419–24.

7 Ballem PJ, Buskard NA, Decary F, Doubroff P. Post-transfusion purpura due to secondary transfer of anti-Pl[A1] by blood transfusion. Br J Haematol 1987;**66**:113–14.

8 Solenthaler M, Krauss JK, Boehlen F, Koller R, Hug M, Lamlle B. Fatal fresh frozen plasma infusion containing HPA-1a alloantibodies. Br J Haematol 1999;**6106**:258–9.

9 von dem Borne AEG, van der Plas-van Dalen CM. Further observations on post-transfusion purpura. Br J Haematol 1985;**61**:374–5.

10 Kickler TS, Ness PM, Herman JH, Bell WR. Studies on the pathophysiology of post-transfusion purpura. Blood 1986;**68**:347–50.

11 Becker T, Panzer S, Maas D et al. High-dose intravenous immunoglobulin for post-transfusion purpura. Br J Haematol 1985;**61**:149–55.

12 Berney SI, Metcalfe P, Wathen NC, Waters AH. Post-transfusion purpura responding to high-dose intravenous IgG: further observations on pathogenesis. Br J Haematol 1985;**61**:627–32.

Further Reading

Waters AH. Post-transfusion purpura. Blood Rev 1989;**3**:83–7.

15 Transfusion-Transmitted Infections

Roger Y. Dodd[1] and Susan L. Stramer[2]

[1] *American Red Cross, Jerome H. Holland Laboratory for the Biomedical Sciences, Rockville, USA*
[2] *American Red Cross, Scientific Support Office, Gaithersburg, USA*

Introduction

Transmission of infectious agents by blood transfusion has been a recognised risk since the identification of transmission and an introduced intervention for syphilis in the 1940s [1]. In particular, in the late 1960s, viral hepatitis was recognised among more than 10% of blood recipients [2]. Since that time, however, there have been continuous advances to the point at which the risk from posttransfusion hepatitis ranges from about one infection per million units transfused for hepatitis B virus (HBV) to one infection per 1.15 million units transfused for hepatitis C virus (HCV) [3–5]. However, many other infections have been found to be transmitted via this route, with HIV being the most notable; the risk of infection with this virus has been reduced to less than one in 1.5 million units transfused [5]. This chapter describes posttransfusion infection and its recognition, details the means that are used to prevent or minimise the risk of such transmission and outlines those infectious agents known to be transmitted by this route. Emerging infections are discussed in Chapter 17, and the problem of bacterial contamination of blood components is reviewed in Chapter 16.

Transmission of Infections by Blood Transfusion

A number of conditions must be met in order for a disease to be transmitted by blood transfusion [6].

- An asymptomatic phase during which the agent is present in the bloodstream.
- Ability of the agent to survive during the collection, processing and storage of the donation.
- Infectivity via the intravenous route.
- A susceptible patient population.
- Development of the disease in at least some infected recipients.

The infections discussed in this chapter are all well recognised as offering risk to transfusion recipients and all are subject to some measures to reduce such risk, but it must be recognised that, to date, no intervention is completely effective. In cases where testing has been implemented, risks are currently extremely low and it is clear that any residual risk is attributable to collection of blood during the so-called early window period after exposure, when the infectious agent may circulate but be undetectable by current methods. Testing has reduced this

Practical Transfusion Medicine, Fifth Edition. Edited by Michael F. Murphy, David J. Roberts and Mark H. Yazer.
© 2017 John Wiley & Sons Ltd. Published 2017 by John Wiley & Sons Ltd.

window period to a few days, reducing residual risk by many orders of magnitude [7,8]. Another threat is the development of new strains or mutations that lead to agents that escape detection, but in most cases, key agents are subject to multiple redundant tests, generally avoiding this problem. This also reduces the risk attributable to laboratory failures (which are themselves very rare). In cases where the principal intervention is a donor question, it is self-evident that a donor's failure to answer the questions correctly may lead to the collection of an infectious unit. It is also not generally possible to craft a question that is completely effective in segregating all those who are infected with a given organism while assuring that there is not an undue loss of donors.

Transfusion-Transmitted Infections: Detection and Management

Clinicians responsible for the care of transfused patients should be alert to the possibility of transfusion-transmitted disease or infection, even though this is now a rare event. Unfortunately, recognition of most transfusion-transmitted infections is not easy, for one or more of the following reasons [6].

- Many transfusion-transmitted infections (TTIs) are asymptomatic.
- If disease symptoms occur, they tend to be non-specific (fever, flu-like illness).
- The incubation period may be prolonged, in some cases extending out to months or even years.
- The patient's underlying disease may mask or modulate evidence of other infections.
- There may be preexisting risk factors for, or infection with, the disease agent that is thought to have been transfusion transmitted.
- Exotic infections may be transmitted by transfusion; they may be unexpected, unfamiliar, or hard to recognise or diagnose.

Effective investigation of a potential transfusion-transmitted infection is relatively complex and time-consuming and does not always lead to a definitive conclusion. Nevertheless, care should be taken to avoid inappropriate designation of the source of an infection temporally linked to transfusion. The following activities may contribute to the proper investigation of a suspected transfusion-transmitted infection.

- Clinical diagnosis of the transfusion-associated disease.
- Use of serological and/or nucleic acid testing to definitively diagnose the disease and to identify the infecting agent.
- Investigation of the patient's pretransfusion blood samples to establish the absence of infection prior to transfusion.
- Investigation of the patient's risk history to eliminate the possibility of alternate routes of infection.
- Investigation of all implicated blood donors for evidence of current or recent infection with the relevant agent; this will require the cooperation of the blood provider.
- Comparison of the agent isolated from the patient with that isolated from the donor by nucleic acid sequencing.
- Alert or consult with infectious disease specialists and/or public health agencies as appropriate.
- Early reporting of cases to the blood provider is critical and is usually required, so that other blood components from the implicated donor can be identified and recovered.

This chapter is concerned with those infections known to be transmitted by transfusion, the individual agents responsible and the diseases that they cause. However, it is worth noting that the presentation of a disease in a transfused patient may offer some clues. A patient may react very rapidly (e.g. even during administration) to the transfusion of a blood component that is contaminated with significant levels of bacteria; this topic is discussed in Chapter 16.

Viruses

Early manifestations (a few days to three weeks) are not common and if they occur, they most likely reflect transmission of a virus that causes acute infection, such as West Nile virus or even dengue virus [9,10]. Such an event is most likely associated with a known outbreak of the disease in question [11]. The most common symptoms are likely to be fever and headache, muscle pain, malaise, possibly with more severe manifestations typical of the virus itself [9]. In the case of the B19 parvovirus, infection may result in red cell aplasia or even an aplastic crisis in addition to viral syndromes [12]. Interestingly, infection with HIV can also result in an early acute viral syndrome, although the manifestations of AIDS are not likely to occur until many years after infection.

Hepatitis was, for many years, the most common infectious complication of transfusion, but is now very infrequent. HBV and HCV infections are usually asymptomatic initially and if there is any clinically apparent disease, it will not occur until several months after transfusion [2]. Transfusion-transmitted hepatitis A virus (HAV) is rare but occasional cases have been reported, as is also the case for hepatitis E virus (HEV). These agents tend to have a shorter incubation period and generally cause an acute, rather than chronic form of hepatitis [13].

As with hepatitis viruses, transfusion transmission of retroviruses is also extremely rare. As pointed out above, there may be an acute viral syndrome shortly after infection with HIV-1, but there is no such early response to infection with HTLV-1 or -2. In the absence of treatment, HIV infection almost invariably will lead to the eventual development of AIDS many years after the original infection, but only a minority of those infected with HTLV will develop symptomatic disease (tropical spastic paraparesis or adult T-cell leukaemia).

Thus, detection of transfusion-transmitted retroviral infection, or indeed hepatitis virus infection, is almost entirely dependent on laboratory testing. However, because most blood collection organisations actively trace recipients of prior donations from repeat donors who are newly found to be infected with these viruses, transfusion services may be notified that an earlier blood component may be infectious and are asked to identify and test the affected recipients. This approach has been responsible for the detection of essentially all confirmed transfusion transmissions of HIV and HCV in the United States since 1999, when nucleic acid testing of all blood donors was implemented.

Parasites

A number of protozoan parasites are transmissible by transfusion, most notably *Plasmodium* spp. (the agents of malaria), *Babesia* spp. and *Trypanosoma cruzi* (the agent of Chagas' disease) [13]. Malaria and *Babesia* infection may present with typical flu-like symptoms a few weeks to a few months after transfusion and may progress to the typical manifestations of the disease. Asplenic patients are at particular risk of disease from *Babesia* infection. In many cases, posttransfusion infection with these agents may be detected by examination of blood smears. Posttransfusion *Babesia* infection is not uncommon in the United States, particularly in areas where the parasite is endemic, but is rare elsewhere in the world [14,15]. In the United States, transfusion-transmitted *Babesia* may be mistaken for malaria.

Posttransfusion *T. cruzi* infection may occur in Latin America, where the parasite is endemic (although control programmes are reducing the threat), but is also recognised in areas where there is significant immigration from endemic regions [16]. Transfusion-transmitted *T. cruzi* may be asymptomatic but can result in severe or fulminant disease in immunocompromised patients. The incubation period for acute infection ranges from 20 to 40 days; fever that is unresponsive to antibiotics is the most common symptom, followed by lymphadenopathy and splenomegaly. The parasite may be detectable in blood films in some cases.

Prions

It is now clear from experience in the UK that the prion that causes variant Creutzfeldt–Jakob disease (vCJD) may be transmitted by transfusion and four such transmissions have been clearly documented. There is, as yet, no evidence for transmission of other prions. Detection of transfusion transmission of the vCJD prion was dependent upon a carefully designed surveillance programme and such an event is not likely to be observed in routine clinical practice, as the incubation period is in excess of several years [13,17].

Interventions to Minimise the Impact of Transfusion-Transmitted Infection

A variety of methods and processes are used to control transfusion-transmitted infections. In general, they involve the identification of appropriate donor populations and the selection of safe donors; testing blood donations for markers of infection or infectivity; treatment of the donation; and, in some circumstances, treatment of the blood recipient. Many of these interventions are required by laws and regulations and/or by voluntary standards [18,19].

Donor populations are selected implicitly by location of collection sites and by voluntary nonremuneration policies and explicitly by avoidance of collection from a variety of institutions (particularly prisons). Asking presenting donors questions relating to medical, travel and behavioural histories is used to assess donor suitability. These questions are intended to identify those at higher risk of certain infections. Typically, donors are asked about:

- a history of selected diseases or infections, such as viral hepatitis, HIV/AIDS, selected parasitic diseases
- intimate or family exposure to specific infectious diseases
- exposure to blood or body fluids through illicit injection or routine transfusion

- receipt of potentially infectious vaccines or therapeutic agents
- behavioural risk factors, particularly involving male–male sex or payment or exchange of drugs for sex
- travel to locations or areas offering risk of exposure to (for example) malaria or the vCJD prion [18].

Depending upon the responses to these questions, the presenting donor will be temporarily or permanently deferred from donation and the deferral will be recorded so that the risk may be identified should the donor try to present again during the time of deferral. The efficacy of these measures to select safer donors can be evaluated by comparing the prevalence and incidence of positive TTI test results among donors with those seen in the general population. In the United States, studies suggest that donor prevalence rates for key TTIs are some 6–20-fold lower than those for the general population, while incidence rates may be 4–20-fold lower than community rates [20]. Testing each donation for markers of infection or infectivity using serological and/or nucleic acid tests is a critical step in assuring safety from infections where such tests are available and suitable; this aspect is covered in Chapter 21.

To some extent, routine post-collection processing of blood components may impact their infectivity. There is some evidence that infectivity for some agents may vary by component, with infectivity for malaria and *Babesia* being found primarily (but not exclusively) in red cell concentrates [13]. Conversely, infectivity for *T. cruzi* seems to be confined to platelet concentrates [16], with one recent exception [21]. The infectivity titre for some agents (most notably HTLV-1) clearly declines with product storage, although this is not considered to be a safety measure in its own right. However, leucocyte reduction of blood components clearly reduces the risk of transmission of CMV and likely that of other cell-associated viruses, including HTLV [13]. Most promising, of course, is the application of formal pathogen reduction methods, which are currently available in many countries for the treatment of platelet concentrates and plasma for transfusion [6]. Methods for whole blood and for red cell concentrates remain under development.

Transfusion-Transmitted Infectious Agents

Viruses

Hepatitis A Virus

Hepatitis A virus is a small (27–32 nm diameter), nonenveloped virus with a single strand of positive sense RNA, 7.5 kb in length, family Picornaviridae, genus *Hepatovirus*. The primary transmission route is faecal–oral, sometimes through food or water or close personal contact. Single-source outbreaks are not uncommon. The incidence of infection in the general population tends to be relatively low at less than 7 per 100 000 annually, although seroprevalence rates are 29–34% in the United States [13]. The incubation period is 10–50 days, with a mode of one month.

The course of disease is almost always acute, typically with anorexia, relatively mild fever, fatigue and vomiting, leading to typical hepatitis with varying degrees of transaminase elevation and icterus. Overall, disease tends not to be severe, with fulminant or fatal cases infrequent – usually much less than 1%. There is a 7–14-day period of viraemia prior to the appearance of symptoms and during this time, blood is likely to be infectious via transfusion. Tests for IgG and IgM antibodies and for viral RNA are available.

A handful of cases of transfusion-transmitted HAV cases have been reported, some with secondary transmission [13]. Testing of whole blood donations is not warranted because transmission is so rare, but plasma for further manufacture is tested for HAV RNA by pooled nucleic acid testing (NAT). Blood donors are usually asked to notify the collection site if they become sick shortly after donation and such postdonation information has led to the identification and recovery of at least some potentially infectious units.

Hepatitis B Virus

Hepatitis B virus is an enveloped spherical virus 42–47 nm in diameter, with a partially double-stranded, circular DNA genome 3.2 kb in length with overlapping reading frames, family Hepadnaviridae, genus *Hepadnavirus*. Transmission routes are primarily sexual, parenteral and perinatal. An unusual feature of HBV infection is the overproduction of excess viral coat material which can circulate at high concentrations, termed hepatitis B surface antigen (HBsAg); its presence is indicative of active infection (acute or chronic) and it is the primary analyte for blood donor screening. Antibodies to HBsAg (anti-HBs) are generally indicative of past infection, but antibodies to the inner core of the virus (anti-HBc) appear earlier and may also indicate some risk of infectivity. IgM anti-HBc in combination with HBsAg are markers of infection within the last six months [22]. Detectable HBV DNA in the plasma is associated with varying levels of infectivity, depending upon the phase of the infection; the early window phase when DNA is the only detectable marker appears to be the most infectious.

The estimated incidence of infection in the United States is approximately 12 per 100 000 whereas the prevalence is 4–5% [23]. Since the introduction of an effective vaccine in the United States, incidence has decreased by 80%. The global burden of chronic HBV infection is as high as 400 million individuals.

The incubation period from exposure to infection is from one week to six months. While many infections are asymptomatic, the range of disease manifestations is extensive, from mild acute symptoms to life-threatening or fatal fulminant cases. Symptoms are generally similar to those described for HAV infection. Chronic infection results more frequently from infection early in life and chronic disease may lead to cirrhosis and/or liver cancer. Diagnostic tests include serum transaminase measurement and detection of HBV antibodies, particularly IgM anti-HBc. Nucleic acid testing may also be of value.

The risk of transfusion transmission varies widely but in the United States has been estimated as approximately one case per million units transfused [3,4]. However, the number of confirmed reported cases is considerably less than would be anticipated from this figure. The major interventions to reduce the risk of transmission include donor questioning for a history of recent viral hepatitis, close contact with a case and risk behaviours for sexual and parenteral exposure. Donations are tested for markers of HBV infection; most important is the use of sensitive immunoassays for HBsAg. In addition, in some countries donors are tested for anti-HBc, which identifies a small number of additional infectious donations among those donors with occult HBV infection (OBI) [22]. Such testing is not practical in areas with a high prevalence of HBV infection, however, because of the high prevalence of anti-HBc. Increasingly, donors are also being tested for HBV DNA, using triplex tests that are also designed to detect HIV and HCV RNA. The incremental impact of such testing on HBV safety has been demonstrated, but appears to be limited, particularly if anti-HBc testing is in place [3].

Hepatitis C Virus

Hepatitis C virus is a small, enveloped spherical (55–65 nm diameter) virus with a single positive strand of RNA, 9.6 kb in length, family Flaviviridae, genus *Hepacivirus*. The transmission route is primarily parenteral. The incidence of new infections in the United States is estimated at approximately six per 100 000 annually and the prevalence is 1.3–1.9% [23]. Most infections are chronic and lifelong; around 20% of infections may resolve. The incubation period is typically 4–12 weeks, with an extended range of 2–24 weeks. Most infections are asymptomatic, but when symptoms occur, they include fever, fatigue, loss of appetite and abdominal pain, among others. Chronic disease may lead to cirrhosis and, in some cases, liver cancer after many years. The incidence has declined significantly over recent years. Although the virus was not specifically identified until 1989, it was recognised as the predominant causative agent of posttransfusion hepatitis [2]. The development, progressive

improvement and universal implementation of tests for anti-HCV in donors have profoundly reduced the impact of this virus on blood safety, with a further significant improvement attributable to the implementation of testing for HCV RNA [24]. Nucleic acid testing has reduced the infectious window period from around 70 days to about seven days [8]. In the United States, the current risk of transmission of HCV by transfusion is one per 1 150 000 units [5]. Fewer cases of posttransfusion HCV infection are observed than would be predicted from this figure. Diagnostic tools include serum transaminase testing, antibody and RNA detection.

Interventions to reduce the transmission of HCV by transfusion include questioning donors about a history of viral hepatitis or exposure to a case and risk behaviours involving parenteral exposure to blood. All donations are tested for antibodies to HCV and in some cases, also to the core antigen of the virus. Nucleic acid testing for HCV has been in place in a number of countries since the late 1990s and has been instrumental in decreasing the residual risk.

Hepatitis D Virus

Hepatitis D virus (HDV) is a very small RNA virus that only infects those with ongoing HBV infection. HDV co-infection increases the severity of disease in those with chronic hepatitis B [13]. Because HDV is dependent on HBV for replication, measures to prevent HBV transmission are also effective against HDV.

Hepatitis E Virus

Hepatitis E virus is a small, nonenveloped icosahedral (30–34 nm diameter) virus with a single, positive strand of RNA, 7.2 kb in length, family Hepeviridae, genus *Hepevirus*. There are four major serotypes with varying geographical distribution and pathogenicity for humans. The transmission routes for types 1 and 2 are primarily faecal–oral, often water-borne, but types 3 and 4 are zoonoses that are frequently food borne, with cases attributable to consumption of raw or undercooked pork [13]. Incidence data are not readily available, but prevalence rates of 20–40% are reported from endemic regions. However, similar rates have been observed in the United States and other nonendemic regions: it is likely that these high rates are attributable to serotypes of low human pathogenicity. The incubation period is usually 3–8 weeks and infection may result in a wide spectrum of disease from unapparent to fulminant, with apparently increased severity in pregnant women [13].

Transfusion transmissions have been shown prospectively in a very large study recently conducted in the United Kingdom in which 225 000 routine blood donors were evaluated. Of these, 79 (or 1:2848) had detectable HEV RNA and 18 of 43 (42%) of traced recipients of their components had evidence of recent HEV infection, of which 10 developed prolonged infection, another three infections occurred in immunosuppressed individuals requiring treatment to clear the virus, and clinical hepatitis developed in another [25]. In the United States, a seroprevalence of 7.7% was found and there was a RNA detection rate of one per 9500 [26]. Transfusion transmission has been noted rarely in nonendemic areas, and with some frequency in endemic areas, such as Hokkaido in Japan [13]. Nucleic acid testing of presenting donors has been implemented as a preventive measure in some areas of concern and, in some cases, for plasma for further manufacture but there seems to be little enthusiasm for widespread application of this intervention.

Human Immunodeficiency Virus

Human immunodeficiency virus is an enveloped, more or less spherical (106–183 nm diameter) virus, with two linear, positive sense strands of RNA, 9.2 kb in length, family Retroviridae, genus *Lentivirus*. There are two major species, HIV-1 and HIV-2, although HIV-2 is much less common and less virulent than HIV-1. HIV-1 has multiple distinct clades [13]. The predominant transmission routes are sexual, perinatal and parenteral. Prevalence and incidence rates vary widely, with rates as high as 20% and 1–2%

in parts of sub-Saharan Africa. Prevalence in the United States is estimated at about 0.4% and incidence rates are about 16 per 100 000 annually [27]. Rates in Western Europe and other highly developed countries are generally somewhat lower. The incubation period to the acute retroviral syndrome averages about 21 days, but may range from five to 70 days. It is now known that HIV RNA becomes detectable around nine days after infection using current NAT assays. Sensitive tests for antibodies to HIV will become positive about three weeks after infection [8]. These periods represent the window periods for nucleic acid and antibody testing.

Most infections are asymptomatic and the acute retroviral syndrome, when it occurs, tends to be relatively mild, with a short (a week or two) period of fever, fatigue and possibly lymphadenopathy and rash. Typically, patients recover and are asymptomatic for many years thereafter, until the symptoms of full-blown AIDS emerge. Diagnosis of infection may be based upon tests for antibodies to HIV and/or the presence of HIV RNA in the plasma.

Currently, the risk of transmission of HIV by transfusion has been estimated as approximately one case per 1 500 000 units [5]. Again, however, transfusion-transmitted HIV infections are not recognised as frequently as this risk estimate would suggest. It is of interest to note that two of the five transmission events noted in the United States since 1999 have involved infection from a transfusable plasma unit, but not from the accompanying red cell concentrate, suggesting that the sensitivity of nucleic acid testing is approaching the infectious dose of HIV offered by a red cell concentrate [24].

While the AIDS epidemic has been a medical and human disaster, it stimulated the current stringent approach to blood safety and continuous quality improvement. All donors are directly asked about a history of AIDS-related symptoms and about possible exposure to infection. Questions about behavioural risk are asked and individuals acknowledging such risk are permanently or temporarily deferred. Some of the questions, particularly those relating to male-to-male sexual activity, have been challenged as discriminatory, particularly when accompanied by permanent deferral. Nevertheless, the rights of the patient to receive safe blood also have to be recognised and policies differ from one country to another, but almost always involve some period of deferral for those considered to be at increased risk of HIV infection. Recently, the United States and Canada have moved away from permanent deferral for male-to-male sexual activity, as have a number of other countries. All donations are, at a minimum, tested for antibodies to HIV and in many areas, also for HIV RNA. Testing for the HIV p24 antigen may be performed as an alternative to testing for RNA, but this approach offers lesser sensitivity.

Human T-Lymphotropic Viruses 1 and 2

Human T-lymphotropic virus is an enveloped, spherical (150–200 nm diameter) virus, with two linear, positive-sense, single strands of RNA, 8.5 kb in length, family Retroviridae, genus *Deltaretrovirus*. There are two different viruses, HTLV-1 and HTLV-2, and at least two additional variants have been described. The primary routes of transmission are sexual and perinatal (via breast milk), and parenteral transmission (particularly via injecting drug use) has been widely documented, especially for HTLV-2. Prevalence rates vary widely, but tend to be very low in developed Western countries. There are pockets of high prevalence in Japan, the Caribbean and Africa (HTLV-1) and among some native populations in the Americas (HTLV-2). Infection is most often asymptomatic; for HTLV-1, there is a lifetime risk of a few percent for the eventual development of adult T-cell leukaemia/lymphoma or tropical spastic paraparesis, but only the latter has ever been associated with transfusion. Less is known about disease associations for HTLV-2.

Transfusion transmission of these viruses has been recognised for many years. In the United States and a number of other countries, donations are tested for antibodies to HTLV-1 and -2, using a single combination test. There is no evidence of residual transmission although it may be estimated that there is a risk of one transmission per several million units [7]. Leucocyte reduction seems to eliminate the risk of transmission, which also declines during refrigerated storage of red cell components.

Cytomegalovirus (Human CMV, HHV-5)

Cytomegalovirus is an enveloped, spherical beta herpes virus 200–300 nm in diameter, with a double-stranded DNA genome of 235 kb pairs, family Herpesviridae, genus *Cytomegalovirus*. Seroprevalence rates vary by age and location but are of the order of 30–40% among blood donors in the United States and Western Europe [13]. There are no good measures of incidence rates, but the presence of antibodies to CMV implies that virus is present, albeit often in latent form. The normal transmission route is by contact, droplets or body fluid exposure, but it is also transmissible from mother to fetus and by blood transfusion and organ transplant. In general, healthy individuals are asymptomatic or show only mild symptoms (fever, lymphadenopathy, mononucleosis-like disease), but vulnerable individuals, including the fetus, low-birthweight infants, transplant patients and those with severe immune deficiencies, may suffer serious or fatal disease, including pneumonia, multiorgan disease, etc. Infection during pregnancy may have profound effects on the fetus, including developmental problems.

Transfusion-transmitted infection is typically recognised 1–2 months posttransfusion. There are two primary interventions to reduce or eliminate posttransfusion CMV infection: leucocyte reduction and/or the use of seronegative blood components for those at risk. Studies have suggested that both methods have similar efficacy in reducing risk but that breakthrough infections may still be seen [28]. There are a number of explanations for such breakthrough cases, including failure of testing or leucocyte reduction, the presence of extracellular virus in early infection and the possibility that at least some hospital-acquired infections may be mistaken for transfusion transmissions. Lastly, reactivation of latent CMV infection triggered by transfusion likely accounts for most reported cases of transfusion-transmitted CMV [29].

Other Human Herpes Viruses

Two other human herpes viruses, Epstein–Barr virus (EBV) and human herpes virus 8 (HHV-8), are known to be transmissible by transfusion [13]. EBV is an almost ubiquitous virus, associated with mononucleosis, and in some locations, especially in Africa, Burkitt's lymphoma and nasopharyngeal carcinoma in Asia. Evidence is increasing for its role in the causation of lymphoproliferative disease among transfused immunocompromised patients, but other than leucocyte reduction, there is little in the way of an intervention, at least in the absence of pathogen reduction. HHV-8 is the causative agent of Kaposi's sarcoma and there is evidence for its transmissibility by transfusion, at least in parts of Africa, where it is endemic. To date, however, there does not appear to be any evidence for transfusion-transmitted HHV-8 disease; reductions in viral loads likely are the result of leucocyte reduction [13].

West Nile Virus

West Nile virus (WNV) is an enveloped, spherical (40–60 nm diameter) virus with a linear, single strand of positive-sense RNA, 11 kb in length, family Flaviviridae, genus *Flavivirus* (Japanese encephalitis complex). The primary transmission route is via (mainly culicine) mosquitoes and the amplifying hosts are primarily birds. Humans are accidental, dead-end hosts, although the virus is readily transmitted via blood transfusion [11]. At the peak of the new epidemic, which emerged in the United States in 1999, several hundred thousand individuals were naturally infected each year; the largest WNV outbreaks ever recorded worldwide occurred in the United States in 2002 and again in 2003; the number of cases has declined and appears to have reached stability. The virus is endemic in parts of Africa, the Middle East and parts of southern Europe where smaller outbreaks frequently occur.

Infection results in a range of outcomes from asymptomatic, through flu-like symptoms occurring in approximately 25% of infected individuals. Symptoms include headache, weakness, new rash, fever, muscle, joint and eye pain, referred to as West Nile fever [9]. More severe neurological disease involving meningoencephalitis, with outcomes sometimes leading to death, occur in between one in 150 and one in 200 infected individuals [9]. The incubation period is 2–14 days with a period of early viraemia of about 7–10 days during which the blood of the patient may be infectious; low levels of viraemia may be detectable for a longer time. In the United States, cases occur mainly between April and October. In 2002, there was a report of 23 well-characterised transfusion-transmitted cases of WNV infections and within less than a year, universal donor screening for WNV RNA by pooled nucleic acid testing was implemented [30]. Experience showed that such testing was insufficiently sensitive to detect all infectious donations so measures were established to perform single donation testing in areas and times with a high incidence of WNV activity [31,32]. Outside the United States, there has not been widespread testing, but donor deferral based upon travel to endemic areas has been implemented in some countries. Testing has been implemented in parts of Europe in response to a number of discrete outbreaks.

Other Arboviruses

West Nile virus illustrated two somewhat unexpected facts: the ability of arthropod-borne viruses (arboviruses) to establish huge, unprecedented outbreaks in previously unaffected areas; and efficient transmission of an acute infection via blood transfusion. Accordingly, unexpected intense outbreaks of infection with chikungunya virus (an alphavirus transmitted by *Aedes* spp. mosquitoes) resulted in specific measures designed to prevent transfusion transmission in some affected areas; however, although explosive outbreaks occurred, transfusion transmission was never documented [6,13]. This continues to be the case even in a large outbreak of chikungunya in the Caribbean and other parts of the Americas. In contrast, seven clusters of transfusion transmission of dengue virus have been reported from Hong Kong, Singapore, Brazil and Puerto Rico [33]. Donor testing has been implemented in Puerto Rico and may be considered elsewhere in the future, particularly in countries in which this virus is not endemic but where outbreaks may occur [10].

Zika virus

Zika virus is a mosquito-borne flavivirus closely related to dengue viruses and is responsible for a large ongoing outbreak first documented in the Americas in Brazil in May 2015. As of September 1, 2016, over 50 countries or areas report active transmission, most in the Americas. http://www.cdc.gov/zika/geo/united-states. html. Zika virus has been proven to cause fetal loss, congenital Zika virus-related syndrome including microcephaly; and, Guillain Barré syndrome and other neurological complications in adults. However, in most cases (~80%) Zika virus infection is asymptomatic.

Zika viral RNA can be recovered from blood donors, and as of September 2016, there have been four probable transfusion transmissions, all reported in Brazil. These occurred from three donors who were identified by post-donation information reports of dengue/Zika virus-like symptoms. None of the recipients developed Zika-related symptoms following transfusion. In addition to mosquito-borne transmission and likely transfusion transmission, sexual transmission has also been documented.

Because of concern about severe disease associations, rapid virus spread in the Americas, recovery of RNA from blood of asymptomatic donors, and reports of transfusion transmission, blood centers in the United States have been screening for travel to or residence in Zika-active areas using a specific question with an associated 28-day deferral. In addition, donors who have had sexual contact with an individual with a Zika virus diagnosis or symptoms, or who has traveled to Zika-active area(s), or donors who have symptoms or a diagnosis of Zika, have been asked to self-defer for 28 days. However, these requirements were superseded by subsequent FDA guidance of August, 2016 for immediate implementation requiring universal, individual donation testing for Zika viral RNA, or the use of approved pathogen reduction technologies.

Human B19 Parvovirus (B19V)

B19V is a small, nonenveloped, icosahedral (23–26 nm diameter) virus with a linear, negative-sense, single strand of DNA, 5.6 kb in length, in the family Parvoviridae, genus *Erythrovirus*. The primary transmission routes are respiratory and transplacental [13]. The virus is transmitted by blood transfusion and, at least in the past, via some plasma-derived products. Levels of viraemia during acute infection can be extremely high, sometimes exceeding 10^{12} DNA copies per mL. The virus is ubiquitous, often causing seasonal outbreaks of mild disease, particularly among children. Seroprevalence rates are around 50% in adults and incidence rates can be 1.5%.

Most infections are asymptomatic, but the virus causes erythema infectiosum (fifth disease) in children and occasional arthropathy in adults. Of particular concern is transient aplastic crisis in patients with shortened RBC survival or haemolytic anaemias; in some cases there may be pure red cell aplasia or pancytopenia. Infection in pregnant women may result in hydrops fetalis. Symptomatic infection from transfusion transmission is extremely rare. Nevertheless, in some countries (such as Germany and Japan), donor blood is routinely screened for viral DNA or by haemagglutination to eliminate the transfusion of components with high titres of virus. Currently, plasma for further manufacture is tested in pools for B19 DNA in order to minimise the levels of virus in manufacturing pools. Such testing is becoming available through rapid, high-throughput procedures and this may lead to expansion of routine blood donation testing.

Bacteria

Currently, the major blood safety risk from bacteria results from contamination of components and subsequent outgrowth, resulting in septic reactions in the patient. This is discussed in Chapter 16. However, a small number of bacterial species may be transmitted from donor to recipient by blood, leading to infection and the development of disease. The best known (but least frequent) example of this is syphilis, although there has been no reported case in the literature since 1960. The rarity of such transmission is likely due to a combination of factors, including donor selection and testing and the fragility of *Treponema pallidum* (the infectious spirochete) in stored components, along with the frequent use of antibiotics among patients.

Recently, there has been concern about the potential for transmission of Q-fever (caused by the small bacterium *Coxiella burnetii*) as a result of large, focused outbreaks of human infection in The Netherlands [13]. The infection resulted from human exposure to airborne bacteria associated with intensive goat farming. Investigations demonstrated bacteraemia in some patients and a small amount of suggestive evidence for rare transfusion transmission. In times and areas of concern, donations were tested for *C. burnetii* by PCR. Veterinary public health measures have, however, essentially eliminated the outbreaks. Other tick-borne *Rickettsia*-like bacteria have engendered some concern, and to date, there have been at least eight reports of transfusion transmission of *Anaplasma phagocytophilum* [13]. There has been no evidence of transmission of *Borrelia burgdorferi* (the agent of Lyme disease) by this route [13].

Parasitic Diseases

Malaria

Human malaria is caused by intraerythrocytic protozoan parasites of the genus *Plasmodium*, namely *P. falciparum*, *P. vivax*, *P. ovale* and *P. malariae*; recently, some cases have also been attributed to the primate parasite *P. knowlesi* [13]. The parasites are transmitted by anopheline mosquitoes. The parasites may be present in the circulation during a prolonged asymptomatic period and are readily transmitted by blood transfusion. Such transmission is thought to be quite common in endemic areas in the tropics, but is also a significant risk in nonendemic countries, as a result of collection of blood from donors infected as a result of travel from endemic areas. Disease symptoms include periodic fever, rigours and chills, headache, myalgias, arthralgias, splenomegaly and haemolytic anaemia. Although the normal incubation period is usually a few weeks, this period may be extended in blood recipients and recognition and diagnosis may not be easy. In general, the most severe forms of the disease are attributable to *P. falciparum*.

Diagnosis may be achieved through microscopic inspection of blood smears, and serological testing; research-level nucleic acid tests are also available. In nonendemic countries, transfusion-transmitted malaria is controlled by questioning donors about a history of malaria and of travel from or residence in malarious areas. Policies differ somewhat but in general, casual travel by residents of nonendemic countries is not a major risk, provided that such travellers are deferred for a few months. On the other hand, those who have resided for long periods in malarious areas may be partially immune and can be infectious for a number of years. Many donors are deferred for travel histories, with a negative impact on blood availability, and in some European countries and in Australia, deferred donors may be tested for antibodies to *Plasmodium* spp. and if non-reactive, are permitted to donate after a shortened deferral period [34].

Babesiosis

Babesia is also an intraerythrocytic protozoan parasite and the causative agent of babesiosis; a variety of species may be found throughout the world [13,15]. *Babesia* spp. are transmitted by ticks and primarily affect mammals, with humans as an accidental host. Babesiosis has symptoms similar to those of malaria, but disease is more severe in the elderly and those patients without a functioning spleen. Transfusion-transmitted babesiosis may be confused with malaria, as the characteristic 'Maltese cross' appearance of the parasite in red cells is quite infrequent. *B. microti* is most often associated with human disease and with transmission by transfusion, which is most often seen in the United States, with a recent report detailing 162 cases (including three from *B. duncani*) since 1979 [14]; the count is now well over 200. Few cases have been reported from any other countries. The disease is generally treatable, but nevertheless, transfusion-transmitted cases have a significant fatality rate. At the time of writing, donor questioning regarding tick bite or clinical disease is insensitive, but investigational donation tests are in limited use in endemic areas. Infection may be diagnosed by serological and nucleic acid tests, or by examination of blood films.

Chagas' disease

Chagas' disease is caused by the protozoan parasite *Trypanosoma cruzi*, which infects numerous mammalian hosts [13][13]. It is transmitted to humans by reduviid bugs, generally as a result of exposure to the parasites in the bug's faecal material, which may be rubbed into mucous membranes or the site of a bite from the bug itself. The parasite is endemic in the Americas, generally between latitudes 40°N and 40°S. Most human infections occur in rural or underdeveloped areas of Latin America where there are more opportunities for interactions between humans and the vector insects, which tend to colonise substandard housing. The parasite often infects infants and children and infection may be lifelong. Infected individuals may be asymptomatic over periods of many years and their blood can transmit the infection via transfusion. Transplacental infection may also occur, sometimes across more

than one generation. Population movements have introduced the infection into nonendemic countries, especially the United States, Canada and Spain.

Initial symptoms after infection may involve localised swelling and mild fever. Over the longer term, hepatomegaly and cardiac or gastrointestinal symptoms may emerge. Fulminant disease may occur in immunocompromised patients, particularly in the case of transfusion transmission. Diagnosis may be achieved through the use of serological tests, although infections are occasionally recognised on examination of blood films. Prevention of transfusion transmission relies primarily upon blood donor testing for antibodies to *T. cruzi*. Such testing is widespread in Latin America and was implemented in the United States in 2007. Subsequent evaluation of the testing programme suggested that selective testing was effective and currently, blood donors are tested only once and if non-reactive, subsequent donations are accepted without any testing. In other countries, notably Canada and Spain, presenting donors are asked about prolonged travel, residence or birth in Chagas-endemic countries and whether their mothers or grandmothers were born in such areas. If so, the donors are tested for *T. cruzi* antibodies and may donate if such tests are non-reactive.

The number of transfusion-transmitted cases is limited and has been described primarily from platelets [16], although there has been a single report of transmission from a red cell concentrate [21].

Prions

Variant Creutzfeldt–Jakob disease (vCJD)

Variant CJD is the human form of bovine spongiform encephalopathy (BSE, mad cow disease), transmitted to humans through ingestion of tissues from infected cattle [13]. The disease was first recognised as a distinct entity in 1996. Although similar to classic CJD, vCJD occurs primarily among younger individuals, presents with psychiatric symptoms and generally has a longer course from diagnosis to death. The pathology typically involves unusual, florid plaques in the brain. About 226 cases have occurred, mostly in the United Kingdom. The frequency of reported cases has been declining over the past five or more years.

Careful review of surveillance data has shown that there have been four instances of transmission of the vCJD agent by transfusion. Three such cases resulted in the development of vCJD in the recipient and the fourth occurred in an individual who died of underlying disease but was found to harbour the agent in the spleen and at least one lymph node [17]. One other possible case of transmission has been reported, attributed to receipt of factor VIII concentrates. Although these events are infrequent, they do reflect a high transmission rate among exposed recipients. Because of concern about such transmissions, a number of preventative measures had been implemented well before the recognition of any transmissions. In the United States, such measures included permanent deferral from donation of individuals judged at risk of exposure to BSE by virtue of residence or prolonged cumulative travel to the United Kingdom and Western Europe and similar measures were taken elsewhere. In the United Kingdom, efforts were made to assure universal leucocyte reduction, elimination of use of domestic plasma for transfusion or fractionation and reduction of transfusion overall. There has been a prolonged effort to develop premortem tests for infection with vCJD, but at the time of writing, no such test was available. To date, there has been no evidence that the classic form of CJD is transmissible by transfusion [13].

KEY POINTS

1) A number of pathogens, including viruses, bacteria, protozoan parasites and one prion, are known to be transmitted by transfusion.

2) Measures are in place to control such transmission, including blood donor selection, deferral, laboratory testing and component treatment.

3) These measures have reduced the incidence of key transfusion-transmitted infections to very low levels, usually less than one case per million components transfused.

4) Transfusion-transmitted infections are difficult to detect and diagnose.

5) Careful studies involving the patient and all implicated donors are necessary in order to confirm that an infection is attributable to transfusion.

6) Transfusion-transmitted infection should be appropriately reported to blood providers and other agencies, as required by regulation or practice.

References

1 Dodd RY. Germs, gels and genomes: a personal recollection of 30 years in blood safety testing, in Blood Safety in the New Millennium (ed. Stramer SL). Bethesda, AABB, 2001, pp. 97–122.

2 Alter HJ, Houghton M. Hepatitis C virus and eliminating post-transfusion hepatitis. Nature Med 2000;**6**:1082–6.

3 Stramer SL, Notari EP, Krysztof DE, Dodd RY. Hepatitis B virus testing by minipool nucleic acid testing: does it improve blood safety? Transfusion 2013;**53**:2448–58.

4 Stramer SL, Wend U, Candotti D et al. Nucleic acid testing to detect HBV infection in blood donors. N Engl J Med 2011;**364**: 236–47.

5 Zou S, Dorsey KA, Notari EP et al. Prevalence, incidence and residual risk of human immunodeficiency virus and hepatitis C virus infections among United States blood donors since the introduction of nucleic acid testing. Transfusion 2010;**50**:1495–504.

6 Stramer SL, Hollinger FB, Katz LM et al. Emerging infectious disease agents and their potential threat to transfusion safety. Transfusion 2009;**49**(Suppl):1S–235S.

7 Dodd RY, Notari EP, Stramer SL. Current prevalence and incidence of infectious disease markers and estimated window-period risk in the American Red Cross blood donor population. Transfusion 2002;**42**:975–9.

8 Busch MP, Glynn SA, Stramer SL et al., for the NHLBI-REDS NAT Study Group. A new strategy for estimating risks of transfusion-transmitted infections based on rates of detection of recently infected donors. Transfusion 2005;**45**:254–64.

9 Zou S, Foster GA, Dodd RY, Petersen LR, Stramer, SL. West Nile fever characteristics among viremic persons identified through blood donor screening. J Infect Dis 2010;**202**:1354–561.

10 Stramer SL, Linnen JL, Carrick JM et al. Dengue viremia in blood donors identified by RNA and detection of dengue transfusion transmission during the 2007 dengue outbreak in Puerto Rico. Transfusion 2012;**52**:1657–66.

11 Pealer LN, Marfin AA, Petersen LR et al. Transmission of West Nile virus through blood transfusion in the United States. N Engl J Med 2003;**349**:1236–45.

12 Dodd RY. B19: benign or not? Transfusion 2011;**51**:1878–9.

13 AABB. Emerging Infectious Diseases Fact Sheets. Available at: www.aabb.org/tm/eid/Pages/default.aspx (accessed 31 October 2016).

14 Herwaldt BL, Linden JV, Bosserman E, Young C, Olkowska D, Wilson M, Transfusion-associated babesiosis in the United States: a description of cases. Ann Intern Med 2011;**155**:509–19.

15 Leiby DA. Transfusion-transmitted *Babesia* spp.: bulls-eye on *Babesia microti*. Clin Microbiol Rev 2011;**24**:14–28.

16 Benjamin RJ, Stramer SL, Leiby DA, Dodd RY, Fearon M, Castro E. *Trypanosoma cruzi* infection in North America and Spain: evidence in support of transfusion transmission. Transfusion 2012;**52**:1913–21.

17 Hewitt PE, Llewelyn CA, Mackenzie J, Will RG. Creutzfeldt Jakob disease and blood transfusion: results of the UK transfusion medicine epidemiological review study. Vox Sang 2006;**91**:221–30.

18 Eder A, Bianco C (eds). Screening Blood Donors. Bethesda: AABB Press, 2007.

19 AABB. Standards for Blood Banks and Transfusion Services, 27th edn. Bethesda: AABB Press, 2011.

20 Dodd RY. Current estimates of transfusion safety worldwide. Dev Biol (Basel) 2005;**120**:3–10.

21 Blumental S, Lambermont M, Heijmans C et al. First documented transmission of Trypanosoma cruzi infection through blood transfusion in a child with sickle-cell disease in Belgium. PLoS Negl Trop Dis 2015;**9**(10):e0003986.

22 Hollinger FB. Hepatitis B virus infection and transfusion medicine: science and the occult. Transfusion 2008;**48**:1001–26.

23 Centers for Disease Control. Viral Hepatitis Surveillance – United States, 2009. Available at: http://www.cdc.gov/hepatitis/Statistics/2009Surveillance/index.htm (accessed 31 October 2016).

24 Stramer SL, Glynn SA, Kleinman SH et al. Detection of HIV-1 and HCV infections among antibody-negative blood donors by nucleic acid-amplification testing. N Engl J Med 2004;**351**:760–8.

25 Hewitt PE, Ijaz S, Brailsford SR et al. Hepatitis E virus in blood components: a prevalence and transmission study in southeast England. Lancet 2014;**384**:1766–73.

26 Stramer SL, Moritz ED, Foster GA *et al.* Hepatitis E virus: seroprevalence and frequency of viral RNA detection among US blood donors. Transfusion 2016;**56**:481–8.

27 Centers for Disease Control Fact Sheets. Available at: http://www.cdc.gov/hiv/library/factsheets/(accessed 31 October 2016).

28 Vamvakas EC. Is white blood cell reduction equivalent to antibody screening in preventing transmission of cytomegalovirus by transfusion? A review of the literature and meta-analysis. Transfus Med Rev 2005;**19**:181–99.

29 Drew WL, Roback JD. Prevention of transfusion-transmitted cytomegalovirus: reactivation of the debate? Transfusion 2007;**47**:1955–8.

30 Stramer SL, Fang CT, Foster GA, Wagner AG, Brodsky JP, Dodd RY. West Nile virus among blood donors in the United States, 2003 and 2004. N Engl J Med 2005;**353**:451–9.

31 Biggerstaff BJ, Petersen LR. A modeling framework for evaluation and comparison of trigger strategies for switching from minipool

to individual-donation testing for West Nile virus. Transfusion 2009;**49**:1151–9.

32 Dodd RY, Foster GA, Stramer SL. Keeping blood transfusion safe from West Nile virus: American Red Cross experience, 2003–2012. Transfus Med Rev 2015;**29**:153–61.

33 Matos D, Tomashek KM, Perez-Padilla J, Munoz-Jordan J et al. Probable and possible transfusion-transmitted dengue associated with NS1 antigen-negative but RNA confirmed-positive red blood cells. Transfusion 2015 doi:10.1111/trf.13288

34 Seed CR, Kee G, Wong T, Law M, Ismay S. Assessing the safety and efficacy of a test-based, targeted donor screening strategy to minimize transfusion transmitted malaria. Vox Sang 2010;**98**:e182–e192.

Further Reading

AABB. Standards for Blood Banks and Transfusion Services, 27th edn. Bethesda: AABB Press, 2011.

Alter HJ, Klein HG. The hazards of blood transfusion in historical perspective. Blood 2008;**112**:2617–26.

Barbara JAJ, Regan FAM, Contreras MC (eds). Transfusion Microbiology. Cambridge: Cambridge University Press, 2008.

Bern C, Kjos S, Yabsley MJ, Montgomery SP. *Trypanosoma cruzi* and Chagas' disease in the United States. Clin Microbiol Rev 2011;**24**:655–81.

Busch MP. Transfusion-transmitted viral infections: building bridges to transfusion medicine to reduce risks and understand epidemiology and pathogenesis. Transfusion 2006;**46**:1624–40.

Eder A, Bianco C (eds). Screening Blood Donors. Bethesda: AABB Press, 2007.

Perkins HA, Busch MP. Transfusion-associated infections: 50 years of relentless challenges and remarkable progress. Transfusion 2010;**50**:2080–99.

Petersen LR, Hayes EB. Westward Ho? The spread of West Nile virus. N Engl J Med 2004;**351**:2257–9.

Petersen LR, Jamieson DJ et al. MA. Zika virus. N Engl J Med 2016;**374**:1552–63.

Stramer SL, Hollinger FB, Katz LM et al. Emerging infectious disease agents and their potential threat to transfusion safety. Transfusion 2009;**49**(Suppl):1S–235S.

Zou S, Stramer SL, Dodd RY. Donor testing and risk: current prevalence, incidence, and residual risk of transfusion-transmissible agents in US allogeneic donations. Transfus Med Rev 2012;**26**:119–28.

16 Bacterial Contamination

Sandra Ramírez-Arcos and Mindy Goldman

Canadian Blood Services, Medical Services and Innovation, Ottawa, Canada

Incidence of Bacterial Contamination

Transfusion-associated septic events have been reduced by the introduction of improved donor screening and skin disinfection methods, as well as implementation of first aliquot diversion and bacterial testing. Recent reports of septic reactions indicate that bacterial contamination of blood components continues to be the predominant transfusion-associated infectious risk in Europe and North America [1,2]. From 2011 to 2015, the US Food and Drug Administration (FDA) reported 14 fatalities caused by blood components contaminated with bacteria [2]. In Canada, the Transfusion Transmitted Injuries Surveillance System Programme Report for 2006–12 described 33 transfusion reactions involving bacterially contaminated blood components [3]. Only one probable transfusion reaction involving a platelet unit contaminated with *Staphylococcus aureus* has been reported in the UK since universal screening of platelet concentrates using an automated culture method was implemented in 2011. However, in this period there have been three near misses where bacterial contamination with *S. aureus* was detected. Transfusion of those units was prevented because the presence of aggregates was noted during visual inspection of the platelet concentrates [1].

Results of platelet screening with automated culture methods have been summarised in a recent review by Benjamin and McDonald [4] and an ISBT Forum on bacterial contamination in platelets [5]. The data were collected from 16 published reports and 18 contributions (from 16 countries), respectively. These studies revealed an incidence of confirmed positive cultures ranging from 0.01% to 0.1%. Septic reactions representing false-negative culture results were reported at rates of approximately 0.007% [4,5].

Blood Components Implicated in Adverse Transfusion Reactions

Platelet Concentrates

Platelet concentrates (PCs) are the blood components most susceptible to bacterial contamination due to their storage conditions being amenable for bacterial growth. PCs have a physiological pH and high glucose content and are stored with constant agitation at $22 \pm 2\,°C$ in oxygen-permeable plastic containers. The initial levels of bacteria in PCs are usually exceedingly low (<10 colony forming units, cfu/PC unit) but clinically significant levels (10^5 cfu/mL) can be reached after 3–5 days of storage, depending on the organism [6].

Clinical sequelae of transfusing bacterially contaminated PCs are variable and may be acute

Practical Transfusion Medicine, Fifth Edition. Edited by Michael F. Murphy, David J. Roberts and Mark H. Yazer.
© 2017 John Wiley & Sons Ltd. Published 2017 by John Wiley & Sons Ltd.

or delayed, depending on the severity of the recipient's medical condition, the type and concentration of the contaminant organism and the timing of transfusion [7,8].

Red Blood Cells

Storage of red cell units at low temperatures (1/2–6 °C) limits bacterial growth and decreases the risk of adverse posttransfusion events. However, psychrophilic (growing optimally at refrigeration temperatures) pathogenic bacteria can proliferate under red cell storage conditions reaching clinically significant concentrations.

Reactions associated with transfusion of bacterially contaminated red cell units are usually severe, due to infused endotoxin (lipopolysaccharide) associated with the cell wall of Gram-negative bacteria. Clinical symptoms may include fever over 38.5 °C, hypotension, nausea and vomiting starting during the transfusion. Septic shock with complications such as oliguria and disseminated intravascular coagulation may occur [8].

Plasma and Cryoprecipitate

The incidence of ATRs due to contaminated plasma or cryoprecipitate is very low. Only a few reports are found in the literature documenting cases of products being contaminated during thawing in water baths. Recipients developed severe infections including endocarditis and septicaemia several days posttransfusion [8].

Contaminant Bacterial Species

Platelet Concentrates

Gram-positive bacteria are the predominant PC contaminants. Although these bacteria have the ability to survive and proliferate during PC storage, most of them are considered to be non-pathogenic. Coagulase-negative staphylococci such as *Staphylococcus epidermidis* and propionibacteria are the predominant contaminants of PCs [5,8,9]. Transfusions with fatal outcomes

due to platelets contaminated with *S. epidermidis* have been reported worldwide [2,10]. Missed detection of *S. epidermidis* is attributed to slow growth under platelet storage conditions and the ability to form slimy bacterial aggregates (biofilms) [11]. Other Gram-positive bacteria often identified as PC contaminants include corynebacteria, *S. aureus*, *Bacillus* spp. and *Streptococcus* spp. [1,8–10]. Most of the PC contaminants are either aerobic or facultative anaerobic bacteria; however, there have been reports of septic reactions associated with strict anaerobic organisms such as *Clostridium perfringens* [9].

Gram-negative bacteria can also be present in PCs and will cause severe and often fatal infections due to the potent septic shock reaction induced by the endotoxin, which elicits an uncontrolled inflammatory response in the recipient. The most frequently identified Gram-negative PC contaminants include *Escherichia coli*, *Klebsiella pneumoniae*, *Enterobacter* spp. and *Serratia* spp. [6–9].

Red Blood Cells

Red cells are the most frequently transfused blood component. The predominant red cell contaminants are Gram-negative bacteria of the family Enterobacteriaceae, with *Yersinia enterocolitica* being the predominant species. *Yersinia* is a psychrophilic organism and proliferates well at 1–6 °C, reaching levels $>10^8$ cfu/mL after three weeks of incubation. Transfusion of red cell units heavily contaminated with *Y. enterocolitica* results in severe septic shock due to high levels of endotoxin [12].

Other red cell Gram-negative bacterial contaminants include *Serratia* spp., *Pseudomonas* spp., *Enterobacter* spp., *Campylobacter* spp., and *E. coli*, all of which have the potential to cause endotoxic shock in recipients [7–9,13].

Plasma and Cryoprecipitate

Burkholderia cepacia (previously known as *Pseudomonas cepacia*) and *Pseudomonas aeruginosa* have been implicated in ATRs due to contaminated plasma and cryoprecipitate [8].

Sources of Contamination

Contaminant bacteria of blood components can originate from the donor or the blood collection and processing procedures.

Blood Donor

The predominant blood component bacterial contaminants are Gram-positive bacteria that are part of the normal skin flora and, more rarely, Gram-negative bacteria that can originate from silent donor bacteraemia or be part of the transient skin flora. It is impossible to completely decontaminate human skin and it has been reported that normal skin flora organisms such as *S. epidermidis* can adhere firmly to human hair despite skin disinfection [8].

Asymptomatic donor bacteraemia may lead to contamination of blood components. Low-level bacteraemia may occur in the incubation or recovery phase of acute infections after procedures such as tooth extraction. Chronic, low-grade infections, such as osteomyelitis, have been associated with contaminated platelet products, as have gastrointestinal disorders such as diverticulosis and colon cancer [8,14].

Blood Collection and Production Processes

Blood collection and production processes can also be sources of bacterial contamination. Three cases of *Serratia marcescens* sepsis following platelet transfusions were linked to contaminated vacuum tubes used for blood collection [8]. *Burkholderia cepacia* and *Pseudomonas aeruginosa* implicated in transfusion reactions due to contaminated plasma and cryoprecipitate were isolated from the water baths used to thaw the products [8].

Investigation of Transfusion Reactions

Symptoms of transfusion-associated septic reactions usually appear during the first four hours after the transfusion was initiated; however, there are reports of delayed symptoms of a transfusion reaction that could go underrecognised [10]. If a septic reaction is suspected, the transfusion should be stopped immediately. Remaining components, intravenous solutions and blood samples from the recipient should be sent for microbiological investigation. Septic transfusion reactions are confirmed if the same bacterium is isolated from the recipient and the implicated blood component. Associated components to the concerned blood component should be recalled and, if available, also cultured. If the contaminant organism is not part of the normal skin flora, the donor should be contacted and followed up. The donor's health should be considered as well as the possibility of recurrent contaminated donations. Depending on the results of the investigation, donor deferral from future donations might be required [14–16].

Prevention Strategies

Strategies used to decrease the levels of bacterial contamination in blood components include donor screening, skin disinfection, first aliquot diversion, pretransfusion detection and pathogen reduction technologies.

Donor Screening

Most transfusion centres have established methods for donor screening to avoid collection of potentially contaminated blood components. Donor screening includes body temperature determination and answering questions related to the donor's general health and potential signs of infection or silent bacteraemia, such as the occurrence of recent dental work, gastrointestinal diseases or malaise.

Skin Disinfection

Since the majority of PC contaminants are part of the skin flora, optimal skin disinfection of the phlebotomy site is essential to maximise the inactivation of contaminant bacteria during blood donation.

Several factors affect the efficacy of skin disinfection, including the type and concentration of antiseptic used and the mode of application. A two-step method involving a scrub with a 0.75% povidone–iodine compound followed by an application of a 10% povidone–iodine preparation solution is outlined in the AABB Technical Manual. A one-step 2% chlorhexidine and 70% isopropyl alcohol skin cleansing kit has been extensively validated and is being used in the UK, USA, Australia and Canada [8].

First Aliquot Diversion

Diversion of the first 30–40 mL of blood at the point of collection has been associated with significant reduction in contamination by skin flora at several blood centres [8,13,17]. The diverted blood sample is usually used for viral and immunohaematology testing.

Single Donor Apheresis Versus Pooled Platelet Concentrates

An increased risk of bacterial contamination has been traditionally associated with pooled platelet concentrates in comparison to single donor apheresis platelet concentrates due to a potential pooling of microorganisms [13]. However, nowadays, apheresis donors may donate by a double or triple platepheresis procedure and therefore multiple contaminated therapeutic units can be produced, counterbalancing the 'pooling' effect of whole-blood-derived platelet concentrates. Studies from other countries such as Canada and Germany have shown that the rate of contamination of apheresis platelet concentrates and buffy coat platelet pools is similar [18,19].

Bacterial Detection Methods

Routine testing of platelet concentrates for bacterial contamination has been implemented worldwide. Detection of bacteria in transfusable blood components is more complex than viral detection since bacterial titers increase over time under routine blood component storage

conditions. Factors that should be considered prior to the implementation of a bacterial screening method include the screening method and the testing protocol. Since initial bacterial loads are usually very low (<1 cfu/mL), a very sensitive technique should be used in the blood collection centre shortly after collection. However, less sensitive methods may be used at the hospital end for blood component screening prior to transfusion.

Pretransfusion Detection Methods Used by Blood Component Suppliers

The BacT/ALERT® 3D system (bioMérieux, Marcy l'Etoile, France) and the Pall enhanced Bacterial Detection System (eBDS, Pall Corporation, New York, USA) are culture systems that have been licensed in Europe and North America to detect bacterial contamination in PCs [4,5,20].

The BacT/ALERT system uses liquid aerobic and anaerobic culture bottles with a colorimetric sensor at the bottom that changes colour from green to yellow when pH decreases as a result of the metabolic activity of growing bacteria. The culture bottles are inoculated with 8–10 mL of PC samples and are incubated at 36 °C for 1–7 days, depending on the centre. This system can detect 1–10 cfu/mL of most common platelet contaminants [4]. When an initial positive culture is confirmed by repeat testing of the implicated blood component, a retention sample and/or samples from the recipient, it is considered to be a true (confirmed) positive. Table 16.1 summarises the rate of contamination in selected blood centres that use the BacT/ALERT system for platelet screening. True positive rates vary from 1/134 to 1/9863.

Despite its high sensitivity, several instances of missed bacteria detection in PCs tested by the BacT/ALERT system have been reported worldwide. Examples of microorganisms that were implicated in false-negative cases include *S. aureus* in the UK [1], *Salmonella*, *S. marcescens*, group A *Streptococcus*, *S. aureus* and

Table 16.1 Prevalence of bacterial contamination in platelet concentrates in selected blood centres [1,8].

Centre	Number of units/ pools tested	Initial positives	True positives Number	True positives Rate per 1000
American Red Cross regional blood centres	1 786 142	1285	351	0.2 (1/5088)
Belgian Red Cross	107 827	1030	803	7.4 (1/134)
Canadian Blood Services	917 321	811	93	0.1 (1/9863)
Copenhagen Transfusion Service	22 165	50	34	1.5 (1/651)
Department of Immunology and Transfusion Medicine, Norway	36 896	88	12	0.3 (1/3074)
Funen Transfusion Service, Denmark	22 057	84	21	1.0 (1/1050)
Welsh Blood Services	54 828	257	38	0.7 (1/1442)
UK, NHS Blood and Transplant	1 020 688	4 185	320	0.3 (1/3189)
Blood Centre of Zhejiang Province (China)	8000	21	5	0.6 (1/1600)
Japanese Red Cross	43 569	80	47	1.1 (1/927)
Australian Red Cross	302 386	3,207	550	1.8 (1/549)
Copenhagen Blood Transfusion Service Centre	22 165	50	34	1.5 (1/651)

Source: Data from McDonald et al. [1] and Ramirez-Arcos & Goldman [8].

coagulase-negative staphylococci in Canada [8,10,17] and *S. aureus*, coagulase-negative staphylococci, *Streptococcus* spp., *S. marcescens*, *E. coli*, *K. pneumoniae*, *Morganella morgannii*, *P. aeruginosa* and *Acinetobacter* spp. in the USA [2]. All of these false negatives resulted in septic transfusion reactions. Attempts to decrease the likelihood of false-negative transfusion reactions include increasing the testing volume, delaying sample testing, retesting components after 3–4 days of storage, transfusing early during storage or treating products with pathogen inactivation techniques.

Most centres routinely test for aerobic bacteria, as the majority of clinically significant organisms belong to this group. Centres using the two-bottle system have reported an increase in the detection rate of bacterial contamination in PCs since anaerobic culture bottles allow the capture of strict anaerobic bacteria such as *Propionibacterium acnes*. Although cases of transfusion-transmitted *P. acnes* have been reported, none of them have resulted in severe transfusion reactions. However, there are reports of severe and fatal ATRs due to the presence of the anaerobes *Eubacterium limosum* and *Clostridium perfringens* [8].

The Pall Bacterial Detection System uses the decrease in oxygen concentration as an indicator of bacterial growth in platelet concentrates. Between 4 and 6 mL of platelet concentrate samples are transferred into an incubation bag. After 24–30 hours of incubation, the oxygen concentration of this bag is measured with an oxygen analyser. A decrease in the percentage of oxygen to ≤19.5% is indicative of bacterial growth. This system only detects aerobic Gram-positive and Gram-negative bacteria at the levels of 100–500 cfu/mL with a sensitivity of 96.5%. The Pall eBDS system has been validated for bacteria detection in both PCs and red cells [7,8,13].

Other methods developed to detect bacterial contamination in PCs include detection of bacterial 16S rRNA genes by reverse transcriptase polymerase chain reaction and pH monitoring [7,8,20].

Bacterial Detection Methods to Be Used Prior to Transfusion

Methods to be used at the hospital can be less sensitive in detecting bacteria in the range of 10^3-10^4 cfu/mL, but such tests need to be rapid and specific. The Pan Genera Detection (PGD) immunoassay from Verax Biomedical (Marlborough, MA, US) and the BacTx colorimetric assay from Immunetics (Boston, MA, US) have been licensed by the FDA for late testing of platelet concentrates [20].

Pathogen Reduction Technologies

Pathogen reduction technologies involve the treatment of PCs as soon as possible after collection to inactivate or reduce the level of contaminating bacteria, viruses, parasites and residual leucocytes. Three technologies, Mirasol® (TerumoBCT, CO, USA), INTERCEPT™ Blood System (Cerus Europe BV, Amersfoort, The Netherlands) and THERAFLEX UV-Platelets technology (Macopharma, Tourcoing, France), have received CE (Conformité Européenne) Mark registration while only INTERCEPT has received FDA approval for use in the US [7,20].

The INTERCEPT process is used within the first 24 hours after collection and utilises a synthetic psoralen, amotosalen HCl, which targets nucleic acid and utilises UVA light (3J/cm^2: 320–400 nm) to form covalent adducts with nucleic acids. INTERCEPT inactivates a broad spectrum of bacterial species associated with transfusion reactions but cannot inactivate bacterial spores. No septic reactions have been reported in countries where the system has been used for several years [7,20].

The Mirasol system uses riboflavin (vitamin B2, 50 μg per 300 mL) with UVC, UVB and a portion of UVA light (265–375 nm). The efficacy of this process is based on the association of riboflavin with nucleic acids and the generation of reactive oxygen species, leading to nucleic acid disruption. The efficacy of Mirasol to inactivate bacteria ranges from 33% to 100% [7,20].

The THERAFLEX system, which utilises UVC light without a photochemical compound, is still in clinical development [7,20].

KEY POINTS

1) Bacterial contamination of blood components poses the most prevalent transfusion-transmitted infectious risk.
2) Platelet concentrates are the blood components most susceptible to bacterial contamination.
3) Interventions such as improved donor screening and skin disinfection, first aliquot diversion, bacterial testing and pathogen reduction technologies have decreased the occurrence of transfusion-associated septic events.
4) Gram-positive skin flora are the predominant blood component contaminants.
5) Gram-negative bacteria are less frequently found as blood component contaminants but they pose the major infectious risk due to their production of endotoxin.

References

1 McDonald CP, Allen J, Roy A et al. One million and counting: bacterial screening of platelet components by NHSBT, is it an effective risk reduction measure? Abstract 4D-S27-02. Vox Sang 2015;**109**(Suppl. 1): 61.
2 Fatalities Reported to FDA Following Blood Collection and Transfusion. Annual Summary for Fiscal Year 2015. Available at: http://www.fda.gov/downloads/BiologicsBloodVaccines/SafetyAvailability/ReportaProblem/TransfusionDonationFatalities/UCM518148.pdf (accessed 9 January 2017).
3 Transfusion Transmitted Injuries Surveillance System. Summary Results for 2006–2012.

Available at: www.phac-aspc.gc.ca/hcai-iamss/ ttiss-ssit/index-eng.php (accessed 11 November 2016).

4 Benjamin RJ, McDonald CP and the ISBT Transfusion Transmitted Infectious Disease Bacterial Workgroup. The international experience of bacterial screen testing of platelet components with an automated microbial detection system: a need for consensus testing and reporting guidelines. Transfus Med Rev 2014;**28**(2):61–71.

5 Pietersz RN, Reesink HW, Panzer S et al. Bacterial contamination in platelet concentrates. Vox Sang 2014;**106**(3):256–83.

6 Jacobs MR, Good CE, Lazarus HM, Yomtovian RA. Relationship between bacterial load, species virulence, and transfusion reaction with transfusion of bacterially contaminated platelets. Clin Infect Dis 2008;**46**(8):1214–20.

7 Corash L. Bacterial contamination of platelet components: potential solutions to prevent transfusionrelated sepsis. Expert Rev Hematol 2011;**4**(5):509–25.

8 Ramirez-Arcos S, Goldman M. Bacterial contamination, in Transfusion Reactions (ed. MA Popovsky), American Association of Blood Banks, Bethesda, 2012, pp.153–181.

9 Walther-Wenke G, Schrezenmeier H, Deitenbeck R et al. Screening of platelet concentrates for bacterial contamination: spectrum of bacteria detected, proportion of transfused units, and clinical follow-up. Ann Hematol 2009;**89**:83–91.

10 Kou Y, Pagotto F, Hannach B, Ramirez-Arcos S. Fatal false-negative transfusion infection involving a buffy coat platelet pool contaminated with biofilm-positive Staphylococcus epidermidis: a case report. Transfusion 2015;**55**(10):2384–9.

11 Greco C, Martincic I, Gusinjac A, Kalab M, Yang AF, Ramírez-Arcos S. *Staphylococcus epidermidis* forms biofilms under simulated platelet storage conditions. Transfusion 2007;**47**(7):1143–53.

12 Guinet F, Carniel E, Leclercq A. Transfusion-transmitted Yersinia enterocolitica sepsis. Clin Infect Dis 2011;**53**(6):583–91.

13 Palavecino EL, Yomtovian RA, Jacobs MR. Bacterial contamination of platelets. Transfus Apher Sci 2010;**42**(1):71–82.

14 Ramirez-Arcos S, Alport T, Goldman M. Intermittent bacteremia detected in an asymptomatic apheresis platelet donor with repeat positive culture for Escherichia coli: a case report. Transfusion 2015;**55**(11):2606–8.

15 Public Health Agency of Canada. Guideline for Investigation of Suspected Transmitted Bacterial Contamination. Available at: www.phac-aspc.gc.ca/publicat/ccdr-rmtc/08vol34/34s1/34s1-eng.php (accessed 11 November 2016).

16 Eder AF, Goldman M. How do I investigate septic transfusion reactions and blood donors with culturepositive platelet donations? Transfusion 2011;**51**(8):1662–8.

17 Robillard P, Delage G, Itaj NK, Goldman M. Use of hemovigilance data to evaluate the effectiveness of diversion and bacterial detection. Transfusion 2011;**51**(7):1405–11.

18 Jenkins C, Ramírez-Arcos S, Goldman M, Devine DV. Bacterial contamination in platelets: incremental improvements drive down but do not eliminate risk. Transfusion 2011;**51**(12):2555–65.

19 Schrezenmeier H, Walther-Wenke G, Müller TH et al. Bacterial contamination of platelet concentrates: results of a prospective multicenter study comparing pooled whole blood derived platelets and apheresis platelets. Transfusion 2007;**47**(4):644–52.

20 De Korte D, Marcelis JH. Platelet concentrates: reducing the risk of transfusion-transmitted bacterial infections. Int J Clin Transfus Med 2014;**2**:24–37.

Further Reading

AABB Association Bulletin #14-04. Available at: www.aabb.org/programs/publications/ bulletins/Documents/ab14-04.pdf (accessed 11 November 2016).

Bacterial Risk Control Strategies for Blood Collection Establishments and Transfusion Services to Enhance the Safety and Availability of Platelets for Transfusion – Draft Guidance for Industry. Available at: http://www.fda.gov/downloads/ Guidances/Blood/UCM425952.pdf (accessed 9 January 2017).

17 Emerging Infections and Transfusion Safety

Roger Y. Dodd

American Red Cross, Jerome H. Holland Laboratory for the Biomedical Sciences, Rockville, USA

Introduction

The Institute of Medicine in the United States has defined emerging infections as those whose incidence in humans has increased within the past two decades, or threatens to increase in the near future. Emergence may be due to the spread of a new agent, the recognition of an infection that has been present in the population but has gone undetected or the realisation that an established disease has an infectious origin. Emergence may also be used to describe the reappearance (or reemergence) of a known infection after a decline in incidence. A proportion of such emerging infections have properties that permit their transmissibility by blood transfusion; perhaps the most notable example has been HIV/AIDS, although there are others, such as West Nile virus (WNV), dengue virus, Zika virus, *Babesia* and malaria. This chapter will explain the basis for emergence of infectious agents and discuss their recognition and management in the context of the safety of the blood supply.

Emerging Infections

There is no single reason for the emergence of infections, although it is possible to establish relatively broad groupings [1].

- Failure of existing control mechanisms, including the appearance of drug-resistant strains,

vaccine escape mutants or cessation of vector control accounts for a large group of agents.
- Environmental change can have profound effects, whether through global warming, changes in land utilisation or irrigation practice, urbanisation or even agricultural practices.
- Population movements and rapid transportation can introduce infectious agents into new environments where they may spread rapidly and without constraint, as has been the case for WNV in the US.
- Human behaviours can contribute in a number of ways: new agents have been introduced into human populations by contact with, or even preparation and consumption of, wildlife; many infections have been spread widely though extensive sexual networks, and armed conflicts have led to extensive disease spread.

Of course, many of these factors may also work in combination. Key points are that new or unexpected diseases can appear in any location at any time and that an appropriate understanding of the epidemiology of such diseases can assist in the development of appropriate interventions.

In order to be transmissible by transfusion, an agent must have certain key properties [2].

- Most importantly, there must be a phase when the agent is present in the blood in the absence of any significant symptoms. Until recently, it was generally thought that such infectivity would reflect a long-term carrier

Practical Transfusion Medicine, Fifth Edition. Edited by Michael F. Murphy, David J. Roberts and Mark H. Yazer.
© 2017 John Wiley & Sons Ltd. Published 2017 by John Wiley & Sons Ltd.

state for the agent in question, as exemplified by HIV, HBV or HCV, although there had been a few cases of transmission of hepatitis A virus, which provokes an acute infection with a relatively short period of asymptomatic viraemia. However, the finding of transfusion transmission of WNV showed that, in epidemic outbreaks, acute infections could be readily transmitted by transfusion.

- A secondary requirement is that the agent must be able to survive component preparation and storage.
- Finally, the agent should have a clinically apparent outcome in at least a proportion of cases of infection, or it will lack clear relevance to blood safety and its transmission will not generally be recognised. There are some examples of transfusion-transmissible agents that do not seem to cause any significant outcomes, such as GB virus type C/hepatitis G virus (GBV-C/HGV) and torque tenovirus (TTV).

Table 17.1 lists a number of emerging infections that are known, or suspected, to be transfusion transmissible and also notes the factors thought to be responsible for their emergence.

Approaches to the Management of Transfusion-Transmissible Emerging Infections

As far as possible, emerging infections that do, or may, impact on blood safety should be managed in a systematic fashion. In general, this will be the responsibility of agencies that are charged with the maintenance of public health, or the management of the blood supply or its regulation. However, there are a number of areas in which individual professionals can contribute. One of these is the first step, which is the recognition of a transfusion-transmitted infection and its subsequent investigation. It is, in fact, unlikely that the first occurrence of an emerging infection will be seen in a transfused recipient, so it is therefore important that there be a system of assessing the threat and risk of emerging

infections for their potential impact on blood safety. This implies a process for evaluating each emerging infection for its transmissibility by this route and for estimating the severity and potential extent of the threat. The risk assessment should help to define the need for and urgency of development and implementation of interventions to reduce the risk of transmission of the agent. Such interventions, if implemented, should be evaluated for efficacy and modified as appropriate.

Increasingly, at least in the United States, there is declining use of blood and financial pressures on hospitals. This appears to be driving decisions on the adoption of blood safety issues towards the hospitals and away from the blood providers. In these circumstances, practitioners responsible for hospital blood services may find that they need to advocate for safety improvements within their hospital's management structure.

Assessing the Risk and Threat of Transfusion Transmissibility

It is important to have a general awareness of the status of new and emerging infections, with particular reference to your own country or area. Such awareness may involve familiarity with a number of sources of information, ranging from news media, through to alerts from local, national and global public health agencies, to specialised resources such as ProMED Mail (an internet list server and website that tracks and comments on disease outbreaks) [3]. Other tools continue to become available; for example, the American Association of Blood Banks (AABB) maintains a listing of potentially transfusion-transmissible infectious agents that has been published in print and on its website; the listing also contains much of the information discussed below, along with a ranking of threat level. Other agencies (for example, the Centers for Disease Control and Prevention and the World Health Organization) provide general, current information about emerging infectious agents on their websites.

Table 17.1 Selected emerging infections potentially or actually transmissible by blood transfusion.

Agent	Basis for emergence	Notes
Prions		
vCJD	Agricultural practice: feeding meat and bonemeal to cattle	Of most concern in UK; apparently coming under control
Viruses		
Chikungunya	Global climate change, dispersion of mosquito vector, travel	Rapid emergence in a number of areas, including Italy, the Caribbean and the Americas. Surveillance indicated
Dengue	Global climate change, dispersion of mosquito vector, travel	Similar properties to WNV; surveillance indicated, limited testing implemented
HBV variants	Selection pressure resulting from vaccination	Mutants may escape detection by standard test methods
HHV-8	Transmission between men who have sex with men and perhaps by intravenous drug use	Transmission by transfusion and transplantation known
HIV	Interactions with wildlife, sexual networks, travel	Classic example of an emerging infection
HIV variants	Viral mutation, travel	May escape detection by standard tests
Influenza	Pandemic anticipated as a result of antigenic change	Possible threat to blood safety, major impact on availability
SARS	Explosive global epidemic, wildlife origin, spread by travel	No demonstrated transfusion transmission, epidemic over
Simian foamy virus	Exposure to monkeys, concern about species jumping and mutation	Regulatory concern over blood safety, intervention in Canada
WNV	Introduction into the US (probably via jet transport), rapid spread across continent	Recognition of transfusion transmission in 2002 led to rapid implementation of NAT for donors
Zika virus	Introduced to Brazil via air transport	Explosive expansion through Americas via *Aedes* spp.; major concern over causation of microcephaly, rapid implementation of multiple interventions
Bacteria		
Anaplasma phagocytophilum	Tick-borne agent expanding its geographic range	At least 8 potential transfusion transmissions reported
Borrelia burgdorferi	Tick-borne agent expanding its geographic range and human exposure	No transfusion transmission reported
Coxiella burnetii	Intensive goat farming in The Netherlands, human exposure	Presumptive evidence of transfusion transmission, donor selection and NAT implemented
Parasites		
Babesia spp.	Tick-borne agent expanding its geographic range and human exposure	More than 200 transfusion transmission cases reported Geographically selective investigational testing
Leishmania spp.	Increased exposure to military and others in Iraq, Afghanistan	Unexpected visceral forms potentially transmissible
Plasmodium spp.	Classic reemergence, in part due to climate change, travel	Reemergence threatens value of travel deferral
Trypanosoma cruzi	Imported into nonendemic areas by population movement	Transfusion transmissible, preventable by donor testing

HBV, hepatitis B virus; HHV, human herpes virus; HIV, human immunodeficiency virus; NAT, nucleic acid testing; SARS, severe acute respiratory syndrome; vCJD, variant Creutzfeldt–Jakob disease; WNV, West Nile virus.

Box 17.1   Key questions to assess risk of transfusion transmissibility of an infectious agent.

1) Have transfusion-transmitted cases been observed?
2) Does the agent have an asymptomatic, blood-borne phase?
3) Does the agent survive component preparation and storage?
4) Are blood recipients susceptible to infection with the agent?
5) Does the agent cause disease, particularly in blood recipients?
6) What is the severity, mortality and treatability of the disease?
7) Are there recipient conditions, such as immunosuppression, that favour more severe disease?
8) Is there a meaningful frequency of infectivity in the potential donor population?
9) Is this frequency declining, stable or increasing?
10) Are there reasons to anticipate any changes in the frequency of donor infectivity?
11) What is the level of concern about the agent and its disease amongst professionals, public health experts, regulators, politicians, media and general population?
12) Are there rational and accessible interventions to eliminate or reduce transmission by transfusion?

Box 17.1 outlines questions that serve to define the risk of transfusion transmission of each agent and the potential extent and severity of that risk. The primary question is whether or not the disease agent can, in fact, be transmitted by blood. As pointed out above, this is dependent on the presence of an asymptomatic phase during which the disease agent is present in the bloodstream. In some cases, of course, there may already be documentation of transfusion transmission of the agent in question, or there may be suggestive evidence, such as transmission by organ transplantation. However, in the latter case, such evidence may not be definitive, as rabies has been transmitted by organ transplantation but is almost certainly not transmissible by blood. The answer to this question is not always readily obtainable, but may often be inferred by considering what is known about the natural transmission route of the infection, or from the properties of closely related organisms. The duration of the blood phase of the infection will have a direct impact on the risk of transmission, reflecting the chance that an individual will give blood during the infectious phase.

The actual risk of transmission is a function of the frequency of the infection in the donor population and the length of the period of blood-borne infectivity [4]. The period of infectivity may not, however, be identical to the period during which the infectious agent can be detected in the blood. For example, in the case of WNV, periods of viraemia in excess of 100 days have been measured occasionally, but the actual infectious period may be limited to the week or two prior to the appearance of IgG antibodies. Another difficulty is that the frequency of disease and the frequency of infection may differ greatly, as is again the case with WNV.

Nevertheless, it is abundantly clear that individuals who do not develop symptoms may be infectious via their blood donations. Consequently, it may be important to estimate the size of the infected (and infectious) population by laboratory testing rather than through disease reporting. Indeed, organised studies of prevalence rates of infection amongst donor populations have been used in many circumstances in order to assess the level of risk and to predict the impact of a testing intervention. Examples of this approach include studies on HTLV, trypanosomes (*T. cruzi*), *Babesia* and more recently, dengue virus, where assessments of the frequency of viraemia are proving valuable.

Another important factor is the dynamics of the outbreak. Is the frequency of infection stable or increasing, and if increasing, is change linear or logarithmic and what is the rate of increase? Obviously, rapid increase, as seen in the case of WNV, would imply a need for a more rapid response than would a slow, linear increase, as in the case of *T. cruzi*.

The severity of disease that may result from a transfusion-transmitted infection is also an important guide to the extent and speed of implementation of any intervention. There are both objective and subjective aspects to such an assessment. Clearly, the severity of the disease and its associated mortality can be defined, but it may also be important to judge the public concern around the disease, which may be disproportionate to its actual public health impact [2]. Another factor that is often presented as important is the extent to which a transfusion-transmitted infection might result in further or secondary infections. In actual fact, transmission of an infection by transfusion will almost certainly not lead to any magnification of an epidemic, but nevertheless, it is something that should be considered.

A word of caution is in order with respect to efforts to use modern laboratory methods to identify previously unrecognised infectious agents. There is increasing enthusiasm for this approach, but it is important to recognise that without any established relationship to a disease state, the results of such searches can be misleading. At this time, for example, it does not appear that either TTV or GBV-C/HGV has any relationship to any disease state and they do not seem to offer risk to blood recipients, despite clear evidence of their transmissibility. It is unclear how many other such orphan viruses are awaiting discovery.

The recent recognition and management of a new retrovirus, XMRV, originally thought to be associated with prostate cancer and chronic fatigue syndrome (CFS), is instructive. It was suggested that this virus was a threat to transfusion safety and an organised programme was put in place to evaluate this possibility [5,6].

A complication was that CFS advocates actively promoted the concept of transfusion risk as a means to establish legitimacy (and perhaps funding) for the disease. A key activity was a careful, blinded evaluation of a number of different tests for XMRV, including those used by the laboratories responsible for the original discoveries. This evaluation, along with other studies, revealed that the available tests could not reliably identify the virus or related ones, either in patient samples or negative controls [7]. The original observations were eventually shown to be due to various forms of contamination and XMRV itself was revealed to be a laboratory artefact. Whilst early intervention for an emerging infection may be necessary and appropriate, care should be taken to avoid reacting to situations involving incomplete or imperfect science.

Recognition of Transfusion Transmission of Emerging Infections

There is no simple formula for recognising that a transfusion-transmitted infection has occurred, particularly in the case of a rare or unusual disease agent. Nevertheless, many such events have been recognised by astute clinicians. Knowledge of the potential for transmission of an emerging infection can be valuable and very likely contributed to the relatively early recognition of transfusion transmission of WNV [8]. Unusual posttransfusion events with a suspected infectious origin should be brought to the attention of experts in infectious diseases or public health agencies for assistance in identification and follow-up. Appropriate investigation of illness occurring a few days or more after transfusion can reveal infections through identification of serological or molecular evidence of infectious agents in posttransfusion samples. However, such detection is by no means definitive. It is helpful if a pretransfusion patient sample is also available, as this will reveal whether the condition predated the transfusion. Also, recall and further testing of implicated donors will reveal whether one or more of them was the likely source of the infection. Ideally, if the responsible organism can be isolated from both donor and recipient, molecular analyses such as nucleic acid sequencing can demonstrate (or exclude) the identity of the agent from the two sources.

Information from the donor may also be a critical source of identification of a transfusion transmission. More specifically, donors are requested to report to the blood collection facility the occurrence of any signs of illness in the few days after donation. This allows the blood components to be recalled or, if already transfused, should lead to investigation of the recipient. The first two reported cases of transfusion-transmitted dengue were identified in this fashion. Similarly, lookback to recipients of prior donations from a donor with a newly recognised infection may identify transmission of a chronic infection. Indeed, all cases of transfusion transmission of HIV in the United States since 1999 were recognised through lookback.

There are significant problems in recognising that infections with a very long incubation period may have been transmitted by transfusion; this was illustrated by HIV/AIDS, which did not result in well-defined illness until many years after exposure. This prevented early recognition of transfusion-transmitted AIDS and further concealed the actual magnitude of the infectious donor population and of the population of infected blood recipients. This implies that, for emerging infections that appear to have lengthy incubation periods, it would be wise to assess transfusion transmissibility by serological or molecular evaluation of appropriate donor–recipient sample repositories, or to engage in some form of active surveillance such as that used to identify the transmission of variant Creutzfeldt–Jacob disease (vCJD) by transfusion in England [9]. Haemovigilance programmes may contribute to the identification of posttransfusion infections, although they are generally designed to identify well-described outcomes.

Interventions

In the event that an emerging infection is found to be transfusion transmissible and public and professional concern implies a need to protect the safety of the blood supply, there are a number of interventions that could be considered.

A possible but rather unsatisfactory approach is to focus on the recipient by diagnosing and treating cases that occur. This, of course, works only for treatable infections. It is *de facto* part of the approach to manage transfusion babesiosis in the United States at this time. In the case of highly localised outbreaks, or where there are alternate sources of blood, it may be possible to stop collection of blood in the affected area.

Most interventions are focused on the donor or the donation. In the absence of a test, it may be possible to devise a question that would identify some proportion of donors at risk of transmitting the infection. Such measures are usually neither sensitive nor specific but may have value, particularly where the disease is localised so that a travel history is sufficient to identify those at risk.

The development and implementation of a test for infectivity in donor blood is usually a more sensitive and specific approach than questioning, and for some infections may be the only valid solution. In the past, serological tests were relied upon but now, nucleic acid testing is also available and may be a better solution, as was the case for WNV. Indeed, a test for WNV RNA was developed and implemented in less than a year in the United States [10]. However, this is not always the optimal solution. For example, some parasitic diseases in particular result in long-term, antibody-positive infection with very low levels of infectious agent in the bloodstream, resulting in only intermittent NAT-positive findings. This is particularly true of Chagas' disease, and as most individuals were infected early in life, antibody tests are preferable for identifying potentially infectious donors [11].

An emerging technology that offers some promise is pathogen reduction, which is a treatment that inactivates infectious agents in blood whilst retaining the biological activities of the blood itself. Methods are currently available for plasma and for platelet concentrates and are in use in some countries. It should be noted that available methods may have differing efficacies for different infectious agents and that they may not be fully successful in eliminating very high levels of infectivity for some agents, although this has not been established in practice. A real disadvantage is that no method is currently available for red cells. A pathogen reduction method was implemented for platelets in the island of La Réunion during a large outbreak of chikungunya virus infection and has been used for recent Zika outbreaks.

The precautionary principle is often cited when interventions to reduce the risk of transfusion-transmitted infections are discussed. In general, it is suggested that, in the absence of any specific information about the efficacy of an intervention, it is appropriate to implement it, as long as it does no harm. This position may be arguable, particularly as commentary on the precautionary principle suggests that it should not be invoked without some evaluation to assure that the measure is not extreme and does not exceed other measures taken in known circumstances. In fact, significant measures were taken to reduce the potential risk of transmission of vCJD even before it was known that it was transmissible by transfusion. It can be argued that subsequent events justified the precautions taken, but this may not always be the case [12].

Making decisions about the implementation of blood safety measures is very complex and requires consideration of many objective and subjective factors. Increasingly, attention is being focused upon the process of risk-based decision making, which has recently been formalised [13].

KEY POINTS

1) Some emerging infections may threaten the safety of the blood supply.
2) Those responsible for maintaining the safety of the blood supply should be familiar with emerging infections.
3) Physicians responsible for the care of transfused patients should be alert for signs of unexpected infections.
4) The nature and extent of the safety threat offered by emerging infections may be assessed by examination of a fairly simple sequence of questions.
5) If interventions are needed, consideration should be given to the use of donor questions and/or laboratory tests.
6) Care must be taken to balance public concern against good science.

References

1 Morens DM, Folkers GK, Fauci AS. Emerging infections: a perpetual challenge. Lancet Infect Dis 2008;**8**:710–19.
2 Stramer SL, Hollinger FB, Katz LM et al. Emerging infectious disease agents and their potential threat to transfusion safety. Transfusion 2009;**49**(Suppl.):1S–233S.
3 www.promedmail.org/
4 Glynn SA, Kleinman SH, Wright DJ, Busch MP, NHLBI Retrovirus Epidemiology Study. International application of the incidence rate/ window period model. Transfusion 2002;**42**:966–72.
5 Klein HG, Dodd RY, Hollinger FB et al., the AABB Interorganizational Task Force on XMRV. Xenotropic murine leukemia virus-related virus (XMRV) and blood transfusion: report of the AABB Interorganizational XMRV Task Force. Transfusion 2011;**51**:654–61.
6 Simmons G, Glynn SA, Holmberg JA et al., for the Blood XMRV Scientific Research Working Group (SRWG). The Blood Xenotropic Murine

Leukemia Virus-Related Virus Scientific Research Working Group: mission, progress, and plans. Transfusion 2011;**51**:643–53.

7 Simmons G, Glynn SA, Komaroff AL et al., for the Blood XMRV Scientific Research Working Group (SRWG). Failure to confirm XMRV/MLV in the blood of patients with chronic fatigue syndrome: a multi-laboratory study. Science 2011;**334**:814–17.

8 Biggerstaff BJ, Petersen LR. Estimated risk of West Nile virus transmission through blood transfusion during an epidemic in Queens, New York City. Transfusion 2002;**42**:1019–26.

9 Hewitt PE, Llewelyn CA, Mackenzie J, Will RG. Creutzfeldt–Jakob disease and blood transfusion: results of the UK Transfusion Medicine Epidemiological Review study. Vox Sang 2006;**91**:221–30.

10 Dodd RY. Perspective: Emerging infections, transfusion safety and epidemiology. N Engl J Med 2003;**349**:1205–6.

11 Benjamin RJ, Stramer SL, Leiby DA, Dodd RY, Fearon M, Castro E. *Trypanosoma cruzi* infection in North America and Spain: evidence in support of transfusion transmission. Transfusion 2012;**52**(9):1913–21.

12 Wilson K, Ricketts MN. The success of precaution? Managing the risk of transfusion transmission of variant Creutzfeldt-Jakob disease. Transfusion 2004;**44**:1475–8.

13 https://allianceofbloodoperators.org/abo-resources/risk-based-decision-making/rbdm-framework.aspx

Further Reading

Alter HJ, Stramer SL, Dodd RY. Emerging infectious diseases that threaten the blood supply. Semin Hematol 2007;**44**:32–41.

Biggerstaff BJ, Petersen LR. Estimated risk of transmission of the West Nile virus through blood transfusion in the US, 2002. Transfusion 2003;**43**:1007–17.

Dodd RY, Leiby DA. Emerging infectious threats to the blood supply. Annu Rev Med 2004;**55**:191–207.

Hewitt PE, Llewelyn CA, Mckenzie J, Will RG. Creutzfeldt–Jakob disease and blood transfusion: results of the UK Transfusion Medicine Epidemiology Review study. Vox Sang 2006;**91**:221–30.

Mackenzie JS, Gubler DJ, Petersen LR. Emerging flaviviruses: the spread and resurgence of Japanese encephalitis, West Nile and dengue viruses. Nat Med 2004;**10**(12)(Suppl.):S98–S108.

Simmons G, Glynn SA, Komaroff AL et al. Failure to confirm XMRV/MLVs in the blood of patients with chronic fatigue syndrome: a multi-laboratory study. Science 2011;**334**:814–17.

Stramer SL, Dodd RY, AABB Transfusion-Transmitted Emerging Infectious Diseases Subgroup. Transfusion-transmitted emerging infectious diseases: 30 years of challenges and progress. Transfusion 2013;**53**:2375–83.

Stramer SL, Fang CT, Foster GA, Wagner AG, Brodsky JP, Dodd RY. West Nile virus among blood donors in the United States, 2003 and 2004. N Engl J Med 2005;**353**:451–9.

Stramer SL, Hollinger FB, Katz LM et al. Emerging infectious disease agents and their potential threat to transfusion safety. Transfusion 2009;**49**(Suppl.):1S–233S.

Tomashek KM, Margolis HS. Dengue: a potential transfusion-transmitted disease. Transfusion 2011;**51**:1654–60.

Weiss RA, McMichael AJ. Social and environmental risk factors in the emergence of infectious disease. Nat Med 2004;**10**(12)(Suppl.):S70–S76.

18

Regulatory Aspects of Blood Transfusion

William G. Murphy[1], Louis M. Katz[2] and Peter Flanagan[3]

[1] Irish Blood Transfusion Service, and University College Dublin, Dublin, Republic of Ireland
[2] America's Blood Centers, Washington, DC, USA; Infectious Diseases, Carver College of Medicine, University of Iowa Healthcare, Iowa City, USA
[3] New Zealand Blood Service, Auckland, New Zealand

Introduction

Blood is an irreplaceable medicine used in life-saving circumstances. Every country's government must ensure that its citizens and visitors have access to an adequate supply of safe and effective blood for transfusion. The World Health Organization (WHO) has identified the importance of a well-legislated and regulated blood transfusion service as a crucial component in assuring safety [1]. Because it is necessary to source blood from biologically and behaviourally heterogeneous humans, absolute uniformity of product and its absolute safety cannot be guaranteed, no matter how extensively we interrogate donors, and test and process their donations. Pragmatic compromises must be reached between adequate safety and adequate supply.

Government, through the regulatory agencies, has explicit responsibility for overseeing the safety of blood for transfusion. Blood suppliers also have an ethical and professional responsibility to go beyond the minimum regulatory or legal requirements in the interests of safety if the regulator does not require sufficient quality, and in any event they have a responsibility to ensure that standards are met in a consistent manner. Government is also ultimately responsible for the adequacy of supply, and must ensure that the compromise between safety and supply is achieved.

The Components of Blood Regulation

Guiding Principles and Law

National or international law, which has the force of justice and humanity, and which is defined and enacted by legitimate representatives of the society concerned, establishes the regulatory framework for blood components in a jurisdiction. A competent system of regulation must be backed by such law, which specifies and limits the scope and power of the regulator. The law should be explicit, and production of blood for transfusion in a state should be expressly governed by statute. For example, within the EU member states, the national statutes are subject to the Blood Directives – a set of laws developed over several years between 1996 and the present that are binding on all the member states of the Union. There is a core or parent Directive [2] and a set of subsidiary ones covering donors and donations and component specifications [3], traceability and haemovigilance [4] and quality systems [5]. Additional updates and modifications may appear in response to emerging threats or technical advances. Elsewhere national, federal, provincial and state laws almost invariably provide a basis for regulation, though in several parts of the world such laws and regulations may be merely aspirations [6].

Guiding principles may be explicit or implicit. For example, the EU specifies 'Principles of Good Practice' [7] as the principles covering the quality systems in blood establishments (Article 11 of 2002/98/EC – the core EU Directive on Blood Transfusion [2], and a recent amendment to the Quality Directive [8]), and furthermore specifies Good Manufacturing Practice (GMP) as an overall guiding principle in the Preamble of Directive 2002/98/EC3. The Preamble also contains other statements of principle, scope and intent, and these may have a legal function in the event of dispute. It states, for example, that the intent of the regulations is to ensure public health, thereby forever giving blood safety in the EU primacy over legitimate commercial interests in the drafting and execution of regulations. The Therapeutics Goods Administration (TGA) in Australia produces a specific Code of GMP for blood and tissues. This includes both quality and technical standards that must be met. The United States Food and Drug Administration (FDA) states that GMPs are the guiding principles in the functioning of blood services. GMPs (generally called just GMP outside North America) are a dynamic and very comprehensive set of overall directions, principles, rules and regulations that reduce the entropy in a complex system, and thereby the likelihood of mishap. Regulators, however, draft regulation as well as enforce it, and can and do increase complexity beyond any possible meaningful improvement in safety. This requires a constant dynamic in the regulatory process in the light of emerging knowledge, science and understanding: see below.

The precautionary principle emerged in the 1980s as a statement of best practice when faced with serious but unquantifiable risks. This principle was enshrined at the 1992 Rio Conference on the Environment and Development: 'Where there are threats of serious or irreversible damage, lack of full scientific certainty shall not be used as a reason for postponing cost-effective measures to prevent environmental degradation'. Since then it has come to be explicitly adopted for health protection, for example in the European Union [9] and in Canada [6,10]. It continues to develop and evolve and to gather increased force of law through case law in Europe and elsewhere.

Most formulations of the precautionary principle include explicit acknowledgment that decisions taken under its aegis are subject to reconsideration and modification as more complete data are accrued. This results in tensions over what constitutes sufficient evidence to undertake amendment of long-standing regulatory decisions.

Standards

Professional advisory bodies as well as technical standards bodies such as the International Standards Organization (ISO) may set product and process standards to be adhered to for accreditation, whereas regulators define rules and regulations that blood component and service providers must comply with to operate within the law. Regulators may, however, mandate accreditation by other bodies as a regulation to be complied with. In this way, ISO standards and national technical standards bodies or of professional bodies such as the American Association of Blood Banks (AABB) and the College of American Pathologists (CAP) in the United States may be explicitly applied to blood component or transfusion service providers and may be given force of law. Standards used for accreditation and regulatory purposes need to be current; they also need a firm, functioning and explicit mechanism of review and change as scientific knowledge accrues, circumstances change and experience informs.

Application and Enforcement of Regulations

A regulation is of limited value if it is not or cannot be enforced because the rule of law is lax, the enforcing agency is weak or the standard is unrealistic or unrealistically expensive. There are three levels of application of regulations and standards in the regulatory setting.

Inspection/Accreditation/Licencing

In most countries with a robust health system, all bodies participating in the business of providing blood for transfusion are required to be visible and accountable through an official process, usually by some combination of registration, accreditation and licencing. Self-inspection, or accreditation by peer review, is generally no longer considered acceptable in isolation. Different scales of licencing requirements often apply to facilities that collect and test blood from donors than to hospital blood banks, who either store blood for transfusion and issue it, or who conduct minimal processing. Licences are time limited and require renewal with reinspection typically every 1–3 years.

Enforcement

The rule of law demands compliance. Regulatory authorities can and do apply fines, sometimes of millions of dollars, to blood establishments that fail to comply with legal requirements. Hospital blood banks may be closed for serious quality failures. Blood transfusion staff may be arrested and jailed, though usually as a result of egregious events rather than for systematic failures detected through routine application of regulatory methods.

Vigilance: Haemovigilance/Feedback/Market Surveillance

Large-scale systematic well-organised surveys of clinical outcomes over tens or hundreds of thousands of recipients are required to track the occurrence and even to establish the existence of problems with the function, safety and quality of medicines, devices or processes. Within blood transfusion practice, this is known as haemovigilance; originally mandated in France and voluntary in the UK, it has evolved to become mandatory in many jurisdictions. In the United States, a formal haemovigilance initiative was integral to the modification of blood donor deferrals for male-to-male sexual behaviours (www.fda.gov/BiologicsBloodVaccines/BloodBloodProducts/QuestionsaboutBlood/ucm108186.htm). In the EU, haemovigilance also extends to adverse effects in blood donors. This will change approaches to donor care as more valid statistics on the incidence of very rare events emerge, and lead to mandatory approaches to such common events as iron deficiency.

Threat Surveillance

Some regulatory agencies have adopted a formal threat surveillance role, by which they generally mean infectious disease threat surveillance. For example, the FDA works closely with the Centers for Disease Control and other agencies in the Department of Health and Human Services in the United States, and in Europe the European Commission works with the European Centre for Disease Control. Haemovigilance systems augment this approach. The Alliance of Blood Operators (ABO) has developed a risk-based decision-making framework to help address emerging threats in a systematic manner [11].

The Regulatory Bodies (Table 18.1)

There are several types of bodies involved in the regulatory framework or structure in blood transfusion. They contribute to the formulation or application of the law and/or the formulation, application or review of standards, or they can enforce the regulations.

National Statutory Bodies with Powers of Enforcement

Most high and medium development index countries have a more or less functioning national medicines agency that sets and applies standards for drugs and biologics being manufactured, imported, sold and prescribed in that country. Similar bodies, in many cases the same body, set and apply standards for labile blood components. They have the force of law and can fine or imprison those who break the law. A person setting up their own blood collection service within the EU, for example, without a licence from the relevant government agency would face serious charges. Examples of such bodies are the FDA in the United States, the Medicines and Healthcare products Regulatory Agency (MHRA) in the UK, Agence Nationale de Sécurité du Médicament et des Produits de Santé (ANSM) in France, the Paul Erhlich Institute (PEI) in Germany, Therapeutic Goods Administration (TGA) in Australia, Health

Table 18.1 Agencies involved in regulatory processes in blood transfusion.

Type of agency	Name	Role	Further information
Multinational agency with statutory powers	The European Commission	Drafts laws for implementation in European Union member states. These laws include technical specifications for blood components, for example. Oversees the application of those laws through national authorities – the 'competent authorities'	Lacks a well-defined structure for scientific analysis of the impact of the laws on healthcare and health economic implications of practices; has a limited but developing ability to adapt to advances in the field
National agency under statutory authority from legislative bodies with regulatory powers, and significant scientific/ developmental/leadership roles	The FDA (United States); Paul Ehrlich Institute (Germany); Agence Nationale de Sécurité du Médicament et des Produits de Santé (ANSM) (France)	Defines national rules and regulations and licences the blood establishments in national or federal setting. Conducts scientific programmes aimed at developing the field of blood banking and the scientific basis of regulation, and publishes its work in a peer-reviewed environment	Within the EU, the member states have to comply with the basic requirements of the EU laws; beyond that they are free to impose other requirements and standards. Germany, through the PEI, licences blood components as medicines, as does Austria. In the US, the FDA establishes minimum requirements for safety, purity and potency and licences and inspects facilities against them and maintains an active research programme in support of good regulation and guidance
National agency under statutory authority from legislative bodies with regulatory powers, but without significant in-house scientific activity, though in some cases they provide scientific leadership through structured partnerships between the regulator, BTS and government agencies	Health Canada, the Therapeutic Good Agency (Australia), MHRA (UK), South Africa, New Zealand, other EU member states, Brazil, etc.	Inspects and licences blood banks and blood transfusion services on its territory in accordance with national laws (in the EU these national laws are subservient to EU law and must include all the EU requirements as a minimum)	
National agency that also manages the blood supply	In several of the old Communist bloc countries, for example, a combined central power base was established at the national blood service provider, who then assumed the role of regulator in the EU setting	Both provider and regulator. Very difficult to avoid the impression of failure of separation of responsibilities	

(Continued)

Table 18.1 (Continued)

Type of agency	Name	Role	Further information
International treaty-defined agency with considerable leverage in national and international blood banking policies and regulations	The World Health Organization/Pan-American Health Organization	The WHO requires member states to develop policies and standards in national blood transfusion systems	The WHO carries considerable force in many parts of the world, but much less so in high development index areas. In several countries dependent on aid for blood transfusion development, the WHO approach has quasi-regulatory status
	The Council of Europe (European Directorate for the Quality of Medicines and Health Care, EDQM)	The Council of Europe has for many years produced an annual technical guideline, which attempted to raise the bar of quality in member states in an iterative fashion. This function has now devolved to the EDQM under the influence of the European Commission. The Guide is now published every two years. Recent editions have begun to separate standards from principles. Increasingly EDQM is positioning itself as the technical organisation managing the technical aspects of the Directives. This in many ways mirrors its work in managing the European Pharmacopeia	This situation is in evolution – the EDQM is developing a more formal link with the European Commission in this function, i.e. providing the technical expertise the Commission needs to maintain regulation in blood transfusion (the only country to date to give the Council of Europe Guide regulatory force is Australia)
Supranational incorporated bodies that have no statutory powers, but seek to provide scientific leadership and define standards of professional practice	AABB, ISBT		
Supranational incorporated bodies that have no statutory powers but have a lobbying and advocacy function	ABC, ABO, EBA, IPPC, IPFA, PPTA, International Federation of Red Cross and Red Crescent Societies		

Patient organisations	Groups representing patients who depend on a safe and adequate supply of blood components for health – including people with haemophilia, thalassaemia, immune deficiencies or antitrypsin deficiency	Organisation to put pressure on blood services, commercial suppliers and politicians to address patients' needs for an adequate supply of good-quality, safe medicines	Can be very powerful campaigners for change in the legislation or regulation of blood components, especially where supply and safety may be compromised
Donor organisations	FIODS (International Federation of Blood Donor Organizations)	Promote voluntary unpaid donation; strong supporters of blood collection programmes	Influence and activity vary considerably from country to country
Other groups who involve themselves in public debates and political activity in relation to blood transfusion	Notably LBGT (lesbian, bisexual, gay and transgender) groups and supporting allied groups such as student unions	Address perceived inequalities and discrimination in donor deferral policies or in access to services and products	In several jurisdictions such groups have been successful in changing restrictions banning men who have sex with men from donating blood

*The Council of Europe is not the European Council – the former is a union to promote humanitarian values and principles in law, rights and health, among other areas, and produces advice and works by recommendation and peer pressure between states; the latter is an administrative arm of the European Union. (The other two administrative arms are the Commission – essentially a very powerful civil service – and the Parliament. While all EU member states belong to the Council of Europe, not all Council of Europe member states belong to the EU.)

Canada in Canada and the various national agencies in the EU and other European countries. They are not all the same – some, notably the FDA, PEI and ANSM, have developed roles as leaders in blood transfusion science and participate actively in developments in the field. In several countries, including some of the old Eastern bloc members of the EU, the agency within the state responsible for regulation (in the EU these agencies are called 'Competent Authorities') is also the national transfusion service, reflecting older Communist structures. In these cases it is very difficult to maintain the perception of avoidance of conflicting interests.

Supranational Agencies with Statutory Powers

The European Commission in the EU – essentially the civil service of the European Union – has very broad powers in the field of consumer safety and citizens' health, including explicit powers under the founding treaty for ensuring blood safety. A series of laws (Directives) have been enacted since 2002 that cover licencing of blood establishments, accreditation of hospital blood banks and technical specifications, from donor qualification to component transportation. In addition, the Directives address traceability and haemovigilance. The Commission has very little in-house expertise in blood transfusion and uses industry expertise, sourced mainly through the Departments of Health in the member states, to provide support.

The FDA in the United States is of a similar scale and scope, insofar as it has a remit across the 50 states, a number of territories and commonwealths and the District of Columbia. The United States carries substantial weight in the industry far beyond other national statutory agencies. It has a very mature and heavily resourced function in defining standards and direction of research and, uniquely, decides which tests or other technologies must and may be applied within its jurisdiction.

Supranational Agencies with Treaty-Defined Powers and Remits

There are two of these – the World Health Organization (including the Pan American Health Organization, PAHO) and the Council of Europe. They may exclude countries from membership, but in reality their power is soft and their function is essentially advisory, though they can provide support with funding or with channelling of funding from others. While the WHO involvement in blood transfusion carries considerable weight in medium and low development index countries, this is not the case in high index ones. The WHO's approach is essentially to promote national policies around a central nationally coordinated blood transfusion service with accountability to government.

Professional Organisations within the Blood Transfusion Community Itself That Set or Define Professional Standards

These bodies have no statutory powers. Examples include the AABB and the International Society of Blood Transfusion (ISBT), and national professional organisations. They have an important regulatory function in providing professional support, including defined professional standards.

Other Agencies

There are other agencies with more limited input into the regulatory process. These include those with an advocacy role at government or international level: the International League of Red Cross and Red Crescent Societies, America's Blood Centers (ABC), the European Blood Alliance (EBA), the ABO and professional trade associations such as the International Plasma Producers Congress (IPPC), the Plasma Protein Therapeutics Association (PPTA) and the International Plasma Fractionation Association (IPFA).

Patient Involvement

The voice of the patient in regulation of blood transfusion, where expressed, is generally through the political process and the governance arrangements for regulators, hospitals and blood suppliers. In addition, several well-organised groups representing users of blood components – people with thalassaemia and sickle cell anaemia – and plasma products – people with haemophilia or primary immune deficiencies – have valid concerns and often provide formal input into regulatory processes [12].

Donor Involvement

Donor associations exist as separate entities to blood transfusion services in several countries and have an international body – the International Federation of Blood Donor Associations. From time to time, these groups may lobby regulators, governments and blood suppliers.

Other Groups

Public bodies, for example lesbian, bisexual, gay and transgender groups and allied groups, may become involved in public debates and issues surrounding blood transfusion from time to time.

The Role of Blood Transfusion Agencies and Health Professionals Vis-À-Vis Regulatory Agencies

Laws, regulations, ethics and social values evolve. What is accepted as ethical and proper in one time and place may not be legal in another. Laws governing gender and sexuality are but one example. So while the law as it is must be observed and respected, it need not be revered as complete, correct or immutable. Neither should it be seen to be outside the sphere of influence of the public to whom it applies. In contrast, it is the civic duty of citizens of a state and the ethical duty of scientists and physicians everywhere to attempt to correct deficits or address shortcomings in the law, whether through contributing to the drafting of new statutes, correcting technical errors, including omissions, in the law itself or advocating repeal when the prevailing conditions render laws obsolete. This must be effected through legal and transparent processes, perhaps ideally through competent and legal organisations for this purpose, including, in blood transfusion, the AABB, ABC, EBA and similar bodies.

In almost no country are the regulatory authorities concerned with improvements in the efficacy of red cells or platelets, or with treatment protocols and guidelines. These remain the preserve of the professionals in the field. Blood remains a problematic medicine; regulation tends by its nature to be very conservative and tends to preserve the status quo at the expense of development. This may give rise to a natural and often constructive tension between regulators and practitioners, to whom it is obvious that there is much to be improved.

Regulatory compliance is always part of professional and scientific integrity and endeavour, but it is never all of it, and much less a substitute for it.

KEY POINTS

1) A well-legislated and regulated blood transfusion service is a crucial component in assuring safety of the blood supply within a country or state, although there are large differences among different jurisdictions in how this is addressed.

2) Regulations should, but do not always, address issues of adequacy of supply and availability of blood within a state, as well as quality, safety and scientific developments.

3) Regulations are based in law, which should be explicit in statute, and are governed by guiding principles, often in practice a version of the precautionary principle and the principles and rules of Good Manufacturing Practice.

4) State regulatory agencies apply standards; these are often set by national accreditation or standards bodies, or by professional bodies within the field.

5) The nature and scope of regulations may be influenced by forces inside or outside blood transfusion – lobbying by professional groups, trade organisations, patients and groups and other interested bodies can apply pressure for change at the political and public levels.

References

1 World Health Organization. Resolutions Relating to Blood Safety Adopted by WHO governing Bodies. Available at: www.who.int/bloodsafety/en (accessed 11 November 2016).

2 Directive 2002/98/EC of 27 January 2003 of the European Parliament and of the Council setting standards of quality and safety for the collection, testing, processing, storage and distribution of human blood and blood components and amending Directive 2001/83/EC. Official Journal of the European Union 2003; L 33/30.

3 Commission Directive 2004/33/EC of 22 March 2004 implementing Directive 2002/98/EC of the European Parliament and of the Council as regards certain technical requirements for blood and blood components. Official Journal of the European Union 2004; L 91/25.

4 Commission Directive 2005/61/EC of 30 September 2005 implementing Directive 2002/98/EC of the European Parliament and of the Council as regards traceability requirements and notification of serious adverse reactions and events. Official Journal of the European Union 2005; L 265/32.

5 Commission Directive 2005/62/EC of 30 September 2005 implementing Directive 2002/98/EC of the European Parliament and of the Council as regards Community standards and specifications relating to a quality system for blood establishments. Official Journal of the European Union 2005; L 256/41.

6 Epstein J, Seitz R, Dhingra N et al. Role of regulatory agencies. Biologicals 2009;**37**:94–102.10.

7 Good Practice Guidelines for Blood Establishments and Hospital Blood Banks Required to Comply with EU Directive 2005/62/EC. Available at: www.edqm.eu/sites/default/files/medias/fichiers/good_practice_guidelines_dec_2013.pdf (accessed 11 November 2016).

8 Commission 2016 Directive 2016/1214 of 25 July 2016 amending Directive 2005/62/EC as regards quality system standards and specifications for blood establishments. Official Journal of the European Union; L199/14.

9 Europa. Summaries of EU Legislation. The Precautionary Principle. Available at: http://eur-lex.europa.eu/legal-content/EN/TXT/?uri=URISERV%3Al32042 (accessed 11 November 2016).

10 Vamvakas EC, Kleinman S, Hume H, Sher GD. The development of West Nile virus safety policies by Canadian blood services: guiding principles and a comparison between Canada and the United States. Transfus Med Rev 2006;**20**:97–109.

11 www.allianceofbloodoperators.org/abo-resources/risk-based-decision-making.aspx (accessed 11 November 2016).

12 O'Mahony B, Peyvandi F, Bok A. Does the orphan medicinal product regulation assist or hinder access to innovative haemophilia treatment in Europe? Haemophilia 2014;**20**(4):455–8.

Further Reading

Commission Directive (EU) 2016/1214 of 25 July 2016 amending Directive 2005/62/EC as regards quality system standards and specifications for blood establishments (Text with EEA relevance). Available at: http://eur-lex.europa.eu/legal-content/EN/TXT/?uri=CELEX%3A32016L1214 (accessed 11 November 2016).

Food and Drug Administration. Good Guidance Practices. 21 CFR 10.115. Available at: www.ecfr.gov/cgi-bin/text-idx?SID=b0b64a301338e214335664f9ef08de6e&mc=true&node=se21.1.10_1115&rgn=div8 (accessed 11 November 2016).

Sunstein CR. The Laws of Fear: Beyond the Precautionary Principle. Cambridge: Cambridge University Press, 2005.

19 The Role of Haemovigilance in Transfusion Safety

Katharine A. Downes[1] and Barbee I. Whitaker[2]

[1] University Hospitals, Cleveland Medical Center Case Medical Center and Case Western Reserve University, Cleveland, Ohio, USA
[2] Research and American Association of Blood Banks Center for Patient Safety, Bethesda, USA

Introduction

The goal of the haemovigilance movement is to improve patient and donor safety and transfusion outcomes [1]. The International Haemovigilance Network (IHN) defines haemovigilance as:

> A set of surveillance procedures covering the entire transfusion chain (from the donation of blood and its components to the follow-up of recipients of transfusions), intended to collect and assess information on unexpected or undesirable effects resulting from the donation of blood and the therapeutic use of labile blood products, and to prevent the occurrence or recurrence of such incidents.

Since transfusion hazards occur anywhere from donor selection to recipient transfusion to consequences beyond transfusion, a haemovigilance system needs a broad scope to capture, identify and define such risks.

Merely collecting data without acting on it does not prompt transfusion system improvements. Establishing problem frequency and documenting process failures help determine priorities and allocate resources towards highest impact opportunities. Thus, haemovigilance systems provide opportunities for improvement in transfusion systems and patient outcomes.

Origin and Structures

Haemovigilance systems arose from events that challenged the safety of blood transfusion. The handling of the HIV risk in the 1980s provided additional impetus for ongoing risk assessment measures. In subsequent years, as transfusion risk from HIV and HCV diminished through concerted interventions, efforts and attention were redirected towards long-standing, incompletely addressed problems.

Over the past 23 years, haemovigilance systems have developed in countries around the globe with legal and organisational structures that vary from country to country (Figure 19.1).

The European Community currently requires implementation of a haemovigilance system in each member state, with reporting to a central office [7]. Systems in other developed nations take a hybrid approach, with some residing within and deriving reporting mandates from a national ministry of health while others are primarily organised collaboratively through professional societies or a nation's blood collection system. Although each country has developed characteristics unique to its own healthcare and transfusion systems, haemovigilance systems bear multiple similarities and yield similar results [8]. Features of successful haemovigilance systems are listed in Box 19.1.

Practical Transfusion Medicine, Fifth Edition. Edited by Michael F. Murphy, David J. Roberts and Mark H. Yazer.
© 2017 John Wiley & Sons Ltd. Published 2017 by John Wiley & Sons Ltd.

Year	Country/Region	Development
1992	Japan	Earliest reported system [2]
1992	France	First European system, mandatory reporting [3]
1996	United Kingdom	First European voluntary system reporting system – Serious Hazards of Transfusion (SHOT) [4]
2003	Europe	European Blood Directives [5]
2003	United Kingdom	Discovery of association between TRALI and female plasma
2010	United States	Voluntary reporting system developed through public-private sector collaboration [6]

Figure 19.1 Timeline of critical haemovigilance events.

Box 19.1 Important features of a haemovigilance system.

Standardised definitions and terminology
Nonpunitive data evaluation
Broad participation, supported by education
Reporting of occurrence using rates
Confidentiality of submitted data
Sufficient detail to make effective recommendations to improve practice(s)
Focus on improved safety and outcomes
Simple, efficient operations
Sustainable organisation

Box 19.2 Benefits of standardised, uniform data and terminology.

Permit use for data capture and reporting
Ensure data integrity for comparative analyses
Enable consistent tracking of internal performance over time
Permit benchmarking across institutions
Allow for assessment of outcomes of process improvements

Definitions and Terminology in Haemovigilance Systems

Analysis of clinical events such as transfusion reactions or near miss incidents requires clear, precise definitions resistant to misinterpretation in order to decrease the chance of misapplying a classification and degrading submitted data. Standardised definitions and categorisation in data capture are necessary for meaningful comparisons in data analysis (Box 19.2).

The IHN recognised early on the importance of data convention standardisation for comparison between systems [9]. Often incorporated into transfusion adverse event definitions are criteria that define the reaction, score its severity and determine the imputability or likelihood that the observed event is attributable to transfusion. The International Society of Blood Transfusion (ISBT) haemovigilance working party developed transfusion reaction definitions that

may be used to achieve commonality and facilitate meaningful comparisons of data between countries. An example of an ISBT transfusion reaction definition is given in Box 19.3.

Some systems interpose a review of the reported event to ensure that it meets the reporting system definitions. Such rigour adds robustness to reporting, but larger systems or those with fewer resources need to depend on participants' adherence to definitions and accurate data entry. Even with clear definitions of adverse events, misapplication of definitions may occur. Some haemovigilance systems adjudicate reported data submitted prior to analysis; for those that lack adjudication, process validation of the application of definitions may be critical at local and national levels [11].

Adverse Event Detection and Reporting

All haemovigilance systems develop and/or apply a system to capture events directly from the site of transfusion or donation. Ensuring that those

---

Box 19.3 International Society for Blood Transfusion haemovigilance definition, severity score and imputability grade examples [10].

Definition: hypotensive transfusion reaction

- This reaction is characterised by hypotension defined as a drop in systolic blood pressure of ≥30 mmHg occurring during or within one hour of completing transfusion **and** a systolic blood pressure ≤80 mmHg.
- Most reactions do occur very rapidly after the start of the transfusion (within minutes). This reaction responds rapidly to cessation of transfusion and supportive treatment. This type of reaction appears to occur more frequently in patients on ACE inhibitors.
- Hypotension is usually the sole manifestation but facial flushing and gastrointestinal symptoms may occur.
- All other categories of adverse reactions presenting with hypotension, especially allergic reactions, must have been excluded. The underlying condition of the patient must also have been excluded as a possible explanation for the hypotension.

Severity

Grade 1 (nonsevere): the recipient may have required medical intervention (e.g. symptomatic treatment) but lack of such would not result in permanent damage or impairment of a body function.
Grade 2 (severe): the recipient required inpatient hospitalisation or prolongation of hospitalisation directly attributable to the event resulted in persistent or significant disability or incapacity; or the adverse event necessitated medical or surgical intervention to preclude permanent damage or impairment of a body function.
Grade 3 (life-threatening): the recipient required major intervention following the transfusion (vasopressors, intubation, transfer to intensive care) to prevent death.
Grade 4 (death): the recipient died following an adverse transfusion reaction.

- *Grade 4 should be used only if death is possibly, probably or definitely related to transfusion. If the patient died of another cause, the severity of the reaction should be graded as 1, 2 or 3.*

Imputability

This is, once the investigation of the adverse transfusion event (ATE) is completed, the assessment of the strength of relation to the transfusion of the ATE.
Definite (certain): when there is conclusive evidence beyond reasonable doubt that the adverse event can be attributed to the transfusion.
Probable (likely): when the evidence is clearly in favour of attributing the adverse event to the transfusion.
Possible: when the evidence is indeterminate for attributing the adverse event to the transfusion or an alternative cause.
Unlikely (doubtful): when the evidence is clearly in favour of attributing the adverse event to causes other than the transfusion.
Excluded: when there is conclusive evidence beyond reasonable doubt that the adverse event can be attributed to causes other than the transfusion.

- *Only possible, probable and definite cases should be used for international comparisons.*

likely to first identify problems with a transfusion will report the occurrence is a critical first step in creating and maintaining a useful, credible haemovigilance system. Some systems identify and train individuals who oversee reporting of events into the system (France, United Kingdom, Quebec) while others with more established transfusion medicine professional presence at the hospital level employ pre-existing hospital transfusion reaction monitoring systems that report to the hospital's transfusion service and committee (United States). Regulatory and accreditation requirements strongly influence many aspects of such transfusion reaction reporting systems in US healthcare organisations.

Haemovigilance System Limitations

Untoward outcomes occurring long after a transfusion will always inherently challenge haemovigilance systems because of the loss of an obvious temporal relationship (Box 19.4). For example, identifying transfusion-transmitted infection requires recognising the lack of other means of transmission to the recipient and relative rarity of the disease entity. The healthcare provider would need to contact the transfusion

---

Box 19.4 Limitations of haemovigilance systems.

Incomplete reporting
Detection of transfusion relationship of late events, including infections
Limited details
Variation in terminology and definitions
Influence of healthcare system's or institution's 'culture' regarding compliance, process improvement and reporting
Acceptance of nonstandard definitions and terminology
Inability to track cases back to their source to ensure that correct and complete reporting has occurred

---

service for investigation and possibly haemovigilance system reporting. Haemovigilance-like investigations led to the detection of transfusion-transmitted West Nile virus (WNV) relatively early in the United States outbreak; linking poor patient outcome and transfusion exposure of an organ donor would have been more difficult if the incubation period had been longer. Additional utility of a haemovigilance system is real-time assessment of regional risk through donor testing and revision of donor testing protocols in response to information. Haemovigilance systems are not constructed to identify emerging infectious agents or other agents that remain unknown.

Scope of Reporting

The scope of haemovigilance systems varies; there are relative advantages and disadvantages to different approaches (Box 19.5). While the UK system limits its focus to only *serious* hazards having the largest potential impact on a particular recipient, such a design may miss events of lesser morbidity that affect a larger number of patients or that may be harbingers of more serious sequelae. The more common approach of seeking to capture all transfusion reactions risks system fatigue with numerous, less informative reports of nonsevere events obscuring major, clinically significant events.

Including incidents not directly associated with a reaction or an untoward outcome is an important means to detect problems in the transfusion system and preventing these from harming patients. Whether called 'incident', 'deviation' or 'error', failures to adhere to standard procedures may represent human limitations, inadequate training, unique features of a patient's situation or a combination of factors that align with weak points in the transfusion system. Most notable among these has been patient and sample identification errors in pretransfusion testing. Inclusion of 'near miss' events where the error is detected and remedied and/or where it does not cause harm to the recipient quickly

Box 19.5 Variations among haemovigilance systems.

Scope	Serious events
	All events regardless of severity including 'near miss' events
	Only events causing harm
Breadth	Labile transfusible components
	Plasma derivative products
	Tissues and/or organs for transplantation (biovigilance)
Analysis	System level
	Institutional level
	Healthcare system level, comparison with all hospitals – locally, regionally, nationally and/or internationally
	Comparison with (anonymous) peer institution subset
	Appropriateness of analysis of incidents and events
	Access to full details of incidents and events

causes such occurrences to become the most commonly reported events in a haemovigilance system. Some haemovigilance systems do not examine product- or process-related incidents unless there is actual harm to the recipient or donor. Although these occurrences may individually appear to be of minor importance, they represent a critical view into the workings of a transfusion system and allow preventive actions to be taken to bolster system safeguards.

Breadth of the System

While the IHN's definition of haemovigilance focuses on labile components, there remains much to be learned about the use of and reactions to plasma derivative products. In some jurisdictions, such as Canada, these are handled through the same transfusion service system. The principles of haemovigilance – including product traceability, learning from one's practice and a commitment to continual improvement – are

applicable to transplantation as transfusion services handle these products in some countries.

Inclusion of donor operations is integral to a haemovigilance system since a system that spans the transfusion process is best positioned to identify system problems and inform policy changes. Already enlightening have been data on the frequency of postdonation reaction rates with different blood volumes collected and delineation of the rate of postdonation death among donors assumed to be healthy. As with the recipient-focused end of the system, established standardised terminology and definitions should be used to ensure comparability of recorded observations [12].

Analysis of Incident Reports

A healthcare system and national review of transfusion system problems and outcomes are important. At the smallest unit of common policies and practice (usually the hospital), transfusion reactions and practice should be analysed and compared to the larger whole, such as national comparators. The individual hospital which participates in a national haemovigilance system that captures these kinds of data can benefit by comparing their experience to that of others working in the same type of system. Understanding where in the transfusion chain differences in practice are occurring may identify steps and practices in the process associated with superior outcomes.

The degree to which an institution focuses on outcome improvement and adherence to policies is probably an important determinant of haemovigilance system acceptance and high rates of reporting compliance. It is more likely that staff will feel comfortable reporting occurrences when 'incidents' are considered system failures rather than failures of personnel. As incidents are part of the transfusion process, they may be linked in some cases with adverse events; a recent study of transfusion-associated circulatory overload (TACO) found that one in five TACO reactions was due to human error [13].

Reporting Requirements Structure

Haemovigilance system reporting requirements may be voluntary or mandatory. Error reporting will suffer in a system where reporting may be 'required' but more frequently leads to punishment of individuals rather than changes to what may be a cumbersome, error-prone system. A nonpunitive approach to reporting – for the reporting individual and the institution itself – is essential for compliance. Even with confidentiality safeguards, voluntary reporting is unlikely to attract respondents unless the value of reporting efforts is understood. All systems note a rise in the number of reports submitted over their first few years as more become aware of the system, its importance and the logistics of reporting. System endorsement by a professional association or the ministry of health may boost participation, particularly if the system is easy to use.

Whether participation is voluntary or mandatory, local preparation is a key success factor. Effective preparation includes detailed review of current processes and procedures for adverse reaction reporting and a gap analysis compared to what will be expected for the haemovigilance programme [14]. Such reviews optimally include representation from all stakeholder groups, including physicians, nurses, laboratory staff and information system support staff, sufficient time for creating locally appropriate policies and procedures and adequate testing and training. Pilot implementation at a hospital may be a useful way to uncover issues for correction prior to data entry into a national haemovigilance system.

Data Management

Reporting simplicity is key to high participation rates. Most haemovigilance systems are converting or have converted to electronic submission systems. An intelligent, web-based data capture system could display only items pertinent to the case report as it unfolded. Such a context-sensitive system could check for completeness or internal congruity in a case and prevent entry errors. The quality of analysis possible from computerised databases depends upon the appropriateness of the definitions of the data elements established in the database, appropriate application of definitions and consistent data entry.

Most haemovigilance systems are not interfaced with a facility's internal error management software, but centrally coordinated healthcare systems may be able to integrate laboratory information, patient medical records, error management and haemovigilance systems to accomplish this. ISBT128 uniform terminology [15] provides the traceability that is key for haemovigilance structures. Ideally, data integration of multiple information system sources (hospital, laboratory, blood bank) reduces complexities and duplication [16].

The more detail of an event captured, the greater impact on policy development reports can offer. Capturing detail about where an incident occurred may help identify high-risk clinical areas and knowing which steps in the transfusion process were vulnerable to error will similarly help direct attention to the part of the transfusion process where improvements may have greatest impact. Capturing the results of root cause analysis and estimating recurrence probability and impact can help focus attention on critical targets.

A critical category of data elements in a haemovigilance system is the denominator of the number of units of each component type transfused or the number of pretransfusion specimens tested which is used to turn reported occurrences into rates. Once a system is mature after a few years with a well-established reporting rate, then quality assurance projects and interventions may be pursued. A comparison of event rates may allow meaningful comparison across institutions and/or countries of different sizes and transfusion activity levels.

Learning from Experience

Haemovigilance systems are sufficiently mature in a number of countries that the medical literature is providing an increasing number of reports of their observations. These observational reports allow interesting insights into the problems faced by different transfusion systems and the risks borne by their donors and recipients.

Common themes from haemovigilance led to recommendations that have improved transfusion safety. Transfusion of the incorrect unit or component is the most potentially serious system problem which may manifest as the patient not receiving precisely the component (sub) type ordered or as a fatal haemolytic transfusion reaction. Inadequate and/or inaccurate patient or sample identification at the time of pretransfusion sampling and at transfusion are frequent problems that defy simple solutions and merit more attention and capable technology. As shown by the Canadian experience, almost half of all high severity incidents were related to pretransfusion sample collection, and a third of all high severity events where harm occurred were associated with transfusion of the incorrect unit.

The greatest mortality risk in most systems currently appears to be transfusion-related acute lung injury (TRALI), although assessment of the frequency of this complication is complicated due to subtle differences in the definitions applied and that significant underrecognition is undoubtedly occurring.

Recognition of the magnitude of the problem posed by TRALI and the high frequency of TRALI cases associated with the plasma of female donors prompted the UK's National Blood Service to reduce the proportion of plasma for transfusion from female donors, resulting in a marked reduction in the number of deaths attributable to TRALI.

Identification in a single reporting period that TACO was the most common cause of post-transfusion mortality in Quebec [1] prompted increased clinician education about this condition, and additional clinical attention to the complication lead to a decline in its frequency.

Data from haemovigilance systems have helped define the frequency of bacterial contamination of platelets, investigate clusters of such incidents and document the effects of patient safety-oriented interventions [17].

Several applications of haemovigilance data from the Serious Hazards of Transfusion(SHOT) system have been particularly noteworthy, improving transfusion safety in the UK system and showing the power of haemovigilance when data are applied thoughtfully through evidence-based recommendations (see Further Reading).

Reports of mistransfusion due to patient/sample misidentification continued unabated until the recognition that descriptions of the problem alone would not effect an improvement. Evolution of the SHOT recommendations included near miss events, not just mistransfusions, that cause patient harm. Subsequent implementation of augmented approaches to patient, sample and unit identification was associated with a decline in the number of reported deaths due to mistransfusions. Similar results of interventions have been reported from other systems, such as in France, where ABO-incompatible transfusions were reduced by three-quarters [18]. SHOT continues to refine its recommendations on this topic to address patient safety concerns [19], demonstrating that improvement to patient safety is an iterative process.

Haemovigilance data have led to some unexpected, intriguing observations. Thirteen fatal cases of graft-versus-host disease (GVHD) [20,21] were reported in a 10-year time span through SHOT, all of them prior to the implementation of universal leucocyte reduction and all but two of them in patients who did not meet the usual indications for use of irradiated components. Universal leucocyte reduction was associated with a marked reduction in the number of posttransfusion purpura (PTP) cases reported and an apparent shift of these from predominantly red cell recipients (57% from 3%) to include more platelet recipients. This information may be useful in exploring the pathophysiology of these reactions and provide information that may be relevant to blood supply systems not currently employing this approach to component production. Without a haemovigilance system operating 'in the background' to amass this experience, these findings might have been missed due to the relative infrequency of GVHD and PTP.

Future Directions

Haemovigilance systems applied locally could address important, unanswered research questions through the large number of tracked events. Even a healthcare subunit may choose to apply haemovigilance definitions to its own practice(s) to better characterise adverse events and their frequency [22,23]. A haemovigilance system's large purview can be applied for postmarketing surveillance to help assess the safety of new interventions, such as pathogen inactivation through targeted studies. As new technologies emerge through tablets and smartphones, opportunities for new reporting tools may be added to haemovigilance's armamentarium.

Intangible Benefits

In addition to evidence-based benefits, haemovigilance programmes bring intangible benefits. Participating in a coordinated, standardised programme aimed at improving patient transfusions engenders confidence in laboratory and clinical staff, and particularly for laboratory staff, greater recognition of the role they play in patient care. The benchmarking inherent in haemovigilance may interest clinical departments and hospital administrators seeking such data. Computerising formerly paper-based processes reduces inefficiencies of manual data entry. Participating in haemovigilance efforts also offers satisfaction from being involved in an even greater good.

KEY POINTS

1) 'If you can't measure it, you can't improve it'; measurement alone will not improve systems. Concerted action to improve transfusion systems and reduce transfusion risks is necessary.

2) Haemovigilance systems are most effective when based on data reported consistently using standardised nomenclature and definitions.

3) Including 'near miss' incidents in haemovigilance reporting provides insights into weak points of the transfusion process and opportunities to improve the system by reducing the potential for human error to cause harm.

4) The most dangerous problem reported across multiple haemovigilance systems is the transfusion of an incorrect blood component, often relating to sample and patient identification errors.

5) Identifying serious problems followed by action(s) directed at their cause can improve transfusion safety, as seen in the steps taken to reduce the frequency of TRALI and ABO-related acute haemolytic events.

6) Haemovigilance systems may be extended to provide important information about haemotherapy decisions and follow-up of new transfusion approaches.

References

1 Engelfriet CP, Reesink HW. Haemovigilance. Vox Sang 2006;**90**:207–41.

2 Juji T, Nishimura M, Watanabe Y, Uchida S, Okazaki H, Tadokoro K. Transfusion-associated graft-versus-host disease. ISBT Sci Ser 2009;**4**:236–40.

3 Rebibo D, Hauser L, Slimani A, Hervé P, Andreu G. The French haemovigilance

system: organization and results for 2003. Transfus Apher Sci 2004;**31**:145–53.

4 Stainsby D, Jones H, Asher D et al, on behalf of the SHOT Steering Group. Serious hazards of transfusion: a decade of hemovigilance in the UK. Transfus Med Rev 2006;**20**:273–82.

5 Directive 2002/98/EC of the European Parliament and of the Council of 27 January 2003 setting standards of quality and safety for the collection, testing, processing, storage and distribution of human blood and blood components and amending Directive 2001/83/EC. Available at: http://eur-lex.europa.eu/legal-content/EN/TXT/?uri=CELEX:32002L0098 (accessed 13 November 2016).

6 Chung, K, Harvey A, Basavaraju, Kuehnert MJ. How is national recipient hemovigilance conducted in the United States? Transfusion 2015;**55**:703–7.

7 Directive 2002/98/EC of the European Parliament and of the Council of 27 January 2003 setting standards of quality and safety for the collection, testing, processing, storage and distribution of human blood and blood components and amending Directive 2001/83/EC. Available at: http://eur-lex.europa.eu/legal-content/EN/TXT/?uri=CELEX:32002L0098 (accessed 13 November 2016).

8 Faber JC. Work of the European haemovigilance network (EHN). Transfus Clin Biol 2004;**11**:2–10.

9 Robillard P, Chan P, Kleinman S. Hemovigilance for improvement of blood safety. Transfus Apher Sci 2004;**31**:95–8.

10 International Society of Blood Transfusion Working Party on Haemovigilance. Proposed Standard Definitions for Surveillance of Non Infectious Adverse Transfusion Reactions. Available at: www.isbtweb.org/fileadmin/user_upload/Proposed_definitions_2011_surveillance_non_infectious_adverse_reactions_haemovigilance_incl_TRALI_correction_2013.pdf (accessed 13 November 2016).

11 AuBuchon JP, Fung M, Whitaker B, Malasky J. AABB validation study of the CDC's National Healthcare Safety Network Hemovigilance

Module adverse events definitions protocol. Transfusion 2015;**54**:2077–83.

12 Standard for Surveillance of Complications Related to Blood Donation. Available at: www.aabb.org/research/hemovigilance/Documents/Donor-Standard-Definitions.pdf/(accessed 15 January 2017).

13 Piccin A, Cronin M, Brady R, Sweeney J, Marcheselli L, Lawlor E. Transfusion-associated circulatory overload in Ireland: a review of cases reported to the National Haemovigilance Office 2000–2010. Transfusion 2015;**55**:1223–30.

14 Dunbar N, Walsh SJ, Maynard KJ, Szczepiorkowski ZM. Transfusion reaction reporting in the era of hemovigilance: where form meets function. Transfusion 2011;**51**:2583–7.

15 Kong C, Meng Z, Lv H, Yan L, Zheng X. Implementation of ISBT128 in China. Transfusion 2010;**50**:80–4.

16 Sharma G, Parwani AV, Raval JS, Triulzi DJ, Benjamin RJ, Pantanowitz L. Contemporary issues in transfusion medicine informatics. J Pathol Inform 2011;**2**:3.

17 Robillard P, Delage G, Ital NK, Goldman M. Use of hemovigilance data to evaluate the effectiveness of diversion and bacterial detection. Transfusion 2011;**51**:1405–11.

18 Renaudier P. The French Hemovigilance Network: from the blood scandal to epidemiologic surveillance of the transfusion chain, in Hemovigilance: An Effective Tool for Improving Transfusion Safety (eds RR de Vries, JC Faber). Wiley-Blackwell, Chichester, 2012, pp.147–58.

19 SHOT Annual Report and Summary 2015. Available at: www.shotuk.org/wp-content/uploads/SHOT-2015-Annual-Report-Web-Edition-Final-bookmarked-1.pdf. (accessed 15 January 2017).

20 Kopolovic I, Ostro J, Tsubota H et al. A systematic review of transfusion associated graft-versus-host disease. Blood 2015;**126**(3):406–14.

21 Williamson LM, Stainsby D, Jones H et al, on behalf of the Serious Hazards of Transfusion Steering Group. The impact of universal leukodepletion of the blood supply

in hemovigilance reports of posttransfusion purpura and transfusion-associated graft-versus-host disease. Transfusion 2007;**47**:1455–67.

22 Oakley FD, Woods, Marcella, Arnold S, Young PP. Transfusion reactions in pediatric compared with adult patients: a look at rate, reaction type, and associated products. Transfusion 2015;**55**:563–70.

23 Li N, Williams L, Zhou Z, Wu Y. Incidence of acute transfusion reactions to platelets in hospitalized pediatric patients based on the US hemovigilance reporting system. Transfusion 2014;**54**:1666–72.

Further Reading

AuBuchon JP, Whitaker BI. America finds hemovigilance! Transfusion 2007;**47**:1937–42.

Callum JL, Kaplan HS, Merkley LL et al. Reporting of nearmiss events for transfusion medicine: improving transfusion safety. Transfusion 2001;**41**:1204–11.

De Vries RR, Faber JC (eds). Hemovigilance: An Effective Tool for Improving Transfusion Safety. Wiley-Blackwell, Oxford, 2012.

De Vries RR, Faber JC, Strengers PF, Board of the International Haemovigilance Network. Haemovigilance: an effective tool for improving transfusion practice. Vox Sang 2011;**100**(91):60–7.

Williamson LM. Transfusion hazard reporting: powerful data, but do we know how best to use it? Transfusion 2002;**42**:1249–52.

Serious Hazards of Transfusion Home Available at: www.shotuk.org/home.

20

Donors and Blood Collection

Marc Germain[1], Ellen McSweeney[2] and William G. Murphy[2,3]

[1] Héma-Québec, Quebec City, Canada
[2] Irish Blood Transfusion Service, National Blood Centre, Dublin, Republic of Ireland
[3] Health Service Executive, Clinical Strategy and Programmes, and University College Dublin, Republic of Ireland

Collecting blood from people for transfusion to others is an essential part of healthcare. A developed healthcare system needs to provide approximately 27–40 therapeutic units of red cells and up to six therapeutic doses of platelets annually per thousand of the population it serves.

Blood Donors: Paid, Directed, Payback and Altruistic

People can be motivated to donate blood in three different ways:

- as a direct response to the needs of an individual they care about
- for an economically valued reward
- as an altruistic act.

All three methods are in wide use today, and all have their drawbacks. However, societies that succeed in establishing a mature programme of altruistic donations generally gain a more secure and stable supply of safer blood for transfusion. There is compelling evidence that the incidence and prevalence of infectious diseases are higher among donors who donate for personal economic gain. Also, individuals who are directly approached by a relative or friend to donate for a particular patient are more likely to withhold critical information about their personal infectious risk history.

Motivation, recruitment and retention of altruistic donors are not easy or cheap. In most developed nations, 5% or less of the population donates per year. Establishing and maintaining a mature altruism-based blood donation and collection programme requires a high degree of social cohesion and an immense effort in education and communication. Many successful national or regional programmes based on altruism were set up around the middle of the twentieth century, at a time of national need in conflict or post-conflict. Countries that did not establish altruism-based blood services to begin with have tended to find it much more difficult to establish one afterwards. Huge efforts are currently being made to redress this throughout the developing world (see Chapter 24).

Paying blood donors will provide a supply of blood, but it requires enough people in the population for whom the payment on offer provides sufficient motivation. In more developed economies, the balance of high demand for blood for transfusion with limited numbers of people who will be motivated by the rewards on offer, often makes paying for donations an inadequate strategy. In addition, paying for blood also undermines the alternative, more successful motivation of altruism in these economies.

Apart from the problems of supply, paid donors are, in general, a less safe source than volunteer donors. In an analysis of 28 published

Practical Transfusion Medicine, Fifth Edition. Edited by Michael F. Murphy, David J. Roberts and Mark H. Yazer.
© 2017 John Wiley & Sons Ltd. Published 2017 by John Wiley & Sons Ltd.

data sets, it was found that while the incidence of disease markers had diminished over the years between 1977 and 1996 for paid and unpaid donors alike, unpaid donors were on average 5–10 times safer than paid donors and that this difference had not changed over time (see van der Poel et al., in Further Reading). It is assumed that people who have no great incentive to donate other than genuine regard for their fellow humans will tend not to withhold risk information. People who need money or items of small economic value at the level they may be offered by blood services are more likely to withhold relevant risk information. In addition, increased at-risk exposure from drug addiction or sex working occurs more frequently at the lower economic margins of a Westernised society.

A system of directed and payback donations, where donors are recruited among the relatives and friends of the patient requiring blood transfusions, also provides some supply. Such an approach will generally be insufficient to support a well-developed healthcare system and is prone in places to covert payments to donors, including professional donors. However, it is believed by some experts that a system relying on donations by family members and acquaintances may offer a viable and safe alternative in developing countries where a fully altruistic model is not yet in place.

European Union (EU) Directive 2002/98/EC (see Further Reading) instructs member states to promote community self-sufficiency in human blood and blood components and to encourage voluntary unpaid donations of blood and blood components.

Even in the altruistic model, the underlying motivations to donate blood are likely to be multifaceted and complex. Fortunately, blood donation behaviour is increasingly being studied by psychologists and sociologists. These insights will help blood collection agencies to attract and retain donors, beyond the well-accepted strategies that successful programmes already apply: active communication with the donor from the beginning, making donation convenient, reducing donor anxiety and adverse reactions, having well-trained and motivated staff and encouraging temporarily deferred donors to return as soon as possible following the expiry of their deferral period [1].

Challenges still remain in recruiting donors from ethnic minorities. Migrant populations have different disease patterns with different transfusion demands. Added to this, data suggest that migrants tend not to become blood donors in their new country. A number of factors may contribute to the proportionally low representation of minorities in the donating population, including culture, lack of social/ethnic identification, fear and lack of information.

Donor Management in Europe

Almost 50 blood establishments from 34 European countries contributed to the development of the DOMAINE Donor Management in Europe Project (see Further Reading) to analyse practices in donor management in Europe. The project compiled a *Donor Management Manual* and developed a training programme to provide tools for blood establishments to optimise practice in their local context. The manual covers all aspects of donor management, from recruitment and retention to donor counselling and ethical issues.

Risks to the Blood Donor

Blood donation is generally very safe. Most people can readily tolerate venesections of approximately 10% of their blood volumes without apparent harm or significant physiological compromise. However, it is not a trivial undertaking and requires considerable care to minimise the risk to the donor, who can almost never expect any health benefit from the donation. The risks associated with blood donation are listed in Table 20.1.

An internationally accepted description and classification of adverse events and reactions was proposed by the European Haemovigilance

Table 20.1 Adverse events or reactions in blood donors.

Type of event or reaction	Incidence
Vasovagal events or reactions	
Dizziness, nausea, simple fainting, severe faint with prolonged loss of consciousness and convulsions; associated trauma from falls or vehicle accidents	1.4–7% moderate reactions rate* 0.1–0.5% severe reaction rate*
Hospitalisation rate	1 per 198 000 donations* Two-thirds of these are due to vasovagal reactions
Needle injury	
Sore arm	12.5% females, 6.9% males*
To the vein, causing pain and bruising, which may be extensive, thrombophlebitis, thrombosis	9–23%*
To the artery, causing extensive bruising, fistula, aneurysm, distal ischemia, compartment syndrome	0.003–0.011%*
To the nerve, causing pain, and motor and sensory loss, which can be prolonged	0.016–0.9%* 0.0022% (disablement)*
To a tendon, causing acute and intense pain	Rare
Serious cardiovascular events or reactions	
Angina, myocardial infarction, cerebrovascular accident	Very rare; may or may not be causally related to the donation; always associated with underlying pre-existing disease
Iron deficiency with or without anaemia	
Even in the absence of anaemia, tissue iron deficiency may be associated with mild disturbance of cerebral function, such as impaired concentration, and with sleep disturbance/ restless legs	Regular blood donors: iron depletion >20%*, absent iron stores 15%* Frequent donors: absent iron stores: males 16.4%, females 27.1%*
Allergic reactions/anaphylaxis	
Reactions may be to the skin preparation materials or adhesives, or to latex in the attendants' gloves	Rare
In apheresis donors in addition to the above	
Citrate toxicity from the anticoagulant	Mild reactions are common 80%* Severe reactions are rare 0.4%*
Thrombocytopenia and protein deficiency from excessive platelet or plasma donations respectively	Rare and easily prevented
Allergic reactions to ethylene oxide used in the sterilisation of the harness	Rare
Haemolysis/air embolus due to errors in the procedure or problems with the manufacturing of the harness	Very rare
For granulocyte donors: allergic reactions to hetastarch if used as a sedimentation agent or adverse drug reactions to steroids or growth factors used to raise the donor's leucocyte count	Mild reactions including bone pain are common with the use of growth factors and steroids in donors. Many blood services do not provide granulocytes by apheresis. Pooled buffy coats provide an alternative that is logistically simpler, safer for the donor and may be equally efficacious

* When marked with an asterisk, the figure is from Amrein et al. [10].

Network (EHN) and the International Society of Blood Transfusion (ISBT) in 2004 and refined in 2008 and 2014. They classified complications into two main categories: those with predominantly local symptoms and those with predominantly generalised symptoms. Complications specific to apheresis procedures were categorised separately. Complications were further graded into mild, moderate and severe and were assigned an imputability score for the likelihood of blood donation being the cause of the reaction.

Some complications are specific to apheresis donations, including citrate reactions, haemolysis, air emboli and allergic reactions to ethylene oxide used in the sterilisation of the harness. Most blood establishments will only report citrate effects if they are severe or if they result in the donation being discontinued, the mild reactions being very frequent (metallic taste and tingling in the lips).

Longer term consequences of donation, such as iron depletion, with or without associated anaemia, are not currently reported as complications of donation.

The overall incidence of complications directly related to blood donation is often quoted as being approximately 1%, though the true reaction rate may be higher. One study, where information on adverse events was actively sought on follow-up rather than relying on passive collection of spontaneous reports by donors, reported that from 1000 randomly selected donors, three weeks after donation 36% had had one or more adverse events [2]. Of complications collated by the EHN/ISBT Working Group, 99% belonged to four categories: vasovagal reactions (86% of all complications), haematomas (13%), nerve injuries (1%) and arterial punctures (0.4%) [3].

Rarely, severe complications arise, such as accidents related to vasovagal reactions and nerve injuries with long-lasting symptoms. Vasovagal reactions that occur after the donor has left the session, estimated to represent 10% of all these reactions, are of particular concern and may have on rare occasions lead to accidental deaths. A retrospective analysis of Danish data relating to 2.5 million donations found that severe complications occurred with an incidence of 19 per 100 000 procedures [4].

Young age, first-time donor status and low total blood volume are independent predictors of higher reaction rates. Complication rates of 10.7% in 16 and 17 year olds, 8.3% in 18 and 19 year olds and 2.8% in donors aged 20 years and older have been observed. Syncope occurred in four in 1000 donations and injury in six in 10 000 donations in 16 to 17 year olds and almost half of the injuries that occurred in American Red Cross regions involved whole-blood donors in this age group [5].

It is unlikely that the risks to blood donors can ever be reduced to zero. This places a significant ethical burden on blood services to use their best endeavours to reduce the risks. This includes the careful collation and analysis of data on the incidence and nature of adverse events or reactions, and the sharing and comparison of these data among blood services, with the goal of identifying and promoting best practices. The uneven risk-to-benefit ratio for blood donors also places an ethical responsibility on healthcare givers to avoid wastage and unnecessary use of blood transfusions.

Several strategies can be used to reduce the risk of complications occurring during and after donation, both to ensure the health and well-being of blood donors and also to sustain an adequate blood supply. Even minor reactions discourage donors from donating again and more severe reactions profoundly decrease the return rate of donors. Best practices include good needle insertion techniques, predonation education, optimising the session environment, appropriate selection criteria (particularly as regards estimated blood volume), vigilant supervision of donors, water ingestion before donation, distraction techniques and muscle tension during phlebotomy and postreaction instructions to donors [6].

Donor Selection and Exclusion

Prospective blood donors are subjected to a process, often specified in national legislation, intended to minimise the risks to the donor and to the eventual recipient of the donated blood. This involves a donor history, including any recognisable risk in the donor, for transmitting infectious agents to the recipient. Infectious risks from donors are listed in Table 20.2, along with available mitigation strategies.

In some services, the donor undergoes some cursory form of physical examination, but the value of this examination is doubtful, at least among altruistic donors.

Donors generally undergo a measurement of their haemoglobin level, either prior to the donation or, in some countries, on a sample taken at the same time as the donation. This is either from a skin puncture ('capillary sample') or a venous sample. This measurement of haemoglobin serves two purposes: it provides some

Table 20.2 Infections risks from blood donors.

Categories of risks	Examples of infections	Donor exclusions that may reduce risk
Failure of a test to detect an infectious agent where it should have done so: while this risk is very low, it is not zero and provides a reason to continue strict exclusion practices in the presence of increasingly sensitive testing methods	HIV 1 and 2, hepatitis C, hepatitis B	Excluding at-risk donors identified by questions about risk activities in the past, e.g. drug use or high-risk sexual activity at any time in the past
Window-period infections: a donor is infectious with an agent for which the donation is routinely tested, but the infection was acquired so recently that the donor does not yet have detectable infectivity in the blood	HIV 1 and 2, hepatitis C, hepatitis B	Excluding at-risk donors identified by questions about risk activities in the recent past, e.g. recent at-risk sexual activity, recent tattoos or piercings or recent invasive procedures
Infections for which donors are not routinely tested	Malaria, West Nile virus, Chagas' disease, visceral leishmaniasis, vCJD, dengue	Excluding donors, where possible, on the basis of travel or previous residence. This is very difficult in areas of high prevalence and endemicity, and requires additional testing where possible
	Any recently acquired infection that the donor has not yet cleared and that may have a viraemic or bacteraemic phase	Excluding donors on the basis of a recent history of any febrile illness; excluding donors who have recently had a live virus vaccination
Known diseases in the donor's past that may have an unknown transmissible element	Cancer, autoimmune diseases	Excluding donors with a previous history of cancer, with the exception of some localised and cured forms
		Excluding donors with a history of a multisystem autoimmune disease
Risks from unrecognised, yet-to-emerge infectious agents	In the recent past HIV and HCV were extensively spread by blood transfusions before the true nature of the diseases became apparent. A similar fate could have arisen with vCJD	Excluding donors with a history of conditions strongly associated in the past with the early and extensive spread of emerging diseases with long incubation periods. Such donors include sex workers and intravenous drug users. More contentiously, excluding men who have previously had sex with men at any time in their past

(Continued)

Table 20.2 (Continued)

Categories of risks	Examples of infections	Donor exclusions that may reduce risk
Risk from transmissible spongiform encephalopathies	All prion diseases are considered to have the possibility of an infectious blood phase	Excluding donors who have previously received blood transfusions
		Excluding xenotransplant recipients
		Excluding donors who have a strong family history of spongiform encephalopathy; excluding donors who have been treated with human-derived pituitary hormones or dura mater
		Outside the UK and Europe, exclusion on the basis of residence in higher risk countries during the BSE epidemic
		In some European countries, previous recipients of blood transfusions are excluded to try to limit the risk of transfusion-acquired vCJD

BSE, bovine spongiform encephalopathy; HCV, hepatitis C virus; HIV, human immunodeficiency virus; vCJD, variant Creutzfeldt–Jakob disease.

protection to the donor against having a preexisting anaemia made worse by donating and it helps ensure that the final therapeutic product will have a minimum red cell content. The cut-off levels for the allowable haemoglobin level in the donor vary between blood services and regulatory authorities and are empirically derived. Often, as in the EU rules (Directive 2004/33/EC, see Further Reading), a different level is used for males and females, with the allowable minimum haemoglobin level set higher for males. Haemoglobin levels vary in the same individual between capillary and venous blood [7], with the seasons and the time of day and with posture and activity. In addition, this measurement does not provide protection against nonanaemic iron deficiency.

In some jurisdictions, donor exclusions may be specified by law. In the EU, the specifications are generally interpreted as a minimum requirement by the member states or the national blood services; in the USA and other jurisdictions, in contrast, the specifications are generally regarded as a maximum requirement by the blood service operators. The EU requirements for permanent and temporary exclusion of donors are listed in Box 20.1; these requirements are routinely exceeded, for example based on local epidemiological risks.

Deferral rates vary in different blood services, ranging in the EU from 0.5% to 25.2% of donors, with a mean of 10.9%. The lowest deferral rates are in countries where the public knowledge of blood donation selection criteria is high – where donors may register online and complete an eligibility questionnaire in advance. A low haemoglobin level is typically the most frequent reason for deferral, accounting for nearly 40% of deferrals.

Iron Deficiency in Blood Donors

Blood donation results in a significant iron loss of approximately 200–250 mg per donation. Both iron deficiency causing anaemia and iron deficiency in the absence of anaemia are common among donors, particularly in females of

Box 20.1 Deferral criteria for donors of whole blood and blood components. Reproduced from Commission Directive 2004/33/EC of 22 March 2004 implementing Directive 2002/98/EC of the European Parliament and of the Council as regards certain technical requirements for blood and blood components, OJ L 91, 30.3.2004, http://eur-lex.europa.eu, © European Union, 1998–2012.

Permanent deferral criteria for donors of allogeneic donations

Cardiovascular disease

Prospective donors with active or past serious cardiovascular disease, except congenital abnormalities with complete cure

Central nervous system disease

A history of serious CNS disease

Abnormal bleeding tendency

Prospective donors who give a history of a coagulopathy

Repeated episodes of syncope or a history of convulsions

Other than childhood convulsions or where at least 3 years have elapsed since the date the donor last took anticonvulsant medication without any recurrence of convulsions

Gastrointestinal, genitourinary, haematological, immunological, metabolic, renal or respiratory system diseases

Prospective donors with serious active, chronic or relapsing disease

Diabetes

If being treated with insulin

Infectious diseases

Hepatitis B, except for HBsAg-negative persons who are demonstrated to be immune

Hepatitis C

HIV-1/2

HTLV I/II

Babesiosis (*)

Kala-azar (visceral leishmaniasis) (*)

Trypanosomiasis cruzi (Chagas' disease) (*)

Malignant diseases except *in situ* cancer with complete recovery

Transmissible spongiform encephalopathies (TSEs) (e.g. Creutzfeldt–Jakob disease, variant Creutzfeldt–Jakob disease)

Persons who have a family history that places them at risk of developing a TSE, or persons who have received a corneal or dura mater graft, or who have been treated in the past with medicines made from human pituitary glands. For variant Creutzfeldt–Jacob disease, further precautionary measures may be recommended

Intravenous (IV) or intramuscular (IM) drug use

Any history of nonprescribed IV or IM drug use, including body-building steroids or hormones

(Continued)

Box 20.1 (Continued)

Xenotransplant recipients

Sexual behaviour

Persons whose sexual behaviour puts them at high risk of acquiring severe infectious diseases that can be transmitted by blood

Temporary deferral criteria for donors of allogeneic donations

Infections
Duration of deferral period

After an infectious illness: prospective donors shall be deferred for at least 2 weeks following the date of full clinical recovery. However, the following deferral periods shall apply for the infections listed in the table:

Brucellosis (*): 2 years following the date of full recovery

Osteomyelitis: 2 years after confirmed cured

Q-fever (*): 2 years following the date of confirmed cured

Syphilis (*): 1 year following the date of confirmed cured

Toxoplasmosis (*): 6 months following the date of clinical recovery

Tuberculosis: 2 years following the date of confirmed cured

Rheumatic fever: 2 years following the date of cessation of symptoms, unless evidence of chronic heart disease

Fever > °C†: 2 weeks following the date of cessation of symptoms

Flu-like illness: 2 weeks after cessation of symptoms

Malaria (*):

Individuals who have lived in a malarial area within the first 5 years of life: 3 years following return from last visit to any endemic area, provided person remains symptom free; may be reduced to 4 months if an immunological or molecular genomic test is negative at each donation
Individuals with a history of malaria: 3 years following cessation of treatment *and* absence of symptoms; accept thereafter only if an immunological or molecular genomic test is negative
asymptomatic visitors to endemic areas: 6 months after leaving the endemic area unless an immunological or molecular genomic test is negative
Individuals with a history of undiagnosed febrile illness during or within 6 months of a visit to an endemic area: 3 years following resolution of symptoms; may be reduced to 4 months if an immunological or molecular test is negative

West Nile virus (WNV) (*): 28 days after leaving an area with ongoing transmission of WNV to humans

Exposure to risk of acquiring a transfusion-transmissible infection

Endoscopic examination using flexible instruments
Mucosal splash with blood or needlestick injury
Transfusion of blood components
Tissue or cell transplant of human origin
Major surgery
Tattoo or body piercing
Acupuncture unless performed by a qualified practitioner and with sterile single-use needles

---

Box 20.1 (Continued)

Persons at risk due to close household contact with persons with hepatitis B; defer for 6 months or for 4 months provided a NAT test for hepatitis C is negative

Persons whose behaviour or activity places them at risk of acquiring infectious diseases that may be transmitted by blood; defer after cessation of risk behaviour for a period determined by the disease in question and by the availability of appropriate tests

Vaccination

Attenuated viruses or bacteria: 4 weeks

Inactivated/killed viruses, bacteria or rickettsiae: no deferral if well

Toxoids: no deferral if well

Hepatitis A or hepatitis B vaccines: no deferral if well and if no exposure

Rabies: no deferral if well and if no exposure. If vaccination is given following exposure, defer for 1 year

Tick-borne encephalitis vaccines: no deferral if well and if no exposure

Other temporary deferrals

Pregnancy: 6 months after delivery or termination, except in exceptional circumstances and at the discretion of a physician

Minor surgery: 1 week

Dental treatment:

Minor treatment by dentist or dental hygienist (note that tooth extraction, root filling and similar treatment is considered as minor surgery): defer until next day

Medication: based on the nature of the prescribed medicine, its mode of action and the disease being treated

Deferral for particular epidemiological situations

Particular epidemiological situations (e.g. disease outbreaks):

Deferral consistent with the epidemiological situation (these deferrals should be notified by the competent authority to the European Commission with a view to Community action)

Deferral criteria for donors of autologous donations

Serious cardiac disease: depending on the clinical setting of the blood collection

Persons with or with a history of:

Hepatitis B, except for HBsAg-negative persons who are demonstrated to be immune
Hepatitis C
HIV-1/2
HTLV I/II

Member states may, however, establish specific provisions for autologous donations by such persons
Active bacterial infection

The tests and deferral periods indicated by an asterisk (*) are not required when the donation is used exclusively for plasma for fractionation.
[†] Temperature threshold missing from the original text of the Commission Directive; the definition of fever is usually >37.5 °C.
Source: Reproduced from Commission Directive 2004/33/EC of 22 March 2004 implementing Directive 2002/98/EC of the European Parliament and of the Council as regards certain technical requirements for blood and blood components. Official Journal of the European Union 2004;**L9**:25–39.

childbearing age. Iron depletion below a ferritin level of 12 μg/L can be present even when there is no evidence of iron-deficient erythropoiesis. It may cause poor concentration and sleep disturbances, and has been associated with restless legs syndrome. Iron deficiency can also arise in donors of plasma or platelets by apheresis due to the red cell losses that result from the procedure. A study of Australian blood donors showed that 5.3% of males and 18.9% of females who met the EU criteria for haemoglobin levels were iron deficient, as defined by a serum ferritin level of less than 12 μg/L. Iron deficiency among the general female population in Australia is 5–7% and is negligible among the general male population [8]. Similar findings were noted in a US study [9].

In blood donors who are considered healthier compared to the general population, the true clinical significance of iron deficiency without anaemia has not been studied extensively and remains largely undetermined. One study has found that female blood donors with lowered iron stores, when compared with donors with normal iron stores, are more likely to report pica, the craving and compulsive eating of nonfood substances [11]. However, no association has consistently been found between low iron stores and other potential complications of iron deficiency, including restless legs syndrome and decreased cognitive functions. A recently published Danish study conducted among 16 375 blood donors did not show any association between self-reported health-related quality of life and iron status [12].

Iron deficiency among donors may be prevented or treated by adequate intake of oral iron. However, optimum regimens for blood donors have not been generally defined and practice varies considerably. Options include regular measurement of blood or plasma indices of iron deficiency, routine provision of iron supplements and dietary advice. Due to the risk of serious iron toxicity in children who accidentally take a donor's iron tablets, iron should be dispensed with adequate precautions.

Blood Collection/Donation Process

The entire donation procedure needs to be controlled within a functioning quality system, while maintaining the humanity of the process, and especially the dignity of the donor. The venue must be clean and warm, but not excessively so, uncluttered, bright and without excessive noise. Staff should not be distracted or distressed by extraneous events. There must be appropriate space available for confidential discussions between donors and staff. The flow of the donor from reception through registration, interview, haemoglobin check (if done) and venesection should be orderly and unidirectional.

Several blood services do not take a blood collection from a donor on their first attendance. Instead, they take a sample for blood group, blood count and virus screen. This practice provides some protection against window period donations from people who are donating for the purposes of getting an HIV or hepatitis test. It is, however, very costly, especially when a significant proportion of blood comes from first-time and once-only donors.

Donors may be recruited or retained to donate for apheresis as well as, or instead of, whole blood. Apheresis may be for red cells, usually as a double dose from larger donors, platelets or plasma, or combinations of these. Donor acceptance or rejection criteria are similar to those for whole-blood donors, though plasma donors may be exempted for some infectious risks (see Box 20.1). Platelet and plasma donation intervals are shorter. Since patients receiving apheresis platelets and, to a lesser extent, apheresis red cells receive fewer donor exposures, there is a benefit to using these components as much as possible. Much of the plasma used in the manufacture of blood components comes from apheresis donors, many of whom are paid and who can donate up to twice weekly. Since the early 1990s, blood component manufacture has had a very good safety record regarding transmission of infectious diseases. This has been achieved by increased donor screening and exclusion procedures, advances in testing and effective methods of pathogen removal or inactivation. As things stand at present, the supply of manufactured blood components worldwide could probably not be maintained without paid plasma donation.

Obligations to Donors

Although donors are well and are not seeking care, they are nevertheless subjected to a health-care intervention. The blood service has an ethical obligation to them from the very start of the first attendance. The service's main duty of care is to the recipient of the donation, but it has obligations to the donor that must also be discharged. Donation is not a right, but rights accrue to the donor once the process is embarked upon.

The donor has a right to:

- confidentiality and autonomy
- informed consent
- protection from harm – including not being made to feel unhealthy when they are outside donation specifications
- receive the results of tests when these are of significance to their health

- receive direction and counselling around the results of such tests
- be protected as much as possible from adverse events or reactions.

In turn, donors are required to:

- identify themselves correctly
- be truthful in their answers to the screening questions
- inform the blood service if any change arises in their health after they have donated.

In some services, donors are also given the option of informing the collection agency that they knowingly withheld important information during the screening process. This 'confidential unit exclusion' process is still in use in some countries. The value of this process for making blood safer is doubtful.

Donors also have some rights in relation to the use of their donation – the consent that they give must include the possibility that the donation may not be used for the therapeutic use that they assume, but that it might expire unused or be used for control purposes. Where a unit of blood is collected specifically for control, test or calibration purposes, explicit consent should be sought. Lastly, donors have a right to expect that healthcare providers will ensure ethical and appropriate use of this unique medicinal product.

KEY POINTS

1) The incidence and prevalence of infectious diseases are higher among donors who donate for personal economic gain.
2) Iron deficiency is common among donors; it can occur in the absence of anaemia and even of iron-deficient erythropoiesis and might result in adverse health outcomes, although the true extent of this potential problem has yet to be determined.
3) Assessing the donor is a critical manufacturing step in the preparation of the final therapeutic product.
4) The donor has a right to confidentiality and autonomy, informed consent and protection from harm.
5) Clinicians should take account of the unique nature of blood components as a medicine, to avoid wastage and ensure appropriate use.

References

1 Ringwald J, Zimmermann R, Eckstein R. Keys to open the door for blood donors to return. Transfus Med Rev 2010;**24**:295–304.

2 Newman PH, Roth AJ. Estimating the probability of a blood donation adverse event based on 1000 post donation interviewed whole-blood donors. Transfusion 2005;**45**:1715–21.

3 Sorensen B, Jorgensen J. International bench marking of severe complications related to blood donation. Vox Sang 2010;**99**:294.

4 Sorensen BS, Johnsen SP, Jorgensen J. Complications related to blood donation: a population-based study. Vox Sang 2008;**94**:132–7.

5 Eder AF, Hillyer CD, Dy BA, Notari EP 4th, Benjamin RJ. Adverse reactions to allogeneic whole blood donation by 16- and 17-year-olds. JAMA 2008;**299**(19):2279–86.

6 Eder AF. Improving safety for young blood donors. Transfus Med Rev 2012;**26**:14–26.

7 Tong E, Murphy WG, Kinsella A et al. Capillary and venous haemoglobin levels in blood donors: a 42-month study of 36,258 paired samples. Vox Sang 2010;**98**(4):547–53.

8 Farrugia A. Iron and blood donation – an underrecognised safety issue. Dev Biol (Basel) 2006;**127**:137–46.

9 Bryant BJ, Yau YY, Arceo SM, Daniel-Johnson J, Hopkins JA, Leitman SF. Iron replacement therapy in the routine management of blood donors. Transfusion 2012;**52**:1566–75.

10 Amrein K, Valentin A, Lanzer G, Drexler C Adverse events and safety issues in blood donation – a comprehensive review. Blood Rev 2012;**26**:33–42.

11 Spencer BR, Kleinman S, Wright DJ et al., for the REDS-II RISE Analysis Group. Restless legs syndrome, pica, and iron status in blood donors. Transfusion 2013;**53**:1645–52.

12 Rigas AS, Pedersen OB, Sørensen CJ et al. No association between iron status and self-reported health-related quality of life in 16,375 Danish blood donors: results from the Danish Blood Donor Study. Transfusion 2015;**55**:1752–6.

Further Reading

Council of Europe. Final Report – Collection, testing and use of blood and blood products in Europe in 2003. Strasbourg: Council of Europe Publishing. Available at: www.edqm.eu/medias/fichiers/2003_Report_on_the_collection_testing_and_use_of_blood_and_blood_products_in_Europe.pdf (accessed 13 November 2016).

Crusz TAM. Adverse events of blood donation. Available at: http://onlinelibrary.wiley.com/doi/10.1111/j.1365-3148.2006.00693_43.x/abstract European Commission (accessed 13 November 2016).

Commission Directive 2004/33/EC of 22 March 2004 implementing Directive 2002/98/EC of the European Parliament and of the Council as regards certain technical requirements for blood and blood components. Official Journal of the European Union 2004;**L9**:25–39.

ISBT Working Party on Haemovigilance. Standard for Collecting and Presentation of Data on Complications Related to Blood Donation. 2007. Available at: www.isbt-web.org/documentation (accessed 13 November 2016).

Van der Poel CL. Remuneration of blood donors: new proof of the pudding? Vox Sang 2008;**94**(3):169–70.

Van der Poel CL, Seifried E, Schaasberg WP. Paying for blood donations: still a risk? Vox Sang 2002;**83**(4):285–93.

21 Blood Donation Testing and the Safety of the Blood Supply

Mindy Goldman

Canadian Blood Services, Medical Services and Innovation, Ottawa, Canada

Introduction

This chapter describes laboratory testing of blood donations, including:

- red cell serological testing
- microbiological testing and donor follow-up
- operational and quality control issues.

Red Cell Serological Testing

Every blood donation is tested for:

- ABO blood group
- RhD blood group
- the presence of irregular red cell antibodies.

These tests are necessary for safe transfusion practice in order to reduce the risk of premature destruction of the transfused donor red cells in a recipient's circulation due to immunological incompatibility. Correct ABO blood group typing is critical, since naturally occurring antibodies can cause intravascular haemolysis and severe transfusion reactions if incompatible red cells are transfused. The RhD antigen is highly immunogenic and RhD-negative recipients are usually transfused with RhD antigen-negative red cells to avoid alloimmunisation.

Red cell phenotyping may be performed for other antigens, such as RhC/E, Kell, S, s, Fya/b and Jka/b [1,2]. More extensively phenotyped red cells are needed for transfusion support of patients who have produced alloantibodies or are receiving prophylactically matched units to avoid alloimmunisation (e.g. thalassaemia, sickle disorders). In some countries, such as the UK and The Netherlands, females with childbearing potential are routinely transfused with K- units. Some blood services, such as the National Health Service Blood and Transplant (NHSBT) supplying hospitals in England and North Wales, perform full Rh and Kell phenotyping on all donations; others perform phenotyping on selected units. Increasingly, molecular biology microarray technology is being used to screen donors for multiple blood group systems, or for absence of a high frequency antigen, such as U. Extended phenotyping or genotyping may be performed on selected groups of donors, such as individuals of Afro-Caribbean origin, to meet the needs of sickle cell anaemia patients for antigen-matched units. Additional phenotyping results may be printed on the red cell component label, to assist hospitals in selecting appropriate red cell units.

ABO and RhD Grouping, and Detection of Red Cell Antibodies

Tests are carried out on anticoagulated venous blood samples collected at the time of donation, identified by a unique bar-coded identification system, which in most countries is an

Practical Transfusion Medicine, Fifth Edition. Edited by Michael F. Murphy, David J. Roberts and Mark H. Yazer.
© 2017 John Wiley & Sons Ltd. Published 2017 by John Wiley & Sons Ltd.

International Society for Blood Transfusion (ISBT) 128 number.

Donor red cells are tested with monoclonal anti-A and anti-B capable of detecting clinically relevant subgroups of these red cell glycoproteins (forward grouping). A reverse grouping is performed by testing the donor plasma with A and B reagent cells. RhD grouping is performed by testing donor red cells with two different highly sensitive monoclonal anti-D reagents. In many countries, RhD-negative first-time donors undergo further testing to confirm that they are D-negative. Use of sensitive reagents and repeat testing are carried out to optimise the detection of weak or partial D-bearing red cells, including category D^{VI}. Some of these individuals may be considered as D-negative in a different context, for example, testing done in a prenatal setting.

Blood services use automated testing systems where samples are divided into separate microtitre plate wells, results are read photometrically and the pattern of results obtained analysed by microprocessors to establish the ABO blood group. The forward and reverse ABO testing results must be concordant in order to assign a donor blood group, and for repeat donors, ABO and RhD test results must be concordant with historical records.

Donor samples are screened for the presence of high titres of red cell antibodies that could cause reduced red cell survival or haemolysis when transfused into antigen-positive recipients. Donor plasma is mixed with group O R_1R_2 red cells, positive for clinically significant red cell antigens. In general, only antibodies reacting in the IAT are considered to be clinically significant. Initial screening is performed using an automated testing system; manual testing may then be used to determine antibody specificity and titre. Donations with nonspecific, clinically insignificant or low-titre antibodies may still be released for transfusion, since during component preparation the amount of antibody-containing plasma will be very small and diluted with an additive storage solution.

In some blood services, such as the NHSBT, blood for neonatal transfusion is tested for irregular antibodies to a higher level of sensitivity than standard testing for all other blood in order to further minimise the very small risk of transfusion reactions due to passive transfer of antibodies.

High Titre Anti-A and Anti-B

Some group O donors have high titres of anti-A and anti-B that could cause lysis of A cells and, more rarely, B cells, particularly where large volumes of plasma are transfused [3]. Recipients should receive group-specific or AB plasma to avoid haemolytic reactions. Most recipients receive group-specific red cells. However, group O red cells may be transfused to neonates and patients with no known blood group requiring urgent transfusion. Because most red cell units are stored in additive solutions, the amount of plasma transfused is small, so risks of haemolysis are very low. Some blood services or hospital blood banks screen for high-titre haemolysins for large-volume red cell transfusions for neonates.

Since platelets have a short shelf-life, it is not always possible to provide group-specific transfusions. Cases of haemolysis have been reported, particularly in group A paediatric/neonatal recipients receiving group O platelets. Plasma can be screened for high-titre haemolysins by observing the reactions between donor plasma and a diluted sample of reagent A_1B red cells; products that are under a predetermined cut-off level can be labelled accordingly. This can be done using automated systems; however, there is no standard testing method or clear acceptable cut-off titre shown to prevent all haemolytic reactions.

Supplementary Testing

Occasionally, anomalies appear in serological testing that make interpretation of results difficult. For example, it has been estimated that one in 10 000 blood donors has a positive direct antiglobulin test (DAT), which could interfere with some of the above assays or give a positive result on hospital cross-matching. Donors with positive DAT results on several donations may be deferred.

Testing for HbS may be performed on a subset of units with particular phenotypes likely to be used for transfusion support for patients with sickle cell disease or for neonates during exchange transfusions. The need for a sickle cell screening test depends on the prevalence of HbS within the donor population. Sickle trait (HbAS) blood significantly interferes with the function of some filters currently used for leucocyte reduction and HbAS units do not freeze well using current methods.

Donors with test results that may be of clinical importance should be informed of their results. This includes donors with positive DAT results on several donations and donors with HbAS. Donors with rare blood groups or with red cell alloantibodies are also usually informed by the blood service.

Microbiological Testing of Blood Donations and Donor Follow-Up

Infectious agents transmissible by blood transfusion are described in Chapter 15. Donor selection criteria and deferral of at-risk individuals are important steps in reducing the risk of collecting infectious blood donations. For some agents, no laboratory testing is currently available and donor criteria are the only means of deferring at-risk donors. Where testing is available, donor criteria are still important, particularly for recently infected donors, who may be asymptomatic and have negative test results but are infectious. This interval, when testing is negative but transfusion may transmit infection, is known as the 'window period'. Laboratory screening tests form the core of the process to identify infected blood components prior to transfusion [4–6].

Samples

Tests are carried out on serum or plasma venous samples collected at the time of donation and sent to highly automated centralised donor

testing laboratories. As with samples for serological blood grouping, correct labelling of microbiological samples to ensure traceability of results is extremely important. Most tests are performed on individual donor samples, but nucleic acid testing (NAT) is often performed on pools of samples from 6–24 donors. In some resource-poor countries with a high incidence of infectious donors, point-of-care rapid tests may be used on the clinic site.

Testing Process and Donor Management

Sensitivity and specificity are important test attributes. Sensitivity refers to the ability of the test to identify truly infected individuals correctly. From the perspective of the transfusion recipient, sensitivity is the most important criterion for a screening test, i.e. the test will accurately identify infected donors. Specificity refers to the ability of the test to identify correctly donors who are not infected. Specificity is important both to avoid discarding donations from safe donors and to reduce the resulting confirmatory workload necessary to provide appropriate donor counselling of those whose samples are reactive in a screening assay. Although most currently used screening assays show remarkably high levels of both specificity and sensitivity in countries with low prevalence rates of infection, it is essential that additional assays are available to confirm infection in the donor.

Principles of Investigating a Repeat-Reactive Sample

If an initial screening test is reactive, it will be repeated in duplicate. If both repeat tests are negative, the overall result is considered negative, the blood donation will be used and the donor may continue to donate. If a repeat test is again reactive, the donation will be discarded, and confirmatory or supplementary tests are performed to establish whether the screening test result represents a true positive. Since donors constitute a low-prevalence population, despite the high specificity of screening tests, significant numbers of samples identified as repeatedly reactive on screening are not confirmed positive on supplementary testing (termed false-positive or nonspecific reactions). These individuals are deferred from further donation, although some blood services permit donors with false-positive results to be retested after a defined deferral period. If all further testing in the re-entry protocol is negative, these individuals may be reintegrated as donors.

Blood services must have policies for notifying donors with repeat reactive test results. In some countries, the law requires reporting of an infected person for some infections, such as HBV, to public health authorities. For donors with false-positive test results, it can be difficult to explain that although the test almost certainly represents a false-positive reaction, the individual may be deferred as a blood donor.

When a donor is found to be repeat reactive, components from previous donations that may still be in inventory will be retrieved and discarded as potentially infectious. If the donor is confirmed to be infected, recipients of earlier components from the donor will be identified and offered relevant testing, a process termed 'lookback'. With improvements in testing and shortening of the window period, the likelihood of identifying an infected recipient component/product on lookback investigation has become vanishingly small.

Principles of Infectious Disease Testing

Screening tests may detect the host immune response to the microbial agent (such as antibody to HCV), a microbial antigen (such as the hepatitis B surface antigen, HBsAg) or the nucleic acid of the microbe (NAT). Testing for bacterial growth is covered in Chapter 16.

Immunoassays

Immunoassay principles using enzyme or chemiluminescent techniques of detection form the basis for infectious disease testing. Donor plasma at a fixed dilution is incubated over a solid phase where an antigen–antibody interaction occurs. After incubation and washing, the products of the antigen–antibody interaction are detected by a revealing agent. A conjugate linked to an enzyme such as peroxidase can be detected photometrically after addition of substrate, which produces colour. Alternatively, the optical device may detect photons emitted by a chemiluminescent reaction. Assays may involve detection of antibody, antigen or both antigen and antibody, often referred to as 'Combo assays', in a single well.

All immunoassays depend on the interaction between microbial antigens and antibodies. Monoclonal antibodies with high avidity directed at 'conserved' microbial antigen epitopes are used in test kits, resulting in high specificity. However, mutations in the target epitope may render the antigen undetectable. HBsAg assays must be able to detect known mutants, especially the vaccine escape variant G145R.

Nucleic Acid Testing

In NAT, nucleic acid is extracted from the donor plasma, and an amplification step such as polymerase chain reaction (PCR) or transcription-mediated amplification (TMA) is used to amplify and detect microbial genetic sequences. Testing is usually done on small pools of 6–24 donor samples, termed minipools. Single-donor testing may be considered in particular circumstances to enhance sensitivity. Single-sample testing may also be required for resolution of a reactive pool to determine which donor sample contains the microbial target. Testing may be done individually for each agent or in a multiplex assay to identify several agents (HIV, HBV and HCV) in a single reaction. Newer, completely automated platforms have reduced the operational complexity of testing.

Nucleic acid testing reduces the window period when donors may be infectious but have negative serological testing results. Window periods using serological assays are estimated as 15 days for HIV, 59 days for HCV, 67 days for HBV; and 9.5 days for HIV, eight days for HCV and 38 days for HBV using NAT. The utility of NAT depends on the incidence of these infections in donors, which determines the likelihood of possible serological window period donations. In countries such as the UK, Canada and the USA, where incidence rates are extremely low, the NAT yield, i.e. the number of infectious donations detected by NAT alone, has been extremely low, less than one in 1 million donations [5]. In contrast, the NAT yield has been considerably higher in countries such as South Africa, with a higher incidence of HIV. The changing epizoology of arthropod-borne infections, such as West Nile virus (WNV), is a target for discretionary NAT, the introduction being mandated by disease activity in any location. For WNV, single-donor NAT may be used instead of minipool NAT at the height of an epidemic in a given community.

Screening Tests and Donor–Recipient Matching

Table 21.1 lists the screening tests used in different countries [7]. Some tests are mandatory and used to screen all donations, while others may be discretionary and used on selected higher risk donors or on all donors once. CMV antibody testing may be done on a subset of donations in order to provide CMV seronegative components for patients at risk of severe CMV infection. Pooling of plasma may also require additional NAT testing of the start pool for a range of agents including HAV, HEV and parvovirus B19, that are not effectively inactivated by the fractionation process. The decision to implement a particular screening test in a country depends on consideration of a number of factors, including the incidence and prevalence of the infectious disease in the donor population, the available testing technologies and the known or anticipated morbidity associated with transfusion-transmitted infection. For example, in Australia, donors with geographic risk for WNV will be temporarily deferred, and donors with geographic risk for Chagas' disease will be permanently deferred, rather than performing selective testing for these infections. Regulatory requirements for testing and the availability of test kits specifically licenced for donor screening also play an important role.

Table 21.1 Screening tests on blood donations in five countries as of 2016. *Source:* Adapted from O'Brien et al. [7].

Infection	Test	USA	Canada	France	UK	Australia
HIV-1, -2	HIV antibody	√	√	√	√	√
	HIV NAT	√	√	√	√	√
HCV	HCV antibody	√	√	√	√	√
	HCV NAT	√	√	√	√	√
HBV	HBV surface antigen (HBsAg)	√	√	√	√	√
	HBV NAT	√	√	√	√	√
	Antibody to HBV core antigen (anti-HBc)	√	√	√	Selective	Selective
HTLV-1/2	HTLV antibody	√	√	√	Selective	√
Syphilis	*Treponema* antibody	√	√	√	√	√
Malaria	Malarial antibody	No	No	Selective	Selective	Selective
Chagas' disease	*Trypanosoma cruzi* antibody	Selective	Selective	Selective	Selective	No
West Nile virus	WNV NAT	√	Seasonal	No	Selective	No

√ Indicates testing on all donations.

Quality Framework and Operational Issues

Ultimately, the microbiological and blood group safety of the blood supply depends on the input and interaction of a number of quality and operational factors.

A formal quality management system is an important part of ensuring that blood donation testing is adequately performed. The quality system needs to meet the requirements of a 'Competent Authority' under EU blood safety directives. Inspections are carried out by the Medicines and Healthcare Products Regulatory Authority (MHRA) in the UK. In the USA, there are both Food and Drug Administration (FDA) regulations and extensive requirements from professional accrediting organisations such as the AABB regarding quality requirements (see

Chapter 18). Testing must be performed only by staff trained in approved standard operating procedures (SOPs). Document control systems must be in place to ensure that only current procedures are used and any changes documented and approved. Any errors that occur in laboratory procedures must be logged using a quality incident report (QIR) system, which requires corrective and preventative action to be taken.

Most transfusion services have surveillance programmes for monitoring rates of transmissible infections in donors, while haemovigilance schemes in place in several countries monitor transmission of transfusion-transmissible agents (see Chapter 19). The reporting of serious adverse events and reactions resulting from transfusion is an essential component of blood safety.

KEY POINTS

1) Every blood donation is tested for ABO and RhD and the presence of irregular red cell antibodies.
2) Phenotyping for other red cell antigens may be important for transfusion support of particular recipient groups.
3) Laboratory screening tests form the core of the process to identify infected blood components prior to transfusion.
4) Processes must be in place to communicate infectious disease marker results and other unexpected results of possible consequence to donors.
5) Both immunoassays and nucleic acid testing are used to identify possibly infectious units.
6) A quality framework is important for the accuracy of all laboratory testing.

References

1 Casas J, Friedman DF, Jackson T *et al.* Changing practice: red blood cell typing by molecular methods for patients with sickle cell disease. Transfusion 2015;**55**:1388–93.

2 Chou ST, Liem RI, Thompson AA. Challenges of alloimmunization in patients with haemoglobinopathies. Br J Haematol 2012;**159**:394–404.

3 Berséus O, Boman K, Nessen SC, Westerberg LA. Risks of hemolysis due to anti-A and anti-B caused by the transfusion of blood or blood components containing ABO-incompatible plasma. Transfusion 2013;**53**:114S–123S.

4 Laperche S. Testing for established viruses: from the screening to the confirmation. ISBT Science Series 2013;**8**(1):58–64.

5 Roth WK, Busch MP, Schuller A et al. International survey on NAT testing of blood donations: expanding implementation and yield from 1999 to 2009. Vox Sang 2012;**102**:82–90.

6 Zou S, Stramer S, Dodd R. Donor testing and risk current prevalence, incidence, and residual risk for transfusion-transmissible agents in US allogeneic donations. Transfus Med Rev 2012;**26**:119–28.

7 O'Brien SF, Zou S, Laperche S, Brant LJ, Seed CR, Kleinman SH. Surveillance of transfusion-transmissible infections – comparison of systems in five developed countries. Transfus Med Rev 2012;**26**:38–57.

Further Reading

AABB Standards for Blood Banks and Transfusion Services, 29th edn. Bethesda: AABB Press, 2014.

Council of Europe. Guide to the Preparation, Use and Quality Assurance of Blood Components, 18th edn. Strasbourg: Council of Europe Publishing, 2015.

Galel SA. Infectious disease screening, in AABB Technical Manual, 18th edn (ed. Fung MK). Bethesda: AABB Press, 2014, pp.179–212.

Guidelines for the Blood Transfusion Services in the UK, 8th edn. Available at: www.transfusionguidelines.org.uk/red-book (accessed 1 November 2016).

Joint United Kingdom Blood Transfusion and Tissue Transplantation Services Professional Advisory Committee Guidelines. Available at: www.transfusionguidelines.org.uk/uk-transfusion-committees/national-blood-transfusion-committee (accessed 1 November 2016).

Production and Storage of Blood Components

Marissa Li[1], Rebecca Cardigan[2], Stephen Thomas[3] and Ralph Vassallo[4]

[1] *United Blood Services, Ventura, USA*
[2] *NHS Blood and Transplant, Cambridge, UK*
[3] *NHS Blood and Transplant, Watford, UK*
[4] *Perelman School of Medicine, The University of Pennsylvania, Philadelphia*

Whole Blood and Its Processing to Components

Guidelines from the UK, Council of Europe, Health Canada, AABB and the United States Code of Federal Regulations (CFR) variously define a whole blood donation as 450–500 mL (±10%) of blood collected into citrate anticoagulant also containing phosphate and dextrose. The clinical indications for transfusion of whole blood are limited to intrauterine/neonatal exchange transfusion and, increasingly in the United States, massive transfusion. Thus, the vast majority of collected whole blood is processed into components – red cells, plasma and platelet concentrates. Whole blood-derived plasma (sometimes called recovered plasma) is suitable for fractionation to plasma derivatives, freezing as transfusable plasma or further manufacture into cryoprecipitate and cryoprecipitate-depleted plasma.

Component production from whole blood consists of centrifugation to separate plasma and cellular material by size and density, followed by manual or automated transfer of components from the primary collection pack to storage packs. Collection and storage packs are manufactured as a single closed unit to maintain sterility. Whole blood donations from which platelets are to be harvested must be held and processed at 20–24 °C. For other donations, preprocessing storage and centrifugation of whole blood can be at either 20–24 °C or 1–6 °C. Some countries permit overnight holding of whole blood at 20–24 °C prior to component production, yielding components of acceptable quality, allowing the production of platelets from the majority of collections and obviating the need for multiple manufacturing shifts.

Collection of Components by Apheresis

Apheresis involves serial or continuous separation of the donor's blood into components inside disposable kits on specially designed equipment, with harvest of specific blood elements and reinfusion of the remainder [1]. Apheresis technology permits the collection of multiple transfusable doses of components from desired ABO- and RhD-specific groups. This is not possible with whole blood collections which yield a single red cell, plasma and partial platelet dose of the same blood type. Therefore, the collection of two O+, O−, A− or B− red cells or two to three A or AB plasmas and/or two or three full-dose platelets may be obtained. The frequency of apheresis component donations is determined by the guidelines established in each country. Double red cell donation requires

Practical Transfusion Medicine, Fifth Edition. Edited by Michael F. Murphy, David J. Roberts and Mark H. Yazer.
© 2017 John Wiley & Sons Ltd. Published 2017 by John Wiley & Sons Ltd.

longer interdonation intervals (as well as higher haemoglobin cut-offs) while plateletpheresis allows collection of 1–3 adult doses per procedure as often as 24 times per year. Total allowable plasma loss varies by jurisdiction and donor blood volume, but is always less than 15 litres per year.

Apheresis safety has been enhanced by the development of instruments with low extracorporeal volume and smaller, more portable machines have permitted collections on mobile sessions. Most plateletpheresis still occurs at fixed sites since the enhanced efficiency of larger instruments results in greater platelet yields. Single donor-derived platelets (as opposed to pooled whole blood-derived units) may be required to reliably produce increments in patients with antibodies to human leucocyte or platelet antigens. Depending upon the diversity of the population and size of the country, 10–60% apheresis composition of the platelet supply is required to assure the product heterogeneity necessary for specialised support of alloimmunised recipients. While more expensive to produce, apheresis components require no further manufacture to produce an adult therapeutic dose, allowing blood centres to decrease the size of their component laboratories. This may accelerate the trend of 'near-donor processing', which is slowly replacing traditional whole blood donation as a result of increasing pressures for type-specific component collections in some countries.

Regulations, Specifications and Quality Monitoring

Specifications for the key parameters of each component type are generally defined in a national guideline, such as those published by the UK Blood Transfusion Services, AABB and in the United States the CFR. The United States Food and Drug Administration (FDA) and Health Canada, both charged with the oversight of blood safety, publish directives and guideline documents outlining good manufacturing practice. European guidelines published by the Council of Europe are not legally binding but intended to promote improvements in practice. However, in 2005, the European Union (EU) directive 2002/98/EC, 'Setting Standards of Quality and Safety for the Collection, Testing, Processing, Storage and Distribution of Human Blood and Blood Components', became legally binding in the UK as the Blood Safety and Quality Regulations (BSQR) 2005. In the UK, compliance of blood establishments with UK guidelines and the BSQR is regulated by the Medicines and Healthcare products Regulatory Authority (MHRA) – for more details see Chapter 18.

Many countries sample a proportion of blood components for quality monitoring to assess compliance with set specifications. The proportion tested is usually determined by statistical process control, but is typically about 1% of components produced [2]. Statistical process control identifies systems that are capable of performing better and highlights trends towards poor performance at an early stage so that corrective action can be put in place to address the problem.

Red Blood Cell Production and Storage (Table 22.1)

Red cells may be produced either from whole blood donations (Figure 22.1) or by apheresis. For the vast majority of red cell components, an additive solution is introduced following separation to achieve a haematocrit of 50–70% and extend storage from 21–28 days to 35–42 days. In the United States and Canada, red cells can be stored without additive solution with a 21–35-day shelf-life, depending upon the base anticoagulant solution in the collection set. Red cells in additive solution have a 35–42-day shelf-life, according to jurisdictional approval for specific additives. Red cell storage temperatures start at 1–2 °C, extending through 6 °C, with

Table 22.1 Specifications for red cell components.

Preparation	Volume		Haematocrit		Hb Content			Haemolysis		WBC content (/unit)			Other	
	CoE	UK	CoE	AABB	CoE	UK	AABB	CoE	UK	CoE	UK	AABB	CoE	AABB
Red cells (in CPD, CP2D or CPDA-1) ± LR	280 ± 50 mL or TBD for LR	280 ± 60 mL for LR	65–75%	≤80%	≥45 g; ≥40 g for LR	≥40 g for LR		<0.8%	<0.8%	90% <1 × 10^6 for LR	90% <1 × 10^6 for LR	95% <5 × 10^6 for LR		≥85% pre-LR recovery
Red cells, in AS (-1, -3, -5 or -7, SAGM, PAGGSM) ± LR	TBD	280 ± 60 mL for LR	50–70%		≥45 g; ≥40 g for LR	≥40 g for LR		<0.8%	<0.8%	90% <1 × 10^6 for LR	90% <1 × 10^6 for LR	95% <5 × 10^6 for LR		≥85% pre-LR recovery
Red Cells, buffy coat removed ± in AS	250 ± 50 mL	As above	65–75%; 50–70% for AS		≥43 g; ≥40 g for LR			<0.8%	<0.8%	90% <1.2 × 10^9				
Red cells, apheresis ± LR, ± AS	TBD	TBD	65–75%; 50–70% for AS		≥40 g		95% ≥50 g & mean 60 g; 95% >42.5 g & mean 51 g for LR	<0.8%	<0.8%	90% <1 × 10^6 for LR	90% <1 × 10^6 for LR	95% <5 × 10^6 for LR		
Thawed reconstituted red cells, (thawed and washed), cryopreserved	>185 mL	TBD	65–75%		≥36 g	≥36 g		<0.2 g sup. Hb/unit	<2 g sup. Hb/unit	90% <0.1 × 10^9	90% <1 × 10^6 for LR	95% <5 × 10^6 for LR	<340 mOsm/L	≥80% pre-glycerol recovery

AS, additive solution; CoE, Council of Europe; LR, leucocyte-reduced; TBD, to be defined (for the system used); WBC, white blood cell.

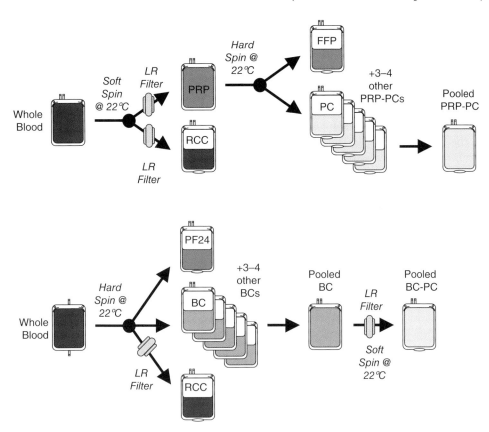

Figure 22.1 (a) Production of leucocyte-reduced (LR) red cell concentrates (RCC), fresh frozen plasma (FFP) and platelet-rich plasma (PRP)-intermediate platelet concentrates (PC). (b) Production of RCCs, plasma frozen within 24 hours of phlebotomy (PF24) and buffy coat (BC)-intermediate PCs. (*See insert for colour representation of the figure.*)

allowance during transport up to 10 °C. To minimise the possibility of bacterial proliferation and maintain viability, red cells should be removed from refrigeration as little as possible.

The most important changes occurring during storage are progressive extracellular leakage of potassium and a decline in red cell recovery to 75–85% of transfused cells at end-expiration. Red cells used for intrauterine transfusions (IUT) and exchange transfusion of neonates are normally stored or reconstituted in compatible plasma. Typically, clinicians will request freshly collected or washed units for potassium-sensitive patients to avoid levels as high as 95 mEq/L of supernatant (5–6 mEq per bag) at the end of storage. For patients who require red cells and have a history of severe or recurrent allergic reactions, or immunoglobulin A (IgA) deficiency with anti-IgA, red cells are washed and resuspended in saline or an approved additive solution. This removes >95% of plasma proteins, removing donor antigens to which patients have preformed antibodies. At least one automated closed system for cell washing is now available, which allows red cells to be stored after washing for up to 14 days instead of the 24 hours allowed after processing in an open system [3]. Red cells from donors with rare phenotypes or autologous units from patients with one rare or multiple common red cell alloantibodies, for whom provision of compatible donor blood is extremely difficult, can be stored frozen for 10 years or longer. Prior to transfusion, frozen red cells are thawed and washed to remove the cryoprotectant used to preserve them.

Platelet Production and Storage (Table 22.2)

Platelets may be separated from whole blood donations and subsequently pooled, or collected by apheresis. Platelet production from whole blood requires two centrifugation steps which differ in their intermediate. In the UK, Europe and Canada, pooled buffy coats (BC) are generated by 'bottom and top' processing, while in the US, platelet-rich plasma (PRP) is the intermediate (see Figure 22.1) [4]. BC and apheresis platelets yield similar increments after transfusion while PRP platelets tend to produce lower post-transfusion increments. This has been attributed to harsher centrifugation against a plastic surface and consequent increased activation for PRP platelets compared to the softer red cell cushion against which BC platelets are concentrated. The significantly lower cost of pooled whole blood-derived platelets contrasts with their marginally greater risk of viral, parasitic and bacterial disease transmission and the inability to match alloimmunised recipients with a larger volume, compatible single donor apheresis unit. Leucocyte reduction (LR) by filtration or by in-line apheresis technology is easily accomplished. An adult therapeutic dose of platelets ($>2.5 \times 10^{11}$) can be consistently manufactured from four or more whole blood donations. In contrast, with the appropriate selection of donors, 1–3 adult therapeutic doses (2.5–11×10^{11}) can be harvested from a single donor during one apheresis collection procedure.

Platelets are stored under agitation at 20–24 °C for five days, which may be extended to seven days if an approved method to detect or inactivate bacterial pathogens is used. Cold-stored platelets were used in the 1960s and 1970s. The markedly decreased circulation times of these platelets because of cold-induced neoantigen formation and reticuloendothelial destruction led to their replacement with agitated 20–24 °C platelets [5]. Cold-stored platelets are under investigation for limited use in actively bleeding patients due to their better immediate haemostatic properties compared with room temperature-stored units in aggregation and patient bleeding time studies. Currently, the use of frozen platelets stored in DMSO is mainly restricted to military blood banks. However, studies are ongoing to assess the suitability of this product in the civilian setting.

Table 22.2 Specifications for platelet components.

Preparation	Volume (CoE)	Platelet content	WBC content (/unit)	Expiry pH$_{22°C}$
Platelets (recovered, single unit) – PRP intermediate	>40 mL per 0.6×10^{11} platelets	CoE: $>0.6 \times 10^{11}$ AABB: 90% $\geq 0.55 \times 10^{11}$ (75% for LR)	CoE: $<0.2 \times 10^{9}$ AABB: 95% $<0.83 \times 10^{6}$ for LR	CoE: >6.4 AABB: 90% ≥6.2
Platelets (recovered, single unit) – BC intermediate	>40 mL per 0.6×10^{11} platelets	CoE: $>0.6 \times 10^{11}$	CoE: $<0.05 \times 10^{9}$	CoE: >6.4
Platelets (recovered), pooled	>40 mL per 0.6×10^{11} platelets	CoE: $\geq 2 \times 10^{11}$ UK: $\geq 2.4 \times 10^{11}$, $\geq 2 \times 10^{11}$ in 100% AS	CoE: $<0.3 \times 10^{9}$ in AS, $<1 \times 10^{9}$ in plasma, $<1 \times 10^{6}$ for LR UK: $<1 \times 10^{6}$ for LR AABB: 95% $<5 \times 10^{6}$ for LR	CoE: >6.4 UK: 95% >6.4 AABB: 90% ≥6.2
Platelets, apheresis ± AS	>40 mL per 0.6×10^{11} platelets	CoE: $\geq 2 \times 10^{11}$ UK: $\geq 2.4 \times 10^{11}$, $\geq 2 \times 10^{11}$ in 100% AS AABB: 90% $\geq 3 \times 10^{11}$	CoE: $<0.3 \times 10^{9}$, $<1 \times 10^{6}$ for LR UK: $<1 \times 10^{6}$ for LR AABB: 95% $<5 \times 10^{6}$ for LR	CoE: >6.4 UK: 6.4 – 7.4 AABB: ≥6.2

AS, additive solution; BC, buffy coat; CoE, Council of Europe; LR, leucoreduced; PRP, platelet-rich plasma; WBC, white blood cell.

With prestorage LR and modern storage plastics, platelets stored for seven days in plasma maintain their *in vitro* function, with 15–20% reductions in recovery compared with five-day stored platelets. During storage, platelets undergo a fall in pH due to accumulation of lactic acid, show increased surface expression of activation markers and lose their normal shape. Many different laboratory assays have been advocated to monitor development of the so-called 'platelet storage lesion' but few have been demonstrated to correlate with *in vivo* survival [6]. pH remains the only quantitative change that must be monitored routinely and must be above 6.2–6.4 at outdate. Visual inspection to look for the 'swirling' effect of discoid platelets has been recommended, but this is highly subjective and changes only when the platelets have been grossly damaged.

For patients with severe allergic reactions, usually due to plasma proteins, it is possible to wash platelets. This results in the loss of >20% of platelet number and function, but does ameliorate reaction rates far more than simple plasma volume reduction.

Platelet additive solutions (PAS) are available worldwide for apheresis platelets and, in some countries, whole blood-derived platelet pools [7]. These solutions contain sodium chloride, acetate, citrate, phosphate or gluconate buffers ± potassium and magnesium. Platelets stored in 65% PAS and 35% plasma are available in a number of countries and can be stored for 5–7 days. This strategy makes more plasma available for transfusion or fractionation, appears to reduce allergic reactions, but may result in lower platelet increments, depending on the additive used. Solutions incorporating glucose and bicarbonate require less plasma carry-over which may further reduce plasma-based reactions.

Plasma Production and Storage (Table 22.3)

Fresh frozen plasma (FFP) from a whole blood donation must be separated and frozen as soon after collection as possible, within eight hours in the United States and Canada and preferably within six in continental Europe. Usual unit volumes are 200–300 mL. FFP can also be derived from apheresis collections in 300–600 mL volumes. It is commonly used as a source of multiple coagulation factor replacement for massive transfusion, disseminated intravascular coagulation, warfarin-induced bleeding and liver disease. It can also be used for plasma exchange in patients with thrombotic thrombocytopenic purpura (TTP) or serve as a single source of one or more deficient factors for which no concentrates are available. The permitted shelf-life (three months to seven years) depends on the storage temperature (≤ -18 to $\leq -65\,°C$). In Europe, FFP must be monitored for levels of factor VIII. FFP is thawed in a protective overwrap in a water bath, a purpose-designed microwave oven or dry heat source. Once thawed, FFP should be used as soon as possible since the levels of labile coagulation factors decline during further storage. Most countries permit thawed plasma to be stored refrigerated for at least one day and up to five days in some if it is relabelled as 'thawed plasma'. Demonstrated to contain lower levels of the labile coagulation proteins FV and FVIII, this does not appear to significantly impact the clinical efficacy of thawed plasma [8].

Frozen plasma (plasma frozen within 24 hours after phlebotomy in the United States) is obtained from whole blood or by apheresis and frozen within 24 hours after collection. Its storage requirements, therapeutic efficacy and clinical use are the same as for FFP. In North America, this component is labelled as a product different from FFP, whereas in Europe this is not the case.

Plasma, cryoprecipitate reduced is a by-product of cryoprecipitated antihaemophilic factor production and is deficient in FVIII, von Willebrand factor (vWF), fibrinogen, FXIII and fibronectin. This component is stored at the same temperature and duration as FFP. Once thawed, it must be used within 24 hours or, as allowed in some countries, stored refrigerated for up to five days after relabeling as thawed plasma, cryoprecipitate reduced. Its sole use is as a replacement fluid during plasma exchange for TTP.

Table 22.3 Specifications for frozen plasma components.

Preparation Storage	CoE ≤−18 to −25 °C: 3 mo., <−25 °C: 36 mo.		UK (75% of components) ≤−25 °C: 36 mo.		AABB ≤−18 °C: 12 mo., ≤−65 °C: 7 yr. (FFP only)
Fresh frozen plasma (FFP)	Platelets RBC WBC FVIII	$<50 \times 10^9$/L $<6 \times 10^9$/L $<1 \times 10^6$/unit if LR ≥0.7 IU/mL, ≥0.5 IU/mL if PR	Platelets RBC WBC FVIII Protein	$<30 \times 10^9$/L $<6 \times 10^9$/L $<1 \times 10^6$/U ≥0.7 IU/mL ≥50 g/L	No requirements
Plasma frozen within 24 hours after phlebotomy (± held at room temperature up to 24 hours)	Same as FFP		Same as FFP		No requirements
Liquid plasma	Not recognised		Not recognised		No requirements
Cryoprecipitate	FVIII Fibrinogen vWF Volume	≥70 IU/unit ≥140 mg/unit ≥100 IU/unit 30–40 mL	WBC FVIII Fibrinogen	$<1 \times 10^6$/unit ≥70 IU/unit ≥140 mg/unit	FVIII Fibrinogen	≥80 IU/unit ≥150 mg/unit
Pooled cryoprecipitate			WBC FVIII Fibrinogen Volume	$<1 \times 10^6$/unit ≥350 IU/unit ≥700 mg/unit 100–250 mL	FVIII Fibrinogen	≥80 IU/unit in pool ≥150 mg/unit in pool
Plasma, cryoprecipitate depleted					No requirements

CoE, Council of Europe; FVIII, factor 8; RBC, red blood cell; WBC, white blood cell.

In the United States, liquid plasma is collected from whole blood, stored between 1 °C and 6 °C and expires in 26–40 days, depending upon the base anticoagulant into which it is collected. Use in Europe and North America is generally limited to 7–14 days because of progressive factor loss. The clinical indication for liquid plasma is limited to initial treatment of massively transfused patients with life-threatening haemorrhage. As a never-frozen product with viable lymphocytes, to prevent transfusion-associated graft-versus-host disease (TA-GVHD), irradiation is recommended.

Cryoprecipitate Production and Storage (see Table 22.3)

Cryoprecipitate is manufactured by slowly thawing single units of FFP at 1–6 °C. Cryoprotein precipitates of factors VIII and XIII, vWF, fibrinogen and fibronectin are concentrated 2–9-fold compared with plasma [9]. Thus it is important to remember that cryoprecipitate is not simply a concentrated form of FFP, as many pro- and anticoagulant factors are not found in cryoprecipitate. In North America, each single unit of cryoprecipitate must contain ≥80 IU and ≥150 mg fibrinogen in approximately

5–20 mL of plasma; ≥70 IU and ≥140 mg respectively (generally in ~40 mL) are required in the UK and Europe. Cryoprecipitate can be stored for 1–3 years, depending on temperature and local regulations. Thawed cryoprecipitate has a shelf-life of 4–6 hours depending upon jurisdiction and open or closed system processing. Although originally developed for factor VIII deficiency (haemophilia A), most cryoprecipitate is now prescribed to treat acquired hypofibrinogenaemia, usually in the context of massive transfusion, disseminated intravascular coagulation or liver disease. An adult dose of 5–10 bags is generally indicated once the fibrinogen level falls below 1.0–1.5 g/L.

Some countries pool five or more bags of cryoprecipitate to facilitate its administration. An alternative product would be a virus-inactivated fibrinogen concentrate, but in many countries this is only licensed for congenital qualitative or quantitative defects. Clinical studies demonstrating efficacy of either cryoprecipitate or fibrinogen concentrate for acquired deficiency are accruing, particularly in the setting of massive haemorrhage resuscitation protocols and orthopaedic or cardiovascular surgery with high risk of bleeding [10].

Granulocyte Production and Storage

The transfusion of granulocyte concentrates is uncommon. They are presently indicated only for severely neutropenic patients (count $<0.5 \times 10^9$/L) with bacterial or fungal infections refractory to appropriate antimicrobial therapy. Granulocytes are primarily collected by apheresis, with buffy coat separation from whole blood as an alternative source. Most regulatory agencies require an adult dose of $\geq 1 \times 10^{10}$ granulocytes, which is usually infused daily. To achieve such doses, apheresis donors' peripheral counts are increased with steroids ± granulocyte colony-stimulating factor (G-CSF). Unstimulated apheresis granulocyte collections

often do not result in a minimally acceptable adult dose. G-CSF mobilisation with ~5 μg/kg G-CSF plus oral dexamethasone 8 mg (which further elevates counts and blunts some of the side effects of G-CSF) 12–24 hours prior to apheresis results in collections of $6–8 \times 10^{10}$ granulocytes, a dose sufficient to elevate patients' circulating counts. At present, use of G-CSF for granulocyte collection is permitted in volunteer donors unrelated to the patient in the United States, but not in other countries. Apheresis donors are also exposed to a sedimenting agent (hetastarch or pentastarch) during apheresis which decreases product red cell contamination.

A large but underpowered randomised controlled trial of the efficacy of high-dose granulocyte transfusion in infected neutropenic patients concluded that granulocytes had no significant impact on survival or improvement of infection at 42 days after randomisation [11]. However, *post hoc* analysis showed that patients receiving higher doses ($>0.6 \times 10^9$ cells/kg) had a survival advantage compared to those receiving lower doses, with a trend towards improvement over untreated controls.

Some European countries transfuse buffy coats as a source of granulocytes. A dose of 1×10^{10} can be achieved from 10 buffy coats. A pooled granulocyte component made from 10 buffy coats has been developed in the UK and its safety assessed in clinical studies [12].

Granulocytes should be transfused as soon as possible after collection due to their 24-hour shelf-life and onset of significant functional deficits within six hours of collection. As a consequence of the short transfusion timeframe, infectious disease test results are not usually available prior to release, so many collectors require pre-qualified donors. Granulocytes must be γ-irradiated to prevent TA-GVHD, and never leucocyte reduced. Granulocytes should be kept at 20–24 °C without agitation. Because of red cell contamination, a cross-match should be performed. Substantial numbers of platelets are also present in granulocytes, usually $>2.5 \times 10^{11}$.

Component Modifications

Many countries have implemented or are progressing towards universal LR of blood components since passenger leucocytes have no known therapeutic effect, but do confer risk for certain reactions and infections. Prestorage LR is usually carried out at the blood centre with filters during component separation of whole blood, or by in-process removal of leucocytes during plateletpheresis. Proven benefits of LR include reduced transmission of HTLV-I/II and herpes viruses (including cytomegalovirus, Epstein–Barr virus and human herpes virus 8), and decreased risk of febrile nonhaemolytic transfusion reactions, and HLA alloimmunisation [13]. While theoretically reducing the risk of prion transmission, LR does not eliminate infectivity. A small amount of cellular loss (<10%) accompanies filtration LR. European requirements are the most stringent, requiring demonstration of $<1 \times 10^6$ leucocytes per component (a greater than 3-log reduction). The AABB requires $<5 \times 10^6$ per component, or in the case of unpooled whole blood-derived platelets, one-sixth this amount. Various percentages of units required to meet specifications and the statistical sampling requirements to demonstrate compliance exist across national regulatory agencies. LR failures do occur randomly in small percentages of units as a result of poor apheresis separation, filter manufacturing defects or, more commonly, donor-related filtration issues like sickle cell trait. Erythrocyte sickling has been shown to block some filters or create channels between fibres, allowing leucocytes to pass more efficiently.

γ-Irradiation of leucocyte-containing/contaminated components with 1500–3000 cGy inactivates donor lymphocytes whose proliferation in recipients with compromised immune systems results in TA-GVHD [14].[14] GVHD has been observed after transfusion from blood relatives or human leucocyte antigen-selected units as well as in fetal and neonatal recipients of intrauterine transfusions. Granulocyte transfusions can and should be irradiated, since granulocytes are relatively radio-resistant, unlike contaminating lymphocytes. Unlike platelets which are also resistant, red cells sustain membrane damage which requires a shortening of shelf-life. This is generally the earlier of 28 days after irradiation or the original expiry date, but nuances exist for various products and γ-ray doses.

Pathogen inactivation technologies have been approved for plasma and platelets in Europe and the US and are under development for red cells. Four systems for producing pathogen-inactivated plasma are available [15]. Three are suitable for single donor plasma: visible light + methylene blue (MB) and UV light + amotosalen or riboflavin. The fourth, solvent-detergent (SD) treatment, is applied to plasma pools. All methods generally offer a ≥4-log reduction (range 2–7) of viruses, bacteria and parasites, but all are associated with 20–30% loss of clotting factors. Amotosalen and MB are removed by adsorption prior to transfusion (the latter not in all European countries) while riboflavin is not. Solvent-detergent treatment of ABO-identical pools of hundreds of donors' plasma destroys lipid-enveloped viruses and many bacteria and parasites, but does not affect nonenveloped viruses. Accordingly, hepatitis A and parvovirus B19 testing is performed to select units for pooling and SD treatment. Some SD processes introduce a prion reduction step, and in the UK this or single donor plasma sourced from countries at low risk for variant Creutzfeldt–Jakob disease (vCJD) is used for individuals born on or after 1 January, 1996 as a primary vCJD risk reduction method. In the United States, enthusiasm for pathogen-reduced plasma, various preparations of which have been FDA-approved since 1998, has been low due to cost and improvements in viral and parasitic safety resulting from progress in testing.

Enthusiasm for platelet pathogen reduction is increasing, despite significantly higher costs, due to the far greater risk of bacterial contamination and sepsis than viral or parasitic disease transmission. Three technologies exist: use of amotosalen + UV-A (INTERCEPT™, Cerus

Corporation), riboflavin + UV-A/B (Mirasol™, Terumo BCT) and UV-C alone (THERAFLEX UV-Platelets™, MacoPharma). The UV-C technology is CE-marked but not in wide use in any country, while the former two have gained various jurisdictional approvals and are in use for platelets stored in either plasma or additive solution. All three technologies produce UV-induced nucleic acid damage, inactivating DNA and RNA in pathogens and the leucocytes that cause GVHD. There is variable protein damage which results in reduction of posttransfusion increments, with variably observed increases in transfusion frequency. Nevertheless, pathogen-reduced platelets are effective in terminating and preventing haemorrhage. Pathogen inactivation of platelets could obviate the need for irradiation and CMV testing and for some systems, permits a seven-day shelf-life which reduces wastage. A broad range of activity against pathogens would also be expected to

confer protection against emerging transfusion-transmitted infections. However, until a red cell pathogen inactivation system is also available, some of these benefits cannot be fully realised.

Red cells present a challenge for pathogen inactivation technologies due to the high degree of light absorption by haemoglobin. A second-generation Cerus system employs S-303, an acridine nitrogen mustard alkylator which remains in phase III trials following the suspension of first-generation trials due to neoantigen formation and red cell alloimmunisation. The Mirasol system can be used on whole blood, albeit relying upon higher energies and treatment time which results in significantly reduced red cell viability. It is likely that it will be 2–5 years before either system is licensed for routine use. A prion filter capable of a 3–4-log reduction in red cells has been available since 2007, but cost-effectiveness has been a barrier to wider implementation [16].

KEY POINTS

1) Whole blood is limited to certain clinical settings, therefore most whole blood is separated into its components for transfusion (red cells, plasma and platelets).
2) Blood components can be produced from whole-blood donations or collected directly from the donor by apheresis technology.
3) Blood component storage conditions vary as a function of the production method, ideal temperature for maximal function and the intrinsic life span of the cells or proteins in the product.
4) Systems are now available in all jurisdictions to inactivate pathogens in plasma or platelet components prior to storage.

References

1 McLeod BC, Weinstein R, Winters J et al. (eds). Apheresis: Principles and Practice, 3rd edn. AABB Press, Bethesda, 2013.
2 Lachenbruch PA, Foulkes MA, Williams AE, Epstein JS. Potential use of the scan statistic in blood product manufacturing. J Biopharm Stat 2005;**15**:353–66.
3 Acker JP, Hansen Al, Yi QL et al. Introduction of a closed-system cell processor for red blood cell washing: postimplementation monitoring of safety and efficacy. Transfusion 2016;**56**:49–57.
4 Vassallo RR, Murphy S. A critical comparison of platelet preparation methods. Curr Opin Hematol 2006;**13**:323–30.
5 Grozovsky R, Giannini S, Falet H, Hoffmeister KM. Regulating billions of blood platelets: glycans and beyond. Blood 2015;**126**:1877–84.

6 Devine DV, Serrano K. The platelet storage lesion. Clin Lab Med 2010;**30**:475–87.

7 Gulliksson H. Platelet storage media. Vox Sang 2014;**107**:205–12.

8 Benjamin RJ, McLaughlin LS. Plasma components: properties differences and uses. Transfusion 2012;**52**(Suppl. 1):9S–19S.

9 Nascimento B, Goodnough LT, Levy JH. Cryoprecipitate therapy. Br J Anaesth 2014;**113**:922–34.

10 Levy JH, Welsby I, Goodnough LT. Fibrinogen as a therapeutic target for bleeding: a review of critical levels and replacement therapy. Transfusion 2014;**54**:1389–405.

11 Price TH, Boeckh M, Harrison RW et al. Efficacy of transfusion with granulocytes from G-CSF/dexamethasone treated donors in neutropenic patients with infections. Blood 2015;**126**:2153–61.

12 Pammi M, Brocklehurst P. Granulocyte transfusions for neonates with confirmed or suspected sepsis and neutropenia. Cochrane Database Syst Rev 2011;**10**:CD003956.

13 Bilgin YM, van de Watering LMG, Brand A. Clinical effects of leukoreduction of blood transfusions. Neth J Med 2011;**69**:441–50.

14 Fast LD. Developments in the prevention of transfusion-associated graft-versus-host disease. Br J Haematol 2012;**158**:563–8.

15 Salunkhe V, van der Meer PF, de Korte D, Seghatchian J, Gutierrez L. Development of blood transfusion product pathogen reduction treatments: a review of methods, current applications and demands. Transfus Apher Sci 2015;**52**:19–34.

16 Teljeur C, Flattery M, Harrington P et al. Cost-effectiveness of prion filtration of red blood cells to reduce the risk of transfusion-transmitted variant Creuzfeldt–Jakob disease in the Republic of Ireland. Transfusion 2012;**52**:2285–93.

Further Reading

Canadian Blood Services. Circular of Information for the Use of Human Blood Components. CBS Publishing, Ottawa, 2015. Available at: blood.ca/en/hospitals/circular-information (accessed 1 January 2017).

Canadian Standards Association. CAN/CSA-Z902-10 (R2015) Blood and Blood Components. CSA Publishing, Mississauga, 2010.

Council of Europe. Guide to the Preparation, Use and Quality Assurance of Blood Components, 18th ed. Council of Europe Publishing, Strasbourg, 2015.

Fung MF, Grossman B, Hillyer C, Westhoff C (eds). AABB Technical Manual, 18th edn. AABB Press, Bethesda, 2014.

AABB, ARC, ABC, ASBP. Circular of Information for the Use of Human Blood and Blood Components. Available at: aabb.org/tm/coi/Documents/coi1113.pdf (accessed 1 January 2017).

Ooley PW, et al. (eds). AABB Standards for Blood Banks and Transfusion Services, 30th edn. AABB Press, Bethesda, 2015.

United Kingdom National Blood Services. Guidelines for the Blood Transfusion Services in the United Kingdom, 8th edn. Stationery Office, London, 2013. Available at: transfusionguidelines.org.uk/red-book (accessed 1 January 2017).

23 Blood Transfusion in Hospitals

Erica M. Wood[1], Mark H. Yazer[2] and Michael F. Murphy[3]

[1] Transfusion Research Unit, Department of Epidemiology and Preventive Medicine, Monash University, Melbourne, Australia; Department of Clinical Haematology, Monash Health, Melbourne, Australia
[2] Department of Pathology, University of Pittsburgh, Pittsburgh, USA; Department of Clinical Immunology, University of Southern Denmark, Odense, Denmark; ITXM Centralized Transfusion Service, Pittsburgh, USA
[3] University of Oxford; NHS Blood and Transplant and Department of Haematology, Oxford University Hospitals, Oxford, UK

Introduction

The aim of transfusion practice is to provide 'the right blood to the right patient at the right time for the right reason'. In the framework of transfusion safety, the focus is on ensuring that, when it is clinically indicated, patients receive transfusion support to meet their particular needs, in a safe, timely and cost-efficient manner, with incidents and adverse reactions recognised, managed and reported effectively and with measures in place to prevent occurrence or recurrence. This chapter discusses the roles and responsibilities of the main participants in transfusion safety in a hospital context (Figure 23.1), and highlights some bedside and administrative techniques that have been implemented around the world to improve transfusion safety.

Transfusion safety is an organisation-wide concern. A focus on safety needs to cascade from the highest levels of hospital management right through to the staff managing the bedside processes. Hospital administrators set the tone by establishing an organisational safety culture and a reporting system for errors and near misses that encourages reporting in order to correct ambiguous or inefficient processes.

The hospital transfusion committee is a vital component in ensuring patient safety. By encouraging open discussion amongst participants about adoption of best practices in all aspects of transfusion medicine, dangerous 'workarounds', or ways to circumvent established processes, can be discovered and solutions can be developed to which staff will adhere. The transfusion committee also needs to audit clinical transfusion practice to ensure that thresholds set for transfusion of blood products are being followed, and at the same time ensuring that undertransfusion – the withholding of a necessary transfusion – is not occurring (see Chapter 34).

Specialists in all branches of medicine and surgery are involved in transfusion, and engagement, cooperation and coordination are required by staff and patients to manage the complex, interacting sequences of the process. Of course, the staff who collect the pretransfusion testing samples and who ultimately administer the transfusions are at the forefront of patient safety and must recognise their responsibilities for correct patient identification and sample labelling practices, and perform these tasks with great care. The hospital transfusion medicine service contributes to patient safety by providing clinical leadership;

Practical Transfusion Medicine, Fifth Edition. Edited by Michael F. Murphy, David J. Roberts and Mark H. Yazer.
© 2017 John Wiley & Sons Ltd. Published 2017 by John Wiley & Sons Ltd.

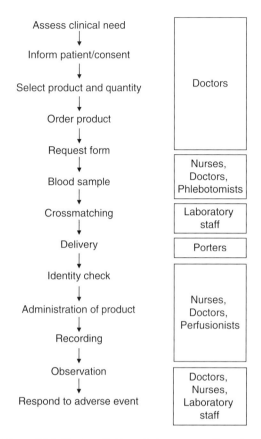

Assess clinical need
↓
Inform patient/consent
↓
Select product and quantity
↓
Order product
↓
Request form
↓
Blood sample
↓
Crossmatching
↓
Delivery
↓
Identity check
↓
Administration of product
↓
Recording
↓
Observation
↓
Respond to adverse event

Doctors

Nurses, Doctors, Phlebotomists

Laboratory staff

Porters

Nurses, Doctors, Perfusionists

Doctors, Nurses, Laboratory staff

Figure 23.1 The hospital transfusion process: Steps in the transfusion process, and the staff predominantly responsible for each step.

by having qualified personnel available to answer transfusion-related questions from staff, patients and families; by investigating suspected adverse events; and by advocating for the best interest of patients when non-evidence-based practice is detected. Thus the responsibility for safe transfusions is found at all levels of a hospital's administrative, medical and nursing staff, bringing complementary skills and expertise and working collaboratively to ensure the final goal is met for every patient, every time.

In many countries, blood for transfusion is not safe, sufficient nor reliably available. In these settings, haemorrhage remains a major direct cause of mortality. However, even in modern healthcare settings with adequate blood supplies,

patients die from transfusion complications [1,2], or from lack of adequate transfusion support: for example, massive haemorrhage is still one of the most common direct causes of maternal death worldwide. Some instances of undertransfusion are due to patient refusal to accept transfusion support, or failure by physicians to recognise and respond to clinical manifestations of bleeding. However, others can be attributed to either lack of knowledge of transfusion protocols or failures of communication within, and between, clinical teams. At the other extreme, patients are frequently overtransfused, and transfusion-associated circulatory overload (TACO) is increasingly recognised as a common serious adverse event [3]. Unnecessary and overtransfusion is also a waste of blood components, which are a scarce resource.

What happens when the culture of safety breaks down and an error happens? Mistransfusion, or 'wrong blood' events, i.e. administering an incorrect unit of blood which either does not meet the patient's special needs or is intended for another recipient, can also have serious consequences, including severe haemolysis due to antigen–antibody incompatibility, and is another well-recognised cause of mortality and morbidity. Human errors leading to mistransfusion can occur at any step in the process, and usually result from failures to comply with clerical or technical procedures, or systems that are either poorly constructed or not understood. Multiple errors are frequently involved in these cases: the so-called 'Swiss cheese' model of error whereby several layers of safeguards are bypassed, leading to the mistransfusion. Some miscollection errors can be detected during the bedside check at the time of administering blood, and this remains a final opportunity to prevent mistransfusion. It has been observed that as many as one in 19 000 red cell units are given erroneously and one in 33 000 will involve ABO-incompatible units [4]. Estimates of mortality due to mistransfusion range from one in 600 000 units to one in 1.8 million.

Enormous investments have been made to reduce the risks of transfusion-transmitted infections but, until recently, there has been much less investment in improving hospital systems required for clinical practice. Consequently, evidence of progress in reducing procedural risks and improving the safety of hospital transfusion practice is slower to accumulate. Some interventions, such as the practice of a bedside ABO group check before transfusion, requiring an ABO group confirmation on a second sample before group-specific blood products are issued to recipients without a historical ABO group on file [5], or the use of physical barriers to transfusion, such as a code to link the patient's wristband, pretransfusion sample and unlock the designated unit of blood from secure storage, are intrinsically attractive. For a variety of reasons, they have been difficult to implement widely [6]. Data to support the effectiveness of many procedural interventions are still limited and many serious (and often preventable) adverse events continue to be reported. However, where haemovigilance programmes have been able to highlight these issues and their causes, and action has been taken to address them, progress has been demonstrated in at least some of these areas [1].

Effective quality frameworks are required to minimise transfusion risks and ensure that the supply of donated blood is managed effectively, minimising unnecessary use and reducing wastage at every step of the process. These in turn require a patient-centred approach to transfusion, committed leadership and adequate resources.

Key Features of Hospital Transfusion Governance

Many countries require blood centres or services (termed 'blood establishments' in Europe) and hospital transfusion laboratories to maintain robust quality systems to ensure good practice, including meeting national or regional standards for good manufacturing, laboratory and/or clinical practice (also see Chapter 18). These requirements are typically overseen by national regulatory authorities and/or professional authorities to ensure compliance. For

example, to meet EU Directives, the UK Blood Safety and Quality Regulations [7] outline requirements for quality management in transfusion laboratories, including staff training, process validation, documentation, storage and handling, traceability and reporting of adverse events. However, these regulations have typically not extended to transfusion practice in clinical areas, and other measures are still needed to ensure that processes and systems that influence the quality and governance of clinical transfusion practice at the hospital level are optimised and working as expected. Recommendations for practice are derived from clinical experience and the peer-reviewed evidence base, along with lessons from haemovigilance and external quality assessment (EQA) schemes. These are translated into policies, standards and guidelines by government agencies and professional groups, who in turn assess implementation and compliance and promote best practice through training, education and communication.

In England, the Care Quality Commission regulates healthcare providers. Many of the national standards for governance and risk assessment are applicable to blood transfusion, including those relating to patient engagement, informed consent, staff training and competency assessment, participation in audit and other quality improvement activities and reporting of incidents. Specifically, the National Patient Safety Agency in England in 2006 issued a safety notice requiring competency-based training and assessment for all staff involved in blood transfusion, a pretransfusion bedside identity check that requires staff to match the blood unit with the recipient's wristband (rather than the compatibility form or case notes), and a formal risk assessment for use of any alternative means of confirming patient identity.

Similar expectations apply in other countries. For example, the Australian Commission on Safety and Quality in Healthcare standard on clinical transfusion practice is part of national safety and quality standards [8] and outlines requirements against which hospitals are assessed for accreditation. In the United States, authorities from state health departments through to national regulators like the Joint Commission on Accreditation of Healthcare Organizations (JCAHO) and the Food and Drug Administration are involved in assessing and regulating transfusion practice.

At an institutional level, executive management is responsible for implementation of standards and policies, including initial and ongoing staff training and appraisal, and for performing and monitoring clinical audits and other quality system activities.

Hospital Transfusion Committees

Hospital transfusion committees (HTCs) are focal points for overseeing transfusion practice at the institutional level. Their roles are outlined in documents such as English NHS 'Better Blood Transfusion' Health Service Circulars, and statements from regulatory bodies like the US JCAHO.

Hospital transfusion committees are essential components of clinical governance, so they must be incorporated into hospital frameworks for clinical governance, performance and risk management and report findings and activities in a timely and meaningful way accompanied by recommendations for action, where appropriate. HTCs have the remit to promote best practice, review clinical transfusion practice, monitor performance of the hospital transfusion service, participate in regional or national initiatives and communicate with local patient representative groups as appropriate (Table 23.1).

To be effective and to deliver on their objectives, HTCs require support from dedicated hospital transfusion teams (see below), at a minimum consisting of a medical specialist, transfusion practitioner(s) and blood transfusion laboratory scientist/manager. Other necessary resources include IT and clerical support to facilitate regular meetings, data retrieval and audit.

Membership of the Hospital Transfusion Committee

A chairperson with understanding and experience of transfusion practice should be appointed by hospital senior management. Ideally, the chairperson should not be the medical specialist responsible for the hospital transfusion service, who could be perceived to have a vested interest. It is very helpful to include representatives from medical and surgical specialties that order blood components (such as from anaesthesia, surgery, critical care, obstetrics and the emergency department), nursing staff from hospital units that are regularly involved in administering blood transfusions (such as haematology/oncology) and from the patient blood management (PBM) programme, to contribute their clinical perspectives.

The following membership is suggested.

- Representatives of all major clinical blood users, including junior medical staff
- Specialist haematologist/pathologist with responsibility for transfusion
- Hospital blood transfusion laboratory senior scientist/manager
- Specialist practitioner(s) of transfusion
- Senior nursing representative
- Representatives from hospital management and clinical risk management
- Local blood centre medical specialist (*ex officio*)
- Other co-opted representatives as required, e.g. from medical records, portering staff, clinical audit, training or pharmacy
- In many settings, participation by a patient representative is encouraged and, in some cases, is a requirement of hospital accreditation

Working Together to Improve the Transfusion Process

The Multidisciplinary Hospital Transfusion Team

This team **works collaboratively to identify and take action on areas for improvement in hospital practice.** Members include:

Table 23.1 Activities of the hospital transfusion committee.

Area or activity	Example
Policies and procedures	Develop and promulgate policies and procedures, including for: • clinical indication and decision to transfuse • establishing and enforcing transfusion thresholds • informed consent process • collection of samples for compatibility testing, including patient identification and specimen labelling requirements • transfusion administration and monitoring • indications for specialised components (e.g. irradiated, CMV-seronegative, phenotype-matched) • Maximum Surgical Blood Ordering Schedule (MSBOS) • blood conservation strategies including use of cell salvage and pharmacological agents • management of patients who decline transfusion • management of adverse reactions
Education, training and assessment	Develop strategy for education, training and assessment of all staff involved in transfusion Monitor implementation and results of education and training activities Develop and/or promulgate information/materials for patients
Audit, monitoring and review	Develop annual audit plans and monitor performance Review adverse event reports Conduct incident, 'near miss' and sentinel event reviews Oversee traceability and record-keeping obligations
System performance	Review: • blood component availability, utilisation and wastage rates • activation of massive transfusion protocol, use of uncrossmatched emergency red cell stocks • performance of institutional transfusion laboratory and blood service ('blood establishment') • participation in regional and national audit, transfusion practice improvement and haemovigilance programme activities • participation in EQA activities Oversee hospital and laboratory accreditation activities relating to transfusion Contingency and disaster planning Function and performance of HTC

• transfusion medicine specialist, to provide medical expertise in clinical and laboratory transfusion practice and clinical leadership for transfusion issues

• biomedical scientist (blood transfusion laboratory manager) in charge of the transfusion laboratory, to bring scientific expertise and oversight of transfusion laboratory activities

• specialist practitioner of transfusion, often with a nursing or biomedical science back-ground, to serve as liaison between clinical areas and transfusion laboratory, including for delivery of education and training; some-times known as a transfusion safety officer [9].

Other contributors may include registrars (fellows) or residents undertaking specialist training in transfusion medicine; personnel with quality management responsibilities in clinical or laboratory areas; or representatives of

PBM, cell salvage or other related clinical programmes; and students, either as regular or occasional invited participants.

Activities depend on organisational needs, and typically focus on problem solving and quality improvement, such as adverse event and incident evaluation, haemovigilance reporting, transfusion policy and procedure development and audit planning and analysis. The group can coordinate transfusion communication, education and research activities and HTC support. Close links with other clinical practice improvement and PBM activities, such as preoperative anaemia management, are important.

To be effective, the hospital transfusion team should meet frequently (weekly or at least monthly) and the HTC should meet as often as it needs to achieve its aims – many hospitals have quarterly HTC meetings. Team meetings also provide teaching opportunities from interesting clinical cases, and may suggest research and quality projects for further development by the group or others.

The Role of the Patient

'Patient-centred care is a dimension of safety and quality' [8]. The concept of patient-centred care recognises the essential role of patients in participating in their own care. Patients are increasingly educated and informed, and can (and should, wherever possible) play important roles in care planning and delivery. For example, individual patients can participate at all stages of the transfusion process, from discussions about what alternatives may be available, to ensuring correct identification at the time of pretransfusion sample collection or bedside administration, and early recognition of adverse events [10].

Patient groups can also play important roles in hospital practice on behalf of their members. For example, community groups representing patients with haemoglobinopathies, bleeding disorders or other major conditions which may require transfusion support, or Jehovah's Witnesses, can provide important input to developing educational materials and ensure these are available, up to date and culturally appropriate.

Informed consent

Communication between patients and clinical staff is essential for healthcare planning and delivery, including for procedures like transfusion which carry potential benefits but also important hazards.

Hospital informed consent processes for transfusion have historically focused on documentation of staff informing patients about the risks of blood components and fractionated products, with little ability to demonstrate that this information is understood by the intended recipients or that the information meets the needs of patients and their families. More recently, the focus has shifted to a process of communication which aims to ensure that patients receive meaningful information relevant to their individual circumstances and in a way that they can understand and use. Definitions and expectations vary between countries and institutions but broadly speaking, for transfusion, patients should understand why transfusion might be necessary, what it would involve and what alternatives are available, including potential benefits and risks of the various options under consideration.

Staff conducting the conversation should have sufficient knowledge of transfusion practice and current risk estimates of infectious and non-infectious hazards to provide accurate information. Ready access to written guidance prepared for clinical staff or patients can facilitate these interactions, as many staff and patients have very limited understanding of the real risks of transfusion. The HTC can be useful in preparing such documents. Many national blood services and practice improvement programmes also provide summaries which are periodically updated with local data. Sufficient time also needs to be allocated for the discussion so that patient questions can be addressed.

For a range of reasons, some patients will not accept transfusion, or will only accept very limited transfusion options. Hospitals must have policies and procedures in place to manage these situations, in line with the principles of respect for patient autonomy and working within organisational and regulatory requirements. For all patients, including those who decline any or some transfusion support, open discussion, clear communication and documentation of agreed plans are essential.

Administration of Blood and Blood Components and Management of the Transfused Patient

This process involves multiple steps.

- Counselling patients regarding the need for blood transfusion and its benefits and risks, when alternative approaches (e.g. treatment of anaemia with iron) are predicted to be insufficient or inappropriate for their circumstances.
- Requesting and prescribing blood products, including any special blood requirements (e.g. for gamma-irradiated blood) and in the appropriate dose.
- Sampling for pretransfusion compatibility testing.
- Collection of the blood product from the storage facility (e.g. the blood transfusion laboratory or a monitored blood refrigerator) and its delivery to the clinical area.
- Pretransfusion bedside checking process, including verifying the prescription for the product and that the product is the right one for the patient.
- Administration of the blood product(s).
- Management of any related procedures for blood collection and reinfusion (e.g. acute

normovolaemic haemodilution, intra- or post-operative cell salvage).
- Patient monitoring, as well as management and reporting of any adverse events.
- Documentation of all steps, including the clinical outcome of the transfusion.

Errors occurring at blood sampling, collection and administration can lead to patient misidentification and mistransfusion. Prescription errors, however, lead either to failure to provide special components to meet recipient special needs or to transfusions which are unnecessary or inappropriate and carry the potential for complications. For example, TACO has occurred when transfusions have been given on the basis of a spuriously low haemoglobin value resulting from samples taken from IV ('drip') arms or measured by gas analysers, or a clerical error where another patient's results are reported. Fatal errors have also occurred in prescribing the wrong volume to transfuse or the wrong rate of transfusion. Failure to monitor transfused patients, particularly in the first 15 minutes of receiving each unit, can lead to life-threatening reactions being overlooked and delays in resuscitation.

Hospitals should have written procedures to cover all these steps, against which relevant staff are trained and regularly assessed, and which are readily available for reference at the bedside. Clinical responsibilities, actions, documents, potential errors and some of their consequences are outlined in Tables 23.2–23.8. Prescription charts, donation numbers of components and batch/lot numbers of fractionated plasma products issued and transfused, nursing observations and recipient vital signs related to the transfusion should be kept in the medical case notes as permanent records. Regulatory and accreditation authorities require a complete audit trail of blood to the patient's bedside. Many hospitals comply with this requirement by returning signed and dated compatibility forms or compatibility labels to the transfusion laboratory. Electronic methods are increasingly replacing hard copy documents with associated improvements in reliability and efficiency.

Table 23.2 Examples of some errors and other problems in the transfusion process, and their potential outcomes.

Problem	Potential outcome
Unnecessary prescription	Patient subjected to unnecessary risks, including transfusion-associated circulatory overload
	Blood component wastage
Prescribed components do not meet patient special requirements	Transfusion complications (e.g. transfusion-associated graft-versus-host disease)
Blood not stored in controlled environment	Blood component wastage Transfusion complications (e.g. risk of bacterial growth)
Pretransfusion samples taken from incorrect patient Sample transposition or other laboratory errors Incorrect unit of blood collected and/or administered	Mistransfusion and potential for ABO- or RhD-incompatible transfusion
Insensitive techniques in pretransfusion testing	Potential for acute and delayed haemolytic transfusion reactions
Poor laboratory management of blood stocks	Blood component wastage
	Inappropriate overuse of group O red cells and potential for consequent shortages of that group
Delay in emergency provision of blood components	Patient morbidity/mortality due to bleeding, hypoxia or abnormal haemostasis

Table 23.3 Prescription of blood components.

Responsibility	Action	Documentation	Examples of potential problems and errors
Medical staff	Ensure patient is aware of need for transfusion and has received, read and understood information related to risks and benefits	Patient information materials Hospital consent form	Staff and patient insufficiently educated about risks/hazards Failure to take account of patient religious beliefs or other patient views
	Prescribe component, any special requirements, quantity/volume and rate/duration of transfusion	Prescription form or chart	Unnecessary prescription, failure to follow hospital guidelines, or as result of error in laboratory test results
			Lack of awareness of, or failure to prescribe, special components
	Document rationale for transfusion	Patient medical record	

Related national and hospital procedures and documents

Guidelines for the use of blood and blood components, including special requirements

Practice guidelines/procedures for individual diseases/treatments

Table 23.4 Requests for blood and blood components.

Responsibility	Action	Documentation	Examples of potential problems and errors
Medical and registered nursing staff	Provide full patient identification, their location and diagnosis and the justification for transfusion along with details of the type and quantity of component and time required Provide previous obstetric and transfusion history when requesting red cells	Written/electronic request form, or laboratory telephone log in an emergency	Incomplete or incorrect patient information leading to failure to recognise historical laboratory record Failure to record requirement for special components or phenotyped units Failure to request special components
Hospital transfusion laboratory staff	Review historical laboratory record to determine if the patient has any special blood requirements and whether a further sample for pretransfusion testing is required	Previous laboratory record	Patient identification error in transcribing telephone request Failure to locate/heed information contained in historical record Failure to request new sample in recently transfused patient with potential to overlook newly developed red cell antibodies

Related hospital procedures and documents

Pretransfusion sampling and testing protocols

Maximum Surgical Blood Ordering Schedules (MSBOS)

Table 23.5 Sampling for pretransfusion compatibility testing.

Responsibility	Action	Documentation	Examples of potential problems and errors
Medical, nursing and phlebotomy staff	Direct questioning of patient to provide surname, first name and date of birth when judged capable Check that details given match those on patient wristband and on request form		Patient misidentification due to failure to positively identify patient, or wristband missing or with incomplete information
	Take blood sample and immediately label at bedside with required patient information	Sample correctly labelled and signed	Patient misidentification as a result of: Sample tube prelabelled or labelled away from bedside with another patient's information Addressograph label affixed from incorrect patient
Hospital blood transfusion laboratory staff	Determine that sample labelling meets requirements for pretransfusion testing; if unacceptable, inform requester of need for another sample	If unacceptable, document reasons	Potential to issue inappropriate unit Failure to provide blood in a timely manner if clinicians unaware of need for another sample

Related hospital procedures and documents

Hospital sample labelling policy (including for unknown patients)

Hospital policies for allocation and maintenance of unique patient identifiers and for resiting wristbands if they are removed, for example during surgery

Table 23.6 Collection and delivery of blood components from transfusion storage facility to clinical area.

Responsibility	Action	Documentation	Examples of potential problems and errors
Authorised and trained staff	Take documentation bearing patient identification to issue refrigerator	Completed prescription form or collection slip	Incorrect unit collected if no documentation bearing patient ID
	Check that unit removed and accompanying transfusion compatibility form bear identical patient identification details		Incorrect unit removed with the potential that it will be transfused if it is not recognised at the bedside
	Record time and sign that correct unit has been collected		Lack of audit trail from failure to sign out unit from issue refrigerator

Related hospital procedures and documents

Hospital blood collection policy

Table 23.7 Administration of blood components.

Responsibility	Action	Documentation	Examples of potential problems and errors
Medical and registered nursing staff	At bedside, direct questioning of patient (if conscious) to provide surname, first name and date of birth when judged capable Check that the stated patient identity is identical with that on the wristband and the compatibility label on the blood pack	Prescription form Compatibility label Patient wristband	Unit transfused to wrong patient if checked away from bedside or no verification of patient identity
	Check blood group is compatible	Compatibility label Base label on blood pack	Incorrect ABO/RhD group transfused if failure to detect laboratory grouping or labelling error
	Check special requirements fulfilled	Prescription chart Blood pack	Inappropriate component transfused if failure to detect laboratory issuing error
	Check unit not past expiry date, is intact with no visual evidence of deterioration		Transfusion of time-expired component Transfusion of potentially bacterially contaminated unit
	Document and sign date and time of commencement and completion	Compatibility form and/ or prescription chart	
	Retain donation number in patient record	Label/sticker on prescription chart or in patient record	Failure to complete audit trail

Related hospital procedures and documents

Hospital blood administration policy

Table 23.8 Monitoring of transfused patients.

Responsibility	Action	Documentation	Examples of potential problems and errors
Authorised and trained staff	Measure and record clinical observations prior to each unit	Observation chart, recording date and time	Without baseline observations, cannot detect changes warning of transfusion reaction
	Explain to patient possible adverse effects to be reported and keep patient under close visual observation in first 15 min of each unit		Patient not aware of symptoms that can warn of transfusion reaction
	Measure temperature and pulse 15 min after start of each unit	Observation chart, recording time	Potential to miss early signs of serious transfusion reaction
	Measure and record clinical observation at end of each unit	Observation chart, recording time	Cannot know whether subsequent changes in patient condition are temporally related to ongoing transfusion

Related hospital procedures and documents

Hospital policies on monitoring transfused patients and management of transfusion reactions

Technologies to Reduce Patient Misidentification Errors in Administering Blood

Additional Manual Systems of Patient Identification (Figure 23.2)

Sets of distinctive (e.g. coloured) labels with the same unique number can be allocated to each pretransfusion blood sample. One of the labels can be incorporated into an additional patient wristband at the time of phlebotomy, and one each affixed to the request form, sample tube and into the current medical notes. After compatibility testing, the unique number can be printed onto the compatibility label which is attached to the blood unit by the blood transfusion laboratory staff. At the time of pretransfusion checking, the additional unique number provides a supplementary means of cross-checking that the blood unit will be administered to the correct patient.

Electronic Bedside Processes for Safe Transfusion Practice (Figure 23.3)

Bedside handheld computers, barcoded staff identity badges, barcoded printed wristbands for patients and portable printers taken to the bedside for sample tube labels provide the means for improving the accuracy of patient identification and thus transfusion safety [11]. For example, at sample collection, the identity of the phlebotomist and patient can be established by scanning their respective identity cards or wristbands, and barcoded labels generated at the bedside containing the patient's full identification details can be attached to the sample tube at the time and place where it is collected. In the laboratory, allocated units are labelled with a compatibility label with a barcode incorporating both the patient's unique identification details and the unit number. At the time of pretransfusion checking, staff are prompted by a handheld computer to scan their own identification barcode, and the barcodes on the patient wristband, the compatibility label and the unit number on the blood component.

Check the laboratory-generated label against the patient's identity band

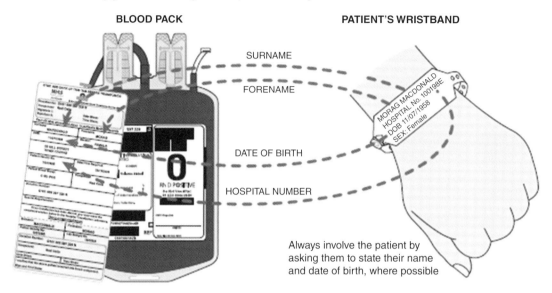

Figure 23.2 How to perform an identity check between the patient and blood component. *Source:* Handbook of Transfusion Medicine, 5th edn, Stationery Office, UK. (*See insert for colour representation of the figure.*)

The computer prompts the staff to verbally check the identity of the (conscious) patient and the barcode scans confirm that the unit is correct for the patient. The user and transfusion laboratory are alerted if there is a mismatch. It also provides prompts to check for special requirements, pre-transfusion observations and the unit expiry date. Documentation of each step is transmitted to the laboratory information system to confirm the traceability of the unit, and to facilitate assessment of the competency of staff in safe transfusion practice.

Electronic bedside systems can be linked to similar systems controlling release of blood from remote blood refrigerators to provide full electronic process control, and to facilitate electronically controlled remote issue (see later in this chapter, and [12]).

Electronic systems for blood transfusion are increasingly being implemented, although further studies are needed to confirm their cost-effectiveness. The acceptance of their use would be even greater if they were integrated with other processes requiring patient identification, such as medication administration.

Influencing Clinical Practice

Potential factors influencing transfusion practice and decision making include:

- physician knowledge, and perception based on clinical experience and review of the literature
- peer pressure and feedback
- effectiveness of hospital governance frameworks
- educational prompts and directions (e.g. through online ordering system settings) at the time of decision making
- patient knowledge and preferences [10]
- financial pressures or incentives
- public and political perceptions and fear of litigation.

Improving transfusion practice within a hospital community requires a planned, consistent approach, endorsed and implemented through clinical governance frameworks, supported over time and monitored for effect. In this endeavour, the HTC can be very useful in disseminating the latest evidence-based information and in auditing and ensuring prescriber compliance with hospital policies and procedures.

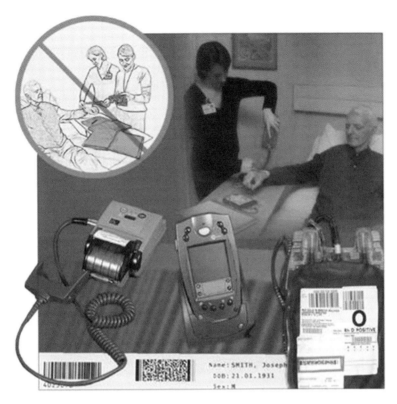

Figure 23.3 Bedside checking using an electronic system. The traditional method of pretransfusion bedside checking requires two nurses and checks of multiple items of written documentation. With barcode technology, a handheld computer reads a barcode on the patient wristband containing full patient details. The handheld computer checks that the patient details on the wristband barcode match those on the barcode (in the red box) on the compatibility label attached to the unit after pretransfusion testing. This barcode also contains the unique number of the unit, and is matched with the barcode number of the unit (top left of the bag) to ensure that the blood transfusion laboratory has attached the right compatibility label. *Source:* Reproduced with permission from Wiley–Blackwell. (*See insert for colour representation of the figure.*)

Guidelines, Algorithms and Protocols

Guidelines are systematically developed statements to assist practitioner and patient decision making about appropriate healthcare for specific clinical circumstances. A list of websites with some examples of guidelines is included at the end of this chapter. Data from randomised controlled trials are generally not available to assess the impact of professional guidelines, but even the promulgation of national guidelines rarely leads to change without local implementation and dissemination strategies, and these require time and resources.

Developing an institutional strategy to implement guidelines is a useful opportunity to gain ownership and participation. For example, educational opportunities arise from examining the evidence basis for the guidelines, and dissent and other local barriers to implementation, such as limited staff or IT resources, or effects on laboratory turnaround times can be identified and resolved.

Institutions should adopt recommendations from authoritative professional guidelines and from well-designed clinical trials. The data and recommendations should be carefully reviewed in light of the need for any customisation for local use. This may involve separating guidelines into sections and/or incorporating some recommendations into other local protocols for specific conditions, such as fresh frozen plasma guidelines incorporated into protocols for management of disseminated intravascular coagulation and massive haemorrhage. These local documents should be incorporated into transfusion policies and disseminated, with training, for all involved staff. A multidisciplinary approach to designing the local guidelines and thresholds allows for the input of the product users, so that their concerns are addressed.

Experience in other medical fields has demonstrated that embedding guideline recommendations into materials used during decision-making and administration processes can significantly improve compliance. Examples include:

- listing clinical indications for special blood components on transfusion request forms or electronic request screens
- using electronic warning systems to alert prescribers when, based on laboratory values, planned transfusions do not meet guidelines (see below)
- listing, on specific transfusion observation charts, actions to be taken in the event of reactions
- detailing checks to be made on the compatibility form prior to administering blood.

Intraoperative algorithms for the use of platelets and plasma to correct microvascular bleeding during and after cardiac bypass surgery have also been successful in reducing inappropriate use of these components, especially when combined with near-patient testing and rapid availability of results.

Clinical Audit

Clinical audit is a quality improvement process that seeks to improve patient care and clinical outcomes, through systematic review of care against explicit criteria or standards, followed by the implementation of change. Analysis of audit findings can lead to recommendations for improvements when deficiencies or nonguideline-based practices are identified, in turn generating cycles where feedback and clarification of hospital policies lead to improved practice.

Audits can be conducted retrospectively or concurrently. Retrospective transfusion audits are often performed under the auspices of the HTC. Some regulatory agencies require a certain percentage of all transfusions to be reviewed by the HTC and those felt to have been administered without reasonable justification brought to the committee's attention. If, from available data, a transfusion is felt to be egregious, further information should be requested from the responsible physician. If the explanation is inadequate or if the physician fails to reply, other steps, such as letters to department chairs, can also be taken. Advantages of this type of review are that communications from the HTC carry additional weight, and they can be educational tools to inform physicians of institutional protocols. The main disadvantages are the limited number of transfusion episodes that can be audited, and, because audits are performed after the event, educational opportunities are lost if the staff who ordered the transfusion cannot be located or cannot recall the event. Retrospective audits also cannot influence clinical practice for the episodes being audited (but might influence prescribing behaviour in the future).

Audits performed concurrently with blood component ordering, but before product issue, can take several forms. A simple example involves transfusion laboratory staff comparing component orders with hospital guidelines; if criteria are not met, the ordering physician is contacted, the reasons for ordering the transfusion discussed and plans established. Intervention by transfusion medicine physicians has been demonstrated to be effective in reducing unnecessary transfusions [13]. Audits of this type have been criticised for potentially causing delay in providing necessary products, although they would also prevent unnecessary transfusions before they were administered.

Significant time, effort and good communication are required to make these audits effective.

Another approach to concurrent audit involves automation to warn clinicians at the time of ordering that the transfusion might not be necessary. Where a hospital uses computerised order entry, and institutional guidelines are in place, warnings can appear on the screen when physicians try to order blood for patients whose laboratory values suggest that transfusion is not indicated. Figure 23.4 demonstrates the response where a physician attempts to order red cells for a patient whose latest haemoglobin value is above the threshold set by the HTC. The warning appears, giving the physician the option of either cancelling the order or proceeding, depending on the patient's current clinical situation (which might not be accurately reflected in a historical laboratory value). The experience of the University of Pittsburgh Medical Center (UPMC) large multihospital healthcare system is that about 10–15% of the orders in which an alert appears are cancelled. This might not seem like a success, but it does contribute to a reduction in unnecessary blood product transfusions and provides some education around evidence-based transfusion thresholds. The ability to track individual physicians and hospital locations that generate the greatest

number of warnings also supports provision of focused education.

Many countries have regional or national clinical audit programmes, with participation being either voluntary or, increasingly, mandated by accreditation or governmental agencies. Participation provides opportunities to benchmark performance between similar institutions, and to promote engagement in practice improvement activities more broadly. The UK national audit programme and several of the practice improvement collaboratives in Australia have made their audit tools available to invite collaboration, comparisons of practice and sharing of resources.

Surveys

Many activities which fall under an 'audit' banner are not comparing practice with a standard, but are monitoring or surveying practice. These activities, many of which can be quantified, often provide information and baseline data which can lead to the development of quality or performance indicators. Trend analysis, or comparison of organisations or blood users with each other, is a powerful means of exerting peer pressure and influencing practice (benchmarking, as above).

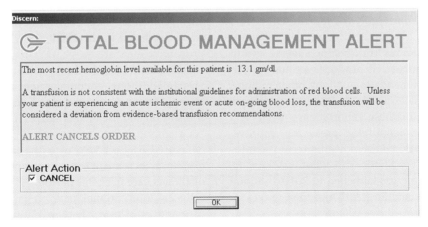

Figure 23.4 Warning message displayed when a physician at a University of Pittsburgh Medical Center (UPMC, Pittsburgh, PA) hospital attempts to order red cells using the computerised order entry system for a patient whose most recent haemoglobin value is in excess of the institutional guidelines.

Performance indicators can be applied to:

- *clinical and laboratory practice issues*: for example: the proportion of medical records with evidence of patients having received written pretransfusion information; percentage of primary hip or knee arthroplasties requiring allogeneic transfusion; proportion of patients receiving platelets after coronary artery bypass grafting; red cell use by surgical procedure (by surgeon or unit); or percentage of anaemic patients being investigated, correctly diagnosed and managed appropriately to minimise unnecessary transfusions
- *process issues*: percentage of mislabelled samples received in the laboratory; patient wristband errors; numbers of units crossmatched to units transfused (C:T) ratio; hospital blood wastage; percentage of group O red cells used.

National Schemes

Many countries now have national schemes to monitor transfusion practice and promote practice improvement. These may be voluntary or mandatory, and institutions may be anonymous or identified. The programmes can be used to influence policy at national and local level, and to educate clinicians. Examples include the following.

- *Haemovigilance programmes*: the UK SHOT scheme is a voluntary system for collecting data on serious transfusion adverse events and near misses. It produces annual reports with recommendations. Many other regional and national examples exist, and experiences presented in these reports have been very valuable in identifying areas for improvement. A national haemovigilance programme in the United States with voluntary hospital participation was launched in 2010 as a joint effort between the AABB and the Centers for Disease Control (see Chapter 19).
- *EQA schemes*: these programmes periodically provide clinical material to be tested by transfusion laboratories. Results are returned for analysis and collated reports disseminated to participants.
- *Utilisation and wastage schemes*: such as the UK Blood Stocks Management and the Australian BloodNet schemes, which collate and publish details of blood stock inventory and wastage, and allow participants to benchmark against comparable hospitals.

Public and Political Perceptions and Fear of Litigation

Transfusion-transmitted human immunodeficiency virus (HIV) led to substantial reductions in allogeneic red cell use in many countries after 1982. These declines are even more significant considering population growth and ageing during this period. Over the same interval, autologous donations increased greatly. Some physicians were sued when transfused patients contracted HIV and the transfusions had not been clinically indicated.

The potential for transfusion-transmitted variant Creutzfeldt–Jakob disease (vCJD) was one of the concerns that led the UK Department of Health in 1998 to require that all hospitals should have HTCs, implement good transfusion practice and explore the feasibility of cell salvage. Universal leucocyte reduction of blood was introduced in the UK in 1999 as a further preventive measure for vCJD. This resulted in a significant increase in the price of blood, which was an additional encouragement for hospitals to implement more judicious approaches to transfusion and use of alternatives to transfusion. As a consequence, red cell use in the UK has decreased by over 25% over the last 15 years, despite an increase in the volume and complexity of clinical care over this period.

Recent international focus on patient-centred care and PBM (see Chapter 34), partly arising from risk and cost concerns as described above, has simultaneously driven active and collaborative activities, involving patients, clinicians (general practitioners and hospital staff), hospital management and government health authority engagement in active and collaborative processes to promote alternatives to transfusion, for example by better management of anaemia and minimising blood loss.

Local Investigation and Feedback Following 'Near Misses' and Serious Adverse Events

SHOT defines a 'near miss' as any error which, if undetected, could result in the determination of a wrong blood group, or the issue, collection or administration of an incorrect, inappropriate or unsuitable component but which was recognised before transfusion took place [1]. In Europe, 'serious adverse events' must also be reported to the competent authority. These events are defined as any untoward occurrences associated with the collection, testing, processing, storage and distribution of blood or blood components, that might lead to death or life-threatening, disabling or incapacitating conditions for patients, or which result in, or prolong, hospitalisation or morbidity. Systematic root cause analyses of these incidents provide opportunities to detect and understand system and process weaknesses and take corrective action to minimise recurrence. Typical weaknesses identified through root cause analyses include inadequate training; human factors such as fatigue, misconceptions and ignorance of relevant policies; environmental factors such as distractions or interruptions, time pressures or access to equipment and IT support; and defective or risky processes.

Sample errors, most importantly those where the tube is labelled with the intended patient's details but contains blood from another patient, 'wrong blood in tube' (WBIT) events, are some of the most common detectable errors reported to haemovigilance programmes. These inevitably

arise as a result of failures to systematically and positively identify the patient at the bedside [14]. However, investigations almost always uncover other contributing factors, which need to be understood and addressed.

- Failure to positively identify the patient. Healthcare workers have often not been trained in and are unfamiliar with hospital policies and procedures, or policies and procedures may be inconsistently implemented – for example, requiring inpatients but not outpatients to wear wristbands during treatment, including transfusion; some staff may also perceive this activity as unimportant or suggesting an inadequate knowledge of patients under their care.
- Reduced junior doctors' hours and shift patterns of those involved in direct patient management, and inadequate communication and documentation, leading to unfamiliarity with patients.
- Admission and discharge practices, which may lead to patients having samples taken for pretransfusion testing before case notes are available or wristbands applied, leading to the potential for misidentification.

Exposure to avoidable patient morbidity or fatality often triggers patient, clinical and management awareness of transfusion hazards and can instigate procedural changes. Corrective action should involve counselling and educating individuals who failed to comply with procedures, but focusing on addressing important, underlying system issues identified above, and supporting patients and staff in often traumatic situations [15].

Education and Continuing Professional Development

Education of all individuals in the transfusion process has traditionally been difficult, but UK experience shows it to be achievable when made an integral part of mandatory hospital training programmes and subject to external inspection. However, it requires considerable dedicated resources, a flexible and pragmatic approach to accommodate shift patterns and staff turnover and availability of staff, including temporary staff and those who work 'after hours'. Observational competency assessment is more readily achieved with the help of clinical 'champions'. Training and knowledge-based assessments can be facilitated by web-based programmes (such as the e-learning modules of the Australian BloodSafe programme, for which over 400,000 staff nationally and internationally have registered) which also permit management oversight of participation.

Education is an essential component of strategies to gain clinician compliance with procedures and guidelines and to modify practice. Educational interventions are more successful when they are interactive, focused on a specific objective and directed at groups of individuals with reflections on their own practice. Continuing professional development schemes for the various groups of staff involved in transfusion encourages knowledge acquisition with documentation (typically via participant portfolios) of accredited activity in educational, professional and vocational areas.

Centralisation of Transfusion Services

The medical and patient safety benefits of a centralised transfusion service (CTS) vary depending on its organisation [16]. The CTS in Pittsburgh, United States (city population 306 000; catchment population 2.1 million), operates as follows. The main blood supplier, the Central Blood Bank (CBB), delivers blood products to a central laboratory. This centrally located facility also houses the red cell reference laboratory and performs most of the automated, batched pretransfusion testing. The laboratory then distributes products to over 25 CTS-networked hospitals in a 'hub-and-spoke' manner. Each hospital has an on-site transfusion laboratory, and is staffed and stocked with products in accordance with the acuity of patients treated and volume of transfusions performed. Each

hospital laboratory performs routine pretransfusion testing and basic immunohaematology, thawing of plasma and cryoprecipitate and some platelet pooling and leucocyte reduction (most is performed centrally).

Perhaps the most important patient safety benefit of a CTS is the ability to access patient records between different hospital sites. Since patients can visit different hospitals within the network, recipient immunohaematology and component modification requirements are available electronically at each hospital's blood transfusion laboratory, reducing the need for reinvestigation and ensuring that any special component modifications are fulfilled for each patient whenever and wherever transfusion support is required. Having records of recipient historical ABO groups provides additional opportunities to detect WBIT errors. In 16 cases where recipient historical ABO groups on file at the Pittsburgh CTS did not match the ABO group of specimens submitted for pretransfusion testing, 6/16 were detected based on an historical ABO group that had been previously collected at a different hospital [17]. Requiring a second ABO group to be performed on a separate specimen before ABO-specific red cells are issued on recipients without an historical ABO group on file would achieve the same end, but requires considerable effort to implement. A recent study of two CTS systems in the United States demonstrated that some sickle cell disease patients with clinically significant antibodies were transfused at many different hospitals. Without the benefit of the CTS's recipient database, haemolytic reactions could have occurred as in many cases, these patients' antibody screens were negative at the time the transfusion was ordered [18].

Other advantages of a CTS include availability of transfusion medicine expertise for community hospitals without experts on staff. CTS transfusion physicians participate on HTCs of all networked hospitals, supporting rapid implementation of evidence-based practice and benchmarking. Consolidating technical expertise into one reference immunohaematology laboratory permits rapid and expert service provision. There are also numerous opportunities for cost savings, through greater efficiency from technical and nontechnical employees, economies of scale and use of automation. Blood supplier logistics are greatly simplified by delivery to one central location, and lower inventory levels can be supported due to the ability to circulate blood products between hospitals to reduce wastage.

Maximum Surgical Blood Ordering Schedule (MSBOS)

This is a table of elective surgical procedures that lists the extent of pretransfusion testing that is routinely required before the case begins (Table 23.9). The MSBOS is prepared taking into account the likelihood of transfusion and

Table 23.9 Example of Maximum Surgical Blood Order Schedule (MSBOS, general surgery).

Operation	Red cells crossmatched or group & screen (G&S)
Lumbar spine disc replacement	No pretransfusion testing required
Caesarean section	No pretransfusion testing required
Colonoscopy with polypectomy	No pretransfusion testing required
Tonsillectomy	No pretransfusion testing required
Spinal laminectomy and decompression	G&S
Carotid endarterectomy	G&S
Lung biopsy	G&S
Mammoplasty reduction	2
Splenectomy	2
Coronary artery bypass graft	
Total hip arthroplasty	2
Resection/repair ascending aortic aneurysm	4
Heart transplant	6
Liver transplant	10

the response time for having blood available, following an immediate spin crossmatch or electronic issue. An MSBOS reduces the workload of unnecessary crossmatching and issuing of blood, and can improve stock management and reduce wastage.

The successful implementation of an MSBOS depends on all parties agreeing to the schedule, education of blood prescribers, confidence of senior staff that there is a robust system for accessing blood promptly when there is unexpected blood loss and ability to override the schedule when there are reasons indicating that greater blood loss will occur. The schedule is constructed by:

- analysing each surgical procedure in terms of C:T ratio
- routinely managing procedures with a C:T ratio greater than 2 (i.e. a low probability of transfusion) with a group and screen, and issuing blood only when there is a need for transfusion
- allocating an agreed number of units for procedures with a C:T ratio of less than 2.

An overall C:T ratio of 1.5 for elective surgery is achievable when the laboratory is centrally issuing blood in accordance with the MSBOS. However, lower ratios are possible with use of electronic crossmatch and/or remote electronic issue from blood refrigerators in theatre suites.

In addition to reducing the number of allocated, crossmatched red cells for specific surgical patients, which increases the number of available units in general inventory, another benefit of adhering to recommendations of the MSBOS is that fewer patients with unexpected antibodies will be taken to surgery without appropriate transfusion support. As the MSBOS indicates the extent of pretransfusion testing that should be performed before surgery, adherence to its recommendations will lead to antibody screening being performed on patients with a reasonable chance of requiring intraoperative transfusion, thereby allowing the transfusion service to locate and crossmatch compatible units before the case begins, should unexpected antibodies be detected.

In recipients with red cell alloantibodies who require transfusion, consideration should be given to the time taken to acquire and cross-match antigen-negative units, and the treating clinical team should be informed.

Acknowledgement

This chapter updates the material in the previous editions based on contributions by Sue Knowles and Geoff Poole.

KEY POINTS

1) The transfusion process is unique as it links blood donors with patients in an altruistic, potentially life-saving activity. For many patients, there is still no substitute for donated blood components.
2) Prescribers of blood components have a duty of care to their patients to ensure that the benefits of the transfusion outweigh the risks, and a moral obligation to donors to ensure that their donations are used appropriately.
3) The transfusion process is multistep and complex, involving patients and many different staff across the broad spectrum of clinical practice and settings, often working under challenging conditions. In this context there are many opportunities for human error to occur.
4) Investments in quality infrastructure, computerisation and automation and training in the clinical and laboratory aspects of transfusion practice are essential to minimise or, ultimately, prevent errors in the transfusion process.

References

1 PHB Bolton-Maggs (Ed) D Poles et al. on behalf of the Serious Hazards of Transfusion (SHOT) Steering Group. The 2015 Annual SHOT Report (2016). http://www.shotuk.org/wp-content/uploads/SHOT-2015-Annual-Report-Web-Edition-Final-bookmarked-1.pdf (accessed 9 January 2017).

2 US Food and Drug Administration. Fatalities reported to FDA following blood collection and transfusion. Annual summary for Fiscal year 2015. Available at: http://www.fda.gov/downloads/BiologicsBloodVaccines/SafetyAvailability/ReportaProblem/TransfusionDonationFatalities/UCM518148.pdf (accessed 9 January 2017).

3 Narick C, Triulzi D, Yazer MH. Transfusion-associated circulatory overload after plasma transfusion. Transfusion 2012;**52**(1):160–5.

4 Linden JV, Wagner K, Voytovich AE, Sheehan J. Transfusion errors in New York State: an analysis of 10 years' experience. Transfusion 2000;**40**:1207–13.

5 Goodnough LT, Viele M, Fontaine MJ et al. Implementation of a two-specimen requirement for verification of ABO/Rh for blood transfusion. Transfusion 2009;**49**:1321–8.

6 Murphy MF, Stanworth SJ, Yazer M. Transfusion practice and safety: current status and possibilities for improvement. Vox Sang 2011;**100**:46–59.

7 UK Blood Safety and Quality Regulations. Available at: www.transfusionguidelines.org.uk (accessed 1 November 2016).

8 Australian Commission on Safety and Quality in Health Care. National Safety and Quality Health Service Standards. Sydney: Australian Commission on Safety and Quality in Health Care, 2011.

9 Miller K, Akers C, Davis AK et al. The evolving role of the transfusion practitioner. Transfus Med Rev 2015;**29**(2):138–44.

10 Davis RE, Vincent CA, Murphy MF. Blood transfusion safety: the potential role of the patient. Transfus Med Rev 2011;**25**(1):12–23.

11 Turner CL, Casbard AC, Murphy MF. Barcode technology: its role in increasing the safety of blood transfusion. Transfusion 2003;**43**:1200–9.

12 Staves J, Davies A, Kay J et al. Electronic remote blood issue: a combination of remote blood issue with a system for end-to-end electronic control of transfusion to provide a "total solution" for a safe and timely hospital blood transfusion service. Transfusion 2008;**48**:415–24.

13 Tavares M, DiQuattro P, Nolette N et al. Reduction in plasma transfusion after enforcement of transfusion guidelines. Transfusion 2011;**51**: 754–61.

14 Bolton-Maggs PH, Wood EM, Wiersum-Osselton JC. Wrong blood in tube – potential for serious outcomes: can it be prevented? Br J Haematol 2015;**168**(1):3–13.

15 Stainsby D, Russell J, Cohen H, Lilleyman J. Reducing adverse events in blood transfusion. Br J Haematol 2005;**131**(1):8–12.

16 Simpson M. Strategies for Centralized Blood Services. Bethesda: AABB Press, 2006.

17 MacIvor D, Triulzi DJ, Yazer MH. Enhanced detection of blood transfusion laboratory sample collection errors with a centralized patient database. Transfusion 2009; **49**:40–3.

18 Harm SK, Yazer MH, Monis GH et al. A centralized recipient database enhances the serologic safety of RBC transfusions for patients with sickle cell disease. Am J Clin Pathol 2015;**141**:256–61.

Further Reading

Department of Health. Better Blood Transfusion. HSC 2007/001. London: HMSO, 2007.

Dzik WH, Corwin H, Goodnough LT et al. Patient safety and blood transfusion: new solutions. Transfus Med Rev 2003;**17**:169–80.

Eisenstaedt RS. Modifying physicians' transfusion practice. Transfus Med Rev 1997;**11**:27–37.

Klein HG, Anstee D (eds). Mollison's Blood Transfusion in Clinical Medicine, 12th edn. Oxford: Wiley-Blackwell Publishing, 2014.

Norfolk D (ed.). Handbook of Transfusion Medicine, 5th edn. Norwich: Stationery Office, 2014. Available at: www.transfusionguidelines. org (accessed 1 November 2016).

Saxena S (ed.). The Transfusion Committee: Putting Patient Safety First, 2nd edn. Bethesda: AABB Press, 2013.

Guidelines and Other Resources

For a range of guidelines and other resources on laboratory and clinical hospital transfusion practice: AABB: www.aabb.org/resources

Australian and New Zealand Society of Blood Transfusion: www.anzsbt.org.au

British Committee for Standards in Haematology: www.bcshguidelines.com

Canadian resources: www.transfusion.ca, www. transfusionontario.org, and www. transfusionmedicine.ca

International Society of Blood Transfusion: www.isbtweb.org

Joint Commission on Accreditation of Healthcare Organizations: www. jointcommission.org

Network for Advancement of Transfusion Alternatives: www.nataonline.com

World Health Organization: www.who.int/ bloodsafety

24 Blood Transfusion in a Global Context

David J. Roberts[1], Alan D. Kitchen[2], Stephen P. Field[3], Imelda Bates[4], Jean Pierre Allain[5] and Meghan Delaney[6]

[1] *University of Oxford and NHS Blood and Transplant and Department of Haematology, John Radcliffe Hospital, Oxford, UK*
[2] *National Transfusion Microbiology Laboratory and NHS Blood and Transplant, Colindale, London, UK*
[3] *Welsh Blood Service, Pontyclun, Wales, UK*
[4] *Liverpool School of Tropical Medicine, Liverpool, UK*
[5] *NHS Blood and Transplant and Division of Transfusion Medicine, Department of Haematology, University of Cambridge, Cambridge, UK*
[6] *Bloodworks Northwest and Department of Laboratory Medicine and Paediatrics, University of Washington, Seattle, USA*

Introduction

Approximately half of all blood donations are collected in high-income countries, home to 15% of the world's population.
(WHO Global Blood Safety Report).

Inequality in the provision of 'safe blood' around the world mirrors the unequal distribution of almost all other resources crucial for effective health services. Unfortunately, in many countries, providing safe blood is made more difficult by lack of blood donors and their high frequency of transfusion-transmissible infection. At the same time, the problems are compounded by the frequent need for urgent life-saving transfusions, such as following childbirth, in children with malaria, trauma, cancer care and other chronic medical conditions.

The purpose of this chapter is to inform a wider audience of the problems faced in the development of transfusion services in low- or medium-resource countries, predominantly focusing on sub-Saharan Africa.

Safety and Supply

A safe supply of blood is an essential part of medical services. An unsafe blood supply is costly in both human and economic terms. Transfusion of infected blood not only causes direct morbidity and mortality, but also undermines confidence in modern healthcare. Those who become infected through blood transfusion may also contribute to a secondary wave of infections. Investment in safe supplies of blood is cost-effective for every country, even those with few resources. At the same time, an insufficient supply costs lives because severely anaemic patients do not survive unless transfused [1,2]. Where should the priority be? The shockwave of the HIV epidemics put overwhelming emphasis on blood safety, but now the supply of blood should resume its legitimate place as a priority. An adequate and sustainable blood supply would go a long way to reducing mortality in developing countries, especially among women and children.

The World Health Organization (WHO) has identified four key objectives for blood services to ensure that blood is safe for transfusion.

Practical Transfusion Medicine, Fifth Edition. Edited by Michael F. Murphy, David J. Roberts and Mark H. Yazer.
© 2017 John Wiley & Sons Ltd. Published 2017 by John Wiley & Sons Ltd.

- Establish a coordinated national blood transfusion service that can provide adequate and timely supplies of safe blood for all patients in need.
- Collect blood only from voluntary non-remunerated blood donors from low-risk populations and use stringent donor selection procedures.
- Screen all blood for transfusion-transmissible infections and have standardised procedures in place for grouping and compatibility testing.
- Reduce unnecessary transfusions through the appropriate clinical use of blood, including the use of intravenous replacement fluids and other simple alternatives to transfusion, wherever possible.

The WHO also emphasises that effective quality assurance should be in place for all aspects of the transfusion process, from donor recruitment and selection, through to infection screening, blood grouping and blood storage, to administration to patients and clinical monitoring for adverse events.

Testing Blood Products

Local blood transfusion services encounter many problems, including lack of funding, insufficient training, poor management, frequent failure in supply of reagents and consumables and breakdown of the cold chain (mostly related to frequent power cuts). Since 2000, a lot of investment has gone into providing HIV, HBsAg and to some extent HCV tests in Africa. In particular, there have been enormous efforts to ensure that blood collected in Africa is tested for HIV. The residual risk of HBV infection remains substantial because of donations containing undetected low levels of HBsAg or occult HBV DNA. Estimates of the residual risk of HIV transmission in the pre-seroconversion window period are 1:2600–6000, hepatitis C 1:400–1500 and hepatitis B 1:300–500, when using enzyme immunoassay (EIA) screening [3,4].

In India, a large proportion of blood donors have historically been commercial or replacement donors. A survey of blood collection services across India showed that 87% of the donor units were screened for HBV, 95% for HIV, 94% for syphilis, 67% for malaria and 6% for HCV. Only 13% of blood banks used ELISA kits for HBsAg. Notification of the occurrence of transfusion-associated hepatitis was provided less than 40% of the time.

Test sensitivity is critical in the face of high prevalence rates for HIV, HBV and HCV (Box 24.1) [5–7]. Nucleic acid testing (NAT) is highly effective and has been introduced in South Africa and a few centres elsewhere [8]. However, widespread use of NAT is out of reach for most countries; cheaper, simpler methods to perform NAT testing would be useful.

Blood Donors

Recruiting voluntary donors from the community is complex and expensive and depends on regular education programmes, collection teams, vehicles and cold storage. It is proving very difficult to expand the number of volunteer donors in poorer counties [14]. Some potential donors are fearful of HIV testing. There are also cultural beliefs surrounding blood donation that inhibit donors coming forward. Some of these appear to be misinformation about donating blood (e.g. 'men will become impotent if they donate blood'; 'HIV can be caught from the blood bag needle'). There are, however, other cultural beliefs related to understanding the value of blood to the individual and to society, for example blood is related to kinship or personal health. Understanding local beliefs surrounding blood and blood donation is likely to be important in developing effective services. It is worth noting that similar problems were a barrier to widespread acceptance of blood donation in London over 70 years ago.

As volunteer donors are in short supply, family members are frequently used to provide blood for their relatives in hospital. In 2002, in

---

Box 24.1 Epidemiology of blood-borne infections in sub-Saharan Africa.

HIV

The overall prevalence of HIV antibody in sub-Saharan Africa ranges between 0.5% and 16%. In donors, it tends to be below 5% in West Africa, below 10% in East and Central Africa and above 10% in southern Africa [5–7,9].

Hepatitis B

Chronic hepatitis B prevalence, indicated by the presence of circulating HBsAg, ranges between 5% and 25% of the population including blood donors. This high prevalence is due to (vertical) transmission at birth or (horizontal) infection in infancy and the virtual absence of national vaccination programmes. Infection after the age of 10 is uncommon. HBsAg is more prevalent in West Africa (10–25%) than in East or Central Africa (5–10%); the lowest prevalence is found in southern Africa (5% or less).

Hepatitis C

Antibody to HCV is not routinely screened for in many parts of Africa, but the prevalence of this infection ranges between 0.5% and 3% and reaches 10–15% in Egypt. The prevalence may be high locally, suggesting the importance of

specific factors such as various types of injections and past diagnostic or vaccination campaigns contributing to spread the infection.

Other infections

Most countries in sub-Saharan Africa do not screen for HTLV since the prevalence is low (<2%). Although the risk of acquiring syphilis from infected blood is low, most blood banks in sub-Saharan Africa do screen for *Treponema pallidum*. Fresh blood is potentially infectious for syphilis, but storage at 4 °C can inactivate the bacterium.

Malaria can be transmitted by transfusion. In areas of low or no malaria transmission, screening for the parasite is important, as recipients are likely to have no immunity. In countries where malaria is highly endemic, the prevalence of *Plasmodium* in donor blood is often very high (16–55%) [10]; excluding donors with low-grade parasitaemia is often impracticable and preemptive treatment of patients receiving transfusion with antimalarial drugs is common practice [11].

Bacterial contamination of blood components is under-recognised and may reach 10% of products at the time of issue [12,13].

Africa as a whole, the WHO estimated that over 60% of blood originated from replacement/family donors. In sub-Saharan Africa, the proportion of blood derived from replacement donors is certainly higher. Most viral infections such as HIV, HBV and HCV have similar prevalence in age-matched replacement and volunteer donors. The ultimate aim should be to maximise conversion of voluntary and replacement donors into regular donors since those who are successful repeat donors have the best safety profile.

Use of Blood Products

In contrast to Europe, most transfusions in sub-Saharan Africa are given for life-threatening emergencies. Transfusions are administered to children predominantly for malaria-related anaemia. Many clinical guidelines, albeit based on consensus opinion rather than well-defined evidence, suggest transfusions for children are indicated if Hb <40 or 50 g/L with symptoms of decompensation [1,15]. Pregnant women are the second most common recipients of blood, particularly for haemorrhagic emergencies.

Significant quantities of blood are also used in trauma, often related to motor vehicle accidents, surgery and general medicine. There are neither systematic reviews nor international guidelines covering the use of blood and blood products in these specific contexts, and few audits of blood use. The scope for improving clinical practice and reducing unnecessary transfusion is probably substantial.

The problems surrounding the rapid supply of safe blood have led to the use of autologous blood transfusion in some settings for elective procedures. There are logistical and training problems to be overcome; however, this appears to be a potential route to decrease the barrier of elective transfusion in certain settings. However, small programmes have been established for autologous transfusion of elective surgery patients at district hospitals.

As low- and middle-income countries (LMICs) improve their public and primary healthcare, chronic medical illnesses, such as cardiac disease, diabetes and cancer, become more of a priority for healthcare services. To be able to provide therapies for these disorders, especially for cancer, transfusions are needed to support patients through bone marrow suppression. Unfortunately, in some instances, the unreliability of blood supply to support elective blood transfusion may force treating physicians to choose less rigorous chemotherapeutic regimens, which can affect long-term outcomes. Initiatives to improve cancer care and cardiac surgery in LMICs must also include attention to blood supply and safety to support patients through intensive treatments.

Systems

Taken together, the low availability of blood donors, cold chain and pathogen testing leads to low stocks of blood and blood products, which ultimately affects patient care and outcomes. Patients in poorer countries usually present late in the course of their disease, and the need for urgent transfusion coupled with shortages of blood mean that patients may die before a blood transfusion can be organised. In situations where blood must be donated by relatives before a patient can be transfused, by the time a donor has been found, screened and venesected, and the blood is transfused into the patient, several hours or even days can elapse. The process can be speeded up if relatives are asked to donate after the patient has been transfused with blood from the hospital's stocks. In this way, a combination of voluntary donations to maintain some emergency stocks with post-transfusion donations from patients' relatives may provide a practical solution to blood shortages. Even in tertiary centres, many patients with anaemia die within a few hours of admission before they can be transfused.

Focus on Sub-Saharan Africa

It is axiomatic that transfusion medicine should be incorporated into national health plans. The WHO has provided a recommended structure of national blood transfusion services. It suggests that at the national level, the transfusion service should have a medical director, an advisory committee and clear national transfusion policies and strategies with the appropriate statutory instruments to ensure the national coordination and standardisation of blood testing, processing and distribution (see Further Reading). Notwithstanding these recommendations, transfusion activities must be integrated with other services at local and national levels.

There has been some progress to realise the WHO's recommendations for a national blood programme. In Africa in 2002, the WHO estimated that among the 46 member states in the African continent, only 14 had a national blood policy and just six had a policy to specifically encourage and develop a system of voluntary non-remunerated donation. In the most recent survey in 2007, 40 out of 41 of African states surveyed had a national blood policy, but only 56% (23 out of 41) countries were able to implement their policies.

It is worth reflecting on why the development of national transfusion services has not been achieved. A key reason is that it is expensive and logistically complex. Management skills to run such services are insufficient and the cost of blood transfusion is high in relation to disposable income and healthcare budgets.

When a transfusion service is provided by individual hospitals, it places an enormous burden on laboratory resources. One survey showed that in a typical district hospital in southern Africa, the overall cost of the transfusion service, including consumables, proportional amounts for capital equipment, staff time and overheads, was 36% of total laboratory costs. In hospital-based systems that depend on replacement donations, it is the patient's family that bear the cost of donor recruitment.

The cost of a national service is even greater because of the additional costs of quality assurance, local education programmes, dedicated collection team(s), vehicles and cold storage. In addition, a national service has to solve the very real practical problems of maintaining regular distributions of blood to remote facilities. A unit of blood in a centralised service costs around four times as much as one from a hospital-based system that uses family replacement donors; this does not include capital costs. Blood is therefore an expensive commodity in relation to the annual per capita budget for healthcare in these countries and it remains to be seen if blood from centralised systems, which in poorer countries are predominantly externally funded, can be sustained without external support. Precise cost–benefit analyses for the use of blood have not been carried out.

A perennial problem in healthcare systems is the availability of skilled technical staff; this may be compounded by internal migration of technical staff from hospitals to national or regional centres. There is a severe lack of training and career advancement opportunities for technical and clinical blood service staff. Training programmes to increase capacity for the processing, testing and issue of blood are therefore an integral part of service development.

Improvements

Putting the WHO Objectives into Practice in Sub-Saharan Africa

Some countries have used external funds to establish an integrated national service, but few have been able to make the transition to a sustainable, national transfusion service in the absence of external funding and even fewer have been able to reach an adequate blood supply. However, some recent success has been achieved in developing a transfusion service in several centres in Nigeria (Box 24.2). The alternative is that transfusion services have to be optimised within the existing general hospital budget. Whatever sums are available, the problems surrounding the supply, safety, cost and use of blood must be addressed. There has to be a balance between providing an ideal, integrated national service and the more pragmatic solutions afforded by local services.

Improving the Blood Supply

Careful donor selection is crucial not only to improve the supply of blood but also to reduce transfusion-transmitted infection risk. The selection of volunteer donors from lower risk populations is considered the most effective approach and considerable effort has been devoted to promoting voluntary, repeat donations. In practice, these are often secondary school students with median age ranging between 16 and 20 years. They are younger and have a greater proportion of females than replacement donors but there are some concerns that although these younger donors have a lower prevalence of transfusion-transmitted infections than older donors, they may have a higher incidence of new infections. Experience has shown that while recruiting volunteer donors in schools can be relatively inexpensive, making them into repeat donors is difficult and expensive. Encouraging both volunteer non-remunerated and family replacement donors to donate blood repeatedly is the challenge for sub-Saharan African blood services in order to provide safer blood [16,17].

Box 24.2 Towards development of a national transfusion service in Nigeria.

In 2004, Nigeria, the most populous country in Africa, had a highly fragmented hospital-based transfusion system. There was little coordination from central government and most of the blood came from replacement and paid donors. Testing for transmissible disease markers was inconsistent and poorly controlled. The current practice of family replacement donors in a hospital-based blood service is the most economical option, but in the face of high child and maternal mortality rates, the blood supply has proved to be insufficient. There was therefore a need to change practice.

The Safe Blood for Africa Foundation, with a grant from USAID and later PEPFAR, established a demonstration blood service in the capital Abuja. This service collected its blood from voluntary unremunerated donors in the local community. The blood was tested for HIV, hepatitis B and C and syphilis and distributed to the local hospitals. A simple but effective quality management system was established with standard operating procedures written and followed. The objective of this project was to be the model for other centres throughout the country. The Federal Ministry

of Health has established six zonal transfusion centres under the umbrella of the national blood transfusion service. In addition, 10 states have opened transfusion centres and there is one that serves the needs of the military forces.

The Federal Minister of Health also established an expert committee which drafted a national blood policy and national guidelines for standards of transfusion practice in Nigeria. The Safe Blood for Africa Foundation has to date provided technical assistance for the establishment of these centres and provided training to the staff in all elements of transfusion.

The major problem was recruiting blood donors. The youth were encouraged to donate with the establishment of a Club 25 programme. There was active promotion through the media and the initiative was highlighted by a televised donation by the President on the occasion of the official opening of the Abuja centre. One problem encountered was the high number of donors presenting with haemoglobin levels below the required standard of 125 g/L. This is probably a reflection of the poor health status within the community.

Several strategies have been devised to encourage repeat donors and thus reduce the risk of virus carriage. In Zimbabwe, Pledge 25 Club, a programme using education and incentives to attract school students to give blood 25 times, has been successful. Similar, less ambitious schemes, for example a 'Club 5', could also be effective. The WHO slogan of 'Safe blood starts with me' has also resulted in educational programmes around the world. These schemes can be complemented by strategies to recruit donors from faith-based organisations or collaborating with radio stations to organise and promote blood donations. Specific strategies intending to encourage family replacement donors to become repeat donors are being developed.

The best use of fluid replacement, pressure devices and pharmaceuticals, such as tranexamic acid for severe haemorrhage, is

under study. Several studies have shown the use of placental blood to prevent neonatal anaemia, particularly in malarious areas. The high haematocrit from the placental blood and easy availability may make it suitable for small-volume emergency transfusions. However, the logistics and infrastructure needed to collect placental blood free of bacterial contamination, to obtain consent from women in labour, and test and distribute these small volumes of blood should not be underestimated.

Improving Screening for Blood-Transmitted Infections

New approaches to blood donor testing for transfusion-transmitted diseases have been adapted to local situations and appear promising. In small blood banks, the expensive microtitre plate systems used post-donation can be replaced by cheaper, more cost-effective, high-performance rapid tests performed pre- or post-donation. Pre-donation testing provides the advantages of reducing material waste with on-site communication with deferred donors who could not otherwise be reached [18]. Some new technology is on the horizon. Rapid immuno-chemical and nucleic acid dipsticks are being developed for blood-borne pathogens and may cut the cost of pre- and post-donation testing to a tenth of present costs. The WHO has established systematic evaluations of both ELISA and rapid tests to guide developing countries in their choice of tests. These evaluations include test costs. Many rapid tests for anti-HIV and HBsAg and fewer for anti-HCV are available, but sensitivity and specificity, ease of use and cost vary greatly. Some of these tests are performed in one single step with results obtained in 10–20 minutes using whole blood, plasma or serum samples. The best assays have sensitivity similar to ELISA for anti-HIV, detect 0.2 ng/mL of HBsAg and have >99% sensitivity for anti-HCV and >99% specificity.

Blood safety has often focused on the risk of viral infection in donors but bacterial contamination of units is also a substantial problem. Two studies have highlighted the considerable risk of bacterial infection in nearly 10% of whole blood units [12,13]. Contamination appears to be of environmental rather than of donor origin and reducing these hazards will be an important challenge in the future.

Meeting the Financial Requirements of Transfusion Services

The challenge for poorer countries is that enough safe blood should be available for health services and individuals even when resources are extremely limited. The high cost of providing blood makes it impossible to recoup the cost of blood by user fees alone and blood services will require internal or external public funding for the foreseeable future [19]. Developing systems that rely more on local resources means

that in the long term they may be more flexible, productive and sustainable.

Improving the Clinical Use of Blood: Guidelines for Transfusion Practice

The use of guidelines can reduce unnecessary transfusions and many institutions in sub-Saharan Africa and Asia have developed guidelines to promote rational use of blood transfusions and blood components (see Further Reading). The scope for improvement in clinical practice is great. For example, strict enforcement of a transfusion protocol in a Malawian hospital reduced the number of transfusions by 75% without any adverse effect on mortality.

The principles underlying most transfusion guidelines are similar and combine a clinical assessment of whether the patient is developing complications of inadequate oxygenation, with measurement of their haemoglobin (as a marker of intracellular oxygen concentration). In the United States, anaesthetists suggest that transfusions are almost always indicated when the haemoglobin concentration is less than 60 g/L, whereas in many Sub-Saharan African countries transfusions are recommended for children at haemoglobin concentrations less than 40 g/L, provided there are no other clinical complications. Moreover, the lack of fractionated blood products and the reliance on whole blood should be considered in context. Using whole blood for many of the common emergency indications for transfusion in Africa may be advantageous, as it supplies critical coagulation factors for patients facing haemostatic challenge, such as in the setting of post-partum haemorrhage and following significant trauma.

Ensuring that the transfusion guidelines are implemented is extremely difficult without formal monitoring and auditing systems. This is particularly problematic if the quality of haemoglobin measurements is not assured as clinicians may rely entirely on clinical judgement to guide transfusion practice, with inevitably a high proportion of inappropriate transfusions. As the cost of providing a unit of blood is approximately 40 times the cost of a quality-assured haemoglobin test, investment in improving haemoglobin testing is likely to not only improve practice but also reduce the cost.

The Ebola Pandemic in West Africa

The outbreak of Ebola virus in three West African countries killed many thousands of people. At the time of the outbreak, there was no proven therapy for the disease; however, 40–65% patients made a full recovery. Those who survived have a developed immunity and it has been hypothesised that antibody-containing plasma recovered from these individuals could be used as a passive therapy for Ebola-infected patents. The epidemic has highlighted the needed for well-organised hospital services and it may be that blood centres could play a significant role in providing treatment if it is proven that plasma harvested from convalescent patients is efficacious in treatment of acutely ill patients.

Conclusion: The Future of Blood Transfusion in a Global Context

Fulfilling the first WHO objective of establishing 'a coordinated national blood transfusion service that can provide adequate and timely supplies of safe blood for all patients in need' has proved to be very difficult in many countries, even given substantial external funding. Nevertheless, some countries have made progress and have recently established national transfusion services. On the other hand, progress has been made by developing local services and there has to be a balance between providing an ideal integrated national service and the more pragmatic solutions afforded by local services. There remains considerable scope to optimise fluid management and other ancillary treatments, and to reduce unnecessary transfusions through the appropriate clinical use of blood and products.

Increased blood supply depends on the recruitment of all types of non-remunerated donors, whether volunteer non-remunerated donors or family replacement donors, and the development of innovative strategies to encourage both groups of donors to give blood regularly.

Resources must be made available by governments to ensure that the essential supplies are available, such as blood bags, grouping reagents and test kits, and laboratory and blood bank management systems also need to be improved to ensure effective testing and processing and the maintenance of the cold chain. Hospitals and other health facilities could cooperate to directly purchase cheap, high-quality tests adapted to their needs. Significant efforts need to be made to ensure that blood services in poorer countries are underpinned by feasible and sustainable internal financing mechanisms so they can operate independently of external donors.

There is currently a feeling of guarded optimism about the future of blood supply and safety in developing countries. The recent increase in allocation of resources for the prevention of HIV across the world, including the investment by governments of wealthy countries and contributions from international and private agencies, has begun to indicate the importance of reducing HIV transmission through blood but runs the risk of neglecting other basic laboratory services, such as blood grouping and haemoglobin measurements. Parallel to the price reduction for antiviral drugs, the cost of screening tests supplied to developing countries has also decreased. The high cost of anti-HCV testing should now be reduced as the patent has expired in Europe. More effective and efficient methods for testing blood are to be welcomed and pathogen reduction methods applicable to whole blood would be an enormous relief, if affordable. The real challenge will be to integrate improvements in the supply and safety of blood in sustainable, coordinated national transfusion services.

KEY POINTS

1) In the last five years, nearly all African states have created a national blood policy, but only just over half have been able to implement their policies.

2) The main obstacles to implementation are a lack of trained staff, the high cost of blood in relation to the healthcare budgets and recruitment of donors.

3) In the absence of centralised services, facilities rely on blood collected by hospitals from family or replacement donors.

4) The high rate of chronic viral infections in the populations implies that the residual risk of infection of HIV and hepatitis B infection remains substantial with ELISA testing.

5) Several initiatives are being trialled to improve the supply and/or safety of blood by encouraging repeat voluntary donors, reviewing donor testing strategies, developing systems that rely more on local resources, using umbilical cord blood, researching methods for low-cost NAT testing and improving clinical practice through guidelines and audits of the use of blood.

References

1 Lackritz EM, Campbell CC, Ruebush 2nd TK et al. Effect of blood transfusion on survival among children in a Kenyan hospital. Lancet 1992;**340**:524–8.

2 Bates I, Chapotera GK, McKew S, van den Broek N. Maternal mortality in sub-Saharan Africa: the contribution of ineffective blood transfusion services. Br J Obstet Gynaecol 2008;**115**:1331–9.

3 Chaudhuri V, Nanu A, Panda SK, Chand P. Evaluation of serologic screening of blood donors in India reveals a lack of correlation between anti-HBc titer and PCR-amplified HBV DNA. Transfusion 2003;**43**:1442–8.

4 Basavaraju SV, Mwangi J, Nyamongo J et al. Reduced risk of transfusion-transmitted HIV in Kenya through centrally co-ordinated blood centres, stringent donor selection and effective p24 antigen-HIV antibody screening. Vox Sang 2010;**99**:212–19.

5 Tagny CT, Diarra A, Yahaya R. Characteristics of blood donors and donated blood in sub-Saharan Franco-phone Africa. Transfusion 2009;**49**:1592–9.

6 World Health Organization. Status of Blood Safety in the WHO African Region: Report of the 2004 Survey WHO Regional Office for Africa. World Health Organization, Brazzaville, 2007, pp.1–25.

7 Tagny CT, Owusu-Ofori S, Mbanya D, Deneys V. The blood donor in sub-Saharan Africa: a review. Transfus Med 2010;**20**:1–10.

8 Vermeulen M, Lelie N, Sykes W et al. Impact of individual donation nucleic acid testing on risk of human immunodeficiency virus, hepatitis B virus and hepatitis C virus transmission in South Africa. Transfusion 2009;**49**:1115–25.

9 Cunha L, Plouzeau C, Ingrand P et al. Use of replacement blood donors to study the epidemiology of major blood-borne viruses in the general population of Maputo, Mozambique. J Med Virol 2007;**79**: 1832–40.

10 Owusu-Ofori AK, Parry C, Bates I. Transfusion-transmitted malaria in countries where malaria is endemic: a review of the literature from sub-Saharan Africa. Clin Infect Dis 2010;**51**:1192–8.

11 Rajab JA, Waithaka PM, Orinda DA, Scott CS. Analysis of cost and effectiveness of pre-transfusion screening of donor blood and anti-malarial prophylaxis for recipients. East Afr Med J 2005;**82**:565–71.

12 Adjei AA, Kuma GK, Tettey Y et al. Bacterial contamination of blood and blood components in three major blood transfusion centers, Accra, Ghana. Jpn J Infect Dis 2009;**62**:265–9.

13 Hassall O, Maitland K, Pole L et al. Bacterial contamination of pediatric whole blood transfusions in a Kenyan hospital. Transfusion 2009;**49**:2594–8.

14 Bates I, Manyasi G, Medina Lara A. Reducing replacement donors in sub-Saharan Africa: challenges and affordability. Transfus Med 2007;**17**(6):434–42.

15 Akech SO, Hassall O, Pamba A et al. Survival and haematological recovery of children with severe malaria transfused in accordance to WHO guidelines in Kilifi, Kenya. Malar J 2008;**7**:256.

16 Allain JP. Moving on from voluntary non-remunerated donors: who is the best donor? Br J Haematol 2011;**154**:763–9.

17 Allain JP, Sarkodie F, Boateng P, Asenso K, Kyeremateng E, Owusu-Ofori S. A pool of repeat blood donors can be generated with little expense to the blood center in sub-Saharan Africa. Transfusion 2008;**48**:735–41.

18 Owusu-Ofori S, Temple J, Sarkodie F et al. Pre-donation screening of blood donors with rapid tests: implementation and efficacy of a novel approach to blood safety in resource-poor settings. Transfusion 2005;**45**:133–40.

19 Hensher M, Jefferys E. Financing blood transfusion services in sub-Saharan Africa: a role for user fees? Health Policy Plan 2000;**15**:287–95.

Further Reading

African Society of Blood Transfusion. Available at: www.afsbt.org/(accessed 14 November 2016).

Bates I, Mundy C, Pendame R et al. Use of clinical judgement to guide administration of blood transfusions in Malawi. Trans R Soc Trop Med Hyg 2001;**95**:510–12.

Choudhury N. Blood transfusion in borderless South Asia. Asian J Transfus Sci 2011;**5**:117–20.

English M, Ahmed M, Ngando C, Berkley J, Ross A. Blood transfusion for severe anaemia in children in a Kenyan hospital. Lancet 2002;**359**:494–5.

Fairhead J, Leach M, Small M. Where techno-science meets poverty: medical research and the economy of blood in The Gambia, West Africa. Soc Sci Med 2006;**65**:1109–20.

Hassall O, Ngina L, Kongo W et al. The acceptability to women in Mombasa, Kenya, of the donation and transfusion of umbilical cord blood for severe anaemia in young children. Vox Sang 2007;**94**(2):125–31.

Kapoor D, Saxena R, Sood B, Sarin SK. Blood transfusion practices in India: results of a national survey. Indian J Gastroenterol 2000;**19**:64–7.

World Health Organization. Universal Access to Safe Blood Transfusion. Available at: www.who.int/bloodsafety/universalbts/en/(accessed 14 November 2016).

World Health Organization. Developing a National Blood System. Available at: www.who.int/bloodsafety/publications/am_developing_a_national_blood_system.pdf (accessed 14 November 2016).

25 Inherited and Acquired Coagulation Disorders

Irina Chibisov[1,2] *and Franklin Bontempo*[1,2]

[1] *University of Pittsburgh Medical Center, Pittsburgh, USA*
[2] *Institute for Transfusion Medicine, Pittsburgh, USA*

Normal Haemostasis

Haemostasis is a series of complex events involving the interaction of blood vessel wall, platelets, coagulation factors, coagulation factor inhibitors and fibrinolytic enzymes which maintain the integrity of the circulatory system. In a normal individual there is a balance between procoagulant and anticoagulant activities and any disruption may lead to bleeding or clotting disorders.

The generation of thrombin is the key to successful haemostasis. Historically, a 'cascade' model developed in the mid-1960s described the intrinsic and extrinsic pathways where inactive clotting factors present in blood were converted step by step to active enzymes which ultimately led to generation of thrombin, which in turn converted fibrinogen to fibrin (Figure 25.1). Although this model explained laboratory coagulation assays, it was inadequate to explain many clinical problems.

The 'cell-based model' better explains *in vivo* coagulation process. In this model of haemostasis, coagulation takes place in three overlapping phases: *initiation*, *amplification* and *propagation* (Figure 25.2).

Initiation of coagulation occurs on damaged tissue factor (TF)-bearing cells which leads to the generation of activated factor VII (FVIIa) and formation of TF–VIIa complex which activates factors IX (FIXa) and X (FXa) and trace amounts of thrombin are generated. Concurrent with this, platelets adhere to the subendothelial matrix and are activated, providing a phospholipid surface for coagulation factor activity. Von Willebrand factor (VWF) is bound to and released from endothelial cells, leading to further platelet recruitment and activation.

During *amplification and propagation*, the small amounts of thrombin generated activate factors V, VIII and XI. This allows formation of the 'tenase' complex (FIXa/FVIIIa) to generate further FXa and the 'prothrombinase' complex (FXa/FVa), which leads to generation of large amounts of thrombin and, ultimately, by activation of fibrin and FXIII, production of a cross-linked stable clot [1,2].

To prevent excessive, inadequate thrombosis, there are inbuilt mechanisms to control the procoagulant response. These include tissue factor pathway inhibitor (TFPI), which inactivates the TF–FVIIa complex; antithrombin, which complexes with and inactivates FIXa, FXa, FXIa and thrombin; the protein C and S pathways, which inactivate FVa and FVIIIa; and thrombomodulin, which binds to thrombin and promotes activation of protein C which cleaves factors Va and VIIIa. Fibrinolysis is also part of the normal haemostatic response. Fibrinolysis is largely carried out by plasmin which breaks down cross-linked fibrin to form D-dimers and other fibrin degradation products (FDP).

Practical Transfusion Medicine, Fifth Edition. Edited by Michael F. Murphy, David J. Roberts and Mark H. Yazer.
© 2017 John Wiley & Sons Ltd. Published 2017 by John Wiley & Sons Ltd.

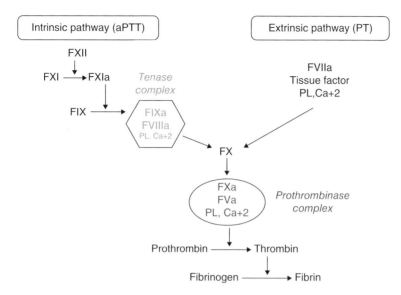

Figure 25.1 'Cascade' model of coagulation. (*See insert for colour representation of the figure.*)

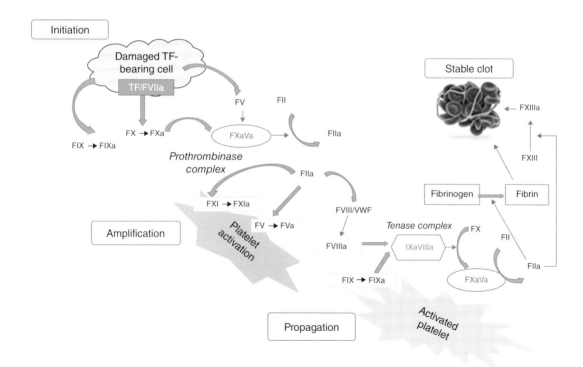

Figure 25.2 Cell-based model of coagulation. Coagulation is initiated on the surface of tissue factor (TF)-bearing cell, generating small amounts of thrombin (FIIa). In the amplification phase, platelets and factors V, VIII and XI are activated. In the propagation phase, large amounts of thrombin are generated, leading to activation of fibrin and factor XIII and production of cross-linked stable clot. (*See insert for colour representation of the figure.*)

Investigation of Abnormal Haemostasis

The most important element in the evaluation of patients with haemostatic abnormalities is a careful personal and family history, their symptoms and clinical signs, including type of bleeding, bleeding following dental work, surgery or childbirth and objective evidence of bleeding such as development of anaemia, requirement for transfusion or surgical intervention. Abnormalities in the haemostatic system may be congenital or acquired. Clinical presentation can vary from mild to life-threatening haemorrhage.

The initial laboratory investigation should include a full blood count with platelet count, prothrombin time (PT), activated partial thromboplastin time (aPTT) and blood film. Additional screening tests that can also be performed are listed in Table 25.1.

Thromboelastogram (TEG®) is a point-of-care test for evaluation of global haemostasis. TEG measures all stages of clot development and dissolution and is used to monitor coagulopathy in trauma patients or surgical patients undergoing liver transplantation or cardiopulmonary bypass (Table 25.2). It assesses haemostasis using whole blood. TEG results need to be correlated with clinical evaluation for patient management. Five major coagulation parameters are measured (Figure 25.3).

Inherited Haemostatic Defects

Haemophilia A

This is an X-linked recessive disorder, but family history may be absent in up to 30% due to spontaneous mutations. This disorder results in reduced or absent activity of factor VIII, whereas there is reduced or absent factor IX activity in haemophilia B.

Haemophilia A is classified into mild, moderate or severe according to factor VIII activity (FVIII:C) (Table 25.3). The effective level for haemostasis is generally about 25–30%. Female carriers usually have >50% FVIII activity, but some female carriers may be symptomatic.

Laboratory abnormalities seen in haemophilia A:

- prolonged aPTT
- reduction of FVIII:C
- normal VWF activity (it is important to measure VWF activity in order to exclude von Willebrand's disease (vWD) where factor VIII levels are also low).

Table 25.1 Laboratory haemostasis screening tests.

System	Test	Factor deficiency
Coagulation	↑PT, normal aPTT	VII
	↑ aPTT, normal PT	VIII, IX, XI, XII, vWF
	↑TT	Fibrinogen, heparin
	Fibrinogen (Clauss assay)	Fibrinogen
Platelets	Platelet count	
	Blood film inspection	
	Platelet function (PFA-100™) Light transmission platelet aggregometry	
Fibrinolysis	D-dimers	
	Euglobulin clot lysis time	
Global haemostasis	Thromboelastogram	

Table 25.2 TEG parameters, selected abnormalities and treatment.

Parameters	Situations in which they are changed	Treatment
R	Prolonged in coagulation factor deficiency	Fresh frozen plasma
MA	Depressed in thrombocytopenia, platelet dysfunction	Platelets, DDAVP
K	Prolonged in platelet dysfunction, thrombocytopenia, coagulation factor deficiency, fibrinogen deficiency	Based on combination of other parameters
Alpha angle	Depressed in hypofibrinogenaemia, dysfibrinogenaemia	Cryoprecipitate
LY30	Shortened in excessive fibrinolysis	Anti-fibrinolytics (tranexamic or aminocaproic acid)

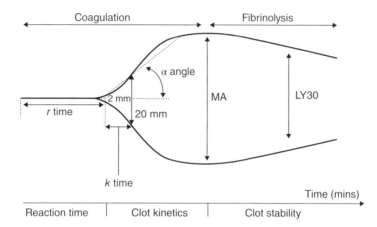

Figure 25.3 Schematic representation of thromboelastography (TEG®). 1. The R value (clotting time) represents the time it takes to initiate clot formation. It is a reflection of coagulation factor activity. 2. The alpha angle represents the thrombin burst and conversion of fibrinogen to fibrin. 3. The MA is maximal amplitude or clot strength derived from platelet function. 4. The K value (kinetics of clot formation) is the time from the end of R until the clot reaches 20 mm and represents the speed of clot formation. 5. LY30 lysis time measures the degree of fibrinolysis.

Management

The mainstay of treatment is to raise the FVIII:C sufficiently to prevent or arrest spontaneous and traumatic haemorrhages or to cover surgery. There are a number of products available, including:

- recombinant factor VIII preparations
- plasma-derived factor VIII concentrates (which vary in degree of purity)
- DDAVP (for mild disease – baseline factor VIII above 15%)
- tranexamic or aminocaproic acid.

Recombinant products are the product of choice to prevent spontaneous joint haemorrhages in children with severe haemophilia (prophylaxis), as well as the treatment of haemorrhages because of the lack of risk of transmission of infection [3]. Plasma-derived factor concentrates undergo donor screening and viral inactivation procedures, but transmission of some nonencapsulated viruses, such as human parvovirus B19, and new emerging infections, such as prion disease, remain a theoretical risk.

There is ongoing debate over whether there is a higher incidence of inhibitor development in patients treated with recombinant factor VIII products versus plasma-derived concentrates which remains unresolved, but recombinant products are still the recommended first line for previously untreated patients.

Table 25.3 Clinical manifestations and treatment of haemophilia A and B.

Factor level (% normal)	Clinical manifestation	Treatment
<1% (severe disease)	Usual age of onset <1 year Spontaneous bleeding common (haemarthrosis, muscle haematoma, haematuria) Bleeding post surgery and dental extraction Posttraumatic bleeding Crippling joint deformity if inadequate treatment	Regular FVIII or IX prophylaxis in children and some adults Factor VIII or IX to treat bleeds Factor VIII or IX for surgery or invasive procedures +/− tranexamic acid
1–5% (moderate disease)	Usual age of onset <2 years Occasional spontaneous bleeding Bleeding post surgery and dental extraction Posttraumatic bleeding	Some patients may need regular factor VIII or IX prophylaxis Factor VIII or IX to treat bleeds Factor VIII or IX for surgery or invasive procedures +/− tranexamic acid
6–40% (mild disease)	Usual age of onset >2 years Bleeding post surgery and dental extraction Posttraumatic bleeding Spontaneous bleeding is rare	Regular prophylaxis usually not required Treatment of haemorrhages or cover for surgery/invasive procedures: haemophilia A: DDAVP, tranexamic acid, factor concentrate haemophilia B: tranexamic acid, factor concentrate

Patients with moderate/severe haemophilia will require factor VIII concentrates for bleeding, prior to invasive procedures, surgery, etc. One unit of factor VIII/kg bodyweight will result in an increase in plasma factor VIII level by 2%. The amount of factor VIII concentrate required is calculated according to the formula:

$$\text{Units of factor VIII required} = \text{weight}\,(\text{kg}) \times \text{desired FVIII : C level}\,(\%) \times 0.5$$

The plasma half-life of factor VIII is 8–12 hours, and repeated doses at 12-hourly intervals are usually needed. Alternatively, a continuous infusion of factor VIII can be given for surgery.

For major soft tissue haemorrhages, levels above 50% are generally sufficient; however, for major surgery, a preoperative level of 100% is necessary and thereafter levels of 50–100% are sufficient for wound healing. Factor VIII:C can be measured before and after doses of concentrate to ensure appropriate levels.

When available, long-acting recombinant factors could be used. Recombinant factor VIII Fc fusion protein has a mean half-life of 19.0 hours and requires administration every 3–5 days for prophylaxis in most patients [4].

Mild haemophilia A should be treated with DDAVP (with or without antifibrinolytics) where possible [3]. DDAVP (0.3 µg/kg bodyweight) is given intravenously or alternatively a 300 μg dose can be administered via intranasal spray. This dose typically increases the levels of factor VIII and VWF 3–5 times above baseline. Hyponatraemia and water intoxication are side effects of this drug, and hence it is not recommended for patients with cardiac failure or children under two years of age. It should be used with caution in the elderly or those with known vascular disease due to thrombogenic potential. The response to DDAVP should be assessed in all patients prior to its use to treat bleeding or cover invasive procedures to ensure that an adequate increase in factor VIII levels is achieved.

Antifibrinolytics reduce fibrinolysis and are of particular use in patients with bleeding from mucosal surfaces, such as epistaxis, oral bleeding or menorrhagia. It is given as an adjunct to DDAVP to reduce bleeding. It should be avoided in patients with haematuria to avoid the complication of clot retention. It is usually given for 7–10 days to allow adequate healing.

Haemophilia B

This X-linked recessive disorder results in a deficiency of factor IX. The clinical manifestations are similar to those of haemophilia A (see Table 25.3).

Laboratory abnormalities seen in haemophilia B:

• prolonged APTT
• reduction of factor IX coagulant activity.

Management
Current products for treatment include:

• recombinant factor IX products
• high-purity plasma-derived factor IX concentrates.

The product of choice for prophylaxis, treatment of bleeding or cover for surgical procedures in previously untreated patients is recombinant factor IX [3]. If unavailable, then high-purity plasma-derived factor IX concentrates should be used.

The dosage of factor IX required can be calculated according to the formula:

$$\text{Units of factor IX required} = \text{weight}\,(\text{kg}) \times \text{desired level}\,(\%) \times 1.0$$

The plasma half-life of factor IX is 18–30 hours so repeated doses are needed and given every 12–24 hours or by continuous infusion.

Long-acting recombinant factor IX is now also available. The half-life of factor IX Fc fusion protein is 82 hours with dosing intervals of 10–14 days. Patients who transitioned from prophylaxis with recombinant factor IX to prophylaxis with factor IX Fc fusion protein had fewer bleeding episodes despite reduced infusion frequency and overall factor consumption [5,6]. Treatment regimens have also been developed for the long-acting products with dose adjustment based on the severity of haemorrhage and clinical response.

Treatment of Patients with Inhibitors
Patients with haemophilia can develop inhibitory antibodies to factor VIII or less commonly IX. Inhibitor development is often heralded by increased frequency of bleeding or loss of response to factor VIII. It is diagnosed by measuring factor VIII levels before and after a dose of factor VIII concentrate and by a Bethesda inhibitor assay.

For patients with haemophilia A, if the inhibitor is of low titre (i.e. <5 Bethesda units), bleeding episodes can be treated with higher than normal doses of human factor VIII [7]. If the inhibitor is of high titre (i.e. >10 Bethesda units), human factor VIII is ineffective to control bleeding and the use of recombinant FVIIa or FEIBA® (Baxter) is recommended. For major haemorrhage, recombinant FVIIa (dose of 70–90 μg/kg initially every two hours) is generally recommended as first-line therapy. Eradication of inhibitors with 'immune tolerance induction' using factor VIII concentrates alone or together with immunosuppression is considered the best long-term treatment option for these patients [7].

For patients with haemophilia B, recombinant factor VIIa is used for bleeding [7]. Immune tolerance using factor IX concentrates can be attempted, although this is more difficult than in haemophilia A.

Von Willebrand Disease

This is the most common inherited bleeding disorder, up to 1% of the population, and is due to a quantitative and/or qualitative defect in the VWF protein. VWF promotes adhesion of platelets to the subendothelium by binding to the platelet receptor glycoprotein Ib and protects factor VIII:C from degradation by activated protein C. Patients who are blood group O have lower levels of VWF than other blood groups.

Von Willebrand disease is classified into three types (Table 25.4) [8]. Clinical symptoms vary from asymptomatic to haemophilia-like bleeding.

Laboratory abnormalities seen in VWD include (variably) (Table 25.5):

- prolonged PFA-100™ closure time
- prolonged aPTT
- reduction of VWF antigen (VWF:Ag)
- reduction of VWF ristocetin co-factor activity (VWF:RiCoF)
- reduction of FVIII:C (which can cause prolonged aPTT)
- abnormal VWF multimers in some type 2 subtypes.

The goal of therapy in patients with VWD is to improve platelet adhesion and raise low FVIII levels. Treatment differs for the various types of VWD [9].

- *Type 1*: DDAVP is the treatment of choice and a dose of 0.3 μg/kg bodyweight is usually given intravenously. Intranasal doses (300 μg for adults or 150 μg for children) can also be given.

Table 25.4 Variants of von Willebrand disease.

Variant	
Type 1	Autosomal dominant inheritance
	Partial quantitative deficiency of VWF
	Normal VWF multimers
	Mild bleeding disorder which decreases during pregnancy, elderly
Type 2	Autosomal dominant inheritance
	Qualitative deficiency of VWF
	Subtypes: 2A: decreased platelet-dependent VWF function with lack of large multimers 2B: increased affinity of VWF to GPIb and loss of large and medium multimers
	2M: decreased platelet-dependent VWF function with normal multimers 2N: markedly decreased VWF affinity for FVIII
Type 3	Autosomal recessive inheritance
	Severe quantitative deficiency of VWF
	Severe haemophilia-like bleeding disorder

Table 25.5 Comparative laboratory findings in types of von Willebrand disease.

Type vWD	vWF:Ag	vWF:RCo	FVIII:C	VWF multimers
1	↓	↓	↓	Normal distribution, all diminished
2				
2A	N or ↓	↓↓	N or ↓	Lack of large multimers
2B	↓	↓↓	N or ↓	Lack of large and medium multimers
2M	↓	↓↓	N or ↓	N
2N	N or ↓	N or ↓	↓↓↓	N
3	↓↓↓	↓↓↓	↓↓↓	Absent multimers

These doses give a two- to threefold increase in endogenous vWF and FVIII:C levels. It is important to test an individual's response to DDAVP prior to surgical procedures. Tranexamic or aminocaproic acid is often also given, either alone for minor bleeding/procedures or in conjunction with DDAVP.

- *Types 2 and 3*: virally inactivated plasma-derived VWF concentrates are required, because no recombinant VWF concentrates are available.

Cryoprecipitate is no longer recommended for treatment since it is not virally inactivated.

Other Inherited Disorders

Hereditary deficiencies of other coagulation factors are rare. Factor XI deficiency is particularly common amongst Ashkenazi Jews and is inherited as an autosomal recessive trait. There is a poor correlation between factor XI levels and bleeding tendency, which usually presents following surgery or dental procedures. If available, factor XI concentrates should be given to treat bleeding; if not, then fresh frozen plasma (FFP) should be administered. There have been concerns about the potential thrombogenicity of factor XI concentrates, so peak levels should ideally not exceed 70 IU/dL [10].

Cryoprecipitate can be used for fibrinogen deficiency/dysfibrinogenaemias, but fibrinogen concentrates should be used in preference if they are available because they undergo viral inactivation steps [3]. Deficiencies of factors II, V, VII, X and XIII can all be treated with FFP, but if more specific therapies are available they should be used in preference. Currently, there are specific factor concentrates for factors VII and XIII. Prothrombin complex concentrates (PCCs) contain factors II, IX and X with variable amounts of VII and are used in conditions associated with deficiencies of one or more of these factors (e.g. treatment of overdosage with warfarin).

Patients with deficiencies of 'contact factors' (factor XII, prekallikrein and high molecular weight kininogen) do not bleed excessively and do not require any treatment.

Acquired Haemostatic Defects

Disseminated Intravascular Coagulation

This is a complex disorder resulting from inappropriate activation of the haemostatic system that can be manifested by both thrombotic and haemorrhagic complications. DIC may be acute (uncompensated), with decreased levels of haemostatic components, or chronic (compensated), with more normal coagulation parameters.

The main triggering mechanism for DIC is the exposure of blood to a source of tissue factor that initiates coagulation, for example on the surface of endothelial cells or monocytes stimulated by endotoxins/cytokines as a result of sepsis, on the surface of damaged cells (placental abruption, cerebral trauma) or from malignant cells leading to thrombin generation and fibrin formation. This may cause microthrombus formation (e.g. gangrene of fingers and toes and renal failure). Secondary activation of the fibrinolytic pathway occurs with subsequent lysis of fibrin and the formation of cross-linked complexes such as D-dimers. Raised levels of these FDPs further add to the bleeding diathesis as they inhibit the action of thrombin and also inhibit platelet function.

Hepatic synthesis is unable to compensate fully for the ongoing consumption of clotting factors, so there is a reduction in their levels. In addition, a consumptive thrombocytopenia develops. This combination of coagulation factor deficiency, thrombocytopenia and the inhibitory actions of raised FDPs causes the generalised and continued bleeding tendency characteristic of DIC. The main causes of DIC are listed in Table 25.6.

The following laboratory abnormalities are seen in DIC [11]:

- fall in platelet count/thrombocytopenia
- increased FDPs: raised D-dimers, increased fibrin monomers
- prolonged PT and APTT
- reduced fibrinogen levels

Table 25.6 Main causes of DIC.

Condition	Examples
Infection	Septicaemia, viraemia
Malignancy	Leukaemia (especially acute promyelocytic)
	Metastatic carcinomas
Obstetric disorders	Septic abortion
	Placenta praevia and abruptio placentae
	Eclampsia
	Amniotic fluid embolism
Trauma	Extensive surgical trauma
	Fat embolism
Shock	Burns
	Heat stroke
Liver disease	Acute hepatic necrosis
Transplantation	Tissue rejection
Extracorporeal circulation	Cardiac bypass surgery
Extensive intravascular haemolysis	ABO-incompatible transfusion
Certain snake bites	
Vascular abnormalities	Kasabach–Merrit syndrome

- anaemia, fragmented red cells (schistocytes), raised reticulocyte count.

In order to help with the diagnosis of DIC in the clinical setting, scoring systems such as that from the International Society for Thrombosis and Haemostasis (ISTH) have been devised [12] (Box 25.1).

Treatment of the underlying disease is the most important aspect of management of patients with DIC. Obstetric emergencies should be attended to immediately. The current British Committee for Standards in Haematology (BCSH) guidelines suggest the following therapies if the patient is bleeding, at high risk of bleeding or requires surgical intervention [11].

- Platelet concentrates if the platelet count is $\leq 50 \times 10^9$/L.

Box 25.1 International Society of Thrombosis and Haemostasis diagnostic scoring system for overt DIC.

Risk assessment

Does the patient have an underlying disorder known to be associated with overt DIC?

If **yes**: proceed

If **no: do not use this algorithm**

Order global coagulation tests (PT, platelet count, fibrinogen, fibrin-related marker)

Score the test results:

Platelet count: $>100 \times 10^9$/L = 0, $<100 \times 10^9$/L = 1, $<50 \times 10^9$/L = 2

- Elevated fibrin marker (e.g. D-dimer, fibrin degradation products): no increase = 0, moderate increase = 2, strong increase = 3
- Prolonged PT: <3 s = 0, >3 but <6 s = 1, >6 s = 2
- Fibrinogen level: >1 g/L = 0, <1 g/L = 1

Calculate score:

≥ 5 compatible with overt DIC: repeat score daily

<5 suggestive for nonovert DIC: repeat next 1–2 days

- Fresh frozen plasma if the PT or APTT is prolonged. Almost all procoagulant factors and inhibitors are contained within FFP. Standard doses of 15 mL/kg should be given, but patients often need up to 30 mL/kg. Prothrombin complex concentrates (PCCs) can be considered if the patient is at risk of fluid overload.
- Fibrinogen replacement with either cryoprecipitate or fibrinogen concentrates if plasma fibrinogen levels are <1 g/L. Cryoprecipitate contains fibrinogen in a 'concentrated' form and each unit will increase fibrinogen by 0.5–1 g/L. Fibrinogen concentrates are virally inactivated plasma-derived preparations that also have the advantage of being highly concentrated; 3–4 g of concentrate will raise the fibrinogen level by 1 g/L.

Following initial replacement therapy, any further treatment should be guided by the clinical and laboratory response with suggested

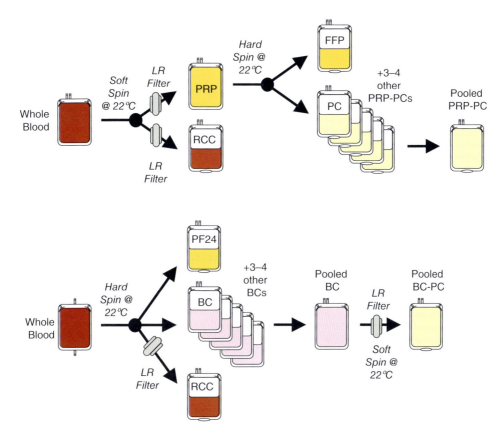

Figure 22.1 (a) Production of leucocyte-reduced (LR) red cell concentrates (RCC), fresh frozen plasma (FFP) and platelet-rich plasma (PRP)-intermediate platelet concentrates (PC). (b) Production of RCCs, plasma frozen within 24 hours of phlebotomy (PF24) and buffy coat (BC)-intermediate PCs.

Practical Transfusion Medicine, Fifth Edition. Edited by Michael F. Murphy, David J. Roberts and Mark H. Yazer.
© 2017 John Wiley & Sons Ltd. Published 2017 by John Wiley & Sons Ltd.

Check the laboratory-generated label against the patient's identity band

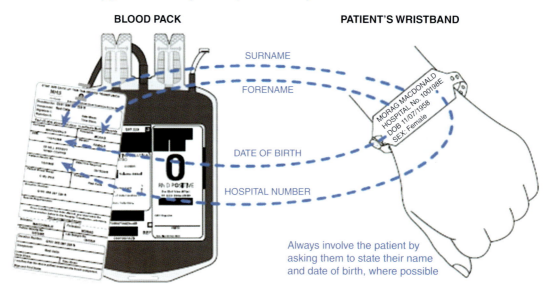

BLOOD PACK **PATIENT'S WRISTBAND**

SURNAME

FORENAME

DATE OF BIRTH

HOSPITAL NUMBER

MORAG MACDONALD
HOSPITAL No. 100198E
DOB 11/07/1958
SEX: Female

Always involve the patient by
asking them to state their name
and date of birth, where possible

Figure 23.2 How to perform an identity check between the patient and blood component. *Source*: Handbook of Transfusion Medicine, 5th edn, Stationery Office, UK.

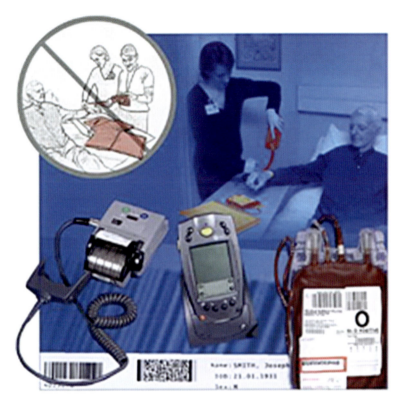

Figure 23.3 Bedside checking using an electronic system. The traditional method of pretransfusion bedside checking requires two nurses and checks of multiple items of written documentation. With barcode technology, a handheld computer reads a barcode on the patient wristband containing full patient details. The handheld computer checks that the patient details on the wristband barcode match those on the barcode (in the red box) on the compatibility label attached to the unit after pretransfusion testing. This barcode also contains the unique number of the unit, and is matched with the barcode number of the unit (top left of the bag) to ensure that the blood transfusion laboratory has attached the right compatibility label. *Source*: Reproduced with permission from Wiley–Blackwell.

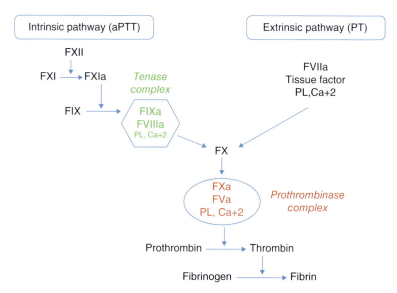

Figure 25.1 'Cascade' model of coagulation.

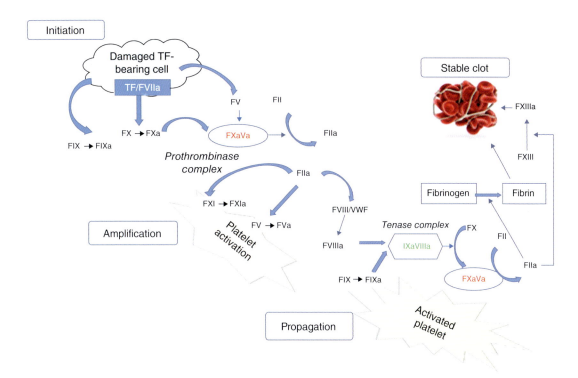

Figure 25.2 Cell-based model of coagulation. Coagulation is initiated on the surface of tissue factor (TF)-bearing cell, generating small amounts of thrombin (FIIa). In the amplification phase, platelets and factors V, VIII and XI are activated. In the propagation phase, large amounts of thrombin are generated, leading to activation of fibrin and factor XIII and production of cross-linked stable clot.

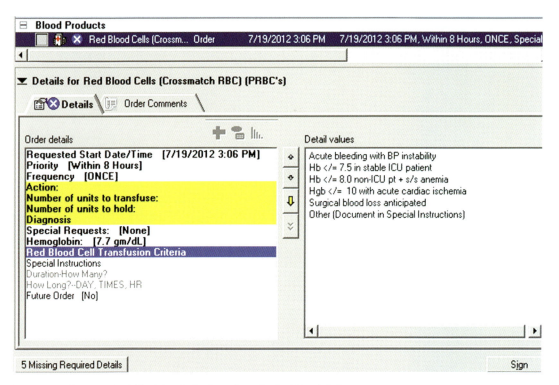

Figure 34.1 Computerised Physician Order Entry Page for Red Blood Cells.

Facility	Total orders	Total alerts	Alerted orders not placed	Percent orders alerted	Percent alerts heeded
PUH	248	182	23	73.4%	12.6%
SHY	208	138	21	66.3%	15.2%
HAM	198	77	21	38.9%	27.3%
PAS	144	74	10	51.4%	13.5%
SMH	146	59	7	40.4%	11.9%
EAS	73	37	10	50.7%	27.0%
HZN	58	28	4	48.3%	14.3%
MER	275	27	4	9.8%	14.8%
NOR	39	23	0	59.0%	0.0%
MWH	103	20	2	19.4%	10.0%
MCK	62	12	3	19.4%	25.0%
BED	15	10	3	66.7%	30.0%

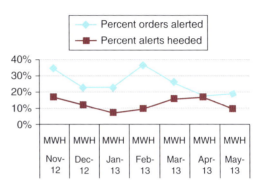

Total orders = Crossmatch Red blood cells, Red blood cells (Crossmatch RBC)
Percent orders alerted = Total alerts / Total orders
Percent alerts heeded = Alerted orders not placed / Total alerts

MWH unheeded RBC order alerts
May 2013

Figure 34.2 Transfusion variance report.

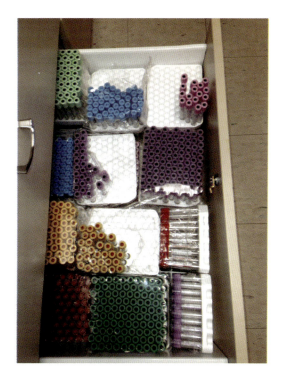

Figure 34.3 The rainbow draw.

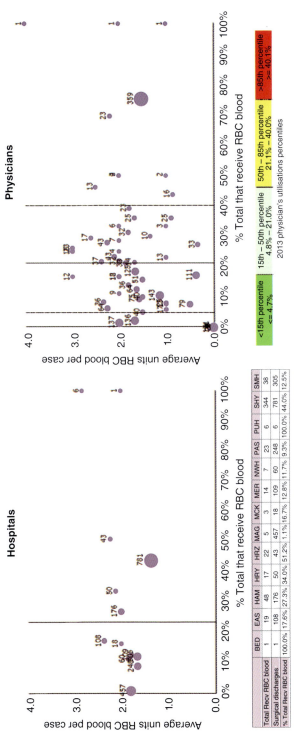

Hospitals

	BED	EAS	HAM	HRY	HRZ	MAG	MCK	MER	NWH	PAS	PUH	SHY	SMH
Total Recv RBC blood	1	19	48	17	22	5	3	14	7	23	6	344	38
Surgical discharges	1	108	176	50	43	457	18	109	60	248	6	781	305
% Total Recv RBC blood	100.0%	17.6%	27.3%	34.0%	51.2%	1.1%	16.7%	12.8%	11.7%	9.3%	100.0%	44.0%	12.5%

Physicians

<15th percentile <= 4.7%	15th – 50th percentile 4.8% – 21.0%	50th – 85th percentile 21.1% – 40.0%	>85th percentile >= 40.1%

2013 physician's utilisations percentiles

	2013/Apr	2013/May	2013/Jun	2013/Jul	2013/Aug	2013/Sep	2013/Oct	2013/Nov	2013/Dec	2014/Jan	2014/Feb	2014/Mar
Surgical discharges	192	182	206	155	197	189	222	224	179	208	193	215
Total receiving RBC blood	58	48	51	39	34	52	53	50	34	39	48	41
% Total that receive RBC blood	30.2%	26.4%	24.8%	25.2%	17.3%	27.5%	23.9%	22.3%	19.0%	18.8%	24.9%	19.1%
Avg units RBC blood per transfused case	1.83	1.77	1.59	1.41	1.91	1.27	1.79	1.66	1.50	1.33	1.31	1.54
Total receiving TXA	103	98	106	79	95	100	126	130	112	132	137	143
% Total that receive TXA	53.6%	53.8%	51.5%	51.0%	48.2%	52.9%	56.8%	58.0%	62.6%	63.5%	71.0%	66.5%
Avg units TXA per transfused case	1.07	1.07	1.07	1.08	1.17	1.07	1.08	1.08	1.14	1.21	1.26	1.24
ALOS w blood	3.4	3.3	3.1	3.2	3.6	2.8	3.0	2.6	2.5	2.3	2.9	3.0
ALOS w/o blood	2.9	2.8	3.0	2.8	2.9	3.0	2.8	2.7	2.7	3.0	2.7	2.8
% Autologous	0.0%	0.0%	3.9%	2.6%	2.9%	0.0%	1.9%	0.0%	0.0%	0.0%	0.0%	0.0%

Figure 34.5 Benchmarking report.

	1st Pillar **Optimise erythropoiesis**	2nd Pillar **Minimise blood loss & bleeding**	3rd Pillar **Harness & optimise physiological reserve of anaemia**
Preoperative	• Detect anaemia • Identify underlying disorder(s) causing anaemia • Manage disorder(s) • Refer for further evaluation if necessary • Treat suboptimal iron stores/iron deficiency/anaemia of chronic disease/iron-restricted erythropoiesis • Treat other haematinic deficiencies • Note: Anaemia is a contraindication for elective surgery	• Identify and manage bleeding risk • Minimising iatrogenic blood loss • Procedure planning and rehearsal • Preoperative autologous blood donation (in selected cases or when patient choice) • Other	• Assess /optimise patient's physiological reserve and risk factors • Compare estimated blood loss with patient-specific tolerable blood loss • Formulate patient-specific management plan using appropriate blood conservation modalities to minimise blood loss, optimise red cell mass and manage anaemia • Restrictive transfusion thresholds
Intraoperative	• Timing surgery with haematological optimisation	• Meticulous haemostasis and surgical techniques • Blood-sparing surgical techniques • Anaesthetic blood conserving strategies • Autologous blood options • Pharmacological/haemostatic agents	• Optimise cardiac output • Optimise ventilation and oxygenation • Restrictive transfusion thresholds
Postoperative	• Stimulate erythropoiesis • Be aware of drug interactions that can increase anaemia	• Vigilant monitoring and management of post-operative bleeding • Avoid secondary haemorrhage • Rapid warming/maintain normothermia (unless hypothermia specifically indicated) • Autologous blood salvage • Minimising iatrogenic blood loss • Haemostasis/anticoagulation management • Prophylaxis of upper GI haemorrhage • Avoid/treat infections promptly • Be aware of adverse effects of medication	• Optimise anaemia reserve • Maximise oxygen delivery • Minimise oxygen consumption • Avoid/treat infections promptly • Restrictive transfusion thresholds

Figure 35.1 The three-pillar, nine-field matrix of perioperative patient blood management. This matrix, designed for the Western Australia Patient Blood Management Program, highlights the multiple patient blood management strategies that may be considered in the perioperative period in a patient/procedure-specific context. GI, gastrointestinal. *Source*: Adapted from Hofmann A, Friedman D, Farmer S. Western Australian patient blood management project 2008–2012: analysis, strategy, implementation and financial projections. Western Australia Department of Health, Canberra, 2007.

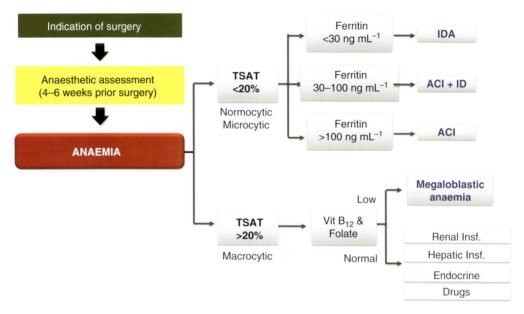

Figure 35.2 Flowchart for anaemia classification. ACI, anaemia of chronic inflammation; ID, iron deficiency; IDA, iron deficiency anaemia; TSAT, transferrin saturation. *Source*: Munoz et al. 2015 [10]. Reproduced with permission of Oxford University Press.

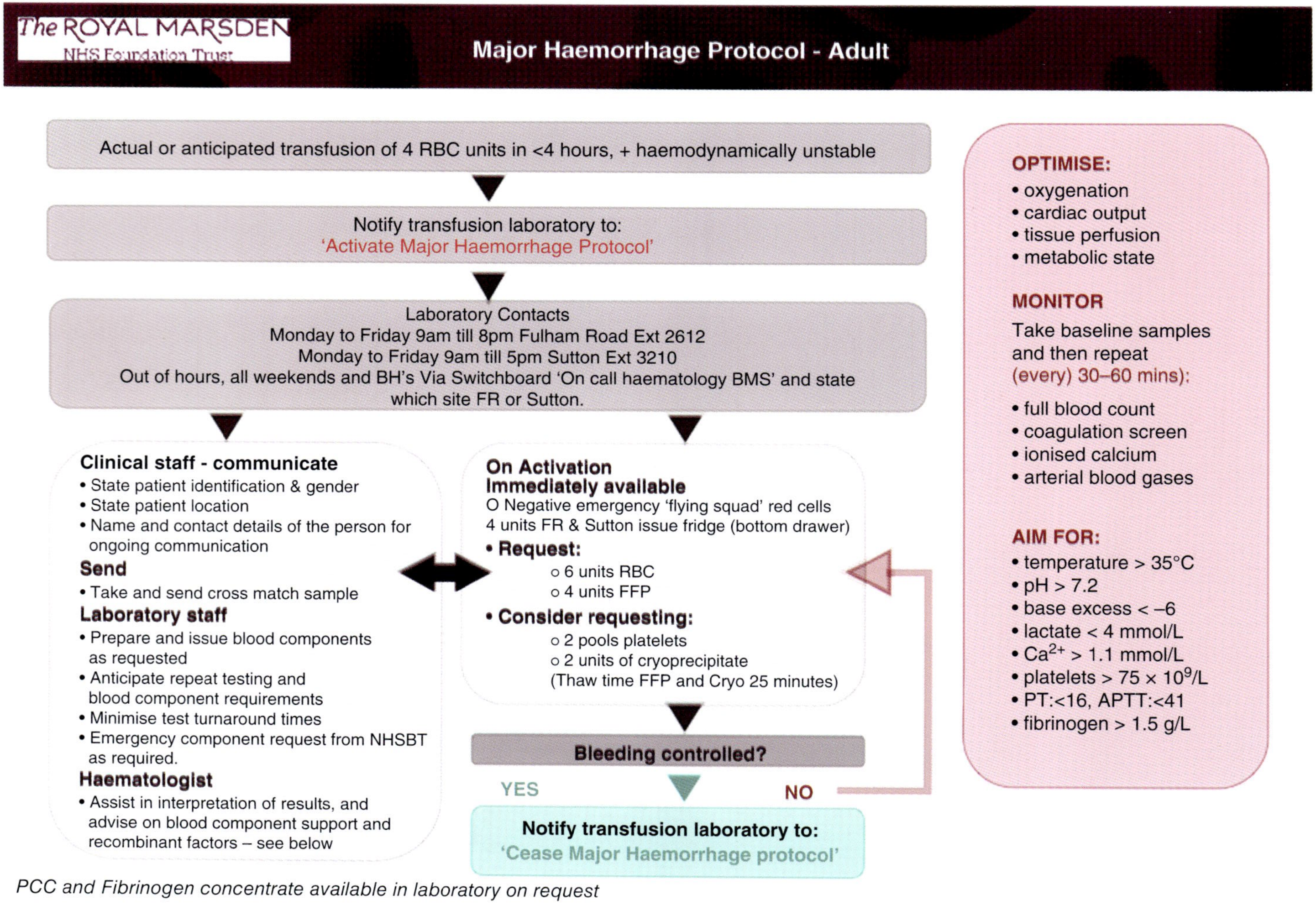

The ROYAL MARSDEN
NHS Foundation Trust

Major Haemorrhage Protocol - Adult

Actual or anticipated transfusion of 4 RBC units in <4 hours, + haemodynamically unstable

Notify transfusion laboratory to:
'Activate Major Haemorrhage Protocol'

Laboratory Contacts
Monday to Friday 9am till 8pm Fulham Road Ext 2612
Monday to Friday 9am till 5pm Sutton Ext 3210
Out of hours, all weekends and BH's Via Switchboard 'On call haematology BMS' and state which site FR or Sutton.

On Activation
Immediately available
○ Negative emergency 'flying squad' red cells
4 units FR & Sutton issue fridge (bottom drawer)
- **Request:**
  ○ 6 units RBC
  ○ 4 units FFP
- **Consider requesting:**
  ○ 2 pools platelets
  ○ 2 units of cryoprecipitate
  (Thaw time FFP and Cryo 25 minutes)

Clinical staff - communicate
- State patient identification & gender
- State patient location
- Name and contact details of the person for ongoing communication

Send
- Take and send cross match sample

Laboratory staff
- Prepare and issue blood components as requested
- Anticipate repeat testing and blood component requirements
- Minimise test turnaround times
- Emergency component request from NHSBT as required.

Haematologist
- Assist in interpretation of results, and advise on blood component support and recombinant factors – see below

Bleeding controlled?

YES

NO

Notify transfusion laboratory to:
'Cease Major Haemorrhage protocol'

OPTIMISE:
- oxygenation
- cardiac output
- tissue perfusion
- metabolic state

MONITOR
Take baseline samples and then repeat (every) 30–60 mins):
- full blood count
- coagulation screen
- ionised calcium
- arterial blood gases

AIM FOR:
- temperature > 35°C
- pH > 7.2
- base excess < –6
- lactate < 4 mmol/L
- Ca^{2+} > 1.1 mmol/L
- platelets > 75×10^9/L
- PT:<16, APTT:<41
- fibrinogen > 1.5 g/L

PCC and Fibrinogen concentrate available in laboratory on request

Figure 35.3 Major haemorrhage protocol (Royal Marsden NHS Foundation Trust). *Source:* Dougherty 2015. Reproduced with permission of John Wiley and Sons.

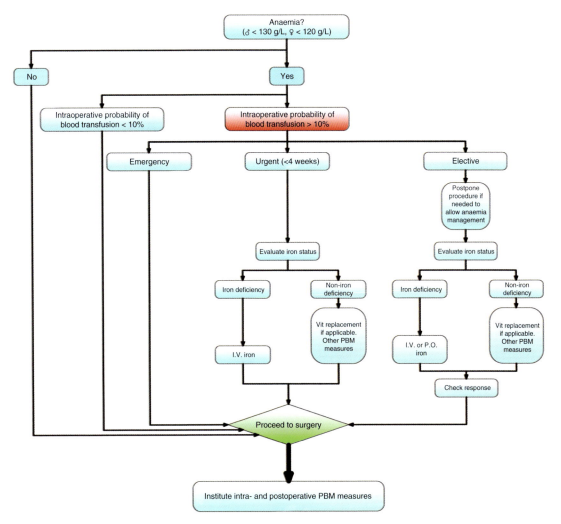

Figure 35.4 Pathways to surgery for patients with preoperative anaemia. IV, intravenous; PBM, patient blood management; PO, per os.

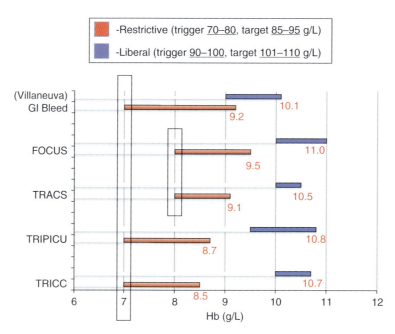

Figure 37.1 Haemoglobin (Hb) triggers (the Hb before transfusion) and Hb targets (the Hb after transfusion) are shown from the five large randomised trials [2,4,19–21] that compared restrictive and liberal transfusion strategies. Although the trial results advocate for the use of a restrictive transfusion strategy, with Hb triggers of 70–80 g/L for most patients, the Hb target concentration in the restrictive group was 85–95 g/L. When this finding is considered in the Functional Outcomes in Cardiovascular Patients Undergoing Surgical Hip Fracture Repair (FOCUS) trial, for example, the two groups compared (Hb trigger 80 versus 100 g/L) had actual daily average Hb concentrations that were 95 in the restrictive group and 110 g/L in the liberal group.

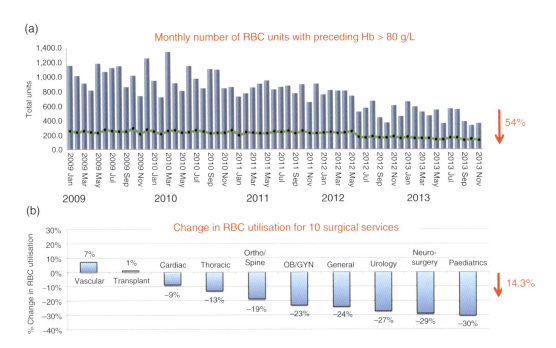

Figure 37.2 Effect of a patient blood management programme (PBM) on red blood cell utilisation. (a) The number of red cell units/month that were ordered with a preceding haemoglobin (Hb) >80 g/L is shown over a five-year period. With a multifaceted PBM programme that includes education, and computerised provider order entry with clinician decision support and a best practice alert, we achieved a 54% decrease in out-of-guideline red cell transfusions between the months of January 2009 and November 2013. (b) We also saw an overall decrease in red cell utilisation for eight out of 10 surgical services and an overall decrease in surgical blood utilisation of 14.3% over the same time period. *Source:* Modified from Zuckerberg et al. 2015 [8]. Reproduced with permission of John Wiley and Sons.

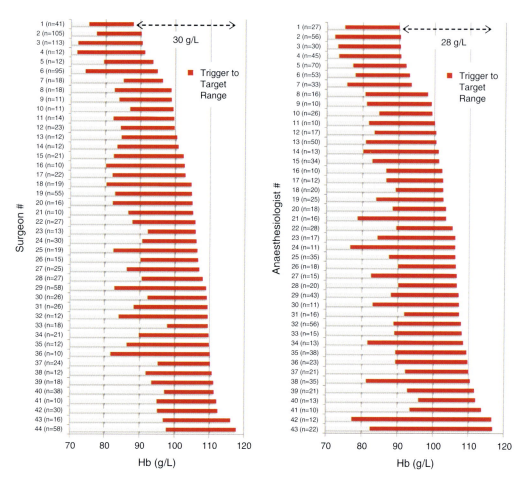

Figure 37.3 Comparison of mean transfusion haemoglobin (Hb) triggers and targets for all surgeons and anaesthesiologists who had 10 or more patients in the anaesthesia information management system (AIMS) database. The mean Hb triggers are designated by the left edge of the red bars and the mean Hb targets by the right edge of the red bars. The span between the lowest and highest Hb triggers was 26 g/L for surgeons and 24 g/L for anaesthesiologists. The span between lowest and highest Hb targets was 30 g/L for surgeons and 28 g/L for anaesthesiologists. *Source*: Modified from Frank et al. 2012 [7]. Reproduced with permission of Wolters Kluwer Health Inc.

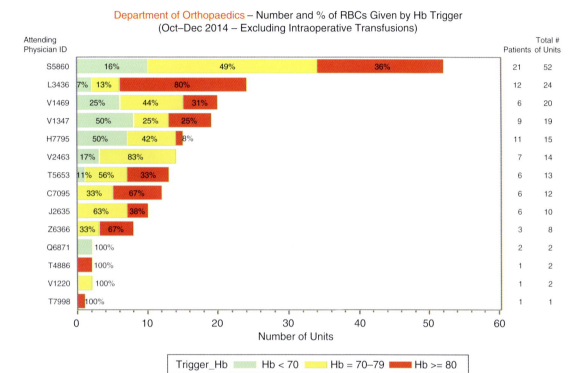

Figure 37.4 These data were taken from the computerised provider order entry system. Individual physicians (y-axis) were compared by the number of red blood cell orders placed (x-axis) over a three-month time period, along with the percentage of orders placed by haemoglobin (Hb) trigger. The proportion of orders for which the most recent Hb preceding the order was <70 g/L is shown in green, 70–79 g/L in yellow and ≥80 g/L in red. An accompanying table for each department is provided showing the five-digit codes on the y-axis correspond to the names of attending physicians.

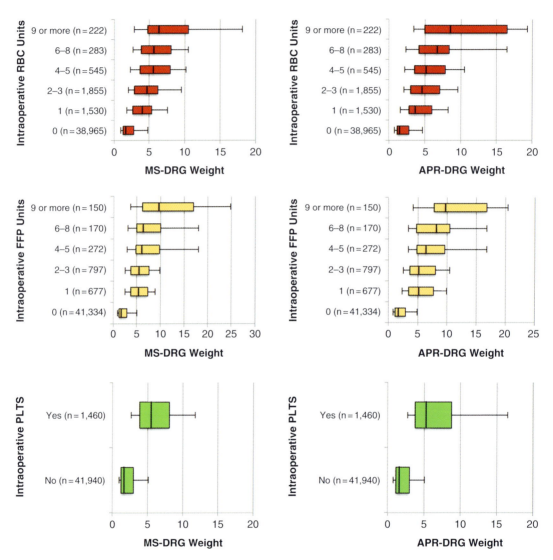

Figure 37.5 Intraoperative blood component requirements are plotted as a function of Case Mix Index (CMI). Left side: CMI is represented by the weighted Medicare Severity Diagnosis-Related Group (MS-DRG Weight). Right side: CMI is represented by the weighted All Patient Refined Diagnosis-Related Group (APR-DRG Weight). The data show a clear relationship between a higher CMI value and greater intraoperative transfusion requirements for red blood cells, fresh frozen plasma (FFP) and platelets (PLTS). Differences in CMI values among transfusion requirement groups are significant for all six analyses shown (P < 0.0001). *Source*: Modified from Stonemetz et al. 2014 [5]. Reproduced with permission of John Wiley and Sons.

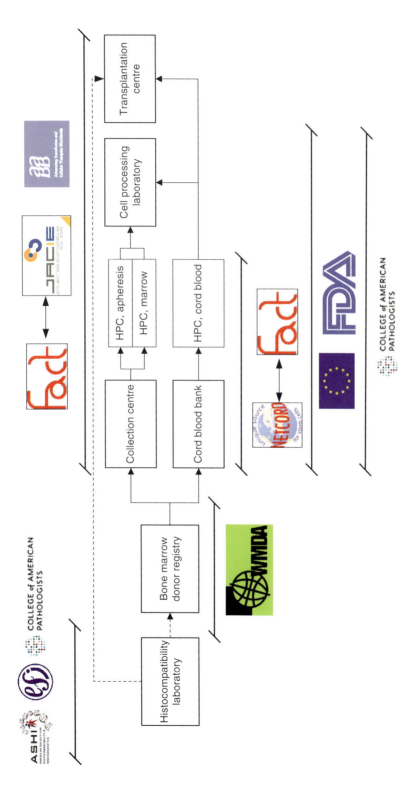

Figure 38.3 Regulatory environment for haematopoietic stem cell transplantation. Note that this figure does not reflect all potential regulatory reporting requirements for transplantation centres.

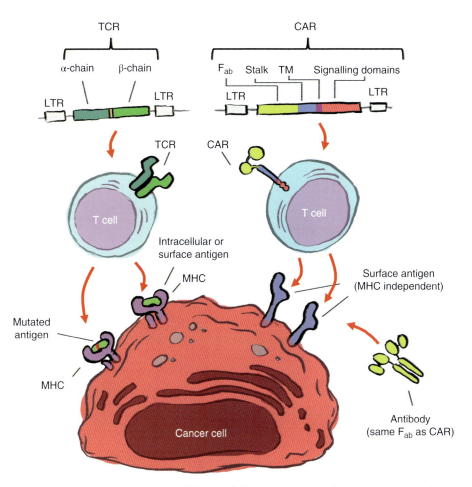

Figure 43.1 Generation of CAR or TCR gene-modified T-cells for cancer immunotherapy. Retroviral and lentiviral vectors encoding CAR or TCR molecules can be used to redirect the specificity of human T-cells. CAR molecules recognise proteins that are expressed on the surface of cancer cells. TCR molecules can recognise peptides that are derived from intracellular proteins, including mutated proteins.

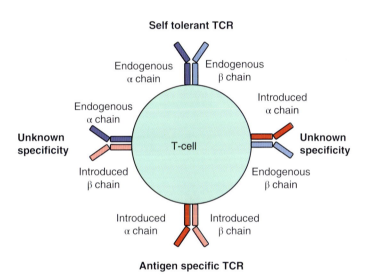

Figure 43.2 Schematic illustrating mispairing with endogenous TCR chains by the introduced TCR chains following retroviral TCR gene transfer.

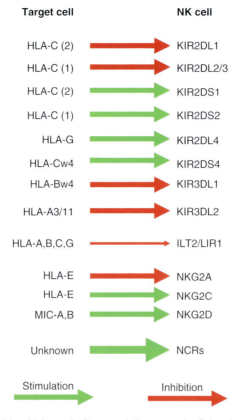

Figure 43.3 Ligands controlling NK cell activation and triggering.

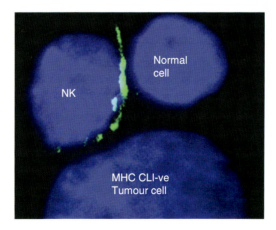

Figure 43.4 Capping of KIR molecules on NK cell. Anti-KIR antibody (*green*) shows co-localisation of KIR and MHC class I molecules at the synapse between the NK and autologous normal cell. In contrast, the MHC-negative tumour cell fails to initiate capping of the KIR molecules.

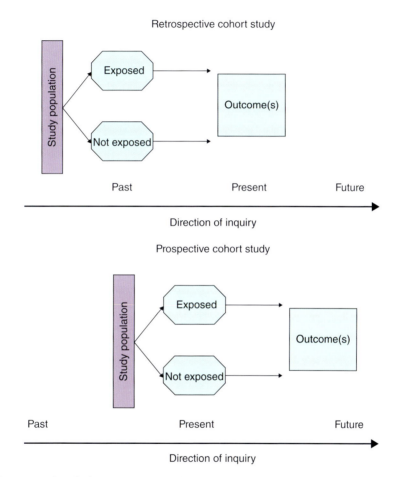

Figure 45.1 Observational study designs: case–control and cohort studies. *Source*: Adapted from Tay and Tinmouth 2007 [22]. Reproduced with permission of John Wiley & Sons.

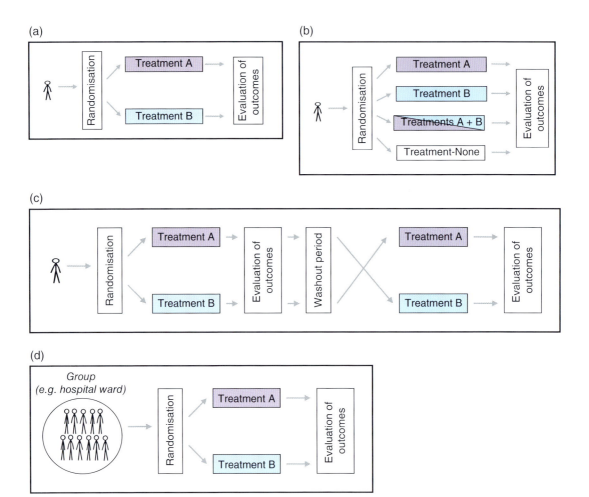

Figure 45.2 Design approaches for randomised controlled trials. (a) Randomised two-group parallel design: subjects randomly assigned to treatment A or B. (b) Factorial design: all subjects randomly assigned to treatment A, treatment B, treatment A + B or no treatment. (c) Randomised crossover design: subjects randomly assigned to treatment A followed by treatment B (after wash-out period) or treatment B followed by treatment A. (d) Randomised cluster design: all subjects in one group/area (e.g. by physician, by hospital, by ward) are assigned to treatment A or B. *Source*: Adapted from Tinmouth and Hebert 2007 [23].

threshold values of platelets $>50 \times 10^9$/L, fibrinogen >1 g/L and the maintenance of the PT and APTT <1.5 times the mean control.

Heparin anticoagulation may also be useful when DIC is complicated by microvascular thrombosis or large vessel thrombosis. Low-dose continuous intravenous therapy (500–1000 IU/h) is one suggested regimen. Critically ill patients with DIC who are not bleeding should receive heparin thromboprophylaxis.

Antithrombin concentrate may have a role in the management of certain groups of patients (e.g. those who do not respond to simple replacement therapy, overwhelming sepsis and meningococcaemia).

Trauma

Uncontrolled haemorrhage is responsible for 30–40% of deaths from trauma. By the time the patient reaches hospital, a coagulopathy has often begun and needs to be corrected promptly to prevent further haemorrhage and allow treatment of injuries. The coagulopathy is multifactorial, with the leading causes being:

- consumption of clotting factors and platelets
- dilution of clotting factors due to fluid resuscitation/massive transfusion
- acidosis leading to clotting factor dysfunction
- hypothaermia leading to clotting factor dysfunction
- DIC, particularly in those with brain injuries.

The combination of acidosis, hypothaermia and coagulopathy is referred to as the 'lethal triad'. Early recognition of the condition is imperative using standard coagulation testing, but there are limitations in this setting and the value of global haemostasis measures, such as TEG and ROTEM®, is being explored. Blood component replacement remains the cornerstone of management. The target for red cell replacement is usually Hb >8 g/dL and for platelets is >50–75×10^9/L. FFP transfusion is likely to be needed once one blood volume has been transfused and is usually given at a dose of 15 mL/kg. In addition, if the fibrinogen level is <1 g/L then fibrinogen concentrates or cryoprecipitate can be given.

Recombinant FVIIa has also been used in cases of refractory trauma-induced coagulopathy to supplement use of FFP. There is only evidence for its benefit in blunt trauma in clinical studies [13]; in more rigorous trials, no mortality benefit has been shown. In addition, the results of the CRASH-2 trial have showed that early administration of tranexamic acid to trauma patients significantly reduces mortality from bleeding without an increase in vascular occlusive events [14].

Liver Disease

All coagulation factors (except VWF) and protease inhibitors are synthesised by hepatocytes. In liver disease, a hypocoagulable state may result from a number of mechanisms: reduced synthesis of coagulation factors; cholestasis and subsequent malabsorption resulting in vitamin K deficiency; and an acquired 'dysfibrinogenaemia'. The platelet count is often reduced due to hypersplenism.

Laboratory abnormalities seen in liver disease include prolonged PT, APTT and thrombin time (TT); the latter may result from low fibrinogen or dysfibrinogenaemia. A prolonged reptilase time in spite of a normal fibrinogen implies a dysfibrinogenaemia or elevated D-dimers.

Coagulation abnormalities occur frequently in patients with severe liver disease, but they are not always associated with bleeding. Bleeding is often precipitated by an event such as surgery or liver biopsy and is rarely attributable to the haemostatic defect alone. If there is bleeding or strong risk for bleeding, then FFP is indicated. Large volumes of FFP are often required to control the bleeding/correct the defect, and this can be problematic in patients who may already have an expanded plasma volume. Complete normalisation of a prolonged PT is often not possible and the use of PCCs may be considered. However, one must be aware of the potential risks of inducing thrombosis or DIC in these patients, particularly since they already suffer from impaired clearance of activated clotting factors and reduced levels of antithrombin. Vitamin K in doses of 10–20 mg may produce some improvement in the coagulation abnormalities. Since thrombocytopenia and platelet function defects are also a feature of hepatic disease, platelet concentrates may also need to be given to maintain a platelet count above $50 \times 10^9/L$. For patients undergoing liver biopsies, the prothrombin time should be corrected to within 2–3 seconds of the upper limit of normal.

Uraemia

The haemostatic defect is mainly due to platelet dysfunction and a defect in platelet–vessel wall interactions, but laboratory abnormalities of platelet function do not appear to correlate well with clinical bleeding. It is also thought that plasma from uraemic patients contains an inhibitor that interferes with normal VWF–platelet interaction.

Dialysis is useful in reversing the haemostatic defects in uraemia, although it may not correct them entirely. Anaemia (particularly when the haematocrit is <20%) should be corrected by either blood transfusion or erythropoietin as this improves platelet function and shortens bleeding time. Infusions of DDAVP (0.3–0.4 µg/kg) have been used successfully to provide short-term correction of the bleeding time and decrease symptoms of bleeding.

Complications of Anticoagulant and Thrombolytic Drugs

Vitamin K Antagonists

Coumarin and phenindione derivatives act by blocking the gamma-carboxylation of glutamic acid residues of vitamin K-dependent coagulation factors, resulting in decreased biological activity of factors II, VII, IX and X, as well as proteins C and S. The international normalised ratio (INR) monitors their effect on the haemostatic system.

Management of excessive anticoagulation depends on the INR level and whether there is minor or major bleeding [15]. In the absence of haemorrhage, warfarin should be stopped for a few days and recommenced when the INR falls into the desired range. Small doses of vitamin K (1–2.5 mg) may be given intravenously/orally if the INR >5.0, as there is a significantly greater risk of serious haemorrhage at this level.

If the patient is bleeding, the anticoagulant effect should be reversed. Vitamin K 5–10 mg should be given intravenously and will have an initial onset of action after 4–6 hours. The action of vitamin K is, however, not maximal for at least 24 hours and therefore additional measures are required.

- Prothrombin complex concentrates: Kcentra (CSL Behring), Beriplex® (CSL Behring) and Octaplex® (Octapharma), which contain factors II, VII, IX and X, are now recommended as the first line for warfarin reversal in case of life- or limb-threatening bleeding, when available. Dosing depends on patient INR at the time of bleeding and PCC used. The disadvantage of these concentrates is that they carry the potential risk of inducing thromboembolism; however, they have much less risk of thromboembolism compared to activated PCC. When using these products, caution should be exercised, especially in high-risk groups.
- In the absence of PCCs, FFP (15–20 mL/kg) will immediately supply the necessary coagulation factors. However, very large amounts of plasma may need to be infused in order to correct the coagulopathy, which may lead to volume overload in some patients.

Red cell and platelet transfusion may become necessary if major bleeding occurs. Platelet transfusion should also be considered if the patient is also treated with antiplatelet therapy.

New Oral Anticoagulants

Several new oral anticoagulants have recently been introduced that have the advantage of not requiring routine monitoring. Drugs currently available include the direct thrombin inhibitor dabigatran and the FXa inhibitors rivaroxaban, apixaban and endoxaban [16]. They have no food interactions and fewer drug interactions than warfarin. Idarucizumab (Praxbind), a humanized monoclonal antibody fragment (Fab), has been approved for reversal of the anticoagulant effect of dabigatran in life-threatening or uncontrolled bleeding or for emergency surgery or procedure. There is no antidote available yet in case of bleeding for patients on FXa inhibitors, although it may become available soon. For drugs with no specific reversal agents, supportive care of bleeding patients should be provided with haemodynamic support and transfusion of blood products in cases of significant haemorrhage. Dialysis has not worked for Xa inhibitors due to high protein binding. PCCs have been used to treat bleeding with Xa inhibitors and rVIIa has been used to treat bleeding with both IIa and Xa inhibitors; however, data are limited and concern for thrombosis remains. There are no ideal tests for evaluation of bleeding patients; the dilute thrombin time, ecarin clotting time or anti-Xa assay using the relevant drug can be used if available.

Thrombolytic Agents

These agents generally cause a state of systemic lysis. Laboratory tests such as the thrombin time and fibrinogen levels will detect the presence of a systemic lytic state, but they do not predict the likelihood of haemorrhage, and most current protocols use fixed-dose schedules.

Haemorrhage complicating these agents is most commonly local (e.g. at the site of catheterisation in the groin); however, intracranial or gastrointestinal bleeding may occur. Measures such as pressure packs will often control local bleeding; more serious bleeding usually necessitates discontinuing thrombolysis. Most agents have a short half-life (minutes) and so the fibrinolytic state will reverse within a few hours of drug cessation. In the case of life-threatening haemorrhage, infusions of cryoprecipitate or FFP can be given to reverse the hypocoagulable state. Antifibrinolytic drugs such as epsilon-aminocaproic acid may or may not provide some additional benefit.

Vitamin K Deficiency

Conditions that impair vitamin K absorption (e.g. biliary tract obstruction) as well as haemorrhagic disease of the newborn can result in a coagulopathy similar to that seen with warfarin overdosage. Any serious/life-threatening bleeding should be treated in the same manner.

Cardiopulmonary Bypass

Haemostatic disturbances that occur during cardiopulmonary bypass (CPB) are multifactorial and related to large doses of heparin, haemodilution, activation and consumption of platelets and coagulation factors by plastic tubing of the CPB circuit, increased thrombin generation and fibrinolysis. The use of TEG or ROTEM may help in guiding replacement therapy in bleeding patients, improve the use of blood products and factor concentrates and is reported to be cost-effective [17].

Acquired Prothrombotic Conditions Treated with Plasma Products

Thrombotic Thrombocytopenic Purpura

Patients with thrombotic thrombocytopenic purpura (TTP) require therapeutic plasma exchange (TPE) with FFP to achieve remission. FFP contains ADAMTS-13, the metalloproteinase enzyme that is deficient or inhibited in TTP. ADAMTS-13 degrades ultralarge multimers of VWF that cause platelet activation and consumption. If TPE is not readily available, simple infusion of plasma should be initiated. FFP and cryoprecipitate-poor plasma can be used interchangeably. Patients with acute idiopathic TTP sometimes require immunosuppression to maintain remission. Rituximab is increasingly being used in TTP and reduces the total amount of plasma received by patients by reducing the number of relapses [18].

Inherited Deficiencies of Coagulation Inhibitors

Previously, FFP has been used as a source of antithrombin III (AT III); however, now specific concentrates or recombinant AT III are available and should be used in perioperative or peripartum setting in patients with congenital AT III deficiency. Patients with AT III deficiency may also be resistant to heparin and may also require AT III concentrate to achieve therapeutic effects of heparin. In some countries, protein C concentrate is also approved as replacement therapy for patients with congenital protein C deficiency. FFP should be used when specific factor concentrates are not available.

Acknowledgement

We would like to acknowledge Vickie McDonald from University College London Hospitals NHS Foundation Trust, London, and Samuel J. Machin from the Haemostasis Research Unit, Department of Haematology, University College London, London, for their authorship of the fourth edition of this chapter which was used as the basis for the current update.

KEY POINTS

1) Clinical history is the most important component in evaluation of patients with bleeding symptoms.
2) Initial laboratory investigation of haemostasis should include a full blood count with platelet count, prothrombin time, activated partial thromboplastin time and blood film.
3) In inherited bleeding disorders, recombinant products should be used where available.
4) The mainstay of DIC treatment remains management of the underlying cause. In bleeding patients, prompt administration of FFP and cryoprecipitate with regular laboratory monitoring is required.
5) Appropriate guidelines (e.g. those provided by the British Committee for Standards in Haematology) should be followed when managing major haemorrhage, aiming for the following parameters: Hb >8 g/dL; platelets $>50 \times 10^9$/L; PT and APTT $<1.5 \times$ mean control; fibrinogen >1 g/L.
6) PCCs should be the first choice for urgent reversal of vitamin K antagonists in cases of life- or limb-threatening bleeding.
7) Patients with TTP should receive therapeutic plasma exchange.

References

1 Hoffman M. A cell-based model of coagulation and the role of factor VIIa. Blood Rev 2003;**17**(Suppl. 1):S1–S5.
2 Versteeg HH, Heemskerk JWM, Levi M, Reitsma PH. New fundamentals of hemostasis. Physiol Rev 2013;**93**:327–58.
3 Keeling D, Tait C, Makris M. Guideline on the selection and use of therapeutic products to treat haemophilia and other hereditary bleeding disorders. A United Kingdom Haemophilia Center Doctors' Organisation (UKHCDO) guideline approved by the British Committee for Standards in Haematology. Haemophilia 2008;**14**:671–84.
4 Mahlangu J, Powell JS, Ragni MV et al. Phase 3 study of recombinant factor VIII Fc fusion protein in hemophilia A. Blood 2014;**123**:317–25.
5 Powell JS, Pasi KJ, Ragni MV et al. Phase 3 study of recombinant factor IX Fc fusion protein in hemophilia B. N Engl J Med 2013;**369**:2313–23.
6 Powell J, Shapiro A, Ragni M et al. Switching to recombinant factor IX Fc fusion protein prophylaxis results in fewer infusions, decreased factor IX consumption and lower bleeding rates. Br J Haematol 2015;**168**:113–23.

7 Hay CR, Brown S, Collins PW, Keeling DM, Liesner R. The diagnosis and management of factor VIII and IX inhibitors: a guideline from the United Kingdom Haemophilia Centre Doctors' Organisation. Br J Haematol 2006;**133**:591–605.

8 Laffan M, Brown SA, Collins PW et al. The diagnosis of von Willebrand disease: a guideline from the UK Haemophilia Centre Doctors' Organisation. Haemophilia 2004;**10**:199–217.

9 Pasi KJ, Collins PW, Keeling DM et al. Management of von Willebrand disease: a guideline from the UK Haemophilia Centre Doctors' Organisation. Haemophilia 2004;**10**: 218–31.

10 Bolton-Maggs PH, Perry DJ, Chalmers EA et al. The rare coagulation disorders – review with guidelines for management from the United Kingdom Haemophilia Centre Doctors' Organisation. Haemophilia 2004;**10**:593–628.

11 Levi M, Toh CH, Thachil J, Watson HG. Guidelines for the diagnosis and management of disseminated intravascular coagulation. British Committee for Standards in Haematology. Br J Haematol 2009;**145**:24–33.

12 Toh CH, Hoots WK. The scoring system of the Scientific and Standardisation Committee on Disseminated Intravascular Coagulation of the International Society on Thrombosis and Haemostasis: a 5-year overview. J Thromb Haemost 2007;**5**:604–6.

13 Hauser CJ, Boffard K, Dutton R et al. Results of the CONTROL trial: efficacy and safety of recombinant activated Factor VII in the management of refractory traumatic hemorrhage. J Trauma 2010;**69**:489–500.

14 Shakur H, Roberts I, Bautista R et al. Effects of tranexamic acid on death, vascular occlusive events, and blood transfusion in trauma patients with significant haemorrhage (CRASH-2): a randomised, placebo-controlled trial. Lancet 2010;**376**:23–32.

15 Keeling D, Baglin T, Tait C et al. Guidelines on oral anti-coagulation with warfarin – fourth edition. Br J Haematol 2011;**154**:311–24.

16 Garcia D, Libby E, Crowther MA. The new oral anti-coagulants. Blood 2010;**115**:15–20.

17 Besser MW, Ortmann E, Klein AA. Haemostatic management of cardiac surgical haemorrhage. Anaesthesia 2015;**70**:87–e31.

18 Scully M, McDonald V, Cavenagh J et al. A phase 2 study of the safety and efficacy of rituximab with plasma exchange in acute acquired thrombotic thrombocytopenic purpura. Blood 2011;**118**:1746–53.

Further Reading

British Committee for Standards in Haematology. Guidelines for the use of fresh frozen plasma, cryoprecipitate and cryosupernatant. Br J Haematol 2004;**126**:11–28.

British Committee for Standards in Haematology. Guidelines on the assessment of bleeding risk prior to surgery or invasive procedures. Br J Haematol 2008;**140**:496–504.

Laffan MA, Lester W, O'Donnell JS et al. The diagnosis and management of von Willebrand disease: a United Kingdom Haemophilia Centre Doctors' Organisation guideline approved by the British Committee for Standards in Haematology. Br J Haematol 2014;**167**(4):453–65.

Paediatric Working Party of the UK Haemophilia Doctors' Organisation. The management of haemophilia in the fetus and neonate. Br J Haematol 2011;**154**: 208–15.

Sucker C, Zotz RB. The cell-based coagulation model, in Perioperative Hemostasis: Coagulation for Anesthesiologists (eds Marcucci C, Schoettker P). Heidelberg: Springer, 2015, pp. 3–11.

Richards M, Williams M, Chalmers E et al., for the Paediatric Working Party of the UK Haemophilia

Doctors' Organisation. Guideline on the use of prophylactic factor VIII concentrate in children and adults with severe haemophilia A. Br J Haematol 2010;**149**:498–507.

Scully M, Hunt BJ, Benjamin S et al., for the British Committee for Standards in Haematology. Guidelines on the diagnosis and management of thrombotic thrombocytopenic purpura and other thrombotic microangiopathies. Br J Haematol 2012;**158**(3):323–35.

Srivastava AK, Brewer EP, Mauser-Bunschoten NS et al. Guidelines for the management of haemophilia. Haemophilia 2013;**19**(1): e1–47.

Tripodi A, Mannucci PM. Mechanisms of disease: the coagulopathy of chronic liver disease. N Engl J Med 2001;**365**:147–56.

26 Massive Blood Loss

John R. Hess

Departments of Laboratory Medicine and Hematology, University of Washington School of Medicine, and Harborview Transfusion Service, Seattle, USA

Definition and Burden of Massive Blood Loss

Massive blood loss has been defined in many ways, from acute haemorrhagic death to ongoing bleeding requiring variously three blood components in one hour, five units of red blood cells (RBCs) in six hours or 10 units of RBCs in 24 hours. However defined, massive blood loss is not a rare event, occurring in between one in 2000 and one in 4000 individuals yearly in developed and peaceful countries [1]. Haemorrhage is the second most common cause of injury death and the most common cause of maternal death. Successful treatment requires planned responses and immediately available resources. Improvements in the management of massive blood loss following injury using hypotensive and haemostatic or 'damage control' resuscitation to support surgical or transvascular control of bleeding have reduced the mortality of grade V liver injury by at least 70% in the last 30 years [2]. This demonstrated ability to save lives with damage control resuscitation has led to new standards and accreditation requirements for hospitals and their blood services [3,4]. Reducing mortality for trauma is also driving efforts to extend blood product-based resuscitation into

prehospital care and to other, nontrauma causes of uncontrolled haemorrhage.

Recently, Sweden and Denmark have been able to gather information on 97 000 massive transfusion episodes occurring in their joint 15 million populations over the 24-year period between 1987 and 2010 [1] (Box 26.1). Fifty six percent of these were acute episodes, defined as patients given 10 or more units of RBCs in two consecutive calendar days, and the remainder were more prolonged subacute bleeding episodes with 10 units given over a seven-day period. For the acute bleeding episodes, 35% occurred in the course of cardiovascular surgery, 16% followed trauma, 11% with cancer surgery, 23% during other surgery, 10% during general nonoperative medical care, 2% with obstetric emergencies and 1% each with uncontrolled bleeding in haematological and nonhaematological cancers. Overall, 30-day mortality was 25% and the average number of RBC units given was 25, suggesting that massive transfusion is a highly effective and cost-effective therapy. A smaller review of 1360 ultra-massive transfusions, defined as the transfusion of more than 20 units of RBCs over two consecutive calendar days, collected from nine hospitals in six developed countries, again showed that 35% occurred during cardiovascular

Practical Transfusion Medicine, Fifth Edition. Edited by Michael F. Murphy, David J. Roberts and Mark H. Yazer.
© 2017 John Wiley & Sons Ltd. Published 2017 by John Wiley & Sons Ltd.

Box 26.1 Trauma resuscitation strategies have changed in last 10 years.

- There is an acute coagulopathy of trauma. Volume resuscitation with crystalloid will make it worse. Early administration of haemostatic blood components for volume resuscitation appears to improve outcome.
- Clinical judgement of massive haemorrhage risk is poor. Assessment scores, such as the Assessment of Blood Consumption (ABC) score, improve prediction. The ABC score gives one point each for systolic BP <90, pulse >110, penetrating mechanism, evidence of free intraabdominal blood by focused abdominal sonography for trauma (FAST). Score ≥2 has a 50% risk of massive haemorrhage.
- Patients in deep shock go straight to OR for attempted haemorrhage control. Those who can tolerate delay get CT scanning to further define extent of injury and sites of bleeding.
- The Critical Administration Threshold of 3 blood components in 1 hour (CAT1) should not be exceeded before declaring a massive

transfusion and initiating a massive transfusion protocol.
- Administering blood components initially in a 1:1:1 unit ratio of plasma:platelets:RBCs insures early coverage of all likely deficits. This requires early access to thawed universal donor plasma, type AB or type A with low-titre B.
- Tranexamic acid limits fibrinolysis, improving haemostasis, reducing blood use and improving survival.
- Resuscitation should be goal directed to correct laboratory-defined deficits as soon as possible. Emergency haemorrhage panels (Hct, Plt, PT and fibrinogen) can be obtained quickly and guide RBC, platelet, plasma and cryoprecipitate administration respectively. The use of TEG/RoTEM is less accurate and less directly correlated with blood component needs.
- It is the author's experience that haemostatic management of bleeding is poorly taught and remains poorly managed in many areas.

---

surgery, 20% transplant surgery, 15% trauma and 2% obstetric emergencies [5]. In this group of mostly elderly patients, 30-day mortality averaged 40%.

This chapter will review:

- the epidemiology of haemorrhage-related mortality following injury
- the acute coagulopathy of trauma and the need for haemostatic resuscitation
- the limitations of conventional blood products and of their ability to provide haemostatic resuscitation
- the effect of blood product ratios in massive haemorrhage resuscitation
- the applicability of this information to patients with surgical and obstetric bleeding
- the special considerations involved in resuscitating infants and children raised by their small blood volume relative to the volume of conventional blood components.

Haemorrhage-Related Mortality Following Injury

Among civilian injury-related deaths that occur after reaching the hospital, over half are the result of profound neurological injury and a third result from uncontrolled haemorrhage [6]. Usually, the remaining deaths are due to multiple organ failure. High energy blunt trauma, such as that sustained in a motor vehicle accident, is the major cause of such injuries, and the critical bleeding sites are largely truncal and buried within the body, involving vascular tears and organ disruption. Injury patterns are frequently complex, and care in specialised trauma centres equipped for and practiced in evaluating and dealing with such patients is associated with markedly better outcomes. In recent studies, half of all haemorrhage deaths in trauma patients in level 1 trauma centres occurred during the first two hours of care, emphasising the importance of early access to haemostatic resuscitation and high-level care [6]. In the Boston Marathon bombings, all patients who reached the hospital alive survived [7].

For battlefield casualties, most of which involve penetrating injury, the fraction of haemorrhagic deaths is higher and time to death is even shorter; 80% of battlefield deaths occur before casualties reach a hospital. Among 6000 fatal US battle casualties in Vietnam, 40% died essentially instantly, 65% were dead within five minutes, 80% in 30 minutes and 90% within two hours of injury [8]. As many of these injuries involved the arteries of the extremities, 50% of the mass and surface area of the body, combat mortality has decreased with increased use of tourniquets and haemorrhage control bandages.

Coagulopathy after Injury

Blood loss and dilution, acidosis and hypothermia and platelet and coagulation factor consumption and fibrinolysis all contribute to coagulopathy (Box 26.2) [9]. As injury severity measured by the injury severity score (ISS) increases, the probability that most of these mechanisms will be active increases. As a result, there is an acute coagulopathy of trauma that manifests as abnormal coagulation tests shortly after injury and is present in about 10% of those patients who are severely injured (ISS >15) and in about 30% of profoundly injured (ISS >24) patients at admission to a trauma centre. Prolongation of the prothrombin time (PT) is the most frequently observed abnormality, followed by reduced fibrinogen, prolongation of the partial thromboplastic time (PTT) and reduced platelet counts [10].

Having this acute coagulopathy of trauma was associated with a fourfold excess risk of dying when the condition was first described a decade ago [11]. Early recognition and treatment of the acute coagulopathy of trauma have become goals in systems of goal-directed trauma care. How best to accomplish these goals remains controversial. Early recognition is limited as the injuries in victims of blunt trauma are often internal and imaging and laboratory tests take time to process and report. Treatment is limited by the cryptic nature of the extent of injury and the frequent lack of immediately available haemostatic blood products.

Box 26.2 Causes of coagulopathy in trauma patients.

- Blood loss: 30–40 + % of blood volume can be lost in patients with stage 3 or 4 shock before resuscitation begins.
- Blood dilution: physiological vascular refill and nonplasma fluid administration dilute plasma coagulation factors and platelets.
- Hypothermia: reduces plasma coagulation enzyme activity by 10% per °C. Coupling between platelet adhesion and activation is lost between 30 °C and 34 °C.
- Acidosis: reduces coagulation factor complex assembly and, therefore, enzyme activity.

Activity is 50% at pH 7.2, 30% at pH 7.0 and 20% at pH 6.8.
- Coagulation factor and platelet consumption: coagulation factors and platelets exist in the normal body in limited amounts. The amounts can be severely depleted by large endothelial area injury and local cycles of local activation and inactivation.
- Fibrinolysis: protein C inactivation of plasminogen activator inhibitor can allow clot breakdown, emphasising the importance of tranexamic acid.

The Limits of Resuscitation with Conventional Blood Products

Patients with massive haemorrhage often need several different blood components at once. However, giving RBCs to maintain oxygen transport while giving plasma and platelets to restore coagulation functions means that the administered products compete with each other for space in the blood volume as the plasma dilutes the RBCs and the additive solution in the RBCs dilutes the plasma. This effect can be seen when whole blood is 'reconstituted' from blood components by mixing back together the unit of RBCs, unit of plasma and unit of platelets made from a single whole blood donation (Figure 26.2). The original whole blood had a haematocrit of around 40%, a platelet count of about $250 \times 10^9/L$, and plasma coagulation factors of averaging $1\,U/mL$. But when the components are added back together, the resulting haematocrit is 29%, the platelet count about $90 \times 10^9/L$ and the concentration of clotting factors about $0.65\,U/mL$ [12]. The seeming losses result from dilution with $70\,mL$ of anti-

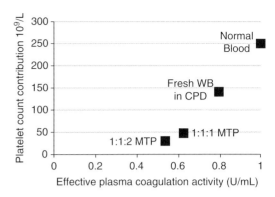

Figure 26.2 Losses of platelet concentration and plasma coagulation factor activity with pooling blood components in ratios.

coagulant and $110\,mL$ of RBC additive solution, along with real losses of cellular components and plasma in the leucocyte reduction filters and bag-to-bag transfers in processing steps. Further, recovered blood cell counts are lower than administered blood cell counts; about 90% of the transfused RBCs and 70% of the transfused platelets are recovered because of storage-related cellular injury that limits *in vivo* recovery. The end result is that giving massively bleeding patients only blood components in a

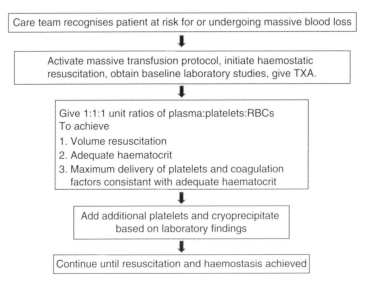

Figure 26.1 Proposed schema for a massive transfusion protocol.

Box 26.3 Results of blood product administration.

- RBCs: one unit increases the Hb by 1 g and Hct by 3% in a 70 kg individual.
- Platelets: one adult dose increases the platelet count by $\approx 30 \pm 15 \times 10^9/L$ in an afebrile, non-obese, nonbleeding patient.
- Plasma: one 250 mL unit increases plasma coagulation factors by 2.5%. Six to eight units

are needed for a 15–20% correction in critically ill or injured patients.
- Cryoprecipitate: one 5 U pool will deliver 1.5 g of fibrinogen and increase fibrinogen concentration by 0.3–0.4 g/L.

1:1:1 ratio of units of plasma, platelets and RBCs as their sole resuscitation fluids barely keeps the haematocrit above 25%, the platelet count above $50 \times 10^9/L$ and the PT and PTT below 1.5 times normal. Giving additional amounts of any one product dilutes the other two and giving additional crystalloid or colloid fluid dilutes all three. Transitioning as quickly as possible to goal-directed therapy, whereby specific products are administered to correct specific deficits as dictated by laboratory testing, should be a focus in managing patients with massive haemorrhage (Box 26.3).

Efficacy of Damage Control Resuscitation

As trauma surgeons adopted resuscitation strategies that markedly limited the amount of crystalloid fluids given and replaced lost intravascular volume with 1:1:1 ratios of blood component units, they noticed several effects. First, the rates of pulmonary oedema and gut swelling that required prolonged intensive care unit (ICU) stays for ventilation and abdominal closure diminished. Second, when they reviewed their experience, mortality was markedly lower in patients who received higher ratios of plasma to RBCs. Finally, overall rates of haemorrhagic mortality and blood use declined. Among critics of plasma use, there has been a tendency to concentrate on the second finding, where in the retrospective studies, it has been impossible to separate the effects of administered plasma on

improved survival from the effects of injury severity on survival. This problem, known as 'survivor bias', confounds many retrospective studies in the field.

Survivor bias is less of an issue in large consecutive series. Johansson and Stensbele described a 30% decrease in the mortality of massive transfusion at the University of Copenhagen hospital with the institution of balanced resuscitation. Cotton and colleagues reported improved survival and lower blood use in a large series of damage control laparotomies comparing periods before and after the institution of 1:1:1 resuscitation. The Dutch military has described survivorship increasing from 44% to 84% in their military casualties after they shifted to 1:1 resuscitation in 2007. The seven US academic trauma centres involved in the Host Response to Injury Large Scale Collaborative Programme noted a 50% decrease in the rate of patients who received one unit of RBCs going on to receive 10 units as the fraction of total plasma and platelets administered in the first hours after admission increased. Finally, the marked improvement in survivorship after grade V liver injury from 24% to 94% was already noted.

The Pragmatic Randomized Optimal Plasma and Platelet Ratios (PROPPR) trial is the only randomised trial to address the question of ratio-based transfusion [13]. However, the trial was underpowered for the observed 30-day mortality of 24%, and the differences in mortality between arms resuscitated with 1:1:1 versus 1:1:2 unit ratios of plasma:platelets:RBCs were not different at the primary safety endpoints of 24 hours or 30 days. However, at secondary endpoints more patients achieved anatomical haemostasis, and more haemorrhaging patients were alive with 1:1:1-based therapy. At the end of the study, the absolute differences in haemorrhagic mortality between the arms remained as equivalent numbers of patients died of CNS injury and multiple organ failure. As a result, the case for damage control resuscitation remains strong, but unsupported by level 1 evidence.

Tranexamic acid for uncontrolled bleeding in trauma is associated with level 1 evidence of efficacy and should be routinely used for all patients at risk of hyperfibrinolysis, such as trauma patients [14]. The benefit appears to be limited to the first three hours after injury in typical patients.

Can the Lessons of Damage Control Resuscitation for Trauma be Extended to Other Massive Haemorrhage Situations?

As noted in the large retrospective reviews of massive transfusion, one-third of patients who die of massive haemorrhage despite receiving massive transfusion die during cardiovascular surgery [1]. Another 20% die during transplant surgery, frequently during liver transplant [5]. Finally, 2% of haemorrhagic deaths that occur despite massive transfusion happen in the puerperium. In each of these situations, massive bleeding is associated with a unique coagulopathy, and all of these situations appear to benefit from timely haemostatic interventions, haemostatically balanced high-volume transfusion and antifibrinolytic therapy.

This means that massive transfusion protocols need to be developed on an institutional basis for all the common situations of massive bleeding, overseen with scientific expertise and managed as critical quality of care resources [15]. The need for better scientific understanding of these situations cannot be overstated, but the need for action for primary and secondary prevention of massive haemorrhage remains a common problem.

Massive Transfusion in Small Children

Massive transfusion in small children is more difficult because the size of conventional blood components approximates to the size of the blood volume of infants. Such children are best managed by giving alternating small aliquots of approximately 10 mL/kg of RBCs and plasma and converting the plasma to platelets in plasma (as opposed to in additive solution) as soon as possible. Because such a regimen is complex and requires special equipment, a specialised paediatric massive transfusion protocol is important and requires frequent practice.

Conclusion

The management of bleeding and coagulopathy in massive blood loss has been an area of major research for the last 10 years and is the subject of major ongoing research. The priority of initial treatment is to maintain perfusion while improving haemostasis. Attention to patient characteristics such as hypothermia is critical to good clinical outcomes.

KEY POINTS

1) Massive haemorrhage is an emergency. Use the administration of three blood components in one hour, the Critical Administration Threshold (CAT1), as a threshold to initiate a massive transfusion protocol.

2) Massive transfusion is complicated. Have a well-developed massive transfusion protocol, practised by clinical teams and transfusion services.

3) In injured patients, massive haemorrhage is frequently accompanied by volume loss, haemodilution, hypothermia, acidosis, factor consumption and fibrinolysis.

4) Massive transfusion protocols using haemostatic resuscitation are highly effective. Start with 1:1 plasma to RBCs to patients exceeding CAT1, and 1:1:1 plasma and platelets to RBCs in trauma patients. Add fibrinogen with obstetric haemorrhage. Convert to goal-directed therapy based on laboratory values as soon as possible. Children need their own protocols.

5) Use a blood warmer. Six blood components at 4 °C will reduce the core temperature of a 70 kg man by 1 °C and increase haemorrhagic mortality by 10%.

6) Measure laboratory parameters frequently, every 30 minutes during massive transfusion. Having an established emergency haemorrhage panel (Hct, Plt, PT and fibrinogen) is ideal as it is easy to order.

7) Tranexamic acid is effective in a variety of settings. It is life saving in injury.

References

1 Halmin M, Chiesa F, Vasan SK et al. Epidemiology of massive transfusion: a binational study from Sweden and Denmark. Crit Care Med 2016;**44**:468–77.

2 Shrestha B, Holcomb JB, Camp EA et al. Damage-control resuscitation increases successful nonoperative management rates and survival after severe blunt liver injury. J Trauma Acute Care Surg 2015;**78**(2):336–41.

3 ACS TQIP. Massive Transfusion in Trauma Guidelines. ACS, Chicago, 2013.

4 AABB Patient Blood Management Standards, Version 1. AABB, Bethesda, 2014.

5 Dzik WS, Ziman A, Cohn C et al, for the Biomedical Excellence for Safer Transfusion Collaborative. Survival following ultra-massive transfusion: an analysis of 1360 cases. Transfusion 2015;**56**:558–63.

6 Dutton RP, Stansbury LG, Leone S et al. Trauma mortality in mature trauma systems: are we doing better? An analysis of trauma mortality patterns, 1997–2008. J Trauma 2010;**69**:620–6.

7 Quillen K, Luckey CJ. Blood and bombs: blood use after the Boston Marathon bombing of April 15, 2013. Transfusion 2014;**54**(4):1202–3.

8 Bellamy RF. Death on the battlefield and the role of first aid. Mil Med 1987;**152**(12):634–5.

9 Hess JR, Holcomb JB, Wolf SE, Cripps MW. Transfusion therapy in the care of trauma and burn patients, in Rossi's Principles of Transfusion Medicine, 5th edn (eds TG Simon TG et al), Wiley-Blackwell, Oxford, 2015.

10 Hess JR, Lindell AL, Stansbury LG, Dutton RP, Scalea TM. The prevalence of abnormal results of conventional coagulation tests on admission to a trauma center. Transfusion 2009;**49**(1):34–9.

11 Brohi K, Singh J, Heron M, Coats T. Acute traumatic coagulopathy. J Trauma 2003;**54**(6):1127–30.

12 Hess JR, Holcomb JB. Resuscitating PROPPRly. Transfusion 2015;**55**(6):1362–4.

13 Holcomb JB, Tilley BC, Baraniuk S et al, for the PROPPR Study Group. Transfusion of

plasma, platelets, and red blood cells in a 1:1:1 vs. a 1:1:2 ratio and mortality in patients with severe trauma: the PROPPR Randomized Clinical Trial. JAMA 2015;**313**(5):483–94.

14 Shakur H, Roberts I, Bautista R et al, for the CRASH-2 Trial Collaborators. Effects of tranexamic acid on death, vascular occlusive events, and blood transfusion in trauma patients with significant haemorrhage (CRASH-2): a randomised, placebo-controlled trial. Lancet 2010;**376**(9734):23–32.

15 Chay J, Koh M, Tan HH et al. A national common massive transfusion protocol (MTP) is a feasible and advantageous option for centralized blood services and hospitals. Vox Sang 2016;**110**:36–50.

Further Reading

Chandler WL, Ferrell C, Trimble S, Moody S. Development of a rapid emergency hemorrhage panel. Transfusion 2010;**50**(12):2547–52.

Ducloy-Bouthors AS, Susen S, Wong CA, Butwick A, Vallet B, Lockhart E. Medical advances in the treatment of postpartum hemorrhage. Anesth Analg 2014;**119**(5):1140–7.

Dyke C, Aronson S, Dietrich W et al. Universal definition of perioperative bleeding in adult cardiac surgery. J Thorac Cardiovasc Surg 2014;**147**(5):1458–63.

Hess JR, Brohi K, Dutton RP et al. The coagulopathy of trauma: a review of mechanisms. J Trauma 2008;**65**(4):748–54.

Hughes NT, Burd RS, Teach SJ. Damage control resuscitation: permissive hypotension and massive transfusion protocols. Pediatr Emerg Care 2014;**30**(9):651–6.

Kacmar RM, Mhyre JM, Scavone BM, Fuller AJ, Toledo P. The use of postpartum hemorrhage protocols in United States academic obstetric anesthesia units. Anesth Analg 2014;**119**(4):906–10.

McQuilten ZK, Crighton G, Engelbrecht S et al. Transfusion interventions in critical bleeding requiring massive transfusion: a systematic review. Transfus Med Rev 2015;**29**(2):127–37.

Novak DJ, Bai Y, Cooke RK et al, for the PROPPR Study Group. Making thawed universal donor plasma available rapidly for massively bleeding trauma patients: experience from the Pragmatic, Randomized Optimal Platelets and Plasma Ratios (PROPPR) trial. Transfusion 2015;**55**(6):1331–9.

Siegal DM. Managing target-specific oral anticoagulant associated bleeding including an update on pharmacological reversal agents. J Thromb Thrombolysis 2015;**39**(3):395–402.

27 Blood Management in Acute Haemorrhage and Critical Care

Gavin J. Murphy[1], Nicola Curry[2], Nishith N. Patel[3] and Timothy S. Walsh[4]

[1] *Cardiac Surgery, School of Cardiovascular Sciences, University of Leicester, Leicester, UK*
[2] *Oxford Haemophilia & Thrombosis Centre, Churchill Hospital, Oxford, UK*
[3] *Cardiac Surgery, School of Clinical Sciences, University of Bristol, Bristol, UK*
[4] *Clinical and Surgical Sciences, Edinburgh University, Edinburgh, UK; Anaesthetics and Intensive Care, Edinburgh Royal Infirmary, Edinburgh, UK*

Introduction

Good blood management emphasises the importance of utilising blood components as part of an overall treatment strategy that is focused on improving patient outcome. Acute haemorrhage and acute anaemia are common in surgical, obstetric and critical care patients. They are also prevalent in nonsurgical patients with upper gastrointestinal (GI) haemorrhage.

These often critically ill patients are characterised by:

- a high red cell transfusion requirement
- usually being cared for in highly monitored environments in which co-interventions with therapeutic adjuncts and the use of evidence-based protocols can reduce the use of conventional blood components
- coagulopathy that requires management to assist correction of cardiovascular instability and anaemia.

This chapter reviews the evidence to guide blood management strategies in patients with critical illness or who are undergoing major surgery with an emphasis on those that have been shown to improve clinical outcomes.

It also specifically considers changes in the management of massive haemorrhage/blood transfusion that have occurred in recent years, as this represents a clinical situation where appropriate blood management is a key determinant of patient outcomes, including survival.

Red Cell Transfusion

Anaemia and Acute Haemorrhage

Anaemia and acute haemorrhage in surgical and critically ill patients accounts for almost 50% of all red cell utilisation. In a UK study [1], the main users of allogeneic red cells were upper GI haemorrhage (13.8%), orthopaedic surgery (6.3%), trauma (5.9%), liver/GI surgery 5.5% and cardiac surgery (5.2%). Over 10% of all red cell transfusions are administered in the intensive care unit (ICU) setting.

In acute haemorrhage, the therapeutic priority is to achieve source control; during this period, the aim is to maintain adequate oxygen delivery to prevent tissue hypoxia and organ dysfunction using fluids, red cells and interventions to prevent or correct coagulopathy. Once haemorrhage has been stopped,

Practical Transfusion Medicine, Fifth Edition. Edited by Michael F. Murphy, David J. Roberts and Mark H. Yazer.
© 2017 John Wiley & Sons Ltd. Published 2017 by John Wiley & Sons Ltd.

management is similar to that for the acutely anaemic patient. This is supported by prospective epidemiological studies in critical care patients where transfusion indicators, i.e. haemoglobin thresholds, are similar in bleeding and nonbleeding patients [2]. Anaemia in the absence of haemorrhage occurs in surgical patients as a result of low preoperative red cell mass or haemodilution, and this may account for the greater proportion of all red cell transfusions. For example, in cardiac surgery, severe haemorrhage occurs in up to 15% of patients, but red cell transfusion occurs in 50–95% of patients, depending on institutional transfusion practice [3].

Acute anaemia is also common in critical care where the aetiology is multifactorial and includes haemodilution, occult blood loss, therapeutic blood sampling and/or impaired haematopoiesis that may be acute, as a result of sepsis for example, or chronic, as a result of chronic renal or other systemic disease. Anaemia is strongly associated with adverse outcomes in the critically ill. Despite the use of multiple interventions and therapeutic adjuncts, such as avoidance of haemodilution, excessive therapeutic blood sampling or other modalities listed below, red cell transfusion is common. Up to 35–45% of patients receive a blood transfusion within five days of ICU admission, of which as many as 90% are administered to reverse anaemia [2].

Indications for Red Cell Transfusion

The most comprehensive guidelines for red cell transfusion were provided by the American Association of Blood Banks (AABB) in 2012 [4]. They make four recommendations.

1) Adhering to a restrictive transfusion strategy (7–8 g/dL) in hospitalised, stable patients (Grade: strong recommendation; high-quality evidence).
2) Adhering to a restrictive strategy in hospitalised patients with preexisting cardiovascular disease and considering transfusion for patients with symptoms or a haemoglobin level of 8 g/dL or less (Grade: weak recommendation; moderate-quality evidence).
3) The AABB cannot recommend for or against a liberal or restrictive transfusion threshold for hospitalised, haemodynamically stable patients with the acute coronary syndrome (Grade: uncertain recommendation; very low-quality evidence).
4) The AABB suggests that transfusion decisions be influenced by symptoms as well as haemoglobin concentration (Grade: weak recommendation; low-quality evidence).

In the UK, the NICE guidelines for transfusion (currently in draft format for consultation) recommend a restrictive transfusion threshold of 70 g/L [5]. For patients with acute coronary syndrome, the guidelines recommend a transfusion trigger of 80 g/L.

However, a recent systematic review challenges some of the assumptions upon which these recommendations are based [6]. This review included 22 randomised controlled trials (RCTs) recruiting over 10 000 patients who were randomised to either a liberal or restrictive transfusion (haemoglobin) threshold. The actual transfusion trigger for each arm varies between trials. Overall, there is no evidence that the risk of short-term mortality differs between patients randomised to liberal or restrictive transfusion strategies (odds ratio (OR) 1.03, 95% confidence interval (CI) 0.84–1.27). This is demonstrated in the forest plot in Figure 27.1. However, stratifying analyses by cardiac disease state suggests that liberal transfusion strategies reduce mortality in RCTs exclusively recruiting patients with active or symptomatic cardiac disease, such as those undergoing cardiac surgery or experiencing myocardial infarction. This suggests that higher thresholds may be beneficial in patients at the limits of their cardiovascular reserve. The absolute threshold remains to be defined. It is also likely that this varies between patients and for individual patients during the course of their illness.

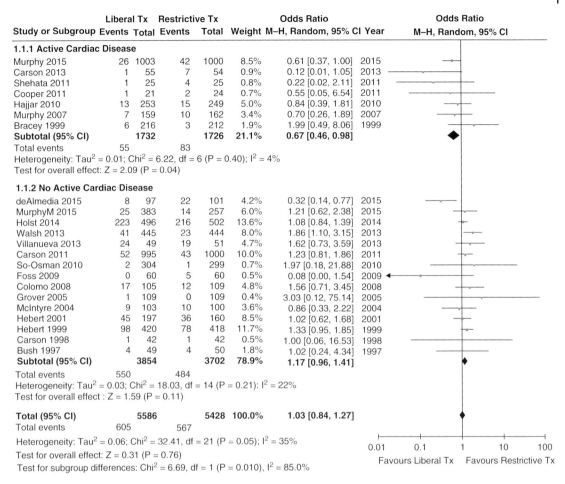

Figure 27.1 Forest plot summarising the odds ratios from RCTs evaluating the relationship between red cell transfusion and 30-day mortality. Upper panel shows odds ratios from RCTs that have compared liberal versus restrictive transfusion thresholds in patients with symptomatic cardiac disease. Lower panel shows odds ratios from RCTs in patients without symptomatic disease. An increasing odds ratio indicates increasing risk of death with transfusion.

Treatment Adjuncts That Reduce Transfusion (see also Chapter 34)

The safety and efficacy of commonly used interventions that reduce transfusion exposure as reported in a series of systematic reviews are summarised in Table 27.1. A limitation of these reviews is that, with the exception of some recent RCTs (BART, CRASH-2), many of the existing trials of blood management interventions included in these analyses have a high risk of bias. This limits the ability of these reviews to provide recommendations for treatment, although they identify important gaps in knowledge that need to be addressed by future trials. A novel feature of more recent reviews is the consideration of combinations of blood management interventions. In many cases, these do not demonstrate an additive benefit from the use of multiple blood management interventions. This is at odds with the 'care bundle' approach,

Table 27.1 Interventions that reduce the risk of acute anaemia and haemorrhage in acute haemorrhage and critical care.

Intervention	Reference	Effect on transfusion risk ratio (95% CI)	Effect on clinical outcome	Risk ratio (95% CI)
Minimise loss of autologous red cells				
Preoperative autologous donation	Henry et al. [7]	0.32 (0.22 to 0.47) 14 trials, 1506 patients	Infection Thrombosis Any transfusion	0.70 (0.34 to 1.43) 0.82 (0.21 to 3.13) 1.24 (1.02 to 1.51)
Acute normovolaemic haemodilution	Davies et al. [8]	0.36 (0.25 to 0.51) 11 trials, n = 1423 patients	Infection Thrombosis	0.70 (0.34 to 1.43) 0.82 (0.21 to 3.13)
Mechanical cell salvage (high-risk patients)	NICE [5]	0.74 (0.58 to 0.93) 4 trials, n = 223 patients	Death Thrombosis Infection	0.97 (0.64 to 1.47) Not estimatable 0.4 (0.18 to 0.87)
Mechanical cell salvage (medium-risk patients)	NICE [5]	0.74 (0.5 to 1.12) 3 trials, n = 384 patients	Death Thrombosis Infection	Not reported
Stimulate erythropoiesis				
IV iron versus placebo or no IV iron (surgery)	NICE [5]	0.77 (0.59 to 0.99) 5 trials, n = 467 patients	Death Thrombosis Infection	1.1 (0.49 to 2.47) - 1.23 (0.63 to 2.42)
Oral iron versus IV iron	NICE [5]	1.2 (0.56 to 2.61) 6 trials, n = 699 patients	Death Thrombosis Infection	1.22 (0.58 to 2.56) - -
Erythropoietin versus placebo (surgery)	NICE [5]	0.59 (0.53 to 0.67) 12 trials, n = 1663 patients	Death Thrombosis Infection	1.55 (0.79 to3.07) 1.37 (0.73 to 2.56) Not estimable
EPO plus IV iron versus placebo	NICE [5]	0.51 (0.39 to 0.67) 2 trials, n = 283	Death Thrombosis Infection	0.33 (0.01 to 7.93) Not estimatable Not estimatable
EPO plus oral iron versus oral iron	NICE [5]	0.06 (0.02 to 0.25) 2 trials, n = 880 patients	Death Thrombosis Infection	0.88 (0.39 to 1.96) 1.71 (0.68 to 4.3) 0.5 (0.05 to 4.98)
Reverse coagulopathy				
Tranexamic acid versus placebo (high-risk surgery)	NICE [5]	0.71 (0.63 to 0.81) 38 trials, n = 4105 patients	Death Thrombosis Infection	0.52 (0.31 to 0.87) 0.62 (0.31 to 1.24) 0.48 (0.18 to 1.23)
Tranexamic acid versus placebo (moderate-risk surgery)	NICE [5]	0.45 (0.38 to 0.52) 25 trials, n = 4577 patients	Death Thrombosis Infection	0.73 (0.15 to 3.66) 0.69 (0.44 to 1.07) 0.93 (0.22 to 3.93)
Tranexamic acid high dose versus low dose (surgery)	Ker et al. [9]	0.62 (0.58 to 0.65) 129 trials, n = 10,488	Death Myocardial infarction Pulmonary embolism	0.61 (0.38 to 0.98) 0.68 (0.43 to 1.09) 1.14 (0.65 to 2.00)
Tranexamic acid versus placebo (trauma)	Ker et al. [10]	0.98 (0.96 to 1.01) 2 trials, 20 367 patients	Death Myocardial infarction Infection	0.90 (0.85 to 0.96) 0.61 (0.40 to 0.92)

(Continued)

Table 27.1 (Continued)

Intervention	Reference	Effect on transfusion risk ratio (95% CI)	Effect on clinical outcome	Risk ratio (95% CI)
Tranexamic plus cell salvage versus cell salvage (high-risk surgical patients)	NICE [5]	0.71 (0.6 to 0.85) 5 trials, n = 514 patients	Death	1.04 (0.07 to 16.41)
Tranexamic plus cell salvage versus tranexamic acid (high-risk surgical patients)	NICE [5]	0.79 (0.43 to 1.45) 1 trial, n = 63 patients	Death	7.71 (0.43 to 137.53)
Aprotinin versus placebo	Henry et al. [11]	0.66 (0.60 to 0.72) 108 trials, n = 11,172 patients	Death Myocardial infarction Renal failure	0.81 (0.63 to 1.06) 0.87 (0.69 to 1.11) 1.10 (0.79 to 1.54)
Aprotinin versus tranexamic acid	Henry et al. [11]	0.90 (0.81 to 1.01) 21 RCTs, n = 4185 patients	Death Myocardial infarction Renal failure	1.35 (0.94 to 1.93) 1.00 (0.71 to 1.42) 1.02 (0.79 to 1.31)
Desmopressin	Carless et al. [12]	0.96 (0.87 to 1.06) 19 RCTs, n = 1387 patient	Death Thrombosis Hypotension	1.72 (0.68 to 4.33) 1.46 (0.64 to 3.35) 2.81 (1.50 to 5.27)
Recombinant activated factor VII	Simpson et al. [13]	0.85 (0.72 to 1.01) 8 RCTs, n = 868 patients	Death Arterial thromboembolic events	1.04 (0.55 to 1.97) 1.45 (1.02 to 2.05)

CI, confidence interval; RCT, randomised controlled trial.

now referred to as patient blood management (see Chapter 34), that has been advocated by enthusiasts of this concept.

Autologous Transfusion Techniques

Preoperative Autologous Donation (PAD)

This involves the patient donating one or more units of his/her own blood preoperatively, often in conjunction with the administration of erythropoietin. This blood is held within the blood transfusion laboratory where it is administered as required during the perioperative stay, as an alternative to allogeneic red cells. PAD is effective at reducing exposure to allogenic blood, but overall exposure to transfused red cells (both autologous and allogeneic) is increased, and PAD is not associated with improved clinical outcomes. Where the local allogeneic blood supply is safe from infectious diseases, PAD may not confer any

overall clinical benefit, so its use should be discouraged. However, it may be advantageous in less developed healthcare systems where transmission of infection by transfusion remains an issue. PAD does not prevent certain reactions like volume overload or febrile nonhaemolytic reactions, nor does it prevent bacterial contamination or the transfusion of an ABO-mismatched unit. PAD is restricted to patients scheduled for elective surgery, requires significant investment in infrastructure for the harvesting, testing and storage of autologous red cells in parallel to the systems in place for allogeneic blood, and its adoption has not been widespread.

Acute Normovolaemic Haemodilution (ANH)

Acute normovolaemic haemodilution involves removing blood from a patient, usually during induction of anaesthesia, replacing it with crystalloid or colloid fluid to maintain circulating volume and storing the blood for reinfusion during surgery as a response to blood loss, or at the end of surgery. Significant haemodilution reduces the red cell mass lost during surgery, and replacement of losses with autologous blood has better homeostatic properties than colloid or crystalloid. ANH may also improve haemostasis by preventing consumption or loss of clotting factors during prolonged procedures or as a result of cardiopulmonary bypass, and has been shown to reduce bleeding rates. ANH also significantly reduces allogeneic red cell exposure, and is inexpensive. It has not been shown to result in specific clinical benefits to patients beyond reducing transfusion exposure. The disadvantages of ANH relate principally to the safety of low haematocrits during surgery, which may increase the risk of neurological, myocardial and renal injury.

Mechanical Cell Salvage

Blood lost as a result of acute haemorrhage during major surgery can be collected (salvaged) using commercially available and widely used devices that wash the blood, removing plasma proteins, cell fragments and other contaminants of the surgical field, allowing reinfusion of washed autologous cells. In high-risk patients, this technique significantly reduces red cell exposure and, more importantly, improves clinical outcomes, including the risk of perioperative infection. There are no apparent benefits in those patients at low risk of bleeding.

Pharmacological Interventions That Stimulate Erythropoiesis

Iron Therapy

The most common cause of anaemia worldwide is iron deficiency, and this represents a risk factor for adverse outcomes in patient undergoing surgery and in the critically ill. Iron therapy (whether oral or intravenous) has been shown to reduce transfusion rates in clinical trials. There appears to be no clinical benefit, however, in terms of reductions in major morbidity and mortality. There is no difference in terms of

efficacy or safety between intravenous and oral iron. Oral iron should therefore be used in preference where possible, as it is much less expensive.

Recombinant Human Erythropoietin (EPO)

Recombinant human erythropoietin is commonly administered along with iron supplementation to reverse chronic anaemia preoperatively in surgical patients, where it has been shown to reduce transfusion exposure without apparent adverse effects. It is suggested that EPO may increase the frequency of thromboembolic complications as a result of higher viscosity, and have an activating effect on platelets. The combination of EPO and iron appears to have a greater transfusion-sparing effect than either treatment in isolation, but there is uncertainty as to whether this has a clinical benefit.

Interventions That Prevent or Reverse Coagulopathy

Antifibrinolytics

The lysine analogues tranexamic acid and ε-amino caproic acid (EACA) act by irreversibly binding to the active site of plasminogen, thereby inhibiting clot lysis. Tranexamic acid reduces transfusion exposure, severe bleeding and, most importantly, mortality in surgical and trauma patients. The mechanism by which it reduces mortality is unclear. It has been suggested that the benefits may be attributed to an anti-inflammatory effect, or alternatively to the prevention of severe bleeding and shock. However, higher doses, which are hypothesised to have additional important anti-inflammatory effects, do not improve outcomes relative to lower doses. Furthermore, head-to-head comparisons of tranexamic acid with the serine protease inhibitor aprotinin show a survival benefit for tranexamic acid, despite the more effective reduction in bleeding with aprotinin. A recent meta-analysis has indicated that tranexamic acid may have a specific cardioprotective effect.

The efficacy of tranexamic acid appears to be greater than that of many other blood management interventions. For example, the overall benefit attributable to the combination of tranexamic acid and cell salvage is influenced largely by the antifibrinolytic. It has therefore been suggested that cell salvage devices should only be used in combination with tranexamic acid.

Desmopressin

Desmopressin is a synthetic analogue of arginine vasopressin that induces the release of the contents of endothelial cell-associated Weibel–Palade bodies, including von Willebrand factor. Its use is indicated in the management of patients with mild haemophilia and von Willebrand disease undergoing minor surgical procedures. The increase in factor VIII and von Willebrand factor concentrations as well as evidence of increased platelet aggregation in response to desmopressin has led to its evaluation as a haemostatic agent in major surgery. A Cochrane review failed to demonstrate any significant reduction in transfusion exposure, or improvement in clinical outcomes attributable to desmopressin use.

Recombinant Activated Factor VII (rFVIIa)

This is a potent pharmacological prohaemostatic agent licenced for use in patients with haemophilia. This has led to the off-label use of rFVIIa for the treatment of severe coagulopathic bleeding in trauma and surgical settings as an adjunct to conventional nonred cell blood components. Its use is associated with a significant (68%) increased risk of major thrombotic complications, especially arterial thrombosis, without a clinically significant reduction in allogeneic red cell requirement in trauma patients.

Coagulopathy

Coagulopathy is a poorly defined term; it may refer to severe impairment of blood coagulation in the setting of trauma or, alternatively, to the laboratory finding of abnormal screening tests of coagulation in a critical care patient. The lack of a clear definition of coagulopathy complicates epidemiological analyses and the development of accurate diagnostic tests and treatments [14]. However, it remains a significant clinical problem and, depending on the definition, affects up to 30% of critically ill patients, 30% of trauma patients, 15% of cardiac surgery patients and 6% of those with acute upper GI haemorrhage.

Coagulopathic patients, whether or not they are actively bleeding, have a worse overall prognosis than similar patients without coagulopathy. This is attributable to the severity of the underlying illness and prior or ongoing significant haemorrhage and shock. It may also be attributable in part, however, to the adverse effects of prohaemostatic therapies; fresh frozen plasma (FFP) and platelets are recognised causes of transfusion complications such as transfusion-related acute lung injury (TRALI), transfusion-associated circulatory overload (TACO), transfusion-associated dyspnoea (TAD) and transfusion-transmitted infection (TTI) [15] (see Chapters 7–17 for more details). Platelets have also been shown in some studies to increase the risk of stroke in patients with cardiovascular disease. These risks, although offset by the risks of ongoing bleeding in coagulopathic patients, may be clinically significant in those without coagulopathy, or when administered to those who are not actively bleeding.

Diagnosis

Effective treatment of coagulopathy, particularly in a bleeding patient, requires accurate and timely diagnosis. The nature of coagulopathy is heterogeneous and is influenced by the patient group, such as severe trauma, liver surgery or cardiac surgery; the type of intervention, such as cardiopulmonary bypass or transplant surgery; and the blood management strategy adopted, for example the use of antifibrinolytics and nonred cell blood components. Specific defects in the coagulation pathway are commonly not detected by standard coagulation screening tests which, by taking as long as 65 minutes, are often considered impractical in the setting of ongoing blood loss. Near-patient testing is increasingly used, but the quality of the evidence surrounding its use in different settings is variable. A recent guideline from the UK National Institute for Health and Care Excellence (NICE) reflects this variation and recommends the use of viscoelastic tests in cardiac surgery, but suggests their use as a research tool only in trauma and obstetrics [16]. Near-patient platelet function analysers and alternative laboratory assays, such as thrombin generation testing, have been shown to accurately predict bleeding and target therapy in small single-centre studies, but wider validation of these techniques is awaited.

Treatment

Without accurate diagnostic tests to identify specific defects in the coagulation pathway that are associated with adverse clinical outcomes, the management of coagulopathy is often empirical, nonspecific and based on the assumption that reversal of coagulopathy is beneficial. The clinical efficacy, safety and cost-effectiveness of this approach are questionable, and this remains an important and under-resourced area of research.

Platelet Transfusion

Acute haemorrhage during surgery is a common indication for therapeutic platelet use. For example, cardiac surgery utilises over 17% of all platelet transfusions in the UK [1]. Indications for, and effective doses of, platelets in the setting of acute haemorrhage are unclear and not supported by evidence outside of haematology/oncology patients. Observational studies report lower mortality rates in trauma patients receiving high-dose platelet transfusion for major blood loss, and a recent US RCT of trauma patients reported that empirical transfusion of higher platelet ratios, in combination with higher plasma ratios, improves haemostasis and leads to fewer deaths from bleeding at 24 hours

[17], although there was no control group not treated empirically with platelet transfusion and no difference between the high and low ratio groups for the actual primary outcomes of this study, including mortality.

Thrombocytopenia in critically ill patients is a risk factor for major bleeding and death, and the prevalence of mild ($<150 \times 10^9$/L) and moderate ($<50 \times 10^9$/L) thrombocytopenia in adult ICU patients is reported at 40% and 8% respectively [18]. There is little evidence from critical care studies that prophylactic correction of thrombocytopenia translates into a survival advantage, or indeed reproducibly raises platelets counts in critically ill patients. Thrombocytopenia increases the risk of haemorrhage during invasive procedures such as central line or spinal catheter insertion, and these are often performed using platelet transfusion 'cover'. Consensus recommendations [19,20] for platelet administration during haemorrhage and in the critically ill are summarised in Table 27.2. These thresholds for platelet transfusions are

Table 27.2 Platelet thresholds for prophylactic and therapeutic platelet transfusion.

Clinical indication	Treatment value ($\times 10^9$/L)
Therapeutic	
Massive transfusion	>50
Massive transfusion and multiple trauma or TBI	>100
DIC and bleeding	>50
Intracerebral bleeding	>100
Prophylactic	
Preinvasive procedure, i.e. LP, CVC, epidural	>50
Presurgery	>50–75
Presurgery at high-risk sites, i.e. brain/eye	>100

CVC, central venous catheter; DIC, disseminated intravascular coagulation; LP, lumbar puncture; TBI, traumatic brain injury.
Source: Adapted from Hunt et al. [19] and Spahn et al. [20].

empirical, have been derived largely from studies in haematooncology patients and do not account for alterations in platelet function or clinical status, which limits their utility.

Fresh Frozen Plasma Transfusion

Nearly half of all FFP administered in the UK is given to critically ill patients: 12% cardiac, 9% liver disease and liver transplant, 7% GI haemorrhage, 6% vascular surgery, 6% haematology, 3% trauma and 2% obstetrics [1]. A UK study reported that 13% of critically ill adult patients received FFP during an ICU admission [21]. Half of these transfusions (48%) were for bleeding; the remainder were for preprocedural prophylaxis (15%) or prophylaxis alone (36%). One-third was given to patients with normal prothrombin time (PT) values. However, the clinical efficacy of FFP has not been clearly demonstrated, for either treatment or prophylaxis. Indeed, it has been reported that standard FFP doses (12–15 mL/kg) are insufficient to significantly increase individual coagulation factor levels. A recent systematic review examining 80 RCTs highlighted that there are few well-supported indications for

FFP administration [22] (Table 27.3) but despite this, numbers of FFP transfusions are increasing.

Fibrinogen Replacement

Traditionally, fibrinogen is replaced during major blood loss or as part of the management for disseminated intravascular coagulation (DIC) once the Clauss fibrinogen value falls below 1 g/L. Fibrinogen is one of the earliest coagulation factors to fall in major bleeding and adequate, timely replacement of fibrinogen is hypothesised to result in improved haemorrhage control. Recent guidelines reflect this shift in practice and recommend 1.5 g/L [19,20] as the transfusion trigger in all forms of major haemorrhage, except obstetric haemorrhage where a 2.0 g/L trigger is advised [19], although these recommendations are based on weak evidence.

Cryoprecipitate is the first-line treatment in the UK for acquired hypofibrinogenaemia, and a standard adult dose (of pool size ranging from 5 to 6 units) raises the plasma fibrinogen level by 1 g/L. Despite the recognition that fibrinogen levels fall rapidly in major haemorrhage, a large UK epidemiology study highlighted consistent

Table 27.3 Summary of FFP RCTs in critically ill patient groups.

Patient group	Total no. RCTs	Total no. patients	Therapeutic RCTs (no.)	Prophylactic RCTs (no.)	Findings
Cardiac surgery	19	948	4	15	No significant benefit from FFP
Liver disease	10	381	3	7	No significant benefit from FFP
Liver failure	1	118	1*	0	↑ survival with plasma exchange and haemofiltration
Thrombotic thrombocytopenic purpura	7	317	7	0	2 RCTs found ↑ response rates/survival
Severe closed head injury	1	44	0	1	↑mortality, ↑ AEs, ↑ delayed IC haematoma with FFP arm
Massive haemorrhage	1	41	1	0	No significant difference in clinical bleeding
Haematooncology	0				

* This trial evaluated plasma exchange in patients with liver failure.
AE, adverse event; IC, intracranial; RCT, randomised controlled trial.
Source: Adapted from Yang et al. [22].

delays in administration of cryoprecipitate to bleeding trauma patients across 22 hospitals in England and Wales [23]. The median time to delivery of cryoprecipitate was 184 minutes from hospital admission (interquartile range (IQR): 84–330), with a median time from injury to admission of 60 minutes. A recent small RCT has demonstrated the feasibility of administering cryoprecipitate early to adult patients with severe trauma haemorrhage [24]. Further work is required in this area to evaluate the clinical effectiveness of cryoprecipitate in active bleeding.

In addition to the interest in higher and earlier doses of cryoprecipitate, there is increasing interest in the use of fibrinogen concentrates. These are currently not licensed in the UK but have obvious advantages in light of their reduced infection risk and standardised fibrinogen concentration (Table 27.4). RCTs in a variety of surgical settings have reported positive outcomes following administration of fibrinogen concentrate (Table 27.5), but more evidence is needed, as the studies are small. A recent Cochrane review reported that fibrinogen concentrate did not affect mortality but led to a significant reduction in allogeneic transfusion, without an increase in thrombotic complications [25]. Larger studies, which will require significant international collaboration, are needed to demonstrate clinical effectiveness of either form of fibrinogen supplementation in major haemorrhage.

Prothrombin Complex Concentrates (PCCs)

These are plasma-derived coagulation factor concentrates that contain three or four vitamin K-dependent factors at high concentration, including factors II, VII, IX and X, as well as variable amounts of anticoagulants and heparin. PCCs are recommended for the treatment of serious or life-threatening bleeding related to oral anticoagulant therapy. Studies have shown that PCCs are safe and effective and normalise international normalised ratio (INR) values

Table 27.4 Comparison of FFP and PCC, cryoprecipitate and fibrinogen concentrate.

Coagulation factor replacement		Fibrinogen replacement	
FFP	PCC	Cryoprecipitate	FgC
Pooled product – nonstandardised	Pooled product – standardised	Pooled product – nonstandardised	Pooled product – standardised
All coagulation factors	Factors II, VII, IX, X, proteins C and S	FVIII, FXIII, vWF, FN, Fg	Fg
Frozen −30 °C Requires thawing	Room temperature (<25 °C)	Frozen −30 °C Requires thawing	Room temperature (<25 °C)
Large volume (often 800–1200 mL)	Small volume – 2000 IU in 80 mL	2 pools ∼ 350 mL	Small volume – 2 g in 100 mL
Standard FFP – no viral inactivation	Yes – pasteurisation and a nanofiltration step for virus removal	No viral inactivation	Yes – pasteurisation 60 °C for 20 hours; Fg adsorption/ precipitation removes virus
TRALI, TACO, TTI, TAD	Thrombosis, DIC	TRALI, TTI	TTI, thrombosis
£112 for 1 litre	£1200 for 2000 IU	£362 for 2 pools	£1000 for 2 g

DIC, disseminated intravascular coagulation; FFP, fresh frozen plasma; Fg, fibrinogen; FgC, fibrinogen concentrate; FVIII, factor VIII; FXIII, factor XIII; FN, fibrinonectin; IU, international units; PCC, prothrombin complex concentrate; TACO, transfusion-associated circulatory overload; TAD, transfusion-associated dyspnoea; TRALI, transfusion-related acute lung injury; TTI, transfusion-transmissible infection.

Table 27.5 Studies evaluating the safety and efficacy of fibrinogen concentrate in major surgery.

Patient group	Study type	Intervention	Comparator	Outcome
Cystectomy	RCT	FgC 45 mg/kg (n = 10)	Placebo (n = 10)	Significant increased MCF ↓ post-operative red cell use at 48 h
Cardiac surgery	RCT	FgC 2 g (n = 10)	No FgC (n = 10)	1 MI & 1 PE in intervention group No significant difference in transfusion need
Cardiac surgery	RCT	FgC median 8 g (dose directed by ROTEM) (n = 29)	Placebo (n = 31)	Significant reduction in transfusion No difference in AE
Cardiac surgery	RCT	FgC mean 3.6 g (dose directed by ROTEM) (n = 58)	Placebo (n = 58)	Significant lower rate of allogeneic blood product transfusion Significant reduction in post-operative blood loss
Cardiac surgery	RCT	FgC 1 g preoperatively (n = 30)	Placebo (n = 30)	No difference in operative red cell use Significant reduction in post-operative blood loss
Hip arthroplasty	RCT	FgC 30 mg/kg preoperatively (n = 15)	Placebo (n = 15)	No difference in perioperative blood loss
Paediatric cardiac surgery	RCT	FgC 60 mg/kg (n = 30)	Cryoprecipitate (n = 33)	No difference in 48-h blood loss or allogeneic blood transfusions Fibrinogen levels rose to a similar degree
Paediatric craniosynostosis and scoliosis surgery	RCT	Craniosynostosis surgery FgC 30 mg/kg (directed by a ROTEM FIBTEM MCF <13) (n = 17)	Craniosynostosis surgery FgC 30 mg/kg (directed by a ROTEM FIBTEM MCF <8) (n = 14)	Significant reduction in perioperative red blood cells
		Scoliosis surgery FgC 30 mg/kg (directed by a ROTEM FIBTEM MCF <13) (n = 12)	Scoliosis surgery FgC 30 mg/kg (directed by a ROTEM FIBTEM MCF <8) (n = 14)	No significant differences
Postpartum haemorrhage	RCT	FgC 2 g (n = 124)	Placebo (n = 125)	No significant differences in red cell transfusion at 6 weeks
Cardiac surgery	RCT	FgC 4 g	1 unit apheresis platelets	No differences in post-operative blood loss or red cell transfusion

AE, adverse event; FFP, fresh frozen plasma; FgC, fibrinogen concentrate; MCF, maximal clot firmness; MI, myocardial infarction; MOF, multiorgan failure; PCC, prothrombin complex concentrate PE, pulmonary embolism; RCT, randomised controlled trial; TRISS, trauma score – injury severity score.

rapidly when compared to FFP. Outcome data examining the effect of PCCs on bleeding rates and mortality are not yet available. PCCs are currently licenced for treatment and perioperative prophylaxis of haemorrhage in patients with congenital and acquired deficiency of factors II, VII, IX or X, if purified specific coagulation factors are unavailable. PCCs are increasingly being considered as a substitute for FFP (Table 27.4 summarises the differences between products) for use in coagulopathy associated with hepatic failure and traumatic haemorrhage. There is currently insufficient evidence to support these indications.

Massive Blood Transfusion

Strategies to manage massive blood transfusion have undergone major changes over the last few years, driven primarily by dismal outcomes observed in these patients using current treatment algorithms and evidence emerging from observational studies in battle casualties that higher volumes of FFP and platelets (approaching ratios of 1:1:1) lead to increased survival in massively transfused patients. Survivor bias was a major confounder of these studies. Building on these data, a large US-led RCT was conducted, randomising 680 adult trauma patients with major haemorrhage to blood product ratios of either 1:1:1 (FFP:platelets:RBC) or 1:1:2 [17]. The study was powered to detect a 10% difference in 24-hour mortality and a 12% difference in 30-day mortality. No significant differences in these primary outcomes were found, although there was a significant reduction in death from exsanguination at 24 hours (9.2% versus 14.6% in 1:1:2 group; P = 0.03) and greater numbers of patients achieved the subjective secondary endpoint of anatomical haemostasis in the 1:1:1 group (86% versus 78%; P = 0.006). This RCT does have limitations; in particular, separating the effects of higher FFP doses from higher platelet doses is impossible and only a small proportion of participants received tranexamic acid, which may reduce the relevance of the PROPPR findings in the UK where tranexamic acid is routinely given.

These results, prior data from many observational studies, and the finding that 25–33% of trauma patients are coagulopathic (elevated INR, PTT) upon presentation to hospital, have led to the development of empirical early delivery of FFP and platelets in major haemorrhage protocols, with guidance of transfusion by coagulation testing later in the process. Major haemorrhage is of course not limited to trauma patients, but there is very little evidence to inform practice in other clinical settings. There are differences between patient groups; many GI haemorrhage patients are elderly, have limited cardiovascular reserve and may be susceptible to fluid overload. Massive haemorrhage protocols for trauma should not be applied to other clinical areas without significant consideration of patient co-morbidities.

Major Haemorrhage Protocols

Between October 2006 and September 2010, delays in the provision of blood in UK hospitals led to 11 deaths and 83 incidents of harm being reported to the National Patient Safety Agency. In light of this, a Rapid Response Report concerning the transfusion of blood in an emergency was produced which recommended the adoption of major haemorrhage protocols in every hospital [26]. Furthermore, the use of 'drills' to test local policies and ongoing education of all staff likely to be involved in massive haemorrhage protocols are advised. Following data from the CRASH-2 study [27], tranexamic acid should be given to all adult trauma patients at risk of bleeding, so long as administration can be given within three hours of injury. And following data in trauma patients, early empirical use of high-ratio FFP:RBC is recommended, with recourse to transfusion guidance from laboratory testing as soon as results are available [19]. In trauma haemorrhage, the use of early platelet transfusions should also be considered [19].

Conclusion

The timely administration of blood components to patients with acute haemorrhage and in the critically ill is often life saving; however, the clinical status of these patients also means that they are highly susceptible to organ dysfunction, and inappropriate transfusion, with its associated risks, may also have important adverse effects on clinical outcomes. Recent systematic reviews have identified important aspects of blood management that improve outcome as well as identifying gaps in knowledge that need to be addressed by future research. Most trials have focused on modifying blood use or short-term outcomes, and many are at high risk of bias. Few data are available regarding the cost-effectiveness of different interventions, in either isolation or combination. Restrictive transfusion practice is safe in critically ill patients without active cardiovascular disease. Conversely, liberal red cell transfusion thresholds appear to reduce mortality in patients with symptomatic cardiovascular disease. Therapeutic adjuncts such as tranexamic acid that reduce transfusion and improve outcomes are well defined and the wider application of these techniques will drive quality improvement. Coagulopathy associated with acute haemorrhage remains underresearched, with no clear understanding of the underlying pathogenesis, accurate diagnostic tests or evidence-based treatments. The significant proportion of blood components utilised by these patients, their poor outcomes and significant utilisation of healthcare resources are arguments for greater investment in this field.

KEY POINTS

1) Blood management focuses on improving patient outcomes in the setting of acute haemorrhage and acute anaemia in critically ill patients.

2) Restrictive use of allogeneic red cell transfusion is safe in patients without cardiovascular disease. There is evidence to suggest that more liberal transfusion may improve outcomes in patients with cardiovascular disease.

3) The use of techniques that enable red cell salvage and autotransfusion will reduce red cell transfusion and in the case of cell salvage will improve clinical outcomes and be cost-effective in patients at high risk of bleeding.

4) Tranexamic acid effectively reduces transfusion exposure and in the setting of trauma and major surgery improves survival.

5) Other pharmacological strategies effectively reduce red cell transfusion but the clinical benefits and risks of these interventions remain to be defined by high-quality trials.

6) Critically ill and acute surgical patients often develop coagulopathy. This is poorly defined, and there are currently no validated sensitive and specific diagnostic tests that have been validated clinically, or shown to improve clinical outcome.

7) The current evidence to support the prophylactic use of FFP and platelets in the critically ill is poor.

8) Massive transfusion protocols that place emphasis on communication, preemptive treatment and the initial use of higher FFP:RBC ratios followed by goal-directed therapy improve outcomes.

References

1 Wells AW, Llewelyn CA, Casbard A et al. The EASTR Study: indications for transfusion and estimates of transfusion recipient numbers in hospitals supplied by the National Blood Service. Transfus Med 2009;**19**:315–27.

2 Corwin HL, Gettinger A, Pearl RG et al. The CRIT Study: Anemia and blood transfusion in the critically ill – current clinical practice in the United States. Crit Care Med 2004;**32**:39–52.

3 Bennett-Guerrero E, Zhao Y, O'Brien SM et al. Variation in use of blood transfusion in coronary artery bypass graft surgery. JAMA 2010;**304**:1568–75.

4 Carson JL, Grossman BJ, Kleinman S et al., for the Clinical Transfusion Medicine Committee of the AABB. Red blood cell transfusion: a clinical practice guideline from the AABB. Ann Intern Med 2012;**157**:49–58.

5 www.nice.org.uk/guidance/indevelopment/gid-cgwave0663/documents (accessed 14 November 2016).

6 Patel NN, Avlonitis VS, Jones HE, Reeves BC, Sterne JAC, Murphy GJ. Indications for red cell transfusion in cardiac surgery: a systematic review and meta-analysis of randomised controlled trials and observational studies. Lancet Hematology 2015;**2**:e543–e553.

7 Henry DA, Carless PA, Moxey AJ et al. Pre-operative autologous donation for minimising perioperative allogeneic blood transfusion. Cochrane Database Syst Rev 2002;**2**:CD003602.

8. Davies L, Brown TJ, Haynes S, Payne K, Elliott RA, McCollum C. Cost-effectiveness of cell salvage and alternative methods of minimising perioperative allogeneic blood transfusion: a systematic review and economic model. Health Technol Assess 2006;**10**:iii–iv, ix–x, 1–210.

9 Ker K, Edwards P, Perel P, Shakur H, Roberts I. Effect of tranexamic acid on surgical bleeding: systematic review and cumulative meta-analysis. BMJ 2012;**344**:e3054.

10 Ker K, Roberts I, Shakur H, Coats TJ. Antifibrinolytic drugs for acute traumatic injury. Cochrane Database Syst Rev 2015;**5**:CD004896.

11 Henry DA, Carless PA, Moxey AJ et al. Anti-fibrinolytic use for minimising perioperative allogeneic blood transfusion. Cochrane Database Syst Rev 2011;**3**:CD001886.

12 Carless PA, Henry DA, Moxey AJ et al. Desmopressin for minimising perioperative allogeneic blood transfusion. Cochrane Database Syst Rev 2004;**1**:CD001884.

13 Simpson E, Lin Y, Stanworth S, Birchall J, Doree C, Hyde C. Recombinant factor VIIa for the prevention and treatment of bleeding in patients without hemophilia. Cochrane Database Syst Rev 2012;**3**:CD005011.

14 Hunt H, Stanworth S, Curry N et al. Thromboelastography (TEG) and rotational thromboelastometry (ROTEM) for trauma-induced coagulopathy in adult trauma patients with bleeding. Cochrane Database Syst Rev 2015;**2**:CD010438.

15 Serious Hazards of Transfusion (SHOT). Annual Report and Summary 2014. Available at: www.shotuk.org/shot-reports/report-summary-supplement-2014/(accessed 14 November 2016).

16 National Institute for Health and Care Excellence (NICE). Diagnostics Guidance 13: Detecting, Managing and Monitoring Hemostasis: Viscoelastometric Point-of-Care Testing (ROTEM, TEG and Sonoclot Systems). Available at: www.nice.org.uk/guidance/dg13/resources/detecting-managing-and-monitoring-hemostasis-viscoelastometric-pointofcare-testing-rotem-teg-and-sonoclot-systems-1053628110277 (accessed 14 November 2016).

17 Holcomb JB, Tilley BC, Baraniuk S et al., for the PROPPR Study Group. Transfusion of plasma, platelets, and red blood cells in a 1:1:1 vs a 1:1:2 ratio and mortality in patients with severe trauma: the PROPPR randomized clinical trial. JAMA 2015;**313**:471–82.

18 Arnold DM, Crowther MA, Cook RJ et al. Utilization of platelet transfusions in the intensive care unit: indications, transfusion triggers, and platelet count responses. Transfusion 2006;**46**:1286–91.

19 Hunt BJ, Allard S, Keeling D et al., for the BCSH. A practical guideline for the hematological management of major hemorrhage. Br J Hematol 2015;**170**:788–803.

20 Spahn DR, Bouillon B, Cerny V et al. Management of bleeding and coagulopathy following major trauma: an updated European guideline. Crit Care 2013;**17**:R76.

21 Stanworth SJ, Walsh TS, Prescott RJ et al., Intensive Care Study of Coagulopathy (ISOC) Investigators. A national study of plasma use

in critical care: clinical indications, dose and effect on prothrombin time. Crit Care 2011;**15**:R108.

22 Yang L, Stanworth S, Hopewell S, Doree C, Murphy M. Is fresh frozen plasma clinically effective? An updated systematic review of randomised controlled trials. Transfusion 2012;**52**:1673–86.

23 NIHR. PGfAR 10036: Traumatic Coagulopathy and Massive Transfusion: Improving Outcomes and Saving Blood. Available at: www.nihr.ac.uk/funding/fundingdetails.htm?postid=2122 (accessed 14 November 2016).

24 Curry N, Rourke C, Davenport R et al. Early cryoprecipitate for major hemorrhage in trauma: a randomised controlled feasibility trial. Br J Anaesth 2015;**115**:76–83.

25 Wikkelso A, Lunde J, Johansen M et al. Fibrinogen in bleeding patients. Cochrane Database Syst Rev 2013;**8**:CD008864.

26 National Patient Safety Agency. The Transfusion of Blood and Blood Components in an Emergency. Rapid Response Report. NPSA/2010/RRR017. Available at: www.nrls.npsa.nhs.uk/alerts/?entryid45=83659 (accessed 14 November 2016).

27 Shakur H, Roberts I, Bautista R et al., for the CRASH-2 Trial Collaborators. Effects of tranexamic acid on death, vascular occlusive events, and blood transfusion in trauma patients with significant hemorrhage (CRASH-2): a randomised, placebo-controlled trial. Lancet 2010;**376**:23–32.

Further Reading

Carson JL, Grossman BJ, Kleinman S et al., for the Clinical Transfusion Medicine Committee of the AABB. Red blood cell transfusion: a clinical practice guideline from the AABB. Ann Intern Med 2012;**157**:49–58.

National Institute for Health and Care Excellence (NICE). Diagnostics Guidance 13: Detecting, Managing and Monitoring Hemostasis: Viscoelastometric Point-of-Care Testing (ROTEM, TEG and Sonoclot Systems). Available at: www.nice.org.uk/guidance/dg13/resources/detecting-managing-and-monitoring-hemostasis-viscoelastometric-pointofcare-testing-rotem-teg-and-sonoclot-systems-1053628110277 (accessed 14 November 2016).

28

Point-of-Care Testing in Transfusion Medicine

Matthew D. Neal and Louis H. Alarcon

Departments of Surgery and Critical Care Medicine, University of Pittsburgh School of Medicine, Pittsburgh, USA

Introduction

Multiple diseases of both infectious and sterile inflammatory aetiology are complicated by abnormalities of haemostasis, and rapid detection of impaired coagulation is paramount to goal-directed resuscitation of these patients. Understanding the laboratory testing options for assessing coagulopathy is key for transfusion medicine specialists as well as all clinicians. Given that rapid identification of coagulopathy is necessary in these often critically ill patients, the use of point-of-care (POC) technology has emerged as a key technique for the rapid assessment of abnormalities of haemostasis.

This chapter will provide an overview of POC technologies relevant to the transfusion medicine specialist and acute care clinician. Emphasis will be placed on the utilisation of these tools in critically ill patients, especially following trauma, where a recent explosion of clinical research has led to a paradigm shift favouring POC testing to guide resuscitation, as well as use in the perioperative period where requests for transfusion are most common.

Limitations of Conventional Coagulation Testing

Conventional haemostasis testing includes a number of assays such as prothrombin time (PT), international normalised ratio (INR) and activated partial thromboplastin time (aPTT), as well as quantification of platelet counts and direct measurement of fibrinogen levels. Designed largely as plasma-based assays, many of these tests lack validation in acute care or critical care settings and are more useful in guiding the management of anticoagulation in the case of PT/INR or detecting absolute deficiencies in coagulation factors or platelet number [1]. In addition, these tests were designed to be analysed under a standard temperature (37 °C) and fail to detect coagulopathies induced by hypothermia [1]. These tests are valuable for measuring the initiation of clot, particularly at the level of thrombin generation within plasma. However, they fail to account for any of the contributions of the cellular components of whole blood that are removed prior to conducting the assay. In particular, none of these conventional tests provides an assessment of platelet function, with conventional testing being limited simply to the detection of platelet number.

Given the prevalence of antiplatelet therapy in the general population and the potential benefits of platelet transfusion to reverse the contribution of antiplatelet therapy to bleeding in the acute setting, this presents a major deficiency. Additionally, no currently available means of conventional testing has the means to quantify clot strength and/or fibrinolysis, which are two key components of coagulation and haemostasis. Finally, the above-mentioned tests in standard labs can take upwards of 45–90 minutes to perform with a requirement for centrifugation, limiting their applicability in emergency circumstances when transfusion needs are most often required [1]. Taken together, these deficiencies have led to a focus on more robust, rapid and inclusive means of determining the entirety of clot formation.

Point-of-Care Testing Options

A variety of different testing options exist in a POC setting to encompass the diverse nature of coagulation and haemostasis. Unfortunately, no one assay has emerged as a gold standard for quantifying all aspects of coagulation and haemostasis. A thorough understanding of the available options will allow the provider to choose the best available test for the clinical situation. An additional limitation of POC testing is the lack of well-designed prospective randomised trials for most conditions. Where data exist, this chapter will outline the major studies and limitations; however, the use of POC testing in many clinical scenarios is based on expert opinion and the theoretical benefits over the limitations of conventional testing that are outlined above. Although POC testing exists for chronic, outpatient management of anticoagulation, this is outside the focus of this chapter and will not be discussed. The two main areas of POC testing that we will explore are analysis of platelet function and viscoelastic testing. Data supporting the use of POC in guiding transfusion will also be reviewed.

Analysis of Platelet Function

Point-of-care analysis of platelet function is largely based on quantification of platelet aggregation in response to an agonist. Platelet function is largely driven by activation, adhesion and subsequent aggregation. Conventional activators of platelets include collagen and thrombin to mimic endothelial injury, as well as adenosine diphosphate (ADP) and arachidonic acid, which are used to test the responsiveness of platelets to inhibition by clopidogrel and aspirin, respectively.

Light transmission aggregometry (LTA) is a standard laboratory method utilised for detecting platelet response and quantifying platelet dysfunction; however, LTA relies upon the use of platelet-rich plasma (PRP), and this labour-intensive process limits applicability in POC situations [2]. Therefore, a variety of techniques utilising whole blood have emerged to assess for platelet dysfunction. These technologies utilise the general principles of platelet aggregometry – agonist stimulation in the setting of a shear stress – and subsequent quantification using some measure of aggregate formation, whether it be light or impedance based. Although multiple instruments exist, commonly applied technologies in clinical practice include the Platelet Function Analyser (PFA-100) (Siemens, Deerfield, IL, USA), VerifyNow (Accumetrics, San Diego, CA, USA), Plateletworks (Helena Laboratories, Beaumont, TX, USA) and Multiplate impedance aggregometry (Dynabyte, Munich, Germany). The differences between these instruments are outside the scope of this chapter, although it is important to note that each has a unique method for determining platelet responsiveness and each has its own strengths and weaknesses.

The use of POC platelet testing has been advocated in a number of clinical scenarios. Importantly, POC technology allows for identification of inherited or acquired platelet dysfunction in an acute care setting. Detection of conditions such as von Willebrand's disease (vWD) or Glanzmann's thrombasthenia may markedly change transfusion strategies. Various small studies have demonstrated the ability of POC platelet testing to identify these defects as well as response to antiplatelet therapy [3–5]. Perhaps the clinical setting in which these POC technologies are best studied is cardiac surgery, where both drug-induced and acquired platelet deficits due to cardiopulmonary bypass are very common [6]. POC platelet function has been shown to reliably predict blood loss [7,8] and to guide perioperative platelet transfusion [9][9]. The use of POC technology to reduce transfusion requirements in cardiovascular surgery has been validated in at least one large prospective randomised trial [10].

Strong consideration should be given to the use of POC platelet testing in the perioperative care of these patients, and certainly any patient presenting with a bleeding diathesis after exposure to cardiopulmonary bypass and/or any other type of extracorporeal circuit (such as extracorporeal membrane oxygenation (ECMO) or ventricular assist devices (VAD)) should be considered to be at high risk for platelet dysfunction. Data supporting the application of POC platelet technology to other types of surgery or acute care presentation are limited to single-centre case reports and small retrospective analyses.

Viscoelastic Testing

Three major methods of viscoelastic testing exist for POC analysis: the Sonoclot Analyser (Sienco Inc, Wheat Ridge, CO, USA), thromboelastography (TEG) (Haemonetics, Braintree,

MA, USA) and rotational thromboelastometry (ROTEM) (Pentapharm, Munich, Germany). All three technologies utilise a small aliquot of whole blood which is agitated to simulate flow conditions and stimulate coagulation. Speed and strength of clot formation, as well as the breakdown of clot, or clot lysis, are quantified. TEG and ROTEM are the best studied of the two technologies and are presently the only two viscoelastic technologies approved by the United States Food and Drug Administration; therefore, they will be discussed in additional detail given the high likelihood that the reader will encounter these in clinical practice in the United States and worldwide.

Thromboelastography

An example of a TEG tracing is show in Figure 28.1, and a description of the TEG variables is included in Table 28.1. An activator is required to initiate clot formation as part of TEG, and the choice of activator results in important modifications of the test that must be clearly understood when interpreting the test. Common activators for TEG are kaolin, which is the standard assay (as shown in Figure 28.1), or tissue factor, which speeds the reaction and markedly shortens the reaction time (eliminating the R time), thus the reference to this test as a rapid-TEG (rTEG). In the rTEG, the R time is replaced by the TEG activated clotting time (ACT), which is measured in seconds rather

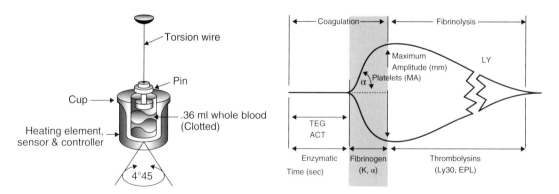

Figure 28.1 Example TEG tracing. *Source:* Allen SR, Kashuk JL. Unanswered questions in the use of blood component therapy in trauma. Scand J Trauma Resus Emerg Med 2011;19:5. Original reprinted with permission from Hemoscope Corporation, Niles, IL.

Table 28.1 Description of TEG parameters.

Parameter	Normal range	Description	Guide for transfusion treatment
R (reaction) time	4–9 minutes	Time to thrombin generation and cleavage of fibrin, factor dependent	Prolonged R treated with FFP
K (kinetics)	1–4 minutes	Measure of the speed to reach 20 mm in amplitude, represents clot kinetics along with alpha	Low K develops from fibrinogen deficiency, impaired thrombin generation, treat with cryoprecipitate, FFP
Alpha angle	47–74 degrees	Rate of increase in clot due to fibrin cross-linking	Low angle develops from fibrinogen deficiency, impaired thrombin generation, treat with cryoprecipitate, FFP
Maximum amplitude	55–73 mm	Clot strength (80–90% platelets, 10–20% fibrinogen)	Reduced MA treated with platelet transfusion
LY 30	0–7.5%	Fibrinolysis	Significant elevation in LY30 (>7.5%) in the setting of ongoing bleeding treated with antifibrinolytics (aminocaproic acid, tranexamic acid)
Coagulation index	+3 to –3	Linear combination of kinetic variables in an equation to calculate overall coagulation status	>3 = hypercoagulable <3 = hypocoagulable

FFP, fresh frozen plasma.

than minutes. rTEG allows for fast progression to assessment of clot strength and ultimately to fibrinolysis, and the shortened reaction time has popularised the use of rTEG in acute care settings. Additional TEG modifications include the use of heparinase cups to neutralise the effect of heparin, whether present systemically or as the anticoagulant in blood collection tubing. The use of heparinase can unmask coagulopathies that are present independent from that achieved by heparin. It has also been used following cardiopulmonary bypass to determine protamine responsiveness. Finally, an additional modification of TEG, called platelet mapping, can be used to determine the degree of pharmacological antiplatelet therapy present from drugs such as aspirin or clopidogrel. Even without the use of platelet mapping, the maximum amplitude (MA) on TEG allows for a robust quantification of platelet function and can be used to guide platelet transfusion.

Thermoelastography was initially invented in the 1940s and popularised for use in liver transplantation. In recent years, the popularity of TEG has grown substantially, and TEG is now commonly used in multiple perioperative settings, including cardiovascular anaesthesia and obstetrics [6], and has been proposed for use in severe sepsis [11]. Multiple prospective studies have shown a reduction in transfusion requirements using TEG-based measurements, particularly following cardiac surgery [6]. The ability to analyse specific components of clot formation as well as to ascertain when adjuncts such as antifibrinolytics are indicated, all within a 30–45-minute window, make TEG a highly useful intraoperative tool. Although evidence-based guidelines fall short of declaring TEG as standard of care in the management of operative transfusion, numerous authors and expert opinion advocate strongly for TEG over conventional haemostasis testing.

Perhaps the most robust literature surrounding the use of TEG is derived from trauma and the resuscitation of massive haemorrhage. Recognition of the existence of a unique, endogenous coagulopathy present in as many as 25% of massively bleeding trauma patients has led to an explosion of retrospective and prospective studies examining the proper ratio of blood components indicated for resuscitation [12,13]. Early in the course of these analyses, it became apparent that conventional coagulation testing was ineffective and inaccurate in measuring coagulation disturbance following severe trauma and haemorrhage. In a landmark study, Holcomb and colleagues demonstrated that TEG was superior to INR in the quantification of coagulopathy following trauma and suggested that TEG should replace INR [14]. rTEG results allow prediction of need for early transfusion in polytrauma patients [15]. Fibrinolysis has been identified as a critical component of the acute coagulopathy of trauma, and a fibrinolytic phenotype is an independent predictor of mortality [16]. TEG allows for rapid quantification of fibrinolysis and can be used to guide antifibrinolytic therapy, setting this viscoelastic testing apart from conventional coagulation testing. TEG-guided resuscitation during massive transfusion is associated with a lower haemorrhage-related mortality in trauma [17].

Rotational Thromboelastometry

Rotational thromboelastometry is a popular form of viscoelastic testing that relies upon changes in clot elasticity over time and is used extensively in Europe but also in a number of US centres since achieving FDA approval in 2011. A comparison of variables measured by TEG and ROTEM is found in Table 28.2. In addition to the modifications of TEG, such as rTEG, the ROTEM assay can be modified using various activators/adjuncts for specific uses (Table 28.3). Multiple, small prospective randomised studies have supported the use of ROTEM to reduce transfusion requirements in cardiac surgery and trauma and, similar to TEG, reports exist on the use of ROTEM in multiple clinical entities, including sepsis [11]. Few well-conducted studies exist comparing TEG and ROTEM head to head so it is impossible, at present, to differentiate between the two for any specific clinical indication.

Despite the enthusiasm for TEG and ROTEM in trauma and massive haemorrhage, the use of these POC tests remains controversial due to the absence of large prospective randomised trials. Two Cochrane systematic reviews have been conducted on the subject, the first in 2011 [18] and the second in 2015 [19]. The objective of the 2011 review was to 'systematically assess the benefits and harms of a TEG or ROTEM

Table 28.2 Comparison of TEG and ROTEM variables.

Variable	TEG	ROTEM
Initial measurement		Reaction time (RT)
Time to maximum thrombin and fibrin cleavage	R time	Clotting time (CT)
Clot kinetics	K, alpha angle	Clot formation time (CFT)
Maximum clot strength	Maximum amplitude (MA)	Maximum clot firmness (MCF)
Time to maximum strength		MCF-t
Clot elasticity	G	MCE
Clot lysis time (CLT)	LY30, LY60	CL30, CL60
Maximum lysis		CLF
Time to lysis	2 mm from MA	CLT

Table 28.3 Modifications to ROTEM and interpretation.

Test	Activator/Inhibitor	Interpretation
INTEM	Phospholipid, ellagic acid	Similar to aPTT
EXTEM	Tissue factor	Similar to PT
HEPTEM	Heparinase	Neutralises heparin
APTEM	Aprotinin	Inhibits fibrinolysis
FIBTEM	Cytochalasin D	Blocks platelet function, allows for selective analysis of fibrinogen
ECATEM	Ecarin	Detects thrombin inhibitors; similar to ecarin clotting time

aPTT, activated partial thromboplastin time; PT, prothrombin time.

guided transfusion strategy in randomised trials involving patients with severe bleeding.' Nine randomised controlled trials (RCTs) were included in the analysis, with only five providing data on the primary endpoint of mortality. Although no data could support the use of TEG or ROTEM to reduce morbidity or mortality, there was a significant reduction in blood loss noted across all trials, potentially attributable to earlier recognition and correction of coagulopathy [18]. The review by Hunt and colleagues draws the conclusion that viscoelastic testing such as TEG and ROTEM in trauma should be limited to research purposes [19]. The review included only three main studies which focused on a comparison between ROTEM and conventional coagulation testing with a great deal of heterogeneity between studies. One of the authors of this chapter (MDN) challenged the review in a rebuttal that was published as an addendum to the Cochrane review [19]. The rebuttal challenges the assertion that the use of conventional coagulation testing has never been rigorously validated as a standard for the measurement of trauma-induced coagulopathy. In fact, correlation with clinical and haemostatic history is necessary for accurate interpretation of conventional coagulation testing, and measurement of PT and INR alone misses major components of coagulation, including the intrinsic pathway, platelet function and the presence of inhibitors. Including only studies using comparison of ROTEM to PT and INR

without any assessment of clinical bleeding inserts a major form of selection bias into the 2015 review by Hunt and colleagues, and it is clear that more robust prospective analyses are needed.

Point-of-Care Testing in Transfusion Algorithms

A recent, large clinical effectiveness review was undertaken to compare POC viscoelastic testing to conventional laboratory monitoring of haemostasis in cardiac surgery, trauma-induced coagulopathy and post-partum haemorrhage [20]. Analysis of the 39 studies concluded that viscoelastic testing reduced red cell, FFP and platelet transfusion compared to standard coagulation testing. This reduction resulted in significant cost savings in cardiac surgery and trauma. However, there appeared to be no overall clinical outcome differences in these heterogeneous studies. Thus, the study concludes that use of viscoelastic testing may be a more effective means of reducing costs and provide a more efficient guide for blood product management in these clinical settings. Importantly, these findings cannot be extrapolated to other clinical scenarios, although it seems prudent to encourage ongoing research in other perioperative settings given the benefits described for cardiovascular surgery and trauma.

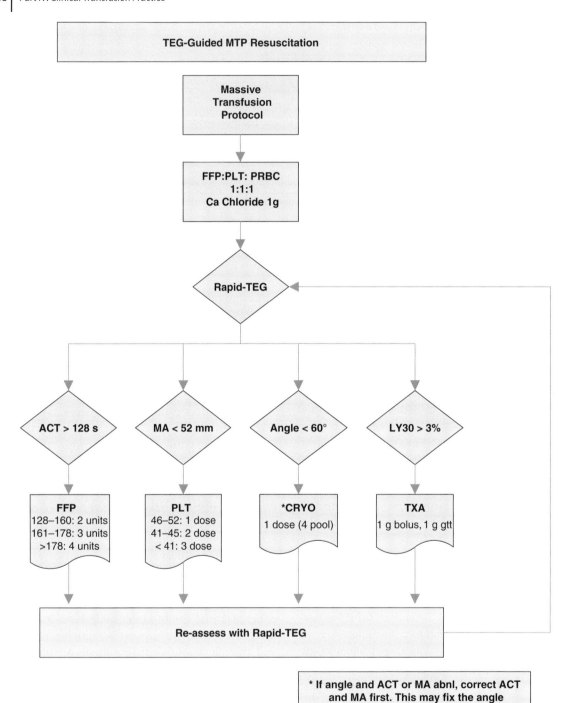

Figure 28.2 University of Pittsburgh Medical Center Massive Transfusion Protocol.

Other authors have devised very specific algorithms for the use of ROTEM to guide the exact administration of blood components in response to viscoelastic changes. In a large German study by Gorlinger and colleagues, the use of ROTEM in cardiac surgery not only reduced blood product use but also reduced the requirement for massive transfusion, unplanned reexploration and thromboembolic events by a significant amount [21]. Similar approaches by Schochl [22] and Theusinger [23] have provided very specific treatment guidelines for blood product transfusion based on the changes noted in viscoelastic testing. These experiences, among others, have led many institutions to utilise TEG/ROTEM-based guidelines for not only their operative transfusion but also their institutional massive transfusion protocols. Although not part of the treatment or resuscitation algorithm, TEG was utilised by most centres in the first prospective randomised controlled trial examining haemostatic resuscitation using fixed ratios of blood components [24] and TEG has become standard of care at many US trauma centres. In fact, the American College of Surgeons Resources for Optimal Care of the Injured Patient 2014 (6th edition) recommends that thromboelastography

should be available at level 1 and 2 trauma centres. Similarly, the National Institute for Health and Care Excellence (NICE) has issued recommendations in favour of using TEG/ROTEM for POC use in cardiac surgery, with recommendations for further research in other areas. Given the increased acceptance of viscoelastic testing and the potential for cost savings and reduction of blood product utilisation, it is likely that many massive transfusion protocols will utilise TEG/ROTEM-based algorithms. Recently, the authors' institution implemented a new massive transfusion protocol based on TEG, included here as Figure 28.2.

In summary, POC testing has evolved as an efficient and cost-effective alternative to conventional laboratory testing that allows for more rapid results in an acute care setting. Studies in cardiovascular surgery, transplantation and trauma suggest that POC testing can effectively guide transfusion of blood components and may improve clinical outcomes, although this remains unproven. Further studies are needed in order to extend these findings into other clinical practices. Future transfusion strategies, including massive transfusion protocols, are likely to be based on validated POC analyses.

KEY POINTS

1) Conventional coagulation tests lack validation in acute care or critical care settings and are more useful in guiding the management of anticoagulation in the case of PT/INR or detecting absolute deficiencies in clotting factors or platelet number.

2) POC platelet technology allows for identification of inherited or acquired platelet dysfunction in an acute care setting, which is not detected by conventional coagulation testing.

3) Prospective studies have validated the use of POC platelet technology to reduce transfusion requirements in cardiovascular surgery.

4) TEG-guided resuscitation during massive transfusion after trauma may be associated with a lower haemorrhage-related mortality in trauma and decreased transfusion of blood and blood components.

5) Viscoelastic testing is cost effective for use in cardiac surgery and following trauma.

References

1 Meybohm P, Zacharowski K, Weber CF. Point-of-care coagulation management in intensive care medicine. Crit Care 2013;**17**(2):218.

2 Paniccia R, Antonucci E, Maggini N et al. Assessment of platelet function on whole blood by multiple electrode aggregometry in high-risk patients with coronary artery disease

receiving antiplatelet therapy. Am J Clin Pathol 2009;**131**(6):834–42.

3 Hayward CP, Harrison P, Cattaneo M, Ortel TL, Rao AK. Platelet function analyzer (PFA)-100 closure time in the evaluation of platelet disorders and platelet function. J Thromb Hemost 2006;**4**(2):312–19.

4 Chakroun T, Gerotziafas G, Robert F et al. In vitro aspirin resistance detected by PFA-100 closure time: pivotal role of plasma von Willebrand factor. Br J Hematol 2004;**124**(1):80–5.

5 Shenkman B, Matetzky S, Fefer P et al. Variable responsiveness to clopidogrel and aspirin among patients with acute coronary syndrome as assessed by platelet function tests. Thromb Res 2008;**122**(3):336–45.

6 Enriquez LJ, Shore-Lesserson L. Point-of-care coagulation testing and transfusion algorithms. Br J Anaesth 2009;**103**(Suppl. 1):i14–22.

7 Cammerer U, Dietrich W, Rampf T, Braun SL, Richter JA. The predictive value of modified computerized thromboelastography and platelet function analysis for postoperative blood loss in routine cardiac surgery. Anesth Analg 2003;**96**(1):51–7.

8 Sucker C, Litmathe J, Feindt P, Zotz R. Platelet function analyzer (PFA-100) as a useful tool for the prediction of transfusion requirements during aortic valve replacement. Thorac Cardiovasc Surg 2011;**59**(4):233–6.

9 Spiess BD, Royston D, Levy JH et al. Platelet transfusions during coronary artery bypass graft surgery are associated with serious adverse outcomes. Transfusion 2004;**44**(8):1143–8.

10 Weber CF, Gorlinger K, Meininger D et al. Point-of-care testing: a prospective, randomized clinical trial of efficacy in coagulopathic cardiac surgery patients. Anesthesiology 2012;**117**(3):531–47.

11 Muller MC, Meijers JC, Vroom MB, Juffermans NP. Utility of thromboelastography and/or thromboelastometry in adults with sepsis: a systematic review. Crit Care 2014;**18**(1):R30.

12 McDaniel LM, Etchill EW, Raval JS, Neal MD. State of the art: massive transfusion. Transfus Med 2014;**24**(3):138–44.

13 Neal MD, Marsh A, Marino R et al. Massive transfusion: an evidence-based review of recent developments. Arch Surg 2012;**147**(6):563–71.

14 Holcomb JB, Minei KM, Scerbo ML et al. Admission rapid thrombelastography can replace conventional coagulation tests in the emergency department: experience with 1974 consecutive trauma patients. Ann Surg 2012;**256**(3):476–86.

15 Cotton BA, Faz G, Hatch QM et al. Rapid thrombelastography delivers real-time results that predict transfusion within 1 hour of admission. J Trauma 2011;**71**(2):407–14; discussion 414–17.

16 Moore EE, Moore HB, Gonzalez E et al. Postinjury fibrinolysis shutdown: rationale for selective tranexamic acid. J Trauma Acute Care Surg 2015;**78**(6 Suppl. 1):S65–9.

17 Johansson PI, Sorensen AM, Larsen CF et al. Low hemorrhage-related mortality in trauma patients in a Level I trauma center employing transfusion packages and early thromboelastography-directed hemostatic resuscitation with plasma and platelets. Transfusion 2013;**53**(12):3088–99.

18 Afshari A, Wikkelso A, Brok J, Moller AM, Wetterslev J. Thrombelastography (TEG) or thromboelastometry (ROTEM) to monitor hemotherapy versus usual care in patients with massive transfusion. Cochrane Database Syst Rev 2011;**3**:CD007871.

19 Hunt H, Stanworth S, Curry N et al. Thromboelastography (TEG) and rotational thromboelastometry (ROTEM) for trauma induced coagulopathy in adult trauma patients with bleeding. Cochrane Database Syst Rev 2015;**2**:CD010438.

20 Whiting P, Al M, Westwood M et al. Viscoelastic point-of-care testing to assist with the diagnosis, management and monitoring of hemostasis: a systematic review and cost-effectiveness analysis. Health Technol Assess 2015;**19**(58):1–228.

21 Gorlinger K, Fries D, Dirkmann D, Weber CF, Hanke AA, Schochl H. Reduction of fresh frozen plasma requirements by perioperative point-of-care coagulation management with early calculated goal-directed therapy. Transfus Med Hemother 2012;**39**(2):104–13.

22 Schochl H, Nienaber U, Maegele M et al. Transfusion in trauma: thromboelastometry-guided coagulation factor concentrate-based therapy versus standard fresh frozen plasma-based therapy. Crit Care 2011;**15**(2):R83.

23 Theusinger OM, Stein P, Spahn DR. Transfusion strategy in multiple trauma patients. Curr Opin Crit Care 2014;**20**(6):646–55.

24 Holcomb JB, Tilley BC, Baraniuk S et al. Transfusion of plasma, platelets, and red blood cells in a 1:1:1 vs a 1:1:2 ratio and mortality in patients with severe trauma: the PROPPR randomized clinical trial. JAMA 2015;**313**(5):471–82.

Further Reading

Afshari A, Wikkelsø A, Brok J, Møller AM, Wetterslev J. Thrombelastography (TEG) or thromboelastometry (ROTEM) to monitor hemotherapy versus usual care in patients with massive transfusion. Cochrane Database Syst Rev 201;**3**:CD007871.

Holcomb JB, Minei KM, Scerbo ML et al. Admission rapid thrombelastography can replace conventional coagulation tests in the emergency department: experience with 1974 consecutive trauma patients. Ann Surg 2012;**256**(3):476–86.

Hunt H, Stanworth S, Curry N et al. Thromboelastography (TEG) and rotational thromboelastometry (ROTEM) for trauma induced coagulopathy in adult trauma patients with bleeding. Cochrane Database Syst Rev 2015;**2**:CD010438.

Mallett SV, Armstrong M. Point-of-care monitoring of hemostasis. Anaesthesia 2015;**70**(Suppl. 1):73–7, e25–6.

Müller MC, Meijers JC, Vroom MB, Juffermans NP. Utility of thromboelastography and/or thromboelastometry in adults with sepsis: a systematic review. Crit Care 2014;**18**(1):R30.

Pearse BL, Smith I, Faulke D et al. Protocol guided bleeding management improves cardiac surgery patient outcomes. Vox Sang 2015;**109**:267–79.

Theusinger OM, Levy JH. Point of care devices for assessing bleeding and coagulation in the trauma patient. Anesthesiol Clin 2013;**31**(1):55–65.

Theusinger OM, Stein P, Levy JH. Point of care and factor concentrate-based coagulation algorithms. Transfus Med Hemother 2015;**42**(2):115–21.

Thiele RH, Raphael J. A 2014 update on coagulation management for cardiopulmonary bypass. Semin Cardiothorac Vasc Anesth 2014;**18**(2):177–89.

Whiting P, Al M, Westwood M et al. Viscoelastic point-of-care testing to assist with the diagnosis, management and monitoring of hemostasis: a systematic review and cost-effectiveness analysis. Health Technol Assess 2015;**19**(58):1–228.

29 Haematological Disease

Lise J. Estcourt[1,3], Simon J. Stanworth[1,2,3] and Michael F. Murphy[1,2,3]

[1] *NHS Blood and Transplant, John Radcliffe Hospital, Oxford, UK*
[2] *Department of Hematology, Oxford University Hospitals, Oxford, UK*
[3] *Radcliffe Department of Medicine, University of Oxford, Oxford, UK*

Introduction

Patients with haematological diseases are major users of blood components. Haematological diseases requiring transfusion support cover a whole spectrum of clinical disorders: fetal, neonatal and paediatric practice (Chapter 33), haemoglobinopathies (Chapter 30), haemophilia (Chapter 25), immune disorders (Chapter 32) and bone marrow failure syndromes, in addition to haematological malignancies.

The haemopoietic system has a dramatic capacity for increasing the production of blood cells, but this capability varies between different diseases. The scenario of anaemia related to marrow ablation following chemotherapy is very different from anaemia in an individual with a well-compensated chronic haemolytic process. Although 18% of all red cell units are transfused to patients with haematological disease, most are given to patients with malignant disorders [1]. The requirement for blood transfusions in this group is related to both the underlying condition itself and the myelosuppressive/myeloablative effects of the specific treatments used.

This chapter considers the following topics:

- the *indications* for red cell, platelet and granulocyte transfusions in haematology patients

- the approaches to the management and prevention of *complications* associated with transfusions in haematology patients, including the use of special types of blood components.

Red Cell Transfusions

The ready availability of red cell components means that anaemia can be easily treated. There are some special considerations in the management of anaemia that are applicable to haematology patients, as well as other clinical groups.

- The cause should be established and treatment other than blood transfusion should be used where appropriate, for instance in patients with iron deficiency or megaloblastic or autoimmune haemolytic anaemia (AIHA). Anaemia of malignancy may be due to the effects of marrow infiltration or therapy, 'inhibitory' cytokine-mediated influences leading to secondary anaemias (of chronic disorders) or low levels of erythropoietin.

- There is no universal 'trigger' for red cell transfusion, i.e. a given level of haemoglobin concentration (Hb) at which red cell transfusion is appropriate for all patients. Clinical judgement balancing factors such as quality-of-life indices plays an important role in the decision to transfuse red cells or not [2].

Practical Transfusion Medicine, Fifth Edition. Edited by Michael F. Murphy, David J. Roberts and Mark H. Yazer.
© 2017 John Wiley & Sons Ltd. Published 2017 by John Wiley & Sons Ltd.

Patients Receiving Intensive Myelosuppressive/Myeloablative Treatment

There are specific considerations relating to the use of red cell transfusion in patients receiving intensive myelosuppressive/myeloablative treatment, including the need to provide a 'reserve' in case of severe infection or haemorrhage, and the convenience of having a standard policy for red cell transfusion in the setting of an acute haematology service, even if this may result in some patients being overtransfused.

The level of Hb used as the 'trigger' for transfusion varies from centre to centre but is usually in the range 70–90 g/L. A restrictive policy is generally advocated because of data from trials in other patient groups indicating the safety of this approach and the well-recognised risks of transfusion [2]. There are no definite data to support the use of a higher level, although studies in animal models of thrombocytopenia and in uraemic patients suggest that correction of anaemia also results in correction of prolonged bleeding times [3].

Red Cell Transfusions and Chronic Anaemias

In patients with chronic anaemia requiring regular transfusions, red cell transfusions should be used to maintain the Hb just above the lowest level not associated with symptoms of anaemia [4]. There is considerable variation in this level depending on the patient's age, level of activity and coexisting medical problems, such as cardiovascular and respiratory disease; for example, some young patients are asymptomatic with an Hb below 70 g/L, while some elderly patients are symptomatic even at an Hb above 100 g/L. Special considerations apply to patients with haemoglobinopathies, and these are considered in Chapter 30.

The Use of Recombinant Erythropoietin in Haematological Disease

The clinical use of recombinant erythropoietin (RhEpo) might be considered in several situations in haematology patients, such as delayed erythroid engraftment after allogeneic bone marrow/peripheral blood progenitor cell transplantation, the treatment of anaemia in patients with myeloma or myelodysplasia, and in the management of Jehovah's Witnesses with haematological disorders. Evidence supports an association between increases in Hb, reduced red cell transfusion requirements and possibly improvement in quality-of-life indices with RhEpo therapy, although the findings concerning quality-of-life measures are more difficult to compare between studies. Uncertainties also remain about the factors predicting responsiveness, since a number of individuals fail to show adequate responses to RhEpo. However, as discussed in Chapter 46, recent systematic reviews have raised concerns about adverse events (increased morbidity and mortality) in patients treated with RhEpo [5,6]. The most recent American guidelines [5] now only recommend using RhEpo in patients with haematological malignancies who are being treated with palliative intent.

Red Cell Transfusions and Immune Blood Disorders

In immune haemolytic anaemia, antibodies bind to red blood cell surface antigens and initiate destruction via the complement system and/or the macrophage system. Immune haemolytic anaemia may be alloimmune, autoimmune or drug induced (Box 29.1).

Autoimmune haemolytic anaemias are uncommon (incidence 1–3 per 100 000 per year). They are characterised by the production of antibodies directed against high-frequency red cell antigens and often exhibit reactivity against donor red cells. The degree of haemolysis depends on a number of factors, including the characteristics of the bound antibody (e.g. class, quantity, specificity, thermal amplitude), the target antigen (e.g. density, expression) and other host-related genetic factors (e.g. markers of macrophage activity). The antibody class in turn will affect the degree of classic complement

---

Box 29.1 Causes of immune haemolytic anaemia.

Alloimmune

Haemolytic disease of the newborn (see Chapter 33)

Haemolytic transfusion reactions

After allogeneic stem cell, renal, liver or cardiac transplantation when donor lymphocytes transferred in the allograft ('passenger lymphocytes') may produce red cell antibodies against the recipient and cause haemolytic anaemia (see Chapter 8)

Autoimmune

Warm autoantibody (antibody maximally active at 37 °C; usually IgG with anti-Rh specificity)

Idiopathic (>30% of cases)

Secondary to lymphoproliferative disease (e.g. chronic lymphocytic leukaemia, lymphoma)

Secondary to autoimmune disease (e.g. systemic lupus erythematosus)

Cold autoantibody (antibody maximally active at less than 37 °C; usually IgM)

Idiopathic

Chronic cold haemagglutinin disease (monoclonal usually with anti-I specificity)

Secondary to infections (polyclonal)

Mycoplasma (anti-I specificity)

Infectious mononucleosis (anti-I specificity)

Secondary to lymphoproliferative disease

Secondary to autoimmune disease

Paroxysmal cold haemoglobinuria (usually polyclonal IgG with anti-P specificity)

Secondary to viral infections, e.g. measles, mumps, chickenpox

Congenital or tertiary syphilis

Drug induced

Hapten mechanism, e.g. high-dose penicillins (greater than 10 million units/day), cephalosporins

Autoantibody mechanism. e.g. α-methyldopa

Immune complex mechanism, e.g. quinine

---

activation (IgM) or binding to splenic and other tissue macrophages via Fc receptors (IgG1 and IgG3 antibodies). The direct antiglobulin test (DAT) is usually positive but can be negative. The threshold of cell-bound antibody detection, using the antiglobulin test, is 200–500 antibody molecules per cell, but fewer than 100 molecules of IgG per cell may significantly reduce red cell survival *in vivo*. In warm antibody AIHA, IgG antibodies predominate and the DAT is positive with IgG alone (20%), IgG and complement (detected as C3d) (67%) or C3d only (13%). In cold antibody AIHA, the antibodies (usually IgM) easily elute off red cells, leaving complement on the red cell surface (DAT is positive with C3d alone).

Warm Antibody AIHA (see Box 29.1)

Therapy of warm antibody AIHA depends on the severity of the haemolysis. Treatment is usually required once symptomatic anaemia develops. Steroids are the first-line treatment (e.g. prednisolone in doses of 1 mg/kg daily) and are effective in inducing remission in about 80% of patients. Steroids reduce both production of the red cell autoantibody and destruction of antibody-coated cells. Splenectomy may be necessary if there is no response to steroids or if remission is not maintained when the dose of prednisolone is reduced. Other immunosuppressive drugs, such as azathioprine and cyclophosphamide, may be effective in patients who fail to respond to steroids and splenectomy. Ciclosporin and rituximab may also be effective in patients who are refractory to all treatment.

Blood transfusion may be required if there is fulminant haemolytic anaemia or severe anaemia not responding to steroids or other therapy. The presence of red cell autoantibodies on the patient's red cells and in the plasma can cause problems in the identification of compatible blood. It is important to exclude the presence of red cell alloantibodies, and autoabsorption of autoantibodies in the plasma using enzyme treatment of the patient's red cells may be necessary to permit the investigation of the plasma for alloantibodies (see Chapter 23).

Cold Antibody AIHA

In cold autoantibody AIHA, the IgM antibodies attach to red cells and cause their agglutination in the cold peripheries/extremities of the body; activation of complement can cause intravascular haemolysis when the cells return to the higher temperatures in the core of the body. This can occur after certain infections (see Box 29.1), producing a mild-to-moderate transient haemolysis, or can be associated with chronic disease.

Chronic cold haemagglutinin disease usually occurs in the elderly, with a gradual onset of haemolytic anaemia. After exposure to cold, the patient develops an acrocyanosis similar to Raynaud's disease as a result of red cell autoagglutination. If possible, the underlying cause of the antibody production should be treated (associated with clonal B-cell lymphocyte proliferation) and patients should avoid exposure to cold. Treatment with steroids, alkylating agents and splenectomy is usually ineffective. Rituximab is increasingly used as a well-tolerated and effective treatment, producing remission in about 50% of patients. Regular blood transfusion is occasionally required to prevent symptoms of anaemia. The laboratory can usually find compatible blood by using prewarmed techniques when performing compatibility testing.

Paroxysmal Cold Haemoglobinuria (see Box 29.1)

Paroxysmal cold haemoglobinuria is a rare condition that is typically seen in children following a viral illness. It is associated with complement-fixing IgG antibodies that are biphasic (typically anti-P specificity), adhering to the red cell membrane in the cold peripheries, with lysis occurring due to complement activation when the cells return to the central circulation. The lytic reaction is demonstrated *in vitro* by incubating the patient's red cells and serum at $0\,^\circ$C and then warming the mixture to $37\,^\circ$C (direct Donath–Landsteiner test). This test can be falsely negative due to a lack of complement so a more accurate test is the indirect Donath–Landsteiner test (Figure 29.1). Haemolysis is self-limiting, but supportive transfusions may be necessary. P-negative blood should be considered if there is no sustained response to transfusion of P-positive crossmatch compatible blood.

The issue of whether it is necessary to use an in-line blood warmer when transfusing patients with cold antibody AIHA is controversial. It is logical to keep the patient warm and a common practice to use a blood warmer if the patient has florid haemolytic anaemia.

Drug-Induced AIHA (see Box 29.1)

There are three basic mechanisms of drug-induced immune red cell injury. In the hapten mechanism, the drug binds strongly to red cell proteins. IgG antibodies are directed against drug epitopes and only react with drug-coated red blood cells. Antibody production usually occurs 7–10 days after starting the drug and the patient typically is receiving high doses of the drug. Many patients will have a positive DAT but do not have haemolysis. When haemolysis occurs, it usually results in a gradual drop in haemoglobin. In the autoantibody mechanism, the drug induces formation of IgG autoantibodies via unknown mechanisms. α-Methyldopa can cause a positive DAT 6–12 weeks after starting the drug but most patients do not have clinical and laboratory signs of haemolysis. In the immune complex mechanism, the drug forms immune complexes with antibody (usually IgM), which then attach to red cell membrane, causing complement-mediated lysis. Classically, it occurs on second or subsequent exposure to the drug and the patient may present with severe

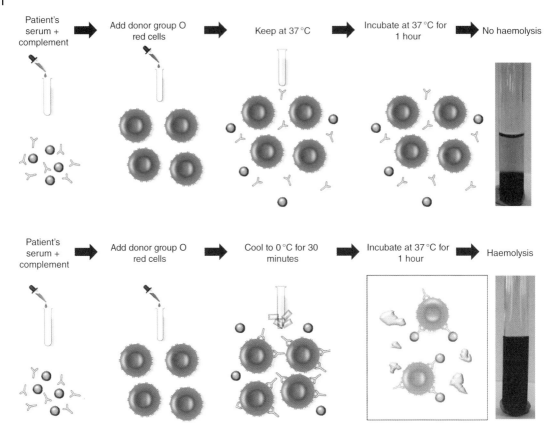

Figure 29.1 The indirect Donath–Landsteiner test for paroxysmal cold haemoglobinuria.

intravascular haemolysis occurring within minutes to hours of drug ingestion.

Paroxysmal Nocturnal Haemoglobinuria

Paroxysmal nocturnal haemoglobinuria (PNH) is a rare, acquired, clonal haematopoietic stem cell disorder due to a mutation in the PIG-A gene producing cells that lack glycosylphosphatidylinositol (GPI)-linked surface proteins. Patients may present with haemolytic anaemia, cytopenias and/or a thrombotic tendency. Haemolysis is caused by the lack of decay-accelerating factor (DAF; CD55) and membrane inhibitor of reactive lysis (MIRL; CD59) that regulate complement activation on the surface of circulating red cells. The only potentially curative therapy for PNH is allogeneic stem cell transplantation; however, this procedure is associated with substantial morbidity

and mortality [7] and, consequently, is not an appropriate therapeutic option for most patients. Transfusion is necessary when therapeutic treatment measures fail to maintain adequate haemoglobin levels. Eculizumab, a humanised monoclonal antibody that inhibits terminal complement activation, has been shown in several trials to be well tolerated and provides a rapid, sustained and clinically significant reduction in haemolysis, fatigue and transfusion requirements, as well as improved quality of life [7].

Platelet Transfusions

In general, platelet transfusions are indicated for the prevention and treatment of haemorrhage in patients with thrombocytopenia or platelet function defects. The cause of the thrombocytopenia should be established before platelet transfusions are used because they are not always appropriate treatment for thrombocytopenic patients, and in some instances are contraindicated, such as in thrombotic thrombocytopenic purpura, haemolytic–uremic syndrome and heparin-induced thrombocytopenia (see Chapter 31).

Bone Marrow Failure

Therapeutic platelet transfusions are established as an effective treatment for patients who are bleeding. However, *prophylactic* platelet transfusion therapy for the prevention of haemorrhage in chronically thrombocytopenic patients with bone marrow failure remains more controversial. Guidelines for platelet transfusion in many countries recommend that the platelet transfusion trigger for prophylaxis is $10 \times 10^9/L$ [8], and most local departmental policies would follow this recommendation, with an acceptance that selected patients with additional risk factors, such as sepsis or invasive infections, might benefit from higher thresholds.

Unfortunately, many audits continue to document that compliance with these general recommendations is poor, and a recent national comparative audit in the UK [9] showed that a large proportion (28%) of platelet transfusions were given inappropriately. One critical question is whether the evidence from published trials, when combined, demonstrates equivalence in terms of the safety of a platelet count threshold of $10 \times 10^9/L$ rather than $20 \times 10^9/L$. A recent systematic review [10] has suggested that there is insufficient evidence to answer this question. However, many of the bleeding events in these studies were relatively minor and platelet transfusions are associated with well-described risks. Hence, there is no evidence to change from the current practice of a platelet transfusion threshold of $10 \times 10^9/L$ unless there are other risk factors for haemorrhage.

A large randomised controlled trial [11] showed there was no significant difference in the number of patients who bled between the low-dose (1.1×10^{11} platelets/m^2), medium-dose (2.2×10^{11} platelets/m^2) and high-dose (4.4×10^{11}/m^2) treatment arms. Overall, a low-dose transfusion policy reduced patients' total platelet requirements but at the expense of a higher number of platelet transfusions. In the UK, the standard adult dose is approximately 2.4×10^{11} platelets, which is close to the low dose used in the recently published large platelet dose trial [11]. There was no difference in the number of platelet transfusion episodes between medium- and high-dose treatment arms, indicating that a high-dose policy decreases neither bleeding nor number of transfusion episodes [12].

A general finding across all prophylactic platelet transfusion trials, including the two largest studies comparing different thresholds [10] or doses [12] mentioned above, has been the lack of any difference in results for haemostatic outcomes between trial arms (i.e. no increased bleeding in the restrictive policy arms for transfusion by lower threshold or dose). This has raised questions about the size of benefit of using platelet transfusions as prophylaxis to prevent bleeding. With this in mind, two randomised controlled trials of prophylactic platelet transfusions have now been completed in adults with thrombocytopenia due to haematological malignancies or their treatment [13,14]. Both found a no-prophylaxis approach led to higher rates of World Health Organization (WHO) grade 2–4 bleeding overall. Platelet usage was markedly reduced in the no-prophylaxis arm in both studies. Prespecified subgroup analyses which compared treatment effects between autologous haematopoietic stem cell transplantation (HSCT) and chemotherapy/allogeneic HSCT patients showed very similar proportions of bleeding between treatment arms in autologous HSCT patients, and a large number of patients would need to be treated with unnecessary prophylactic platelet transfusions to prevent one WHO grade 2 bleed (on average, 43 patients over a 30-day period).

A strategy of transfusing platelets only for therapeutic indications in the context of clinical bleeding may be appropriate for some patients with *chronic* persisting thrombocytopenia due to bone marrow failure syndromes, such as myelodysplasia [8].

Prophylactic platelet transfusions for invasive procedures depend on the type of procedure being performed [8].

- No increase in platelet count required for low-risk procedures: bone marrow aspiration and biopsy, central line insertion.
- Platelet count should be raised to 50×10^9/L: lumbar puncture, transbronchial and liver biopsy and laparotomy.
- Platelet count should be raised to more than 100×10^9/L: surgery in critical sites such as the brain or the posterior segment of the eyes.

Immune Thrombocytopenias

- Autoimmune thrombocytopenias: platelet transfusions should be used only in patients with major haemorrhage [8,15].
- Posttransfusion purpura: platelet transfusions are usually ineffective in raising the platelet count, but may be needed in large doses to control severe bleeding in the acute phase (see Chapter 14).
- Neonatal alloimmune thrombocytopenia: human platelet antigen (HPA)-matched platelet concentrates are the most appropriate treatment for this condition (see Chapter 33).

Massive Blood Transfusion

- Clinically significant dilutional thrombocytopenia only occurs with the transfusion of more than 1.5 times the blood volume of the recipient.
- The platelet count should be maintained above 50×10^9/L in patients receiving transfusions for massive acute blood loss (Chapter 26).

Disseminated Intravascular Coagulation

- In acute disseminated intravascular coagulation (DIC), where there is bleeding associated with severe thrombocytopenia, platelet transfusions should be given in addition to coagulation factor replacement (see Chapter 25).

- In chronic DIC, or in the absence of bleeding, platelet transfusions are not indicated.

Cardiopulmonary Bypass Surgery

- Platelet function defects and some degree of thrombocytopenia frequently occur after cardiac bypass surgery, but prophylactic platelet transfusions are not indicated (see Chapter 27).
- Platelet transfusions should be reserved for patients with bleeding not due to surgically correctable causes.

Granulocyte Transfusions

Severe persisting neutropenia is the principal limiting factor in the use of intensive treatment of patients with haematological malignancies. It may last for two weeks or more after chemotherapy or stem cell transplantation, and during this period the patient is at risk of life-threatening bacterial and fungal infections. The use of haematopoietic growth factors, such as granulocyte colony-stimulating factor (G-CSF), may reduce the duration and severity of severe neutropenia, but they are only effective if the patient has sufficient numbers of haematopoietic precursors. Moreover, the time to response may be several days. Supportive treatment with granulocyte transfusions is a logical approach, although a number of factors have limited its application.

- Difficulties in the collection of neutrophils, which are present in low numbers in normal individuals and which are difficult to separate from red cells because of their similar densities (commercially available long-chain starch solutions now facilitate this separation).
- The short half-life of neutrophils after transfusion, coupled with short storage times and negative effects on function of prolonged storage.
- The frequent occurrence of adverse effects such as febrile reactions, including occasional severe pulmonary reactions and human leucocyte antigen (HLA) alloimmunisation causing platelet refractoriness.

Various methods have been used in the past to increase the number of neutrophils collected for transfusion, including obtaining granulocytes from patients with chronic myeloid leukaemia, treating donors with steroids and using hydroxyethyl starch to promote sedimentation of red cells. There was a further resurgence of interest in granulocyte transfusions as larger doses of granulocytes could be collected from donors using regimens including G-CSF administered 12–16 hours prior to apheresis, together with oral steroids such as dexamethasone to further improve the yields. This acknowledged the accumulating evidence that G-CSF can be safely administered to normal individuals [16].

Randomised controlled trials of granulocyte transfusions have been very challenging to undertake and complete. Recruitment to the Resolving Infections in Neutropenia with Granulocytes (RING) trial did not reach the required target. There was no difference in primary endpoint (a composite 42-day outcome of survival and resolution of infection). It should also be noted that in this trial, just under a third of patients received lower doses than defined in the protocol. Some groups have suggested a potential role for an 'off-the-shelf' component of granulocytes derived from whole blood donations, although the doses of neutrophils are lower [17].

High-dose granulocyte transfusions collected from donors treated with G-CSF might be considered to be indicated in patients of any age with severe neutropenia due to bone marrow failure under the following circumstances:

- proven bacterial or fungal infection unresponsive to antimicrobial therapy or probable bacterial or fungal infection unresponsive to appropriate blind antimicrobial therapy
- neutrophil recovery not expected for 5–7 days
- children and lighter adults might be expected to show better incremental responses to granulocyte transfusions.

Granulocyte transfusions might be considered inappropriate for:

- patients with haematological disease resistant to treatment
- ventilated patients
- patients with known HLA alloimmunisation.

Approach to Complications Associated with Blood Transfusion in Haematology Patients

Transfusion-Transmitted CMV Infection

Clinical Features and Risk Factors

Cytomegalovirus (CMV) infection may cause significant morbidity and mortality in immunocompromised patients, mainly due to pneumonia. Patients who have never been exposed to CMV are at risk for primary infection transmitted by blood components prepared from blood donors who have previously had CMV infection and still carry the virus.

Patients who have been previously exposed to CMV and are CMV seropositive are at risk of reactivation of CMV during a period of immunosuppression. The extent to which CMV-seropositive patients are at risk from reinfection with different strains of CMV remains unknown, but this risk is generally considered to be very low. The patients at risk of transfusion-transmitted CMV infection are shown in Box 29.2 [18]. The use of CMV-seronegative blood components has been shown to reduce the incidence of CMV infection in groups at risk for transfusion-transmitted CMV infection to 1–3%. Incomplete prevention has been suggested to be due to:

- occasional failure to detect low-level CMV antibodies;
- loss of antibodies in previously infected blood donors; and
- transfusion of blood components prepared from recently infected donors.

Cytomegalovirus is transmitted by leucocytes, and a number of studies have found that prestorage leucocyte reduction of blood components is as effective as the use of

Box 29.2 Patients at risk for transfusion-transmitted cytomegalovirus (CMV) infection. [19].

Risk well established

CMV-seronegative recipients of allogeneic bone marrow/peripheral blood progenitor cell transplants from CMV-seronegative donors

CMV-seronegative pregnant women

Premature infants (<1.2 kg) born to CMV-seronegative women

CMV-seronegative patients with HIV infection

Risk less well established

CMV-seronegative patients receiving autologous bone marrow/peripheral blood progenitor cell transplants

CMV-seronegative patients who are potential recipients of allogeneic or autologous bone marrow/peripheral blood progenitor cell transplants

CMV-seronegative patients receiving solid organ (kidney, heart, lung, liver) transplants from CMV-seronegative donors

Risk not established

CMV-seronegative recipients of allogeneic bone marrow/peripheral blood progenitor cell transplants from CMV-seropositive donors

CMV-seropositive recipients of bone marrow/peripheral blood progenitor cell transplants

CMV-seropositive recipients of solid organ transplants

Source: Reproduced from Clark and Miller 2010 [19].

Box 29.3 Indications for the use of cytomegalovirus (CMV)-seronegative or CMV-safe blood components.

Transfusions in pregnancy

Intrauterine transfusions

Transfusions to neonates and to infants in the first year of life

Transfusions to the following groups of CMV-seronegative patients:

After allogeneic bone marrow/peripheral blood progenitor cell transplants where the donor is also CMV seronegative

After autologous bone marrow/peripheral blood progenitor cell transplants

Potential recipients of allogeneic bone marrow/peripheral blood progenitor cell transplants

Patients with HIV infection

CMV-seronegative blood components in the prevention of transfusion-transmitted CMV infection in neonates, patients undergoing remission induction therapy for acute leukaemia and after bone marrow transplantation (the only prospective randomised trial was conducted in transplant recipients using bedside leucocyte reduction filters, which cannot be adequately quality controlled for leucocyte reduction) (Box 29.3). These data suggest that prestorage leucocyte-reduced blood components can be accepted as a substitute for

CMV-seronegative blood components for patients at risk of transfusion-transmitted CMV infection when CMV-seronegative blood components are not available, i.e. that leucocyte-reduced blood components are 'CMV safe'. A consensus conference in Canada recommended that where universal leucocyte reduction has been implemented, both leucocyte-reduced and CMV-seronegative blood should be used for CMV-seronegative pregnant women, intrauterine transfusions and CMV-seronegative allogeneic haematopoietic cell transplant recipients [20]. In the UK, the Advisory Committee on the Safety of Blood, Tissues and Organs (SaBTO) recently concluded that the range of patients provided with CMV-screened blood should be reduced [21]. Specifically it indicated that:

- CMV-seronegative red cells and platelets may be replaced with leucocyte-reduced blood components for adults and children post haematopoietic stem cell transplantation, for all patient groups including seronegative donor/ seronegative recipients.
- Patients requiring transfusions who may require a transplant in the future may also

safely be transfused with leucocyte-reduced products (e.g. seronegative leukaemia or thalassaemia patients).

Transfusion-Associated Graft-Versus-Host Disease

Pathogenesis and Clinical Features

Transfusion-associated graft-versus-host disease (TA-GVHD) is a rare but serious complication of blood transfusion. As discussed in Chapter 13, there is engraftment and proliferation of donor T-lymphocytes and interaction with recipient cells expressing HLA antigens causing cellular damage particularly to the skin, gastrointestinal tract, liver and spleen and the bone marrow. Clinical manifestations usually occur 1–2 weeks after blood transfusion, and early features include fever, maculopapular skin rash, diarrhoea and hepatitis. Haematology patients at risk are those who are undergoing transplantation, have Hodgkin lymphoma or have received therapy with certain drugs, such as purine analogues.

Prevention

The dose of donor lymphocytes sufficient to cause TA-GVHD is unknown, but may be lower than is achievable by current techniques for leucocyte reduction of blood components. However, there have been no case reports of TA-GVHD in the UK since 2001 following the implementation of universal leucocyte reduction of blood in 1999. γ-Irradiation to destroy the proliferative capability of donor lymphocytes remains the usual method of choice to prevent TA-GVHD (see Chapter 11), although it is a radioactive source and requires regular recalibration. An alternative to γ-irradiation is x-ray irradiation, which is used in several European countries. Key considerations in the assessment of methods for the prevention of TA-GVHD are their effectiveness and the avoidance of excessive damage to red cells and platelets. The currently recommended indications for the use of irradiated blood for haematology patients are shown in Box 29.4 [22]. Although

γ-irradiation is currently the accepted method of preventing TA-GVHD, pathogen reduction technologies have been shown to be as effective at inactivating lymphocytes. Pathogen-reduced platelet components are accepted as safe from the risk of TA-GVHD in some countries without the need for further processing such as γ-irradiation.

Ensuring That Patients Receive the Correct 'Special' Blood

An important issue for haematology departments and hospital blood transfusion laboratories is how to ensure that patients receive special blood components (e.g. γ-irradiated) when these products are indicated and that standard blood components are not transfused, as this may have devastating consequences.

Each hospital needs to establish its own procedures so that patients receive the correct special blood components, where they are indicated. These procedures should include the following.

- Education of ward medical and nursing staff about the indications for special blood components and the importance of receiving the correct type of blood component.
- Requests for blood components to include the patient's diagnosis and any requirement for special blood components.
- Storing of individual patient's requirements for special blood components in the blood transfusion laboratory computer.
- The prescription for blood components should include any requirement for special blood components, enabling the ward staff to check that the blood component to be transfused complies with these requirements.

Providing patients with cards indicating their special blood requirements, particularly for those patients receiving shared care between two hospitals and those with a long-term requirement for γ-irradiated blood, e.g. patients with Hodgkin lymphoma.

Box 29.4 Indications for γ-irradiation of blood components in haematology patients.

Indications

Except for stem cell infusions, all donations from first- or second-degree relatives, even if the patient is immunocompetent

Except for stem cell infusions, all HLA-matched components, even if the patient is immunocompetent

All granulocyte components

Allogeneic bone marrow/peripheral blood progenitor cell transplantation: from the time of initiation of conditioning therapy and continuing while the patient remains on GVHD prophylaxis (usually 6 months) or until lymphocytes are $>1 \times 10^9$/L. If chronic GVHD is present or if continued immunosuppressive treatment is required, irradiated blood components should be given indefinitely

Allogeneic blood transfused to bone marrow and peripheral blood stem cell donors 7 days prior to or during the harvest must be irradiated

Autologous bone marrow/peripheral blood progenitor cell transplantation: during and 7 days before the harvest of haematopoietic cells, and then from the initiation of conditioning therapy until 3 months' posttransplant (6 months if total body irradiation is used)

All adults and children with Hodgkin lymphoma should have irradiated red cells and platelets for life

Severe T-lymphocyte immunodeficiency syndromes

Patients treated with purine analogues such as fludarabine, cladribine and deoxycoformycin and newer drugs such as bendamustine and clofarabine

Patients receiving alemtuzumab (anti-CD52)

Patients with aplastic anaemia receiving treatment with antithymocyte globulin

Nonindications

Patients receiving rituximab (anti-CD20).

Non-Hodgkin lymphoma (although this may be reviewed following some recent reports of TA-GVHD in patients with B-cell non-Hodgkin lymphoma)

HIV infection

Source: Reproduced from Treleaven et al [22], with permission of John Wiley & Sons.
TA-GVHD, transfusion-associated graft-versus-host disease.

HLA Alloimmunisation and Refractoriness to Platelet Transfusions [23]

Platelet refractoriness is the repeated failure to obtain satisfactory responses to platelet transfusions and it occurs in more than 50% of patients receiving multiple transfusions.

Various methods are used to assess response to platelet transfusions. If the patient is bleeding, the clinical response is an important indication of the effectiveness of the transfusion. The response to a prophylactic platelet transfusion is assessed by measuring the increase in platelet count after the transfusion. Various formulas have been used to correct for the variation in response dependent on the patient's size and the number of platelets transfused; these include platelet recovery and corrected count increment. However, in practice, a (nonsustained) increase in the patient's platelet count of less than 5×10^9/L at 20–24 hours after the transfusion can be used as a simple measure of a poor response.

Causes

Many causes of platelet refractoriness have been described and can be subdivided into immune mechanisms, most importantly HLA

Box 29.5 Causes of platelet refractoriness.

Immune

Platelet alloantibodies

    HLA

    HPA

    ABO

Other antibodies

    Platelet autoantibodies

    Drug-dependent platelet antibodies

Immune complexes

Non-immune

Infection and its treatment, especially amphotericin B

Splenomegaly

Disseminated intravascular coagulation

Fever

Bleeding

---

alloimmunisation and non-immune mechanisms involving platelet consumption (Box 29.5). Platelet consumption is the most frequent mechanism of platelet refractoriness, usually associated with sepsis. However, immune-mediated platelet destruction remains an important cause of platelet refractoriness; HLA antibodies are the most common immune cause and the other immune causes are rare.

The precise mechanism of HLA alloimmunisation remains uncertain, but primary HLA alloimmunisation appears to be initiated by intact cells expressing both HLA class I and class II antigens such as lymphocytes and antigen-presenting cells. Platelets only express HLA class I antigens and hence leucocyte-reduced blood components cause primary HLA alloimmunisation in fewer than 3% of recipients. Use of prestorage leucocyte-reduced blood components has therefore led to a significant reduction in the incidence of HLA alloimmunisation. However, secondary HLA alloimmunisation does not require the presence of HLA class II antigens, and may occur in patients who have been pregnant or previously transfused with nonleucocyte-reduced blood components.

Investigation and Management

If platelet refractoriness occurs, the following algorithm can be used for investigation and management (Figure 29.2) [23].

1) A clinical assessment should be made for clinical factors likely to be associated with non-immune platelet consumption.

2) If non-immune platelet consumption appears likely, an attempt should be made to correct the clinical factors responsible, where possible, and platelet transfusions from random donors should be continued. If a poor response to random donor platelet transfusions persists, the patient should be tested for HLA antibodies.

3) If non-immune platelet consumption appears to be unlikely, an immune mechanism should be suspected and the patient's serum should be tested for HLA antibodies. If HLA antibodies are present, the specificity of the antibodies should be determined as this may help in the election of HLA-compatible donors. However, HLA antibodies stimulated by repeated transfusions are often 'multispecific' and it is not possible to determine their specificity.

4) Platelet transfusions from HLA-matched donors (matched for the HLA-A, -B antigens of the patient) should be used for patients with apparent immune refractoriness and the response to further transfusions should be observed carefully. Figure 29.3 shows improved responses to HLA-matched platelet transfusions in a patient with platelet refractoriness due to HLA alloimmunisation. If responses to HLA-matched transfusions are not improved, the reason should be sought, and platelet crossmatching of the patient's serum against the lymphocytes and platelets of HLA-matched donors may be helpful in determining the cause and the selection of compatible donors for future transfusions. These matching strategies are based on counting the number of HLA-A and HLA-B mismatches between the patient and donor; this requires a large HLA-typed donor panel and at times no suitable matches can be found. An alternative approach is HLA epitope

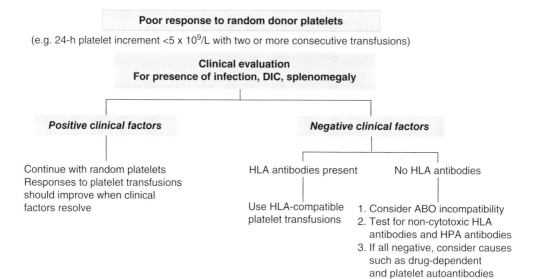

Poor response to random donor platelets

(e.g. 24-h platelet increment <5 x 10⁹/L with two or more consecutive transfusions)

Clinical evaluation
For presence of infection, DIC, splenomegaly

Positive clinical factors

Continue with random platelets
Responses to platelet transfusions
should improve when clinical
factors resolve

Negative clinical factors

HLA antibodies present

No HLA antibodies

Use HLA-compatible
platelet transfusions

1. Consider ABO incompatibility
2. Test for non-cytotoxic HLA
   antibodies and HPA antibodies
3. If all negative, consider causes
   such as drug-dependent
   and platelet autoantibodies

Figure 29.2 Algorithm for the investigation and management of patients with platelet refractoriness. DIC, disseminated intravascular coagulation; HLA, human leucocyte antigen; HPA, human platelet antigen.

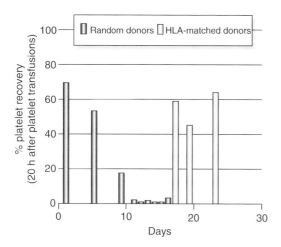

Figure 29.3 Responses to platelet transfusions in a female patient with acute myeloblastic leukaemia undergoing remission induction therapy. There were poor responses to the initial platelet transfusions and the patient was found to have human leucocyte antigen (HLA) antibodies. There were improved responses to platelet transfusions from HLA-matched donors.

matching; this only considers the epitopes on the HLA antigen, whereas standard HLA matching considers the whole HLA antigen.
5) If there are no factors for non-immune platelet consumption and HLA antibodies are not detected, consideration should be given to less frequent causes of immune platelet refractoriness.

- High-titre ABO antibodies in the recipient. This is an unusual cause of platelet refractoriness and can be excluded by switching to ABO-compatible platelet transfusions if ABO-incompatible transfusions have been used for previous transfusions.
- HPA antibodies, which usually occur in combination with HLA antibodies, but sometimes occur in isolation.
- Drug-dependent platelet antibodies, which may be underestimated as a cause for platelet refractoriness.

Alloimmunisation to Red Cell Antigens

Incidence

Alloimmunisation to red cell antigens is another important consequence of repeated transfusions in haematology patients. The incidence of red cell alloimmunisation in adult haematology patients is in the range of 10–15% and is similar to other groups of multitransfused patients, such as those with renal failure. However, a higher proportion of children requiring long-term transfusion support develop red cell alloimmunisation. In sickle cell disease, the incidence is in the range of 20–30% (see Chapter 30). The implications of these observations include the following.

- Patients with sickle cell disease should be phenotyped for Rh, Kell, Fy, Jk and MNS antigens before the first transfusion and patients with thalassaemia and other children requiring chronic transfusion support should be phenotyped for Rh and Kell antigens.
- Blood for transfusion to children requiring long-term transfusion support, including patients with haemoglobinopathies, should be matched for Rh and Kell antigens to prevent alloimmunisation.
- Phenotyping and antigen matching to prevent red cell alloimmunisation are not required for other groups of patients requiring repeated transfusions.

Timing of Sample Collection for Compatibility Testing [24]

In patients with haematological disorders receiving repeated transfusions, an important issue is the timing of blood sample collection in relation to the previous transfusion.

- Where the patient is receiving very frequent transfusion, for example daily, it is only necessary to request a new sample every three days.
- In the UK, if the previous transfusion was 3–14 days earlier, the sample should ideally be taken within 24 hours of the start of the transfusion, although some laboratories stretch this to 48 hours for patients who have been repeatedly transfused without developing antibodies. Other countries, such as Canada, only require a sample within three days of the start of the transfusion.
- Where the previous transfusion was 14–28 days earlier, the sample should be taken within three days of the start of the transfusion.
- Where the previous transfusion was more than 28 days ago, the sample should be taken within one week of the planned transfusion.

Sample collection time frame requirements do vary slightly from country to country.

ABO-Incompatible Bone Marrow/ Peripheral Blood Progenitor Cell Transplants

ABO-incompatible bone marrow/peripheral blood progenitor cell transplants present particular problems (Box 29.6). The transplant may provide a new A and/or B antigen from the donor (major mismatch) or a new A and/or B antibody (minor mismatch). For *pretransplant* transfusions, blood component support should be with the patient's own ABO type. For *posttransplant* transfusions, selection of the appropriate group is more complicated (Figure 29.4) [25]. These recommendations should be followed post transplant until the patient has engrafted, ABO antibodies to the donor ABO group are undetectable and the direct antiglobulin test is negative.

- *Major ABO incompatibility*: the patient's own ABO group should be given. Plasma and platelets should be of the donor-type blood group. The European Group for Blood and Marrow Transplantation (EBMT) also advises that group O red cells can be used.
- *Minor ABO incompatibility*: red cells of the donor ABO group should be given. Plasma and platelets should be of a recipient-type blood group.
- *Major and minor (bidirectional) ABO incompatibility*: give group O red cells, group AB plasma and platelets of the recipient-type blood group.

Studies disagree on whether ABO incompatibility can also affect overall survival, disease-free survival or GVHD. A meta-analysis [26] found no difference in overall survival between recipients of ABO-matched or ABO-mismatched grafts when the donor was related. However, in unrelated donor transplants there was a marginally reduced overall survival in patients who received bidirectional or minor mismatched transplants.

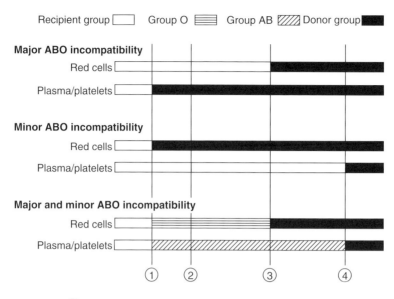

① Begin pre-transplant chemotherapy
② Bone marrow transplant
③ ABO antibodies to donor RBC not detected. Direct antiglobulin test negative
④ RBC of recipient group no longer detected

Figure 29.4 Recommendations for ABO type of blood components in ABO-incompatible bone marrow/peripheral blood progenitor cell transplants. RBC, red blood cell. *Source:* Adapted from Warkentin [25], reproduced with permission of Elsevier.

Box 29.6 Problems associated with ABO-incompatible bone marrow/peripheral blood progenitor transplants.

Major ABO incompatibility (e.g. recipient O, donor A)
Failure of engraftment: risk not increased in ABO-incompatible transplants
Acute haemolysis at the time of reinfusion: avoided by processing donor bone marrow/peripheral blood progenitor cells
Haemolysis of donor-type red cells: avoid by using red cells of recipient type in the early posttransplant period
Delayed erythropoiesis: may be due to persistence of anti-A in the recipient, minimise transfusion of anti-A by using platelets and plasma from group A donors
Delayed haemolysis due to persistence of recipient anti-A: only switch to donor red cells when recipient anti-A undetectable and direct antiglobulin test undetectable

Minor ABO incompatibility (e.g. recipient A, donor O)
Acute haemolysis at the time of reinfusion: avoid by removing donor plasma if the donor anti-A titre is high
Delayed haemolysis of recipient cells due to anti-A produced by donor lymphocytes (passenger lymphocyte syndrome): maximum haemolysis usually occurs between days 9 and 16 post transplant. Rare in T-cell-depleted grafts or when CD34+ cells selected in stem cell processing

Rhesus D-incompatible transplants can also cause difficulties. It is recommended that RhD-negative blood components should be used for RhD-positive recipients with RhD-negative donors. However, no cases of immunisation have been reported when RhD-negative recipients have received RhD-positive transplants, and RhD-positive blood components may be used.

Iron Overload

A major adverse consequence of repeated red cell transfusions over a long period in patients with haemoglobinopathies or myelodysplastic syndromes is iron overload. This important complication is described in detail in Chapter 30.

KEY POINTS

1) Specialist transfusion support and advice is required for many patients with haematological disorders.
2) The need for transfusion, as in other groups of patients, is determined by assessment of individual patient symptoms and blood counts and guided by national and local recommendations for the use of blood.
3) Special blood components are frequently needed to avoid complications such as TA-GVHD.
4) Responses to platelet transfusions should be carefully monitored to identify patients having poor responses, which require clinical and laboratory investigation to determine the most likely cause and the best approach to management.
5) Further work is needed to define the optimal thresholds for red cell and platelet transfusion in patients with haematological malignancies and the role of granulocyte transfusions.

References

1 Tinegate H, Chattree S, Iqbal A, Plews D, Whitehead J, Wallis J. Ten year pattern of blood use in the North of England. Transfusion 2013;**53**:483–9.
2 Goodnough T, Murphy MF. Do liberal blood transfusions cause more harm than good? BMJ 2015;**350**:13–15.
3 Valeri CR, Khuri S, Ragno G. Nonsurgical bleeding diathesis in anemic thrombocytopenic patients: role of temperature, red blood cells, platelets, and plasma clotting proteins. Transfusion 2007;**47**:206S–248S.
4 Killick SB, Carter C, Culligan D et al, for the British Committee for Standards in Hematology. Guidelines for the diagnosis and management of adult myelodysplastic syndromes. Br J Haematol 2014;**164**:503–25.
5 Rizzo JD, Brouwers M, Hurley P et al. American Society of Hematology/American Society of Clinical Oncology clinical practice guideline update on the use of epoetin and darbepoetin in adult patients with cancer. Blood 2010;**116**(20):4045–59.
6 Wilson J, Yao GL, Raftery J et al. A systematic review and economic evaluation of epoetin alfa, epoetin beta and darbepoetin alfa in anemia associated with cancer, especially that attributable to cancer treatment. Health Technol Assess 2007;**11**(13):1–220.
7 Schrezenmeier H, Muus P, Socie G et al. Baseline characteristics and disease burden in patients in the international paroxysmal nocturnal hemoglobinuria registry. Hematologica 2014;**99**:922–9.
8 NICE Guidelines for Blood Transfusion. Available at: www.nice.org.uk/guidance/indevelopment/gid-cgwave0663/consultation (accessed 14 November 2016).
9 Estcourt LJ, Birchall J, Lowe D et al. Platelet transfusions in hematology patients: are we using them appropriately? Vox Sang 2012;**103**(4):284–93.
10 Estcourt LJ, Stanworth SJ, Doree C et al. Comparison of different platelet count

thresholds to guide administration of prophylactic platelet transfusion for preventing bleeding in patients with hematological disorders after myelosuppressive chemotherapy or stem cell transplantation. Cochrane Database Syst Rev 2015;7:CD010983.

11 Slichter SJ, Kaufman RM, Assmann SF et al. Dose of prophylactic platelet transfusions and prevention of hemorrhage. N Engl J Med 2010;**362**:600–13.

12 Estcourt LJ, Stanworth SJ, Doree C et al. Different doses of prophylactic platelet transfusion for preventing bleeding in patients with hematological disorders after myelosuppressive chemotherapy or stem cell transplantation. Cochrane Database Syst Rev 2015;7:CD010984.

13 Stanworth SJ, Estcourt LJ, Powter G et al. A no-prophylaxis platelet transfusion strategy for hematologic cancers. N Engl J Med 2013;**368**:1771–80.

14 Wandt H, Schaefer-Eckart K, Wendelin K et al. Therapeutic platelet transfusion versus routine prophylactic transfusion in patients with hematological malignancies: an open-label, multicentre, randomised study. Lancet 2012;**380**:1309–16.

15 Neunert C, Lim W, Crowther M et al. The American Society of Hematology 2011 evidence-based practice guideline for immune thrombocytopenia. Blood 2011;**117**:4190–207.

16 Price TH. Granulocyte transfusion: current status. Semin Hematol 2007;**44**:15–23.

17 Massey E, Harding K, Kahan BC et al. The granulocytes in neutropenia 1 (GIN 1) study: a safety study of granulocytes collected from whole blood and stored in additive solution and plasma. Transfus Med 2012;**22**:277–84.

18 Sayers M, Anderson KC, Goodnough LT et al. Reducing the risk for transfusion-transmitted cytomegalovirus infection. Ann Intern Med 1992;**116**:55–62.

19 Clark P, Miller JP. Leukocyte-reduced and cytomegalovirus-reduced-risk blood components, in Transfusion Therapy: Clinical Principles and Practice, 3rd edn (ed. P Mintz), AABB Press, Bethesda, 2010.

20 Laupacis A, Brown J, Costello B et al. Prevention of post-transfusion CMV in the era of universal WBC reduction: a consensus statement. Transfusion 2001;**41**:560–69.

21 SaBTO Report of the Cytomegalovirus Steering Group 2012. Available at: www.gov.uk/government/publications/sabto-report-of-the-cytomegalovirus-steering-group (accessed 14 November 2016).

22 Treleaven J, Gennery A, Marsh J et al. Guidelines on irradiated blood components for the prevention of graft-versus-host disease prepared by the British Committee for Standards in Haematology blood transfusion task force. Br J Haematol 2010;**152**:35–51.

23 Dzik S. How I do it: platelet support for refractory patients. Transfusion 2007;**47**(3):374–8.

24 British Committee for Standards in Hematology. Guidelines for compatibility procedures in blood transfusion laboratories. Transfus Med 2004;**14**:59–73.

25 Warkentin PI. Transfusion of patients undergoing bone marrow transplantation. Hum Pathol 1983;**14**:261–6.

26 Kanda J, Ichinohe T, Matsuo K et al. Impact of ABO mismatching on the outcomes of allogeneic related and unrelated blood and marrow stem cell transplantations for hematologic malignancies: IPD-based meta-analysis of cohort studies. Transfusion 2009;**49**(4):624–35.

Further Reading

Education program for the 20th Congress of the European Haematology Association, 2015. Transfusion Medicine: focus on granulocytes

Kopko PM, Warner P, Kresie L, Pancoska C. Methods for the selection of platelet products for alloimmune-refractory patients. Transfusion 2015;**55**(2):235–44.

Nahirniak S, Slichter SJ, Tanael S et al. Guidance on platelet transfusion for patients with hypoproliferative thrombocytopenia. Transfus Med Rev 2015;**29**:3–13.

NICE Guidelines for Blood Transfusion. Available at: www.nice.org.uk/guidance/indevelopment/ gid-cgwave0663/consultation (accessed 14 November 2016).

Silberstein LE, Cunningham MJ. Autoimmune hemolytic anemias, in Blood Banking and Transfusion Medicine: Basic Principles and Practice, 2nd edn (eds C Hillyer, L Silberstein, P Ness, K Anderson, J Roback), Churchill Livingstone, Philadelphia, 2007.

30 Blood Transfusion in the Management of Patients with Haemoglobinopathies

Enrico M. Novelli

Division of Hematology/Oncology, Vascular Medicine Institute, University of Pittsburgh, Pittsburgh, USA

Introduction

Haemoglobinopathies are caused by mutations in the globin genes and are probably the most common single gene disorders in the world. The α-globin and β-globin gene families are located on chromosome 16 and chromosome 11, respectively. Together with haem, they combine to form haemoglobin, which is a tetramer of two α-like and two β-like globins. Developmentally, two different α-globins and four different β-globins are produced, resulting in a variety of haemoglobins (Table 30.1). At birth, there is a gradual switch from fetal to adult haemoglobin, which is largely complete in a year [1]. Quantitative defects in globin chain synthesis cause thalassaemia, whereas qualitative defects result in haemoglobin variants; the most important haemoglobin variant is haemoglobin S (HbS, β^6 glutamic acid-valine), responsible for sickle cell disease (SCD) in homozygotes or compound heterozygotes for other β-globin mutations. Blood transfusion is important in haemoglobinopathies, allowing correction of anaemia, suppression of abnormal erythropoiesis and replacement of abnormal erythrocytes.

α-Thalassaemia syndromes

Most people have four α-globin genes and the common types of α-thalassaemia are due to large deletions of one or more of these genes [2]. Deletion of both α-globin genes on a chromosome can occur, although this is only common in South-east Asia and the eastern Mediterranean. There are three main α-thalassaemia syndromes.

α-Thalassaemia Trait

This is usually due to the deletion of one or two α-globin genes. The haemoglobin is normal with mild hypochromia. Blood transfusion is never needed to treat the condition itself.

HbH Disease

This occurs when there is only one functional α-globin gene. It is typically a mild condition, with haemoglobin of 7–10 g/dL and HbH (tetramers of β-globin) inclusion bodies in erythrocytes. The spleen is moderately enlarged. Blood transfusion is not usually required, but may be necessary following parvovirus B19 infection.

Practical Transfusion Medicine, Fifth Edition. Edited by Michael F. Murphy, David J. Roberts and Mark H. Yazer.
© 2017 John Wiley & Sons Ltd. Published 2017 by John Wiley & Sons Ltd.

Table 30.1 Normal haemoglobins.

Structure	Name	Predominant expression
$\zeta_2\varepsilon_2$	Hb Gower 1	0–10th week gestation
$\alpha_2\varepsilon_2$	Hb Gower 2	5th–10th week gestation
$\zeta_2\gamma_2$	Hb Portland	5th–10th week gestation
$\alpha_2{}^G\gamma_2$	HbF	12th week gestation–4th month
$\alpha_2{}^A\gamma_2$	HbF	12th week gestation–4th month
$\alpha_2\beta_2$	HbA	4th month–death
$\alpha_2\delta_2$	HbA_2	4th month–death

Hb Bart's Hydrops Fetalis

A complete or near-complete absence of functional α-globin genes results in progressive fetal anaemia from the 10th week of gestation. Without intervention, this results in a hydropic fetus and miscarriage at 30–40 weeks, reflecting the importance of α-globin in forming HbF. Occasionally fetal anaemia has been detected and the pregnancy maintained until term with regular intrauterine transfusions. The affected newborns are transfusion dependent and have severe disability. This may either result from the effects of fetal anaemia or be caused by large deletions on chromosome 16. If fetal anaemia is found to be due to Hb Bart's hydrops fetalis, the likelihood of serious and chronic disability should be discussed with the parents prior to starting intrauterine transfusions.

β-Thalassaemia Syndromes

β-Thalassaemia results from a reduced rate of β-globin synthesis, but much of the pathology arises from the resulting excess of α-globin. β-globin is not part of fetal haemoglobin and there are no adverse fetal or neonatal effects. In contrast to α-thalassaemia, most cases of β-thalassaemia are caused by small mutations or deletions in the β-globin gene. More than 300 different mutations have been identified, and the many different combinations result in a phenotypic continuum from asymptomatic to transfusion dependence.

β-Thalassaemia Trait

This results from the inheritance of one mutated β-globin gene. There is minimal anaemia, with hypochromia and microcytosis. Anaemia becomes more marked during pregnancy and occasionally blood transfusion is necessary, although regular or frequent blood transfusions have no role.

β-Thalassaemia Intermedia

This is a clinical term referring to a range of conditions characterised by significant anaemia, splenomegaly and increased iron absorption. Many genetic factors are responsible for thalassaemia intermedia [3] (Box 30.1). Patients typically grow and develop normally without the need for regular blood transfusions, at least for the first few years of life. Anaemia may increase during illness or pregnancy and intermittent transfusions may be necessary. The trigger for blood transfusion is based on clinical signs and symptoms rather than any specific haemoglobin concentration (Hb). Acute symptoms suggesting that transfusion may be beneficial include dyspnoea and fatigue. It can be difficult to decide

---

Box 30.1 Causes of β-thalassaemia intermedia.

Factors lessening severity of predicted β-thalassaemia major
Mild β-thalassaemia mutations, e.g. HbE/β-thalassaemia
Co-inheritance of α-thalassaemia
Co-inheritance of hereditary persistence of HbF
Unexplained
Factors worsening severity of predicted β-thalassaemia trait
Co-inheritance of triplicated α-globin gene
Dominant β-thalassaemia mutation
Unexplained

if someone with severe thalassaemia intermedia would benefit from regular blood transfusions and treatment as for thalassaemia major. In children, this is suggested by poor growth, recurrent illness, marked bony expansion, progressive splenomegaly or evidence of organ damage, such as pulmonary hypertension. Sometimes children require regular blood transfusions to progress through puberty; older adults, who were previously managed without transfusion, may become transfusion dependent due to reduced cardiorespiratory function. Once regular transfusions start, they should be continued long term. Splenectomy may also be indicated. Iron overload can be a problem in thalassaemia intermedia, even in the absence of regular transfusions and iron stores should be monitored regularly and chelation started as necessary [4].

β-Thalassaemia Major

Thalassaemia major is the term used when a patient with β-thalassaemia is treated with regular blood transfusions from an early age. It is usually due to the co-inheritance of severe β-thalassaemia mutations (β° mutations) from both parents, but can be caused by combinations of less severe mutations (β$^+$-thalassaemia) with exacerbation from epigenetic and environmental factors. The clinical problems result from excess α-globin chains, damaging the developing bone marrow erythroid precursors that fail to mature into circulating red cells (ineffective erythropoiesis). The expanded erythroid component of the marrow produces large amounts of growth differentiation factor 15, which reduces hepcidin production by the liver; hepcidin inhibits gastrointestinal iron absorption and the inappropriately low levels result in increased iron absorption. Without transfusions, the child either dies or is seriously ill, with failure to thrive, bony deformity from extramedullary haematopoiesis or a poor quality of life.

The main clinical features of thalassaemia major are therefore:

- severe anaemia
- bone marrow expansion with bony deformity and osteopenia

- hypersplenism and hypermetabolism
- iron overload.

Blood Transfusion in β-Thalassaemia Major

The aim of regular, long-term blood transfusions in thalassaemia major is to:

- reduce or eliminate symptoms of anaemia
- suppress ineffective erythropoiesis to prevent bony deformity
- prevent the development of significant hypersplenism
- suppress extramedullary haemopoiesis.

Studies measuring soluble transferrin receptor levels have shown that erythropoiesis is adequately suppressed by maintaining a pre-transfusion Hb between 9 and 10 g/dL [5]. The post-transfusion Hb is usually kept below 15 g/dL to avoid problems with high blood viscosity and fluid overload. In practice, these parameters are usually achieved by regular, simple transfusions given every 2–5 weeks, the frequency being determined by local resources and pre-transfusion symptoms. Occasionally, more intensive transfusion is used to support cardiorespiratory problems or suppress extramedullary haemopoiesis. Automated exchange transfusions are also used and typically patients have a full-volume exchange every 6–8 weeks. Exchange transfusion has the advantages of decreasing iron loading and less frequent hospital attendances, although it involves more donor exposure with increased risk of alloimmunisation and other adverse reactions; good vascular access is also important and therefore the procedure is more difficult in young children (Table 30.2). It is more expensive than simple transfusion and unavailable in many parts of the world. The insertion of semi-permanent venous access devices is sometimes necessary if venous access is difficult.

With adequate blood transfusion and iron chelation from an early age, the expectation is that children will grow and develop normally, with a good quality of life. Life expectancy should approach the normal range, although

Table 30.2 Advantages and disadvantages of different types of blood transfusion in sickle cell disease.

Simple transfusion	Manual exchange	Automated transfusion
Quick to organise	Slower to organise	Slower to organise and not always available
No additional skills needed beyond those required to administer transfusion	Previous experience and training necessary	Specialist staff and equipment needed
Simple venous access only	Good venous access	Very good venous access at two sites or double-lumen catheter
Quick to complete	Slow to complete	Quick to complete
Limited scope to reduce HbS percentage	Significant decrease in HbS percentage	Very significant decreases in HbS percentage
Fairly predictable final Hb levels and HbS percentage	Unpredictable final Hb and HbS percentage	Predictable final Hb and HbS percentage
Limited donor exposure	Moderate donor exposure	High donor exposure
Significant increase in iron stores	Minimal increase in iron stores	Minimal or no increase in iron stores

chelation failure means that median life expectancy is usually shortened; patients in developed countries born in the 1960s had a median survival of 30 years, but this has progressively increased [6].

Sickle Cell Disease

Sickle cell disease refers to a group of conditions in which the patient is either homozygous for the mutated β^S allele or co-inherits β^S with another β-globin mutation (Box 30.2). The primary pathological event is the polymerisation of deoxygenated HbS, resulting in damage to the red cell membrane, cellular dehydration and increased cytoplasmic viscosity. These abnormal, rigid sickle cells are cleared prematurely leading to a chronic hemolytic anemia and cause vaso-occlusion, first initiated by hyper-adhesion of blood cells to the endothelium of postcapillary venules, and resulting in both acute and chronic ischaemic damage. Clinical consequences of vaso-occlusion are protean and virtually affect every organ. Most common complications include

---

Box 30.2 Types of sickle cell disease.

Severe SCD
  HbSS (sickle cell anaemia)
  HbS β^0-thalassaemia
  HbS O^{Arab}
  HbS D^{Punjab}

Moderate-severe SCD
  HbSC
  HbS β^+-thalassaemia
  HbS Lepore
  HbSE

Mild-moderate SCD
  HbS/hereditary persistence of fetal haemoglobin

---

hyposplenism from splenic auto-infarction, acute vaso-occlusive pain episodes (VOC), acute chest syndrome and acute sequestration of sickle cells in the spleen and liver. Vaso-occlusion also leads to a further cascade of interlinked pathological events, including inflammation, oxidative stress, reperfusion injury, hyper-coagulability, nitric oxide deficiency, hypoxaemia and vasculopathy.

Vasculopathy and endothelial dysfunction seem to be particularly important for some chronic complications, including cerebrovascular disease and stroke, pulmonary hypertension, priapism and leg ulcers. Haemolysis is thought to contribute significantly to the vasculopathy by releasing free haemoglobin into the plasma, which inactivates nitric oxide, resulting in vascular endothelial dysfunction [7].

Blood transfusion plays an important role in combatting many of these pathological processes, including increasing Hb, reducing the number of circulating erythrocytes able to cause vaso-occlusion and reducing intravascular haemolysis. Patients with SCD have increased blood viscosity at normal levels of haemoglobin, so hyper-transfusing to a Hb >10g/dL is potentially harmful as it leads to hyperviscosity and decreased oxygen delivery to tissues and may precipitate acute ischaemic events, particularly in the brain.

When planning a transfusion in SCD, it is important to decide what the target Hb and HbS percentage are, and then plan how best to achieve these, through either a simple top-up transfusion or an exchange transfusion, in which blood is also removed. The advantages of exchange transfusions are more rapid dilution of HbS and maintenance of iron balance. Exchange transfusions are performed most efficiently using automated apheresis (erythrocytapheresis), although this is not always available as an emergency and requires very good vascular access, typically obtained by placement of double-lumen catheters (see Table 30.2).

Indications for Transfusions in Acute Complications of SCD

- *Acute anaemia*: the need for transfusion is dependent on symptoms rather than on haemoglobin level, but is usually necessary when the Hb falls below 5g/dL. A single, simple transfusion aiming to increase the Hb to 8–10g/dL is typically used. Specific causes of acute anaemia include:
  - parvovirus B19 infection: this can be life-threatening in SCD because of transient red cell aplasia and extremely low reticulocyte count. Viral symptoms may be present
  - acute splenic sequestration: high reticulocyte count, enlarging spleen and rapidly falling Hb; potentially fatal without urgent transfusion; it is most common in children under the age of five years and recurrent episodes usually require splenectomy
  - acute hepatic sequestration: rare complication with acute tender hepatopathy and reticulocytosis. Care has to be taken with simple transfusion as red blood cells sequestered in the liver may be released once the crisis has resolved and sudden rises of the Hb into levels associated with hyperviscosity may occur.

- *Acute chest syndrome*: this is defined as radiographic evidence of a new infiltrate in a patient with chest pain, tachypnoea, hypoxia and brisk haemolysis/acute anaemia (although not all symptoms may be present at diagnosis). Five to ten percent of cases deteriorate and require respiratory support if not promptly treated. Early top-up transfusion to increase the Hb to about 10g/dL can prevent deterioration; this also results in a significant reduction in HbS percentage. If deterioration is rapid or mechanical ventilation necessary, the HbS should be reduced to less than 30% with haemoglobin of about 10g/dL, which will often involve an urgent exchange transfusion [8].

- *Stroke*: if acute neurological symptoms occur, urgent blood transfusion should be arranged whilst investigating the cause, which is likely to be cerebrovascular disease. The aim of transfusion is both to reduce HbS to less than 30% and increase Hb to about 10g/dL. This will usually require an exchange transfusion and a retrospective study suggested that outcome is better if an exchange transfusion is used initially rather than a top-up [9]. It is important to correct significant anaemia rapidly with a top-up transfusion before the exchange, to limit the area of brain ischaemia, if there is going to be a delay of more than a few hours before the exchange transfusion can be performed.

- *Multi-organ failure syndrome (MOFS)*: this is a life-threatening complication of SCD with a dire prognosis. It is presumed to be due to massive fat embolisation to end-organs from infarcted bones and may complicate ACS. Exchange transfusion to keep the HbS less than 30% is critical.

Indications for Regular Transfusion in SCD

- *Primary stroke prevention in children with abnormal transcranial Doppler (TCD) scans*: children with increased mean flow velocity of large intracranial arteries by TCD are at high risk of acute stroke. A randomised controlled trial showed that keeping HbS less than 30% with regular transfusions reduced stroke risk by 90% [10]. Current recommendations are to continue transfusions to at least 16 years of age [11] although many clinicians prefer to continue them indefinitely as therapy with hydroxyurea, an alternative disease-modifying strategy, has not been equivalent in preventing secondary stroke [12]. In some centres, the target HbS threshold is increased to 50% later in life to reduce exposure to blood products.
- *Silent cerebral infarct (SIT)*: these are the most common neurological complication in children with SCD and are diagnosed by MRI evidence of small vessel disease in the absence of neurological symptoms or overt stroke. There is growing evidence that SIT is a misnomer since they are associated with poorer cognitive function. A recent trial showed that transfusions reduced the risk of stroke in children with SIT and normal TCD [13].
- *Secondary stroke prevention*: following a first stroke there is a 20–90% chance of further strokes. Retrospective studies suggest that the risk of recurrence is reduced by up to 90% with regular blood transfusions to keep the HbS less than 30%. This requires regular exchange or top-up transfusions, with evidence showing that the high risk of stroke returns once the transfusions stop [14].

- *Progressive organ failure*: hepatic, renal, cardiovascular and pulmonary failure are highly prevalent in older SCD patients, and regular transfusions can help support organ function or prevent further deterioration, although randomised evidence to support this strategy is not available. As survival in SCD improves, there are increasing numbers of older patients and increasing amounts of blood used for this indication.

Conditions for Which Blood Transfusions Are Not Indicated

- *Uncomplicated pain episodes*: current guidelines do not recommend routinely transfusing patients presenting with acute pain episodes/VOC. Nonetheless, a recent retrospective study has renewed interest in using transfusion to improve outcomes in this setting by showing that patients admitted for VOC who were transfused had lower mortality and decreased 30-day readmission rate [15]. Randomised clinical trials to address the benefits of routine transfusion in VOC are currently being planned.
- *Uncomplicated pregnancy*: gestational anaemia may lead to severe anaemia in pregnant patients with SCD and the threshold for transfusion should be based on fetal indications as dictated for women without SCD. Pregnant patients with SCD also experience a higher rate of maternal and fetal obstetric complications and an increased rate of VOC. There is, however, no evidence to support the indiscriminate use of blood transfusion in the absence of complications or severe anaemia.
- *Priapism*: priapism is a painful, sustained erection in the absence of sexual stimulation. There is no established role for transfusion in its prevention or acute treatment. A published case series of exchange transfusion for patients with severe priapism reported a high prevalence of neurological deficits in the transfused patients (ASPEN syndrome) [16]. High post-transfusion Hb leading to hyperviscosity and cerebral ischaemia was the likely culprit.

Preoperative Blood Transfusion in SCD

Patients with SCD tend to experience a high incidence of postoperative complications, including VOC and ACS. Preoperative transfusion has, therefore, been standard of care in SCD for decades, although randomised clinical trial evidence of the beneficial effect of preoperative transfusion has only recently been available [17]. Another prior landmark clinical trial had shown that a conservative top-up transfusion strategy to a Hb of 10 g/dL was as effective as an aggressive exchange transfusion strategy to reduce the HbS to less than 30% in preventing complications [18]. Gray areas, however, still remain as not all types of surgeries may benefit from transfusion and the impact of specific anaesthesia regimens on the risk of postoperative complications is unknown. Most importantly, the best approach to prevent complications in patients with high baseline Hb has not been investigated. These include patients with HbSC disease, which have been excluded from the aforementioned trials, and other patients with high baseline HbS because of hydroxyurea therapy or other mitigating factors such as co-inheritance of α-thalassaemia trait or hereditary persistence of fetal haemoglobin.

Complications of Transfusions in Haemoglobinopathies

In addition to the risks commonly associated with blood transfusion in the general population, patients with haemoglobinopathies are particularly susceptible to red cell alloimmunisation. Transfusional haemosiderosis is also a significant concern because of the high lifetime transfusion burden experienced by a large proportion of patients.

- *Alloimmunisation*: in many countries, including northern Europe and the USA, the thalassaemia and SCD populations are mostly of a different ethnic origin to the majority of the blood donor pool, increasing the risk of alloimmunisation. Red cell alloimmunisation occurs in up to 50% of patients depending on the similarity between the ethnicities of the donor and recipient populations, the patient's underlying inflammatory status and the extent of blood group matching. Alloimmunisation also poses a risk of delayed haemolytic transfusion reactions should the antibody titre fall below detectable levels, or if the patient seeks medical care at hospitals other than where their antibodies had been previously detected. The risk of alloimmunisation can be reduced by choosing blood matched for Rh and Kell groups in both thalassaemia [19] and SCD [20]. Patients who are already alloimmunised should undergo extended red cell phenotypic matching (C, c, D, E, e, K, k, Jka, Jkb, Fya, Fyb, Kpa, Kpb, MNS, Lewis) with some centres also employing red cell genotyping to increase the accuracy of Rh typing, and in locating compatible units. Leucocyte reduction reduces the risk of transfusion reactions, prion transmission and possibly alloimmunisation and should be routinely requested. HbS-negative units only should be transfused.
- *Autoantibody formation/hyper-haemolytic crises*: episodes of brisk haemolysis where bystander red cell haemolysis, in addition to haemolysis of alloantibody-coated red cells, may accompany the development of alloantibodies and occur in up to 25% of thalassaemia major patients and a smaller percentage with SCD. They are associated with non-leucocyte-reduced transfusions and splenectomy and can be characterised by significant autoimmune haemolysis. A direct antiglobulin test may be negative if antibody-coated red cells are rapidly cleared and the reticulocyte count may be relatively depressed because of haemolysis of erythroid precursors. Management includes reserving blood transfusions for life-threatening anaemia, supportive therapy and therapy aiming at controlling the immune response (corticosteroids and immunoglobulins) and boosting red cell production (erythropoietin).

- *Infection*: the prevalence of transfusion-transmitted infections varies widely but is low in most developed countries. Yearly screening for hepatitis B, C and HIV could be considered for all chronically transfused patients. Transfusion transmission of parvovirus B19 is rarely reported, probably because this infection is frequently asymptomatic in healthy recipients. In patients with SCD, parvovirus B19 can, however, cause severe, life-threatening anaemia from acute, transient red cell aplasia (aplastic crisis). Simple transfusions should be administered in these cases.
- *Iron overload*: SCD patients develop haemosiderosis exclusively from red cell transfusions, whilst patients with thalassaemia also suffer from haemosiderosis arising from ineffective erythropoiesis and increased intestinal iron absorption.

Iron Chelation

Regular blood transfusions inevitably cause iron overload. Each unit of transfused blood contains about 200 mg of iron, and typically iron chelation is started after 12 months of regular transfusions or when the ferritin exceeds 1000 μg/L. Without treatment, iron accumulates in and damages the liver, heart and endocrine organs. Cardiac siderosis is a potentially fatal complication, suggested by the development of arrhythmias, heart failure and increasing iron stores on cardiac MRI, and necessitates intensive chelation therapy. In thalassaemia, iron-related heart disease is the major cause of death. In SCD, marked cardiac iron deposition is unusual, although significant morbidity results from hepatic siderosis.

It is important to assess iron stores accurately to monitor chelation therapy (Table 30.3). If there is evidence of progressive iron overload, intensive efforts should be made to improve iron chelation; these will usually focus on improving treatment adherence. Iron chelators include the following.

- *Desferrioxamine (deferoxamine)*: this drug has been available for more than 30 years. Good compliance has been shown to improve survival. Side effects are few but include growth impairment and retinal and cochlear

Table 30.3 Assessment of iron overload.

	Description	Advantages	Disadvantages
Monitoring transfused volume	Annual review of volume of transfused blood	Accurate measure of iron input; inexpensive	Does not assess iron loss through chelation or other means
Serum ferritin	Simple blood test	Inexpensive, widely available; monitors trends in hepatic iron	Increased by inflammation. Variable correlation with liver iron
Liver biopsy	Chemical measurement of liver iron in tissue sample	Accurate quantitation. Also shows liver histology	Invasive. Only small sample of liver analysed
Magnetic susceptometry	Magnetic assessment of liver iron	Noninvasive. Accurate	Very few calibrated machines in the world
T2* MRI	Assessment of liver and heart iron using MRI	Technology widely available. Assesses cardiac iron. Accurate	Variable results from different scanners. Young children need anaesthesia
R2 MRI	Assessment of liver iron using MRI	Widely available. Approved in USA and EU. Results similar between scanners	Cannot assess cardiac iron. Young children need anaesthesia

MRI, magnetic resonance imaging.

toxicity at higher doses. Side effects become increasingly common as iron stores approach normal. Negative iron balance is typically achieved in a transfusion-dependent patient at a dose of 40 mg/kg five nights per week. The main inconvenience with desferrioxamine is its parenteral formulation, usually requiring overnight subcutaneous infusions. Thus, adherence to treatment is poor. In heart failure secondary to iron overload, continuous intravenous desferrioxamine has been shown to be effective [21].

- *Deferasirox*: this oral iron chelator is licensed as a first-line treatment for transfusional iron overload around the world. It appears to be as effective as desferrioxamine with relatively few side effects. The main toxicity involves increases in serum creatinine, which in general have been non-progressive and reversible. Yearly auditory and ophthalmological testing is also recommended in patients receiving this drug. There is emerging evidence that deferasirox effectively chelates cardiac iron [22]. Deferasirox is available as both dispersible or orally administerable tablets that have better gastrointestinal tolerability.

- *Deferiprone*: this oral iron chelator was developed in the 1980s. Side effects include neutropenia and arthritis. The drug has been licensed as a second-line chelator for thalassaemia in Europe for more than 10 years, but was only licensed for use in North America in 2011 because of concern about toxicity and lack of efficacy. Recent studies suggest that it is particularly effective at chelating cardiac iron and various regimes in combination with desferrioxamine have been devised. Because of the risk of agranulocytosis, it is recommended that weekly blood tests are performed on those taking deferiprone [23] and particular caution should be exercised when used in patients on concurrent hydroxyurea therapy.

Acknowledgement

This chapter was based on the chapter in the fourth edition authored by Dr David C. Rees.

KEY POINTS

1) Regular intrauterine transfusions should not be used in fetuses with Hb Bart's hydrops fetalis until the risk of severe handicap has been discussed with the parents.

2) Transfusions should be started in severe β-thalassaemia syndromes on the basis of symptoms rather than a particular Hb level or genotype.

3) Blood transfused to haemoglobinopathy patients should be fully matched for Rh and Kell blood groups, with more extensive phenotypic matching for those already alloimmunised.

4) Urgent blood transfusion is indicated in SCD in acute anaemia, severe ACS, multi-organ failure and acute neurological problems.

5) Regular transfusions are mainly used in SCD for primary and secondary stroke prevention.

6) Preoperative transfusions to a target Hb of 10 g/dL should be administered to patients with SCD undergoing major surgery.

7) Iron chelation should be actively considered after 10–12 blood transfusions.

8) Hepatic iron stores should be monitored in SCD and thalassaemia using a combination of transfusion history, serum ferritin and MRI.

9) In thalassaemia major and severe thalassaemia intermedia, cardiac iron should be monitored using MRI, and intensive chelation started if there is evidence of significant or progressive cardiac iron overload.

References

1 Weatherall DJ. Pathophysiology of thalassaemia. Baillière's Clin Haematol 1998;**11**(1):127–46.

2 Higgs DR, Engel JD, Stamatoyannopoulos G. Thalassaemia. Lancet 2012;**379**:373–83.

3 Danjou F, Anni F, Galanello R. Beta-thalassemia: from genotype to phenotype. Haematologica 2011;**96**(11):1573–5.

4 Taher AT, Musullam K, Cappellini M, et al. Optimal management of beta thalassaemia intermedia. Br J Haematol 2011;**152**(5):512–23.

5 Cazzola M, di Stefano P, Ponchio L et al. Relationship between transfusion regimen and suppression of erythropoiesis in beta-thalassaemia major. Br J Haematol 1995;**89**(3):473–8.

6 Telfer P, Coen P, Christou S et al. Survival of medically treated thalassemia patients in Cyprus. Trends and risk factors over the period 1980–2004. Haematologica 2006;**91**(9):1187–92.

7 Rees DC, Williams TN, Gladwin MT. Sickle-cell disease. Lancet 2010;**376**(9757):2018–31.

8 Vichinsky EP, Neumayr L, Earles A et al. Causes and outcomes of the acute chest syndrome in sickle cell disease. National Acute Chest Syndrome Study Group. N Engl J Med 2000;**342**(25):1855–65.

9 Hulbert ML, Scothorn D, Panepinto J et al. Exchange blood transfusion compared with simple transfusion for first overt stroke is associated with a lower risk of subsequent stroke: a retrospective cohort study of 137 children with sickle cell anemia. J Pediatr 2006;**149**(5):710–12.

10 Adams RJ, McKie V, Hsu L et al. Prevention of a first stroke by transfusions in children with sickle cell anemia and abnormal results on transcranial Doppler ultrasonography. N Engl J Med 1998;**339**(1):5–11.

11 Yawn BP, Buchanan G, Afenyi-Annan A et al. Management of sickle cell disease: summary of the 2014 evidence-based report by expert panel members. JAMA 2014;**312**:1033–48.

12 Ware RE, Helms RW. Stroke With Transfusions Changing to Hydroxyurea (SWiTCH). Blood 2012;**119**:3925–32.

13 DeBaun MR, Gordon M, McKinstry R et al. Controlled trial of transfusions for silent cerebral infarcts in sickle cell anemia. N Engl J Med 2014;**371**:699–710.

14 Adams RJ, Brambilla D. Discontinuing prophylactic transfusions used to prevent stroke in sickle cell disease. N Engl J Med 2005;**353**(26):2769–78.

15 Nouraie M, Gordeuk VR. Blood transfusion and 30-day readmission rate in adult patients hospitalized with sickle cell disease crisis. Transfusion 2015;**55**(10):2331–8.

16 Siegel JF, Rich MA, Brock WA. Association of sickle cell disease, priapism, exchange transfusion and neurological events: ASPEN syndrome. J Urol 1993;**150**:1480–2.

17 Howard J, Malfroy M, Llewellyn C et al. The Transfusion Alternatives Preoperatively in Sickle Cell Disease (TAPS) study: a randomised, controlled, multicentre clinical trial. Lancet 2013;**381**:930–8.

18 Vichinsky EP, Haberkern C, Neumayr L et al. A comparison of conservative and aggressive transfusion regimens in the perioperative management of sickle cell disease. The Preoperative Transfusion in Sickle Cell Disease Study Group. N Engl J Med 1995;**333**(4):206–13.

19 Thompson AA, Cunningham M, Singer S et al. Red cell alloimmunization in a diverse population of transfused patients with thalassaemia. Br J Haematol 2011;**153**(1):121–8.

20 Vichinsky EP, Earles A, Johnson R et al. Alloimmunization in sickle cell anemia and transfusion of racially unmatched blood. N Engl J Med 1990;**322**(23):1617–21.

21 Davis BA, Porter JB. Long-term outcome of continuous 24-hour deferoxamine infusion via indwelling intravenous catheters in

high-risk beta-thalassemia. Blood
2000;**95**(4):1229–36.

22 Tanner MA, Galanello R, Dessi C et al. A
randomized, placebo-controlled, double-
blind trial of the effect of combined therapy
with deferoxamine and deferiprone on
myocardial iron in thalassemia major using

cardiovascular magnetic resonance.
Circulation 2007;**115**(14):1876–84.

23 Pennell DJ, Porter J, Cappellini M et al.
Efficacy of deferasirox in reducing
and preventing cardiac iron overload in
beta-thalassemia. Blood
2010;**115**(12):2364–71.

Further Reading

Olivieri NF, Brittenham GM. Iron-chelating
therapy and the treatment of thalassemia.
Blood 1997;**89** 739–61.

Serjeant GR, Serjeant BE. Sickle Cell Disease, 3rd
edn. Oxford University Press, Oxford, 2001.

Thalassaemia International Federation.
Guidelines for the Clinical Management of

Thalassaemia, 2nd edn. Available at: www.
thalassaemia.org.cy (accessed 15
November 2016).

Weatherall DJ, Clegg JB. The Thalassaemia
Syndromes, 4th edn. Blackwell Scientific
Publications, Oxford, 2001.

31 Heparin-Induced Thrombocytopenia

Andreas Greinacher[1] and Theodore E. Warkentin[2]

[1] Department of Immunology and Transfusion Medicine, Universitätsmedizin Greifswald, Greifswald, Germany
[2] Department of Pathology and Molecular Medicine and Department of Medicine, Michael G. DeGroote School of Medicine, McMaster University, Hamilton, Ontario, Canada; Transfusion Medicine, Hamilton Regional Laboratory Medicine Program and Service of Clinical Hematology, Hamilton Health Sciences, Hamilton, Ontario, Canada

Introduction

Heparin-induced thrombocytopenia (HIT) is an antibody-mediated adverse effect of heparin. It is highly prothrombotic and treatment usually requires substitution of heparin with a rapidly acting non-heparin anticoagulant; vitamin K antagonists (warfarin) are contraindicated during the acute phase of HIT because their use can precipitate limb necrosis due to microthrombosis. Prophylactic platelet transfusions should be minimised. Given these special treatment considerations, the challenge is to distinguish HIT from non-HIT thrombocytopenia. Management of HIT requires knowledge of immunohaematology and haemostasis. Table 31.1 lists the features of HIT with particular relevance for the transfusion medicine specialist.

Pathogenesis

Figure 31.1 illustrates the pathogenesis of HIT [1]. Key features include the following.

- Antigens form when platelet factor 4 (PF4) – a positively charged 31 kd tetrameric member of the C-X-C subfamily of chemokines – forms multimolecular complexes with (negatively charged) heparin when both are present at stoichiometrically optimal concentrations (1:1 to 2:1 ratio of PF4: heparin).

- Both PF4 and heparin bind to platelet surfaces; thus, *in situ* formation of PF4/heparin complexes on platelet membranes localises subsequent formation of PF4/heparin/IgG immune complexes also to the platelet surfaces, i.e. there are no circulating immune complexes in HIT.

- The HIT antigen(s) reside(s) on PF4, rather than on heparin; indeed, non-heparin polyanions (e.g. polyvinyl sulfonate, or PVS- or RNA- or DNA- or RNA-based drugs) can substitute for heparin in forming HIT antigens.

- Ultra-large PF4/heparin complexes are more readily formed with unfractionated heparin (UFH) than with low molecular weight heparin (LMWH), perhaps explaining the 10-fold greater risk of HIT with UFH versus LMWH.

- Heparin causes platelet activation and release of PF4. However, immunisation occurs most often postsurgery and in patients with major trauma (perhaps reflecting PF4 release from activated platelets and/or pro-inflammatory factors).

- Anti-PF4/heparin antibodies become detectable ~4 days (median) after an immunising heparin exposure, with detection of platelet-activating antibodies one or two days later [2,3].

Practical Transfusion Medicine, Fifth Edition. Edited by Michael F. Murphy, David J. Roberts and Mark H. Yazer.
© 2017 John Wiley & Sons Ltd. Published 2017 by John Wiley & Sons Ltd.

Table 31.1 HIT issues relevant to transfusion medicine.

HIT-related item	Transfusion medicine-related comment
PF4/heparin complexes form at optimal stoichiometric ratio	The Coombs test requires an optimal concentration of the antihuman immunoglobulin antibody to achieve agglutination of red cells
Acute HIT activates platelets, monocytes, endothelial cells and the coagulation cascade	Acute haemolytic transfusion reaction activates platelets, leucocytes, endothelial cells and the clotting cascade
Typical-onset HIT (day 5–14)	Timing resembles that of delayed haemolytic transfusion reaction in preimmunised patients
Rapid-onset HIT (<1 day)	Timing resembles that of acute haemolytic transfusion reaction (i.e. due to pre-existing anti-red cell alloantibodies)
'Delayed-onset' HIT antibodies bind to and activate platelets even in the absence of heparin (platelet-derived polyphosphates and chondroitin sulfate substitute for heparin)	In post-transfusion purpura, alloantibodies boosted by transfusing HPA-1a-positive platelets bind to the patient's own (HPA-1a-negative) platelets, causing severe thrombocytopenia (see Chapter 12)
Functional (platelet activation) assays are more predictive for HIT than immunoassays	HLA antibodies that test positive in lymphocytotoxicity tests are more clinically relevant compared to ELISA-only reactive HLA antibodies
Most ELISA-positive patients do not develop HIT	Many individuals with a positive direct antihuman globulin (Coombs) test do not have autoimmune haemolytic anaemia
Particle gel immunoassay	Rapid assay utilising gel card technology commonly used in transfusion medicine
Platelet transfusions (prophylactic)	Relatively contraindicated in HIT
PCCs contain heparin	PCCs are relatively contraindicated during acute HIT
High-dose intravenous IgG (IVIgG)	IVIgG is occasionally used as adjunctive treatment for severe HIT, especially in spontaneous or persisting HIT

ELISA, enzyme-linked immunosorbent assay; HLA, human leucocyte antigen; PCC, prothrombin complex concentrates; PF4, platelet factor 4.

- Anti-PF4/heparin antibodies of IgG and/or IgA and/or IgM can be formed (relative frequency, IgG > IgA > IgM). However, only IgG antibodies have the potential to cause HIT, because platelet activation occurs only when multimolecular complexes of PF4/heparin/IgG result in clustering of the platelet Fc receptors (FcγIIa), causing intravascular platelet activation.
- HIT does *not* exhibit features of a classic primary immune response. Even when HIT occurs during a patient's very first exposure to heparin, IgG antibodies are readily detected after only 4–5 days, whereas IgM antibodies usually are not detected. If IgM antibodies are found, they become detectable at the same time as IgG (i.e. no IgM precedence).
- These atypical features of the HIT immune response could reflect presensitisation due to exposure to bacteria, as negatively charged molecules on bacterial surfaces bind PF4 in a way that exposes HIT antigens [4].
- Platelet activation in HIT includes formation of procoagulant platelet-derived microparticles.

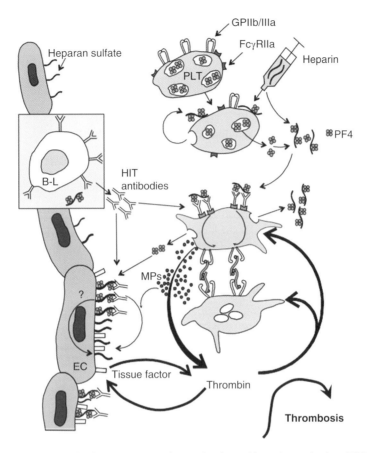

Figure 31.1 Pathogenesis of HIT. Platelet activation, either via binding of heparin to platelets (PLT) or by other mechanisms (e.g. surgery), leads to release of platelet factor 4 (PF4) from platelet α-granules. PF4/heparin complexes form, which in some patients triggers generation of platelet-activating anti-PF4/heparin antibodies ('HIT antibodies'), predominantly of the IgG class. Multimolecular complexes composed of PF4, heparin and IgG are formed on platelet surfaces, leading to cross-linking of the platelet Fc receptors (FcγRIIa). This produces potent platelet activation, including conformational changes in the platelet fibrinogen receptors (GPIIb/IIIa), resulting in platelet aggregation; procoagulant changes in the platelet surface – including generation of procoagulant, platelet-derived microparticles (MPs) – leading to thrombin generation; and further release of granule constituents such as PF4, triggering even more IgG-mediated platelet activation. Further, PF4 binds to endothelial cell (EC) heparan sulfate, resulting in HIT antibody binding to endothelial PF4/heparin complexes and, possibly, EC activation and expression of endothelial tissue factor (open rectangle), contributing further to thrombin generation. Thrombin activates platelets and endothelium, leading to thrombosis. *Source:* Reprinted from Warkentin et al [5], with modifications, with permission.

- Other procoagulant features of HIT include monocyte and endothelial cell activation, and neutralisation of heparin by PF4.
- Sometimes, HIT antibodies strongly activate platelets in the absence of pharmacological heparin (heparin-'independent' platelet activation): this is a feature of 'delayed-onset' HIT [6].

Epidemiology

- The overall frequency of HIT among heparin-exposed inpatients is ∼0.2%.
- The frequency of HIT approaches 5–10% when there are multiple concurrent risk factors for HIT, for example (a) UFH use

(versus LMWH or fondaparinux) for (b) at least 10–14 days (when antibodies peak), (c) postorthopaedic surgery and (d) female sex (1.5–2.0×greater risk of HIT in females versus males) [7].

- HIT occurs more often in post-surgery patients than in medical patients [7]. HIT is rare in pregnancy and in paediatric patients, and probably does not occur in neonates.

- UFH is rarely administered nowadays to postorthopaedic surgery patients. Thus, HIT occurs most often in post-cardiac/post-vascular surgery patients and general surgery patients who receive postoperative UFH thromboprophylaxis.

- Rarely, a transient HIT-mimicking syndrome with thrombocytopenia, thrombosis and high levels of platelet-activating anti-PF4/heparin antibodies can occur without proximate exposure to heparin, but after infection or surgery ('spontaneous HIT') [8].

Heparin-Induced Thrombocytopenia: A 'Clinicopathological' Syndrome

Table 31.2 summarises the major clinical and laboratory features of HIT [9].

Iceberg Model (Figure 31.2)

- HIT occurs in a minority of patients who form anti-PF4/heparin antibodies; anti-PF4/heparin antibodies are detectable in 50–80% of post-cardiac surgery patients, yet HIT occurs in only 1–2% of these patients.

- According to the 'iceberg model', HIT occurs in the subset of patients who form strong heparin-dependent, platelet-activating antibodies of the IgG class; such antibodies are also readily detectable by PF4-dependent enzyme-linked immunosorbent assay (ELISA) [10, 11].

Table 31.2 HIT viewed as a clinical–pathological syndrome.

Clinical	Pathological
One or more of:	**Heparin-dependent, platelet-activating IgG**
• **Thrombocytopenia**	• Positive platelet activation assay (e.g. SRA, HIPA)
• **Thrombosis** (e.g. *venous*: DVT, pulmonary embolism, venous limb gangrene, adrenal haemorrhage, cerebral vein thrombosis, splanchnic vein thrombosis; *arterial*: limb artery thrombosis, stroke, myocardial infarction, mesenteric artery thrombosis, miscellaneous artery; *microvascular*)	• Positive anti-PF4/polyanion-IgG ELISA (implies possible presence of platelet-activating IgG)
• Necrotising skin lesions at heparin injection sites	
• Acute anaphylactoid reactions	
• Disseminated intravascular coagulation (DIC)	
• **Timing**: above event(s) bear(s) temporal relation to a preceding immunising heparin exposure	
• Absence of another more compelling explanation	

DVT, deep vein thrombosis; ELISA, enzyme-linked immunosorbent assay; HIPA, heparin-induced platelet activation (test); PF4, platelet factor 4; SRA, serotonin release assay.

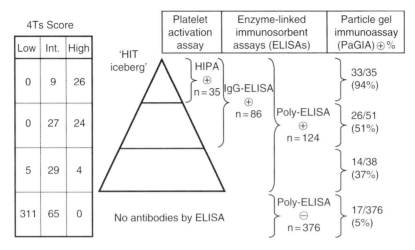

Figure 31.2 Iceberg model using published data [11]. The central 'iceberg' depicts three different antibody reaction profiles, as defined by a platelet activation test (HIPA) and two ELISAs (IgG-ELISA, poly-ELISA). The table on the far left shows the pretest probability scores (4Ts) for the three different antibody reaction profiles, as well as for patients who test negative in both ELISAs (bottom row of 4Ts table). On the far right, the corresponding results in the particle gel immunoassay (PaGIA) are shown. The data demonstrate that the sensitivity of the PaGIA for definite HIT (35 patients depicted as the 'tip of the iceberg') is only 94% (33/35). At the other extreme, ~5% of the patients who have no antibodies by ELISA will test positive in the PaGIA (17/376). ELISA, enzyme-linked immunosorbent assay (or enzyme-immunoassay); HIT, heparin-induced thrombocytopenia; PaGIA, particle gel immunoassay. *Source:* Reprinted from Warkentin & Linkins [10], with permission of John Wiley & Sons.

- Diagnostic sensitivity for clinical HIT of the three major types of assays – ELISA-IgG/A/M, ELISA-IgG, washed platelet activation assay – is similarly high (>99%); however, their diagnostic specificity varies, as follows: platelet activation assays > ELISA-IgG > ELISA-IgG/A/M.

Clinical Picture

Thrombocytopenia

- HIT usually results in mild-to-moderate thrombocytopenia (median platelet count nadir, 60×10^9/L) (~90% have a nadir between 15 and 150×10^9/L) [12].
- In >90% of patients, the platelet count falls by >50% from the peak platelet count that immediately precedes the HIT-associated platelet count fall.

Timing

- 'Typical-onset' HIT indicates thrombocytopenia that begins 5–10 days after an immunising heparin exposure [13].

- 'Rapid-onset' HIT refers to a platelet count fall that begins abruptly (<24 hours) after administration of heparin or a dose increase. Almost invariably, patients have been exposed to heparin within the recent past (past 5–100 days) [13].
- HIT antibodies are remarkably transient, becoming undetectable at a median of 50–85 days (depending on the assay performed) after an episode of HIT [13]. Antibodies have been reported to become substantially weaker within a week – with platelet count recovery – even if heparin is continued [2]. This indicates that a subclass of antibody-producing B-cells is involved in HIT, which differs from classic immunohaematological responses against alloantigens.
- 'Delayed-onset' HIT denotes thrombocytopenia that begins after the immunising heparin exposure has been stopped or that worsens after stopping heparin; patient serum activates platelets *in vitro* even in the absence of

pharmacological heparin (heparin-'independent' platelet activation) and has strongly positive ELISAs [6]. Such patients often have disseminated intravascular coagulation (DIC). The disorder resembles a transient autoimmune reaction.

- 'Persisting' HIT refers to thrombocytopenia that is slow to recover ($\sim$1% of HIT patients take >1 month for the platelet count to rise to >150 × 10^9/L). In these patients, platelet numbers increase in parallel with gradually declining levels of heparin-independent platelet-activating antibodies.

Thrombosis and Other Sequelae

- HIT is strongly associated with venous and/or arterial thrombosis (relative risk, 10–15) [12].
- Thrombosis risk parallels the degree of thrombocytopenia, ranging from $\sim$50% for patients with mild thrombocytopenia ($\sim$150 × 10^9/L) to $\sim$90% for patients with severe thrombocytopenia ($\sim$20 × 10^9/L).
- Limb loss occurs in $\sim$5% of patients with HIT; explanations include limb arterial thrombosis, warfarin-induced venous limb gangrene and DIC-associated microvascular thrombosis [14].
- Venous limb gangrene is acral (distal extremity) necrosis in a limb with deep vein thrombosis (DVT) that occurs despite palpable or Doppler-identifiable arterial pulses. Patients usually have a supratherapeutic international normalised ratio (INR) (>3.5) as a result of anticoagulation with a vitamin K antagonist. A prodromal state is phlegmasia cerulea dolens, i.e. an inflamed, ischaemic, painful limb.
- Venous predominates over arterial thrombosis ($\sim$4:1 ratio) [12], except in patients with arteriopathy ($\sim$1:1 ratio in post-cardiac/post-vascular surgery patients).
- Venous thrombotic events include (listed in descending order of frequency): venous thromboembolism (DVT > pulmonary embolism) > adrenal vein thrombosis > cerebral venous (dural sinus) thrombosis > splanchnic vein thrombosis.

- Adrenal vein thrombosis presents as unilateral or bilateral adrenal haemorrhage; when bilateral, death due to acute adrenal failure can occur (special relevance for critically ill patients).
- Arterial thrombotic events include: limb artery thrombosis > cerebral artery thrombosis > myocardial infarction.
- Overt (decompensated) DIC occurs in 10–15% of patients with HIT, usually with platelet count nadirs < 20 × 10^9/L; laboratory features include relative/absolute hypofibrinogenaemia, elevated INR and/or activated partial thromboplastin time (aPTT) and (rarely) microangiopathy (red cell fragments, elevated lactate dehydrogenase, circulating normoblasts). Clinical features include microvascular thrombosis (e.g. ischaemic limb necrosis despite palpable pulses) and increased risk of treatment failure due to aPTT confounding (discussed below).
- Anaphylactoid reactions occur in $\sim$25% of HIT patients who receive an intravenous UFH bolus and occasionally in patients administered subcutaneous LMWH (Box 31.1). There is an associated abrupt decrease in platelet count that can recover quickly after stopping heparin.

Pretest Probability Scores

- The '4Ts' is a pretest probability score that estimates the likelihood of HIT based upon: *t*hrombocytopenia, *t*iming (of platelet count fall or thrombosis), *t*hrombosis (or other sequelae of HIT) and o*t*her causes for thrombocytopenia (Table 31.3) [15]. Low scores (three or fewer points) are associated with <3% probability of HIT, whereas high scores (6–8 points) indicate $\sim$35–50% frequency of HIT.
- A more recent scoring system is the HIT expert probability (HEP) score, which requires further validation; like the 4Ts system, the HEP score evaluates the extent and timing of thrombocytopenia, the presence of thrombosis (or other HIT sequelae) and other

---

Box 31.1 Anaphylactoid reactions associated with acute (rapid-onset) HIT.

Timing: onset 5–30 minutes after intravenous un-fractionated heparin bolus (less commonly, following intravenous or subcutaneous low molecular weight heparin administration)

Clinical context: recent use of heparin (past 7–100 days)

Laboratory features: abrupt, sometimes rapidly reversible fall in the platelet count

Signs and symptoms:

Inflammatory: chills, rigours, fever and flushing

Cardiorespiratory: tachycardia, hypertension, tachypnoea, dyspnoea, bronchospasm, chest pain or tightness and cardiopulmonary arrest

Gastrointestinal: nausea, vomiting and large-volume diarrhoea

Neurological: pounding headache, transient global amnesia, transient ischaemic attack or stroke

---

potential explanations for thrombocytopenia, but assigns different numerical scores.

- Pretest probability scores are especially useful if interpreted in combination with certain immunoassays so as to predict the post-test likelihood of HIT.
- Critically ill patients with low pretest probability scores may not have HIT even if they test positive [17].

Laboratory Testing

Two general types of assays detect HIT antibodies: platelet activation (or functional) assays and PF4-dependent immunoassays.

- An unusual feature of HIT is that patient serum/plasma-based assays are very sensitive for detecting HIT antibodies, even at the earliest phase of the platelet count decline [3]. In contrast, sensitivity is lower for detecting circulating alloantibodies in delayed haemolytic

transfusion reactions if antigen-positive red cells remain in circulation; in this situation, the direct Coombs test is more sensitive.

- A characteristic feature is *inhibition* of reactivity at very high concentrations of UFH (10–100 U/mL), due to disruption of antigenic PF4/heparin complexes.
- In the absence of new clinical events (e.g. new thrombosis, new platelet count fall), a negative assay for HIT antibodies should *not* be automatically repeated a few days later; this is because a subsequent positive test result is much more likely to indicate subclinical seroconversion than 'true' HIT [3].

Platelet Activation Assays

Washed Platelet Activation Assays

- The best operating characteristics (highest sensitivity/specificity trade-off) are seen with the washed platelet activation assays, the ^{14}C-serotonin-release assay (SRA) and the heparin-induced platelet activation (HIPA) test.
- The SRA is performed in North America, using well-characterised (pedigree) donors, whereas the HIPA test is more widely used in Europe, and is usually performed with (random) donors at blood donation centres (four donors are tested separately to compensate for variable donor-dependent reactivity to HIT sera).
- Quality control manoeuvres include use of: (a) negative and graded (including weak) positive HIT serum controls, (b) Fc receptor-blocking monoclonal antibodies (to confirm platelet activation occurs through platelet Fc receptors and (c) parallel testing in a PF4-dependent ELISA (expected to be positive if the SRA or HIPA is positive – per the iceberg model).

Other Platelet Activation Assays

- Standard platelet aggregometry (using patient platelet-poor plasma tested against normal donor platelet-rich plasma) is not recommended, due to suboptimal sensitivity and specificity and low test/control sample throughput.

Table 31.3 The 4Ts pretest probability score.

	Score = 2	Score = 1	Score = 0
Thrombocytopenia Compare the highest platelet count within the sequence of declining platelet counts with the lowest count to determine the % of platelet fall (**select only 1 option**)	• >50% platelet fall AND a nadir of ≥20 AND no surgery within preceding 3 days	• >50% platelet fall BUT surgery within preceding 3 days OR • Any combination of platelet fall and nadir that does not fit criteria for Score 2 or Score 0 (e.g. 30–50% platelet fall or nadir 10–19)	• <30% platelet fall • Any platelet fall with nadir <10
Timing (**of platelet count fall or thrombosis***) Day 0 = first day of most recent heparin exposure (**select only 1 option**)	• Platelet fall day 5–10 after start of heparin • Platelet fall within 1 day of start of heparin AND exposure to heparin within past 5–30 days	• Consistent with platelet fall day 5–10 but not clear (e.g. missing counts) • Platelet fall within 1 day of start of heparin AND exposure to heparin in past 31–100 days • Platelet fall after day 10	• Platelet fall ≤ day 4 without exposure to heparin in past 100 days
Thrombosis (or other clinical sequelae) (**select only 1 option**)	• Confirmed new thrombosis (venous or arterial) • Skin necrosis at injection site • Anaphylactoid reaction to IV heparin bolus • Adrenal haemorrhage	• Recurrent venous thrombosis in a patient receiving therapeutic anticoagulants • Suspected thrombosis (awaiting confirmation with imaging) • Erythematous skin lesions at heparin injection sites	• Thrombosis not suspected
o**T**her cause for thrombocytopenia† (**select only 1 option**)	• No alternative explanation for platelet fall is evident	**Possible other cause is evident:** • Sepsis without proven microbial source • Thrombocytopenia associated with initiation of ventilator • Thrombocytopenia associated with drugs	**Probable other cause present:** • Within 72 hours of surgery • Confirmed bacteraemia/fungaemia • Chemotherapy or radiation within past 20 days • DIC due to non-HIT cause • Post-transfusion purpura (PTP) • Thrombotic thrombocytopenic purpura (TTP) • Platelet count <20 AND given a drug implicated in causing D-ITP (see list) • Non-necrotising skin lesions at LMWH injection sites (presumed DTH) • Other

Drugs implicated in drug-induced immune thrombocytopenia (D-ITP)
Relatively common: glycoprotein IIb/IIIa antagonists (abciximab, eptifibatide, tirofiban), quinine, quinidine, sulfa antibiotics, carbamazepine, vancomycin
Less common: actinomycin, amitriptyline, amoxicillin/piperacillin/nafcillin, cephalosporins (cefazolin, ceftazidime, ceftriaxone), celecoxib, ciprofloxacin, esomeprazole, fexofenadine, fentanyl, fucidic acid, furosemide, gold salts, levofloxacin, metronidazole, naproxen, oxaliplatin, phenytoin, propranolol, propoxyphene, ranitidine, rifampin, suramin, trimethoprim

* In some circumstances, it may be appropriate to judge timing based upon clinical sequelae, such as timing of onset of heparin-induced skin lesions.

† Usually, oTher scores '0 points' if thrombocytopenia is not present. However, it may be appropriate to judge oTher based upon clinical sequelae, such as whether heparin-induced skin lesions are necrotising (2 points, i.e. a non-HIT explanation is unlikely) or non-necrotising (0 points, i.e. a non-HIT explanation is likely).

DIC, disseminated intravascular coagulation; DTH, delayed-type hypersensitivity; LMWH, low molecular weight heparin.

Source: Reprinted from Warkentin & Linkins [16], with permission of John Wiley & Sons.

- A whole blood aggregometry assay (Multiplate®) seems to have comparable sensitivity to washed platelet assays for detecting platelet-activating HIT antibodies if a highly reactive donor is used.
- Recently, pre-incubation of PF4 was found to increase sensitivity of platelets to activation by HIT antibodies (e.g. in a flow cytometric assay using P-selectin as a marker for platelet activation) [18].

PF4-Dependent Immunoassays (Antigen Assays) (Table 31.4)

Enzyme-Linked Immunosorbent Assays (Solid-Phase Assays)

- Three commercial ELISAs are available to detect anti-PF4/heparin antibodies; reference centres also offer in-house assays. ELISAs are currently the most widely used tests for HIT.
- 'Polyspecific' ELISAs detect antibodies of the three major immunoglobulin classes (IgG/A/M).
- 'IgG-specific' ELISAs are preferred because their sensitivity is as high as the polyspecific assays, with substantially greater diagnostic specificity [10, 11].
- The magnitude of a positive ELISA result, expressed in optical density (OD) units, predicts for greater likelihood of a positive platelet activation test. For an ELISA with a positive OD range of 0.40 to 3.00 OD units, approximate frequencies of positive activation assays are [19]:
  0.40 to 1.00, ~5%
  1.00 to 1.50, ~20%
  1.50 to 2.00, ~50%
  >2.00, ~90%.
- Diagnostic specificity is enhanced somewhat using a high heparin confirmatory step, especially at weak-positive OD values (0.40 to 1.00). However, at higher OD values, lack of high heparin inhibition does not necessarily rule out platelet-activating HIT antibodies.

Fluid-Phase Immunoassays

Two fluid-phase immunoassays have been described; these avoid denaturation of PF4-dependent antigens (as can occur in solid-phase ELISAs), potentially increasing diagnostic specificity.

- *Sepharose G fluid-phase (IgG-specific) ELISA (in-house assay)*: after binding of antibodies to (5% biotinylated) PF4 in the fluid phase, IgG antibodies are captured using Sepharose G. After washing, the amount of biotin-PF4/heparin-antibody complexes immobilised to the beads is measured using peroxidase substrate after initial incubation with streptavidin-conjugated peroxidase.
- *Gold nanoparticle-based fluid-phase ELISA (rapid assay)*: in this 'lateral-flow immunoassay', capillary action causes the test sample to interact sequentially with antigen (ligand-labelled PF4/polyanion complexes), then with (red-coloured) gold nanoparticles coated with anti-ligand and then with immobilised goat antihuman IgG. A positive reaction is a bold-coloured line, which can be read visually or quantitatively with an automated reader. The turnaround time is only 15 minutes after preparation of serum, and the single-assay design facilitates on-demand testing.

Particle-Based Solid-Phase Immunoassays (Rapid Assays)

- *Particle gel immunoassay (PaGIA)*: this assay utilises a gel centrifugation technology system widely used in transfusion medicine. The manufacturer has prepared red, high-density polystyrene beads to which PF4/heparin complexes have been bound. After addition of patient serum/plasma, anti-PF4/heparin antibodies (if present) bind to the antigen-coated beads; a secondary antihuman immunoglobulin antibody is added into the sephacryl gel. Upon centrifugation, agglutinated beads (indicating the presence of anti-PF4/heparin antibodies) do not migrate through the sephacryl gel, whereas non-agglutinated beads (indicating the absence of antibodies) pass through the gel, forming a red band at the bottom. Sensitivity is lower than with the ELISAs (~90–95% versus ~99%) (see

Table 31.4 PF4-dependent antigen assays (immunoassays).

Manufacturer	PF4 (source)	Polyanion	Assay	Ab classes
Commercial immunoassays				
ELISAs				
Diagnostica Stago (Asnières-sur-Seine, France)	Recombinant	Heparin	1) Asserachrom HPIA 2) Asserachrom HIPA-IgG	1) IgG/A/M 2) IgG
Hologic Gen-Probe (Waukesha, WI, USA)	Platelets (outdated)	Polyvinyl sulfonate (PVS)	1) PF4 Enhanced 2) PF4 IgG	1) IgG/A/M 2) IgG
HYPHEN BioMed (Neuveille-sur-Oise, France)	Platelet lysate	Heparin bound to protamine	Zymutest HIA	IgG/A/M, IgG, IgA, IgM
Particle-based assays				
Milenia-Biotec (Giessen, Germany)	Platelets	Heparin	QuickLine HIT Test (lateral flow assay*)	IgG
DiaMed (Cressier, Switzerland)	Platelets	Heparin	PaGIA	IgG/A/M
Akers Biosciences (Thorofare, NJ, USA)	Platelets	None	PIFA Heparin/PF4	IgG/A/M
Instrumentation-based assay				
Instrumentation Laboratory (Bedford, MA, USA)	Platelets	PVS	1) HemosIL HIT-Ab$_{(PF4-H)}$ 2) HemosIL AcuStar HIT-IgG$_{(PF4-H)}$	1) IgG/A/M 2) IgG/A/M or IgG
'In-house' immunoassays (laboratories of the authors)				
Greifswald Laboratory	Platelets	Heparin	PF4/heparin ELISA	IgG, IgA, IgM
McMaster Platelet Immunology Laboratory	Platelets (outdated)	Heparin	1) PF4/heparin ELISA 2) Fluid-phase ELISA	1) IgG, IgA, IgM 2) IgG

* Also has features of a fluid-phase ELISA.

Figure 31.2). The diagnostic specificity is intermediate between that of the (washed) platelet activation assay and ELISA. A positive reaction at 1/4 dilution of patient serum/plasma is more specific for HIT and a positive reaction at 1/32 dilution or greater predicts the presence of platelet-activating antibodies.

- *Particle immunofiltration assay (PIFA)*: this assay utilises a PIFA system, wherein patient serum is added to a reaction well containing dyed particles coated with PF4 (*not* PF4/heparin). The assay performed poorly in two reference laboratories and its use is not recommended.

Instrumentation-Based Immunoassays (Rapid Assays)

Two automated assays that utilise proprietary instruments have recently been developed.

- *HemosIL HIT-Ab$_{(PF4-H)}$*: using an analyser of the ACL TOP® family, this is a latex particle-enhanced immunoturbidimetric assay that detects anti-PF4/heparin antibodies of all classes. In this competitive agglutination assay, the presence of anti-PF4/heparin antibodies within the patient sample will *inhibit* the binding of an HIT-mimicking monoclonal antibody (bound to latex particles) against PF4/PVS in solution. The degree of agglutination is inversely proportional to the level of anti-PF4/heparin antibodies (assessed by a decrease in light transmittance). A positive sample will therefore produce no or minimal increase in absorbance than the negative control samples (the software automatically reports the results in U/mL as the inverse proportion). A positive test is a result $\geq 1.0\,U/mL$. The technology allows for rapid, on-demand single-patient testing.

- *HemosIL AcuStar HIT-IgG(PF4-H)*: using an ACL AcuStar® system instrument, this is a chemiluminescence assay that is also based upon binding of anti-PF4/heparin antibodies within patient serum/plasma to PF4/PVS. Magnetic particles coated with PF4/PVS capture anti-PF4/heparin antibodies present within a patient sample. After incubation, magnetic separation and a wash step, a tracer consisting of an isoluminol-labelled antihuman IgG antibody (or a mixture of three isoluminol-labelled monoclonal antibodies (anti-IgG/A/M)) is added, which binds to the captured anti-PF4/heparin antibodies on the particles. After a second incubation, magnetic separation and a wash step, reagents that trigger the luminescent reaction are added and the emitted light is measured as relative light units (RLUs) by the instrument's optical system. The RLUs are directly proportional to anti-PF4/heparin antibody concentrations. Like the ELISAs, higher assay results indicate a greater likelihood of HIT.

Treatment

The treatment principles of strongly suspected or confirmed HIT are [20]:

- substitute heparin with a rapidly acting non-heparin anticoagulant, usually in therapeutic doses
- avoid/postpone warfarin pending platelet count recovery
- minimise prophylactic platelet transfusions
- test for HIT antibodies
- investigate for lower limb DVT (e.g. ultrasound), even if not clinically apparent.

Rapidly Acting, Non-heparin Anticoagulants

- Anticoagulants for treating HIT can be divided into: (a) long-acting, indirect (antithrombin-dependent) factor Xa inhibitors (danaparoid, fondaparinux) and (b) short-acting direct thrombin inhibitors (DTIs). (Orally active direct factor Xa inhibitors, e.g. rivaroxaban, or DTIs, e.g. dabigatran, seem to be effective for treating HIT, but experience is limited.)
- Table 31.5 compares and contrasts the indirect factor Xa inhibitors versus the DTIs for the management of HIT and suspected HIT [9].
- The reader is referred elsewhere for dosing recommendations for the alternative non-heparin anticoagulants [20].
- HIT-associated consumptive coagulopathy can lead to treatment failure caused by systematic underdosing of the anticoagulant due to PTT-confounding [9, 20].
- Fondaparinux is a reasonable option for treating HIT [21]; further, its proven efficacy and safety in numerous (non-HIT) indications of antithrombotic prophylaxis and therapy are important considerations, given that ∼90% of patients tested do not have HIT.

Prevention of Warfarin-Induced Venous Limb Gangrene

- Warfarin and other vitamin K antagonists are *contraindicated* during the acute thrombocytopenic phase of HIT [20]. This is because their use is strongly associated with the risk of precipitating venous limb gangrene and (less often) central necrosis of skin and

Table 31.5 A comparison of two classes of anticoagulant used to treat HIT.

	Indirect (AT-dependent) factor Xa inhibitors: danaparoid, fondaparinux	Direct thrombin inhibitors (DTIs)*: argatroban, bivalirudin
Half-life	✓ Long (danaparoid, 25 h,[†] fondaparinux, 17 h): reduces risk of rebound hypercoagulability	Short (<2 h): potential for rebound hypercoagulability
Dosing	✓ Both prophylactic- and therapeutic-dose regimens[‡]	Prophylactic-dose regimens are not established
Monitoring	✓ Direct (anti-factor Xa levels); accurate drug levels obtained	Indirect (aPTT): risk for DTI under-dosing due to aPTT elevation caused by non-DTI factors ('aPTT confounding')
Effect on INR	✓ No significant effect; simplifies overlap with warfarin	Increases INR: argatroban > bivalirudin; complicates warfarin overlap
Reversibility of action	✓ Irreversible inhibition: AT forms covalent bond with factor Xa	No irreversible inhibition
Efficacy and safety established for non-HIT indications	✓ Treatment and prophylaxis of VTE (danaparoid, fondaparinux) and ACS (fondaparinux)	Not established for most non-HIT settings
Platelet activation	✓ Danaparoid inhibits platelet activation by HIT antibodies (fondaparinux has no effect)	No effect
Major bleeding risk	✓ Relatively low	Relatively high (~1% per treatment day)
Availability of antidote	No	No
Inhibition of clot-bound thrombin	No effect	✓ Inhibits clot-bound thrombin
Regulatory approval to treat HIT	Danaparoid: yes (although not in the USA); fondaparinux: no	Argatroban: yes. Bivalirudin: no.
Drug clearance	Predominantly renal	Variable (predominantly hepatobiliary: argatroban; predominantly renal and enzymic: bivalirudin)

Check mark (✓) indicates favourable feature in comparison of drug classes.

* Lepirudin was discontinued in March 2012.

† For danaparoid, half-lives of its anti-IIa (antithrombin) and its thrombin generation inhibition activities (2–4 h and 3–7 h, respectively) are shorter than for its anti-factor Xa activity (~25 h).

‡ Although therapeutic dosing is recommended for HIT, availability of prophylactic-dose regimens increases flexibility when managing potential non-HIT situations.

ACS, acute coronary syndrome; aPTT, (activated) partial thromboplastin time; AT, antithrombin; DTI, direct thrombin inhibitor; VTE, venous thromboembolism.

subcutaneous tissues ('classic' warfarin-induced skin necrosis) [14].

- Vitamin K should be given (5–10 mg by slow intravenous injection) if HIT is diagnosed in a patient who is receiving warfarin, especially if DTI therapy is planned (warfarin raises the aPTT and thus risks aPTT confounding of DTI therapy) [9, 20].

- Prothrombin complex concentrates (PCCs) contain small amounts of heparin, and thus their use is relatively contraindicated during acute HIT.

- Argatroban–warfarin overlap is problematic because argatroban prolongs the INR. In a patient who bleeds while receiving argatroban, plasma or PCCs should not be given to reverse a very high INR because the coagulopathy is caused by argatroban rather than because of factor deficiency.

Management of Isolated HIT

- 'Isolated HIT' is defined as HIT recognised because of thrombocytopenia, rather than because of a thrombotic event that draws attention to the possibility of HIT [12].
- Isolated HIT managed by simple discontinuation of heparin is associated with a ~50% risk of symptomatic thrombosis (most often venous thromboembolism (VTE)) and 5% risk of sudden death due to pulmonary embolism [12]; thus, a rapidly acting alternative anticoagulant is recommended when isolated HIT is strongly suspected or confirmed.
- Our practice is to continue therapeutic-dose alternative anticoagulation until there is recovery of the platelet count to a stable plateau within the normal range; we then repeat the venous ultrasound and if it is still negative for DVT, we discontinue anticoagulation.

Adjunctive Therapies

- *Thromboembolectomy* sometimes can salvage an ischaemic limb due to acute large vessel artery occlusion by platelet-rich 'white clots'. Non-heparin anticoagulant protocols, however, are not well established for vascular surgery.
- *High-dose intravenous immunoglobulin (IVIgG)* interferes with HIT antibody-induced platelet activation *in vitro* and reports indicate that its use can result in a platelet count increase in HIT.

However, IVIgG is not an anticoagulant and its use should be considered adjunctive in special circumstances (e.g. severe, persisting HIT).

- *Thrombolytic therapy* may be considered in selected patients with limb- or organ-threatening thrombosis. Concomitant anticoagulation with a non-heparin anticoagulant should be administered if heparin is part of the standard thrombolysis protocol.
- *Inferior vena cava filters* should be *avoided* because their use contributes to local thrombus formation/extension and risks underutilisation of anticoagulation, increasing risk of limb necrosis.

Repeat Heparin Exposure

- The immunology of HIT differs from the 'classic' immune response.
- Antibody titres decrease rapidly with cessation of HIT and in >60% of patients, antibodies are no longer detectable after 100 days.
- In a patient with previous HIT who has become antibody negative, re-exposure to heparin only rarely results in an anamnestic immune response. If repeat immunisation occurs, at least 4–5 days are needed before antibodies are present in sufficient amounts to induce platelet activation.
- The low risk of triggering recurrent HIT allows for deliberate re-exposure to heparin for intraoperative anticoagulation during cardiac or vascular surgery [13, 20]. Usually, heparin is avoided before and after surgery (if antibodies are regenerated, HIT is unlikely to be retriggered in the absence of further postoperative heparin use).

KEY POINTS

1) HIT is a highly prothrombotic, antibody-mediated adverse effect of heparin.
2) Venous thrombosis occurs most often, especially DVT and pulmonary embolism; unusual venous thrombotic events include adrenal haemorrhagic necrosis (secondary to adrenal vein thrombosis) and cerebral

venous (dural sinus) thrombosis. Arterial thrombosis most often involves large limb arteries, cerebral arteries and coronary arteries.
3) The frequency of HIT varies widely and occurs more often in patients who receive UFH (versus LMWH) and are postoperative (versus

medical, obstetric or paediatric); there is minor female predominance.

4) HIT is caused by IgG class antibodies that strongly activate platelets, triggering a procoagulant platelet response; almost always, the antibodies recognise multimolecular PF4/heparin complexes (the antibodies recognise one or more epitopes on PF4; heparin can be substituted by certain other polyanions).

5) Washed platelet activation assays have the highest sensitivity/specificity trade-off for detecting HIT antibodies; although PF4-dependent ELISAs have high sensitivity for detecting HIT antibodies, they lack diagnostic specificity (except when strong positive ELISA results are observed, e.g. >2.00 optical density units in an IgG-specific ELISA).

6) HIT lacks features of a 'classic' immune response, i.e. antibodies of IgG class are detectable 4–5 days following an immunising heparin exposure, without preceding IgM.

7) HIT antibodies are remarkably transient, which explains why rapid-onset HIT only occurs in patients who have been exposed to heparin within the recent past. Also, it explains why heparin re-exposure is appropriate for patients with a previous history of HIT who require cardiac or vascular surgery, provided that platelet-activating antibodies are no longer detectable.

8) Vitamin K antagonists (e.g. warfarin) are contraindicated during the acute phase of HIT because their use can precipitate limb necrosis due to microthrombosis; vitamin K should be administered to a patient diagnosed with acute HIT who is receiving warfarin therapy.

9) Prophylactic platelet transfusions should be avoided during acute HIT, as thrombocytopenic bleeding (e.g. mucocutaneous haemorrhage) is not a feature of HIT and platelet transfusions in theory could increase thrombotic risk.

10) Treatment of HIT should focus on rapidly acting, non-heparin anticoagulants. There are two main classes of therapies: (a) long-acting indirect (antithrombin-dependent) factor Xa inhibitors (danaparoid, fondaparinux) and (b) direct thrombin inhibitors (argatroban, bivalirudin). For the oral direct FXa inhibitors and the oral FIIa inhibitor, early experience is promising (though insufficient for recommendation), while they are a treatment option in stable patients with recent HIT or patients with a history of HIT.

References

1 Greinacher A. Heparin-induced thrombocytopenia. N Engl J Med 2015;**373**(3):252–61.

2 Greinacher A, Kohlmann T, Strobel U, Sheppard JI, Warkentin TE. The temporal profile of the anti-PF4/heparin immune response. Blood 2009;**113**:4970–6.

3 Warkentin TE, Sheppard JI, Moore JC, Cook RJ, Kelton JG. Studies of the immune response in heparin induced thrombocytopenia. Blood 2009;**113**:4963–9.

4 Krauel K, Pötschke C, Weber C et al. Platelet factor 4 binds to bacteria, inducing antibodies cross-reacting with the major antigen in heparin-induced thrombocytopenia. Blood 2011;**117**:1370–8.

5 Warkentin TE, Chong BH, Greinacher A. Heparin-induced thrombocytopenia: towards consensus. Thromb Haemost 1998; 79 (1): 1–7.

6 Warkentin TE, Kelton JG. Delayed-onset heparin-induced thrombocytopenia and thrombosis. Ann Intern Med 2001;**135**:502–6.

7 Warkentin TE, Sheppard JI, Sigouin CS, Kohlmann T, Eichler P, Greinacher A. Gender imbalance and risk factor interactions in heparin-induced thrombocytopenia. Blood 2006;**108**:2937–41.

8 Warkentin TE, Basciano PA, Knopman J, Bernstein RA. Spontaneous heparin-induced thrombocytopenia syndrome: 2 new cases and

a proposal for defining this syndrome. Blood 2014;**123**:3651–4.

9 Warkentin TE. Agents for the treatment of heparin-induced thrombocytopenia. Hematol Oncol Clin North Am 2010;**24**:755–75.

10 Warkentin TE, Linkins LA. Immunoassays are not created equal. J Thromb Haemost 2009;**7**:1256–9.

11 Bakchoul T, Giptner A, Bein G, Santoso S, Sachs UJH. Prospective evaluation of immunoassays for the diagnosis of heparin-induced thrombocytopenia. J Thromb Haemost 2009;**7**:1260–5.

12 Warkentin TE, Kelton JG. A 14-year study of heparin-induced thrombocytopenia. Am J Med 1996;**101**:502–7.

13 Warkentin TE, Kelton JG. Temporal aspects of heparin-induced thrombocytopenia. N Engl J Med 2001;**344**:1286–92.

14 Warkentin TE. Ischemic limb gangrene with pulses. N Engl J Med 2015;**373**:642–55.

15 Linkins LA, Bates SM, Lee AY, Heddle NM, Wang G, Warkentin TE. Combination of 4Ts score and PF4/H-PaGIA for diagnosis and management of heparin-induced thrombocytopenia: prospective cohort study. Blood 2015;**126**(5):597–603.

16 Warkentin TE, Linkins LA. Non-necrotizing heparin-induced skin lesions and the 4T's score. J Thromb Haemost 2010;**8**:1483–5.

17 Selleng S, Malowsky B, Strobel U et al. Early-onset and persisting thrombocytopenia in post-cardiac surgery patients is rarely due to heparin-induced thrombocytopenia even when antibody tests are positive. J Thromb Haemost 2010;**8**:30–6.

18 Padmanabhan A, Jones CG, Bougie DW et al. Heparin-independent, PF4-dependent binding of HIT antibodies to platelets: implications for HIT pathogenesis. Blood 2015;**125**(1):155–61.

19 Warkentin TE, Sheppard JI, Moore JC, Sigouin CS, Kelton JG. Quantitative interpretation of optical density measurements using PF4-dependent enzymeimmunoassays. J Thromb Haemost 2008;**6**:1304–12.

20 Linkins LA, Dans AL, Moores LK et al, for the American College of Chest Physicians. Treatment and prevention of heparin-induced thrombocytopenia: Antithrombotic Therapy and Prevention of Thrombosis, 9th ed: American College of Chest Physicians Evidence-Based Clinical Practice Guidelines.Chest 2012;**141**(2 Suppl.):e495S–530S.

21 Kang M, Alahmadi M, Sawh S, Kovacs MJ, Lazo-Langner A. Fondaparinux for the treatment of suspected heparin-induced thrombocytopenia: a propensity score-matched study. Blood 2015;**125**:924–9.

Further Reading

Cuker A, Cines DB. How I treat heparin-induced thrombocytopenia. Blood 2012;**119**:2209–18.

Cuker A, Gimotty PA, Crowther MA, Warkentin TE. Predictive value of the 4Ts scoring system for heparin-induced thrombocytopenia: a systematic review and meta-analysis. Blood 2012;**120**:4160–7.

Greinacher A, Warkentin TE, Chong BH. Heparin-induced thrombocytopenia, in Platelets, 3rd edn (ed. A Michelson). Elsevier Science and Technology, Oxford, 2012, pp.851–82.

Greinacher A, Pötzsch B, Amiral J, Dummel V, Eichner A, Mueller-Eckhardt C. Heparin-associated thrombocytopenia: isolation of the antibody and characterization of a multimolecular PF4-heparin complex as the major antigen. J Thromb Haemost 1994;**71**:247–51.

Greinacher A, Holtfreter B, Krauel K et al. Association of natural anti-platelet factor 4/ heparin antibodies with periodontal disease. Blood 2011;**118**:1395–401.

Lubenow N, Hinz P, Thomaschewski S et al. The severity of trauma determines the immune response to PF4/heparin and the frequency of heparin-induced thrombocytopenia. Blood 2010;**115**:1797–803.

Warkentin TE. How I diagnose and manage HIT. Hematol Am Soc Hematol Educ Program 2011;143–9.

Warkentin TE, Greinacher A. Heparin-induced anaphylactic and anaphylactoid reactions: two distinct but overlapping syndromes. Expert Opin Drug Saf 2009;**8**:129–44.

Warkentin TE, Greinacher A (eds). Heparin-Induced Thrombocytopenia, 5th edn. CRC Press, Boca Raton, 2013.

Watson H, Davidson S, Keeling D, for the Haemostasis and Thrombosis Task Force of the British Committee for Standards in Haematology. Guidelines on the diagnosis and management of heparin-induced thrombocytopenia: second edition. Br J Haematol 2012;**159**:528–40.

Zheng Y, Yu M, Podd A et al. Critical role for mouse marginal zone B cells in PF4/heparin antibody production. Blood 2013;**121**:3484–92.

32

Immunodeficiency and Immunoglobulin Therapy

Siraj A. Misbah

Oxford University Hospitals, University of Oxford, Oxford, UK

Introduction

The increasing awareness of immunodeficiency and the rapid pace of genetic discovery have helped to ensure that immunodeficiency disorders are no longer viewed as arcane rarities by both clinical immunologists and non-immunologists. In haematology, alongside the major changes in practice that have been driven by advances in fundamental immunology [1], haematologists are also likely to encounter patients with primary immunodeficiency disease due to the frequency of haematological complications associated with this group of disorders. Given that most haematologists will be familiar with the consequences of secondary immunodeficiency, either iatrogenic or associated with lymphoproliferative disease, this chapter will focus principally on primary immunodeficiency disorders (PID) followed by a separate section on immunoglobulin therapy.

Primary Immunodeficiency Disorders

Many PIDs associated with single gene mutations have been aptly called experiments of nature in view of the unique insights that these diseases have provided in unravelling complex immunological functions. Currently, the World Health Organization–International Union of Immunological Societies (WHO/IUIS) Committee on Primary Immunodeficiency Diseases recognises over 250 primary immunodeficiencies for which the underlying molecular basis has been elucidated [2]. As the genetic basis of old and new immunodeficiency disorders is unravelled, it has become clear that the same gene mutation may result in different phenotypes. In investigating and managing patients with PID, it is important to bear in mind this concept of genetic heterogeneity accompanied by equally significant clinical and immunological heterogeneity. For example, the same mutation in the gene encoding the Wiskott–Aldrich syndrome protein (WASP) may result in either full-blown Wiskott–Aldrich syndrome characterised by thrombocytopenia, infections and autoimmunity or a limited phenotype of X-linked thrombocytopenia [3]. Similarly, mutations in recombination activating genes (RAG) may present with a wide range of distinct immunological phenotypes beyond severe combined immunodeficiency. Conversely, a distinct immunophenotypic syndrome may be associated with a wide range of mutations in different genes. Such examples have focused attention on the role of epigenetic changes in influencing disease phenotype, in addition to highlighting the limitations of using immunophenotypic patterns as a guide to underlying molecular defects.

Although PID can affect any part of the immune system, in practice patients with predominant

Practical Transfusion Medicine, Fifth Edition. Edited by Michael F. Murphy, David J. Roberts and Mark H. Yazer.
© 2017 John Wiley & Sons Ltd. Published 2017 by John Wiley & Sons Ltd.

defects of B-cell function and combined B- and T-cell defects constitute the bulk of a clinical immunologist's workload. The immunopathogenesis of antibody deficiency disorders and combined B- and T-lymphocyte deficiency is best understood within the context of B- and T-lymphocyte development. The schematic diagrams set out in Figures 32.1 and 32.2 summarise the major events in B- and T-cell development and the points at which developmental arrest leads to immunodeficiency. The delineation of new immunodeficiencies using whole exome and next-generation sequencing has led to calls for a revised classification of PID, which integrates clinical, immunological and genetic phenotypes [4].

Predominant B-Cell Deficiency Disorders

Common Variable Immunodeficiency

Of the 20 antibody deficiency disorders currently recognised, common variable immunodeficiency (CVID) is the most common acquired PID that is likely to be encountered by haematologists. As its name implies, CVID is characterised by a severe reduction in at least two serum immunoglobulin isotypes associated with low or normal B-cell numbers. In contrast, antibody deficiency disorder associated with severe reduction of all serum immunoglobulin isotypes with absent circulating B-cells is a feature of diseases associated with mutations that interrupt B-cell development (see Figure 32.2).

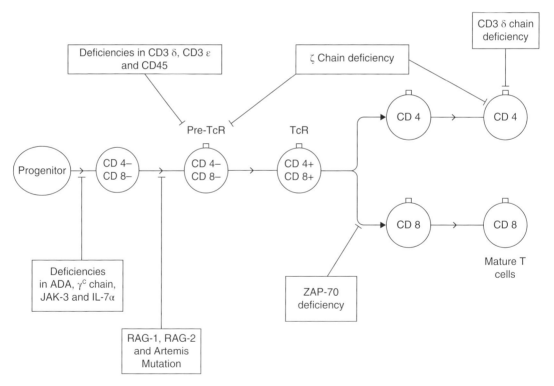

Figure 32.1 Major events in T-cell development and sites of mutations leading to immunodeficiencies. T-cell development in the thymus from a progenitor cell proceeds sequentially from a double-negative state (CD4–, CD8–) to mature T-cells expressing either CD4 or CD8. Stages of T-cell differentiation associated with mutations and deficiencies of proteins are depicted in boxes. *Source:* Adapted from Rudd CE. NEJM 2006;354:1874. ADA, adenosine deaminase; JAK3, Janus kinase 3; RAG, recombination-activating gene; ZAP-70, zeta-chain-associated protein of 70 kd.

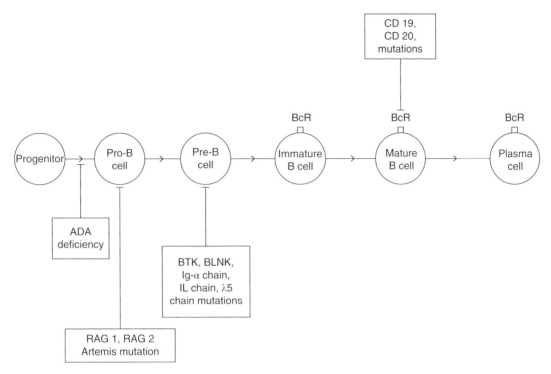

Figure 32.2 Major events in B-cell development and sites of mutations leading to immunodeficiencies. B-cell development in the bone marrow proceeds from a progenitor cell sequentially to plasma cells in the periphery. Stages of B-cell differentiation associated with mutations and deficiencies of proteins are depicted in boxes. *Source:* Adapted from Rudd CE. NEJM 2006;354:1874. ADA, adenosine deaminase; RAG, recombination-activating gene; BTK, Bruton tyrosine kinase; BLNK, mutated B-cell-linked protein.

The term CVID embraces a heterogeneous group of disorders, all of which are characterised by late-onset hypogammaglobulinaemia as the unifying theme [5]. The most common infective manifestation of antibody deficiency is recurrent infection with encapsulated bacteria, particularly *Streptococcus pneumoniae* and to a lesser extent unencapsulated *Haemophilus influenzae*. Many patients develop frank bronchiectasis as a consequence of recurrent chest infections. Despite their inability to mount effective antibody responses to exogenous pathogens, many patients with CVID mount paradoxical immune responses to self antigens, leading to autoimmune disease. In a haematological context, the most frequent of these autoimmune complications are immune thrombocytopenic purpura (ITP) and autoimmune haemolytic anaemia.

A whole host of other organ-specific and systemic autoimmune diseases may also occur, ranging from Addison's disease to systemic lupus erythematosus. Non-infective complications associated with CVID include a curious predisposition to granulomatous disease, lymphoid interstitial pneumonitis and a 100-fold increase in the risk of lymphoma. Although the latter may occasionally be driven by Epstein–Barr virus (EBV), in the majority of cases no underlying infection is evident, raising the possibility that lymphoproliferative disease in these patients is a manifestation of defective immunoregulation.

Despite the inability of B-cells in CVID to produce antibodies, recovery of antibody production has been documented following infection with HCV and HIV, respectively [6]. This observation supports the concept that defective immunoregulation is contributing to poor B-cell function in these patients.

Given the range of infective and non-infective complications associated with CVID, many attempts have been made to produce a clinically useful disease classification based on immunological indices. Recent evidence suggests that a deficiency of switched IgM$^-$ IgD$^-$ CD27$^+$ memory B-cells may correlate with the development of bronchiectasis, autoimmunity and reactive splenomegaly in CVID. The molecular basis for some of the diseases previously included under the umbrella of CVID has recently been elucidated by the detection of mutations in a number of genes associated with B-cell function (Box 32.1). In addition to the molecular defects listed in Box 32.1, there are rare patients with mutations in certain X-linked genes (Bruton tyrosine kinase, CD40 ligand and signalling lymphocyte activation-associated protein) who may present with a clinical phenotype resembling CVID.

The management of CVID revolves around regular Ig replacement optimised to ensure a trough IgG level well within the normal range for effective prophylaxis against bacterial infections. Evidence from a longitudinal study of infection outcomes in 90 patients with CVID followed up over 20 years suggests that the dose of immunoglobulin required to reduce breakthrough infections is individual to a particular patient [7]. Achievement of this goal is therefore likely to be associated with a wide range of trough IgG levels. Early diagnosis and therapeutic intervention with Ig therapy significantly minimise the risk of permanent bronchiectatic lung damage.

X-Linked Agammaglobulinaemia

X-linked agammaglobulinaemia (XLA) was one of the earliest primary immunodeficiencies to be clinically characterised, in the 1950s. Its molecular basis was only elucidated in the 1990s with the discovery of mutations in a protein tyrosine kinase gene, named Bruton tyrosine kinase (Btk).

The Btk gene is located on the long arm of the X-chromosome and encodes for a cytoplasmic tyrosine kinase, which is essential for B-cell signal transduction. Btk mutations are associated with B-cell developmental arrest in the bone marrow. The consequent disappearance of circulating B-cells in association with severe panhypogammaglobulinaemia and poorly developed lymphoid tissue constitute the cardinal immunological features of XLA. Over 400 different mutations in the Btk gene have been recorded to date but there are no significant correlations between genotype and clinical phenotype. The essential role of Btk in B-cell receptor signal transduction, as exemplified by B-cell failure in

---

Box 32.1 Known molecular defects that present with a CVID-like clinical picture.

- Inducible co-stimulatory receptor (ICOS) deficiency
- CD19 deficiency
- Mutations in the transmembrane activator and calcium modulator and cyclophilin ligand interactor (TACI) receptor
- Mutations in the receptor for B-cell activating factor of the TNF family (BAFF)
- Mutations in cytotoxic T-lymphocyte-associated protein (CTLA-4)
- Mutations in nuclear factor - kappa B2 gene (NFKB2)
- Mutations in LPS-responsive vesicle trafficking beach and anchor enhancing (LRBA) gene
- Mutations in phosphatidyl-3-kinase C δ (PIK3CD) gene
- CD20 deficiency
- CD21 deficiency
- CD81 deficiency

XLA, has been exploited by the development of Btk inhibitors (ibrutinib) for the treatment of B-cell lymphomas.

Most boys with XLA present with a history of recurrent sinopulmonary infections on a background of panhypogammaglobulinaemia after the age of six months, once the protective effect of transplacentally acquired maternal IgG has waned. As with CVID, delayed diagnosis of XLA and consequent failure to institute adequate Ig replacement are associated with a high risk of bronchiectasis [8].

In keeping with the absence of a T-cell defect in XLA, infection with intracellular pathogens is generally not a problem. The major exception to this rule is the predisposition to chronic enteroviral infections, including echovirus meningoencephalitis and vaccine-induced poliomyelitis. A clinical phenotype identical to XLA may be caused by mutations in the μ-immunoglobulin heavy chain gene and other components of the B-cell receptor [9].

Severe Combined Immunodeficiency

Severe combined immunodeficiency (SCID) refers to a group of genetically determined disorders characterised by arrested T-cell development accompanied by impaired B-cell function [10]. The incidence of SCID is estimated to be between 1:50 000 and 1:100 000 live births.

Babies with SCID present with recurrent infections associated with lymphopaenia. Among the range of pathogens responsible for infection in SCID, *Pneumocystis jiroveci* (*carinii*), *Aspergillus* species and cytomegalovirus (CMV) predominate in keeping with the profound T-cell deficiency seen in these babies.

To date, at least 18 distinct molecular defects that cause the SCID phenotype have been identified, with eight of the more common defects being listed in Table 32.1. While lymphopenia is characteristic of all forms of SCID, the circulating lymphocyte surface marker profile (see Box 32.1) provides a useful clue as to the underlying genetic defect. For example, deficiency of adenosine deaminase, a key purine enzyme, results in severe lymphopenia affecting T-, B- and NK

Table 32.1 Classification of severe combined immunodeficiency.

Affected gene	Inheritance	Circulating lymphocyte phenotype
Adenosine deaminase (ADA)	AR	T− B− NK−
Common cytokine γ-chain (γc)	X-linked	T− B+ NK−
Jak-3	AR	T− B+ NK−
IL-7α	AR	T− B+ NK+
Recombination activating gene 1, 2 (RAG1/RAG2)	AR	T− B− NK+
Artemis	AR	T−B−NK+
CD3 δ, ζ, ε	AR	T− B+ NK+
CD45	AR	T− B+ NK+

AR, autosomal recessive.

cells leading to its characterisation as T−B−NK− SCID. Based on an analysis of 172 babies with SCID transplanted at a single centre over a 30-year period, three major diagnostic clues have emerged as markers of all molecular forms of SCID: a positive family history was noted in 37%, lymphopenia in 88% and an absent thymic shadow in 92% [11].

Given the profound impairment in T-cell immunity, babies with SCID are at risk of iatrogenic disease with live vaccines and transfusion-associated graft-versus-host disease. For these reasons, immunisation with live vaccines should be regarded as absolutely contraindicated in these babies. Equally, any baby with SCID should only receive irradiated and cytomegalovirus (CMV)-seronegative blood.

The severity of disease and the urgency with which curative haemopoietic stem cell transplantation (HSCT) should be undertaken have led SCID to be regarded as a paediatric emergency. The results of HSCT have improved significantly with early diagnosis and aggressive management of infections and nutritional problems seen in these babies at the time of diagnosis. At present,

HSCT from an HLA-matched sibling donor offers an 80% chance of cure while a fully HLA-matched unrelated transplant offers a 70% chance of cure (Figure 32.3). These results from Europe have recently been confirmed by longitudinal outcome data in 240 infants with SCID transplanted during a 10-year period (2000–2009) in the United States [12]. Neonatal screening for SCID using polymerase chain reaction-based analysis of T-cell receptor excision circles (TRECs – a measure of thymic T-cell output) on Guthrie card blood samples has recently been introduced in parts of the USA [13].

In view of the single gene defects underlying SCID, gene therapy is an attractive option. While offering great promise, the results of gene therapy to date have been mixed. Gene therapy has been successful in some children with adenosine deaminase (ADA) and common cytokine γ-chain deficiency, respectively, with evidence of T-, B- and NK cell reconstitution in the former and T- and NK cell reconstitution in the latter. However, the occurrence of insertional mutagenesis leading to T-cell lymphoproliferative disease in some children with common γ-chain SCID is an important reminder of the obstacles associated with this ground-breaking therapy [14]. This risk has prompted the development of a new generation of self-inactivating and lentiviral vectors which have been used in common γ-chain SCID. To date, there have been no reports of insertional mutagenesis [15].

Investigation of Suspected Immunodeficiency

Although a few patients may have distinctive clues on examination pointing towards a PID, most patients have no physical signs that would specifically point to an immunodeficiency disorder. Conversely, it follows that a

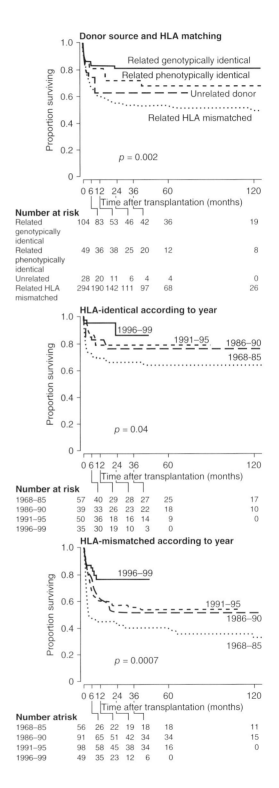

Figure 32.3 Cumulative probability of survival in SCID patients, according to donor source (related or unrelated donor) and HLA matching, and year of transplantation. *Source:* Reproduced from Antoine C et al. Lancet 2003;**361**:556, with permission of Elsevier.

normal physical examination does not exclude immunodeficiency disease.

Immunodeficiency should be included in the differential diagnosis of any patient with severe, prolonged or recurrent infection with common pathogens or even a single episode of infection with an unusual pathogen. The type of pathogen involved provides important clues as to which component of the immune system may be defective and consequently guides the selection of relevant immunological tests (Table 32.2). While this targeted approach has much to commend it in defining immune phenotypes, integration with gene sequencing is increasingly used for definitive molecular diagnosis. Although this chapter is primarily devoted to PID, it is essential to consider and exclude the possibility of HIV infection as a driver for immunodeficiency in many of these clinical scenarios [16].

In view of the complexity of many immunological tests, it is essential that immunological investigations are performed under the guidance of a clinical immunologist to enable appropriate test selection, interpretation and advice on clinical management.

Management of Immunodeficiency

Infections in any immunodeficient patient should be treated aggressively with appropriate antimicrobial therapy. In patients with antibody deficiency, lifelong immunoglobulin replacement remains the cornerstone of management. For children with SCID, HSCT remains the main curative option with the prospect of gene therapy for some forms of SCID. Patients with complement deficiency should be fully immunised with the full range of available vaccines against neisserial, pneumococcal and *Haemophilus* infections. However, it is vital to avoid the use of live vaccines in any patient with immunodeficiency in view of the real risks of vaccine-associated disease, as exemplified by vaccine-induced poliomyelitis in XLA and BCG-induced mycobacterial disease in SCID.

Immunoglobulin Therapy

Therapeutic immunoglobulin is a blood component prepared from the plasma of 10 000–15 000 donors. The broad spectrum of antibody specificities contained in pooled plasma is an essential ingredient underpinning the success of intravenous (IVIg) and, more recently, subcutaneous immunoglobulin (SCIg) in infection prophylaxis in patients with antibody deficiency. Evidence from longitudinal studies in large cohorts of antibody-deficient patients

Table 32.2 Patterns of infection as a guide to selection of immunological tests in suspected immune deficiency.

Type of pathogen	Consider	Relevant immunological tests
A – Encapsulated pathogens	Antibody deficiency Complement deficiency	Serum immunoglobulins, specific antibodies to polysaccharide and protein antigens Haemolytic complement activity
B – Viruses and intracellular pathogens	T-cell defect	Lymphocyte surface marker analysis Lymphocyte transformation
C – Combination of encapsulated pathogens and viruses and other intracellular pathogens	Combined B- + T-cell defect	As for A and B
D – Recurrent neisserial infection	Complement deficiency	Haemolytic complement activity
E – Recurrent staphylococcal abscesses and/or invasive fungal infections	Phagocyte defect	Neutrophil respiratory burst Leucocyte adhesion molecule expression (selected cases)

and a meta-analysis of studies of IVIg replacement have highlighted the inverse correlation between trough IgG levels and the frequency of infection [17]. A similar inverse relationship between incidence of infections and steady-state IgG levels has recently been confirmed in studies of SCIg in patients with PID. In addition to its role in antibody replacement, the success of high-dose IVIg in the treatment of ITP has led to a veritable explosion in its use as a therapeutic immunomodulator in many autoimmune diseases spanning multiple specialties (Table 32.3).

The mechanisms of action of high-dose IVIg in autoimmune disease are complex and reflect the potent immunological actions of the different regions of an IgG molecule. It is helpful conceptually to consider the potential mechanisms of action in relation to the variable regions of IgG (F(ab')2), the Fc region and the presence in IVIg of other potent immunomodulatory substances other than antibody (Figure 32.4). In ITP, the traditional view of Fc receptor blockade as the predominant mechanism by which IVIg is effective has recently been complemented by evidence from murine studies showing that IVIg-mediated amelioration of ITP is crucially dependent on interactions with the inhibitory FcγRIIB as well as the activating receptor, FcγRIII. Evidence from murine studies indicates that up-regulation of FcγRIIB expression occurs via the small sialylated immunoglobulin component of polyclonal IVIg (estimated at 1–3%).

Table 32.3 Use of IVIg as an immunomodulatory agent.

Disorder	Comments
Neurology	
Guillain–Barré syndrome	Treatment of choice and as efficacious as plasmapheresis (RCT, CR)
Multifocal motor neuropathy	Treatment of choice (RCT)
Chronic inflammatory demyelinating polyneuropathy	As an alternative to steroids (RCT)
Dermatomyositis	As an adjunct to immunosuppressive therapy (RCT)
Myasthenia gravis	For myasthenic crises (RCT)
Lambert–Eaton syndrome	For non-cancer-associated cases that have failed to respond to standard therapy (RCT)
Stiff-person syndrome	For severe cases unresponsive to standard therapy (RCT)
Autoimmune encephalitides	As an adjunct to steroids and plasmapheresis
Haematology	
Immune thrombocytopenic purpura	Selected cases unresponsive to standard treatment (RCT)
Parvovirus-associated pure red cell aplasia	Selected cases
Paediatrics	
Kawasaki's disease	Treatment of choice (RCT)
Dermatology	
Toxic epidermal necrolysis	Open studies/case series suggest benefit
Autoimmune blistering disorders	Open studies/case series suggest benefit
Streptococcal toxic shock syndrome	Open studies/case series suggest benefit

The list of indications is not exhaustive but covers those disorders where IVIg is frequently used.
CR, evidence from Cochrane review; RCT, evidence from randomised controlled trials.

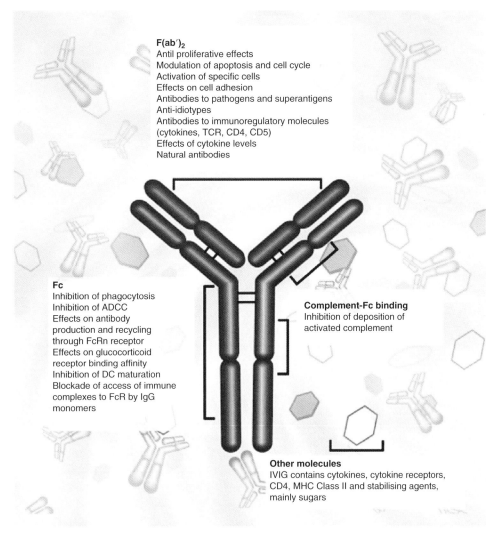

F(ab')$_2$
Antil proliferative effects
Modulation of apoptosis and cell cycle
Activation of specific cells
Effects on cell adhesion
Antibodies to pathogens and superantigens
Anti-idiotypes
Antibodies to immunoregulatory molecules
(cytokines, TCR, CD4, CD5)
Effects of cytokine levels
Natural antibodies

Fc
Inhibition of phagocytosis
Inhibition of ADCC
Effects on antibody
production and recycling
through FcRn receptor
Effects on glucocorticoid
receptor binding affinity
Inhibition of DC maturation
Blockade of access of immune
complexes to FcR by IgG
monomers

Complement-Fc binding
Inhibition of deposition of
activated complement

Other molecules
IVIG contains cytokines, cytokine receptors,
CD4, MHC Class II and stabilising agents,
mainly sugars

Figure 32.4 Immunomodulatory actions of intravenous immunoglobulin. *Source:* Reproduced from Jolles S, Sewell WAC, Misbah SA. Clinical uses of intravenous immunoglobulin. Clin Exp Immunol 2005;**142**:1–11, with permission from John Wiley and Sons.

This observation has led to the hypothesis that the use of small doses of concentrated sialylated immunoglobulin might be as efficacious as the use of conventional high-dose immunoglobulin for immunomodulation [18]. Subsequent *in vitro* and *in vivo* studies in mice and humans on the role of sialylation have proven contradictory, leaving this hypothesis unproven [19].

Immunoglobulin Replacement in Secondary Antibody Deficiency

Intravenous immunoglobulin replacement is beneficial in prophylaxis against infection in selected patients with secondary antibody deficiency associated with B-cell lymphoproliferative disease and myeloma. The predictors of response to IVIg are the presence of hypogammaglobulinaemia accompanied by low concentrations of pneumococcal antibodies and a failure to respond to test immunisation with pneumococcal polysaccharide (Pneumovax). While IVIg is clinically efficacious in patients fulfilling the above criteria, questions remain regarding its overall cost-effectiveness [20]. For this reason, IVIg replacement should be reserved for those patients who have failed a trial of prolonged antibiotic prophylaxis [21]. Despite evidence supporting the use of IVIg in secondary antibody deficiency, in practice its use has not been widespread due to the advent of more immunogenic pneumococcal conjugate vaccines coupled with improved overall management of these haematological malignancies.

Adverse Effects of Intravenous Immunoglobulin Therapy

Immediate Infusion-Related Adverse Effects

Minor to moderate immediate infusion-related adverse effects in the form of headaches, chills, rigours and backache occur in approximately 1% of patients irrespective of the therapeutic dose of immunoglobulin. These adverse effects are largely related to the rate of infusion and/or the presence of underlying infection in the recipient and respond to a combination of a reduction in infusion rate coupled with simple analgesia. Very rarely, some patients with total IgA deficiency and preexisting anti-IgA antibodies may develop anaphylaxis on exposure to IVIg preparations containing IgA. Although this risk may be minimised by the use of an IgA-depleted IVIg preparation in such patients, the exact role of anti-IgA is unclear, since many patients with high-titre antibodies may safely receive IVIg [22]. The recent demonstration of a novel splice variant of FcγRIIA in a patient with anti-IgA who experienced IVIg-induced anaphylaxis raises the possibility that activating receptors for IgG may be a contributory factor in triggering anaphylaxis [23].

Dose-Related Adverse Effects

The increasing use of IVIg for therapeutic immunomodulation has been associated with the development of a range of haematological, neurological, nephrological and dermatological adverse effects that are directly linked to the high doses (2 g/kg) required for autoimmune disease in contrast to the low doses (0.4 g/kg) used for antibody replacement.

Haematological

High-dose IVIg causes a dose-dependent increase in plasma viscosity [24], which is sufficient to precipitate serious arterial and venous thrombosis in patients with preexisting thrombophilia, paraproteinaemia, severe polyclonal hypergammaglobulinaemia and atheromatous cardiovascular disease.

The risk of IVIg-associated acute haemolysis due to passive transmission of anti-blood group antibodies has been greatly minimised by the institution of rigourous quality control measures designed to ensure that the titre of anti-blood group antibodies in IVIg does not exceed 1:64. Despite these measures, there has been a recent resurgence in cases of IVIg-induced haemolysis, which appears to have coincided with the increasing use of more concentrated liquid preparations [25].

Neurological

High-dose IVIg is associated with the development of self-limiting acute aseptic meningitis in a minority of patients (<5%). Patients with background migraine are at higher risk, raising the possibility that meningeal irritation may be due to the interaction of exogenous IgG with meningeal endothelium.

Renal

Nephrotoxicity due to high-dose IVIg is a particular risk associated with sucrose-containing preparations, which trigger osmotic tubular injury, leading to extensive vacuolar changes suggestive of historical cases of sucrose-induced nephropathy. The risk of renal damage is greatly minimised by avoiding the use of sucrose-containing IVIg preparations in patients with preexisting diabetes and renal disease.

Intravenous immunoglobulin should also be avoided or used with caution in patients with mixed cryoglobulinaemia because of the real risk of the IgM component of cryoglobulin, containing rheumatoid factor reactivity, complexing with infused exogenous IgG to cause acute immune complex-mediated renal injury [26].

Dermatological

A variety of cutaneous adverse effects including eczema, erythema multiforme, urticaria and cutaneous vasculitis may be triggered by high-dose IVIg. The relatively small number of cases reported to date does not enable any useful analysis that might help in minimising the development of dermatological adverse reactions.

Risks of Viral Transmission

Viral transmission is a risk with both low- and high-dose IVIg therapy. However, the increasingly stringent screening of donors coupled with the introduction of additional antiviral steps during plasma fractionation has greatly reduced but not eliminated the risk of HCV transmission with IVIg. For this reason, patients on maintenance IVIg should have their liver function monitored along with regular testing for HCV. The lack of any outbreaks of IVIg-associated HCV transmission since the last outbreak in 1993 [27] attests to the success of current viral safety measures. Unlike HCV, HIV and HBV have never been transmitted by IVIg since the process of Cohn-ethanol fractionation specifically inactivates both of these viruses.

While recent reports of the development of variant Creutzfeldt–Jakob disease in recipients of blood from donors with asymptomatic disease have raised concerns of the possibility of prion transmission by blood components, this risk remains largely theoretical with IVIg. Leucocyte reduction and the use of plasma from countries free of bovine spongiform encephalopathy are measures designed to minimise this risk in the UK.

Practical Aspects of Immunoglobulin Therapy – Product Selection and Safe Use

The availability of several different preparations of IVIg (at least six in the UK at present) has raised the question of whether IVIg should be considered a generic product. For the purposes of antibody replacement, it is reasonable to consider the different products as equally efficacious since each product is required to fulfil the stringent criteria laid down by the World Health Organization

for therapeutic immunoglobulin. With regard to the use of high-dose IVIg as an immunomodulator, studies comparing the efficacy of different products in Kawasaki's disease and chronic inflammatory demyelinating polyneuropathy (CIDP) have shown no difference in efficacy. Hence, while it would be reasonable to consider IVIg generic in terms of clinical outcomes [28], because of differences in the manufacturing process and its impact on opsonic activity, Fc receptor function and complement fixation, it is best to regard individual products as distinct entities. In view of this and the potential difficulty in tracking any future outbreak of IVIg-associated viral transmission, it is prudent to maintain patients requiring long-term treatment on the same IVIg product, irrespective of whether IVIg is being used for antibody deficiency or immunomodulation.

Box 32.2 provides a useful checklist for the safe use of high-dose IVIg, including advice on product selection. Advice on individual products should be sought from a clinical immunologist.

Subcutaneous Immunoglobulin

Following comparative trials, the subcutaneous route of immunoglobulin delivery has been shown to be as efficacious as IVIg in infection prophylaxis in patients with primary antibody deficiency [29]. In practice, SCIg has proven to be popular with both patients and clinicians in view of its ease of use in patients with poor venous access and minimal adverse effects, in comparison with IVIg (Table 32.4). Using a weekly infusion regimen, SCIg achieves steady-state IgG levels without the peaks and troughs associated with IVIg. When patients transfer from IVIg to SCIg, the achievement of equivalent or higher steady-state levels with the same dose of SCIg reflects the reduced catabolism with subcutaneous delivery.

The success of SCIg as replacement therapy in antibody deficiency has led to its increasing use for immunomodulation as in inflammatory neuropathy [30,31]. The use of multiple infusion sites in a motivated patient has enabled the delivery of higher doses required for immunomodulation. Using currently available

---

Box 32.2   Checklist for the use of high-dose IVIg.

1. Prior to first infusion:

Check renal and liver function, full blood count, viscosity, serum C-reactive protein, serum immuno-globulins and electrophoresis. Take blood for hepatitis C serology (not necessary to delay treatment while awaiting result) and save aliquot of frozen serum.

Normal renal and liver function and serum IgA	Impaired renal function	Total IgA deficiency (<0.05 g/L)	Partial IgA deficiency	IgM/IgG paraprotein	Patients at risk of hyperviscosity: >4 cp (i.e. serum IgG >50 g/L or with serum IgM >30 g/L) or with background arterial disease
Proceed with any IVIg product	Avoid sucrose-containing IVIg and exercise caution; suggest using 0.4 g/kg/daily for 5 days and slower rate of infusion (suggest halving rate). Check creatinine daily before repeat dose is given	Use IVIg product containing low IgA content Check anti-IgA antibodies (time permitting, not essential)	Proceed with any IVIg product	Consider possibility of mixed cryoglobulinaemia Seek immunological advice before proceeding with IVIg	Exercise caution: use slower rate of infusion (suggest halving rate) and check viscosity at end of course

2. Adhere to the manufacturer's recommendations regarding reconstitution and rate of infusion.
3. Record batch number of product.

Source: Reproduced with permission from Association of British Neurologists. Guidelines on IVIg in Neurological Diseases. www.theabn.org/.

Table 32.4 Adverse effects of intravenous versus subcutaneous immunoglobulin.

	SCIg	IVIg
Local reactions at site of infusion	Common (trivial)	Nil*
Anaphylaxis	—	Very rare*
Viral transmission (HCV)	—	+†
Renal impairment	—	+
Aseptic meningitis	—	+
Thrombosis	—	+

* Possibly related to anti-IgA abs in some cases.
† Last outbreak in early 1990s.

KEY POINTS

1) Over 250 primary immunodeficiency disorders are currently recognised.
2) Common variable immunodeficiency is the most common acquired treatable immunodeficiency.
3) IVIg or SCIg is the mainstay of treatment for patients with antibody deficiency.
4) Haemopoietic stem cell transplantation remains the main curative option for children with SCID.
5) High-dose IVIg is widely used as a therapeutic immunomodulator in a range of autoimmune diseases.

16% SCIg preparations, patients with auto-immune neuropathies are able to self-treat themselves with volumes of 200–220 mL weekly (32–35.2 g). The recent licencing of a 20% SCIg preparation and the future development of hyaluronidase-based preparations will enable the delivery of even higher doses and drive expansion of the immunomodulatory use of SCIg.

References

1 Caligaris-Cappio F. How immunology is reshaping clinical disciplines: the example of haematology. Lancet 2001;**358**:49–55.

2 Herz-Al W, Bousfiha A, Casanova JL et al. Primary immunodeficiency diseases: an update on the classification from the International Union of Immunological Societies Expert Committee for Primary Immunodeficiency. Front Immunol 2014;**5**:162.

3 Buchbinder D, Nadeau K, Nugent D. Monozygotic twin pair showing discordant phenotype for X-linked thrombocytopenia and Wiskott–Aldrich syndrome: a role for epigenetics? J Clin Immunol 2011;**31**:773–7.

4 Maggina P, Gennery A. Classification of primary immunodeficiencies; need for a revised approach? J Allergy Clin Immunol 2012;**131**:292–4.

5 Cunningham-Rundles C. How I treat common variable immune deficiency. Blood 2010;**116**:7–15.

6 Jolles S, Tyrer M, Johnston M, Webster D. Long term recovery of IgG and IgM production during HIV infection in common variable immunodeficiency. J Clin Pathol 2001;**54**:713–15.

7 Lucas M, Lee M, Lortan J et al. Infection outcomes in patients with common variable immunodeficiency disorders: relationship to immunoglobulin therapy over 22 years. J Allergy Clin Immunol 2010;**125**:1354–60.

8 Winkelstein JA, Marino MC, Lederman HM et al. X-linked agammaglobulinemia: report on a United States registry of 201 patients. Medicine (Baltimore) 2006;**85**:193–202.

9 Ferrari S, Zuntini R, Lougaris V et al. Molecular analysis of the pre-BCR complex in a large cohort of patients affected by autosomal recessive agammaglobulinaemia. Genes Immunity 2007;**8**:325–33.

10 Van der Burg M, Gennery AR. The expanding clinical and immunological spectrum of severe combined immunodeficiency. Eur J Paediatr 2011;**170**:561–71.

11 Mcwilliams LM, Railey MD, Buckley RH. Positive family history, low absolute lymphocyte count and absent thymic shadow: diagnostic clues for all molecular forms of severe combined immunodeficiency (SCID). J Allergy Clin Immunol Pract 2015;**3**:585–91.

12 Pai SY, Logan BR, Griffith LM et al. Transplantation outcomes for severe combined immunodeficiency, 2000–2009. N Engl J Med 2014;**371**:434–46.

13 Puck JM. Laboratory technology for population-based screening for severe combined immunodeficiency in neonates: the winner is T cell receptor excision circles. J Allergy Clin Immunol 2012;**129**:607–16.

14 Howe SJ, Mansour MR, Schwarzwaelder K et al. Insertional mutagenesis with acquired somatic mutations causes leukaemogenesis following gene therapy of SCID-X1 patients. J Clin Invest 2008;**118**:3143–50.

15 Hacein-Bey Abina S, Paj S, Gaspar H et al. A modified γ-retrovirus vector for X-linked severe combined immunodeficiency. N Engl J Med 2014;**371** 1407–17.

16 Hanson IC, Shearer WT. Ruling out HIV infection when testing for severe combined immunodeficiencies and other T cell defects. J Allergy Clin Immunol 2012;**129**:875–6.

17 Orange JS, Grossman WJ, Navickis RJ et al. Impact of trough IgG on pneumonia incidence in primary immunodeficiency: a meta-analysis of clinical studies. Clin Immunol 2010;**137**:21–30.

18 Anthony RM, Ravetch JV. A novel role for the IgG Fc glycan: the anti-inflammatory activity of sialylated IgG Fcs. J Clin Immunol 2010;**30**:S9–S14.

19 Von Gunten S, Shoenfeld Y, Blank M et al. IVIG pluripotency and the concept of Fc-sialylation: challenges to the scientist. Nature Rev Immunol 2014;**14**:349.

20 Raanani P, Gaffer-Gvili A, Paul M et al. Immunoglobulin prophylaxis in chronic lymphocytic leukaemia and multiple myeloma: systematic review and meta-analysis. Leuk Lymphoma 2009;**50**:764–72.

21 Dhalla F, Lucas M, Schuh A et al. Antibody deficiency secondary to chronic lymphocytic leukaemia: should patients be treated with prophylactic replacement immunoglobulin? J Clin Immunol 2014;**34**:277–82.

22 Rachid R, Bonilla FA. The role of anti-IgA antibodies in causing adverse reactions to gamma-globulin infusion in immunodeficient patients: a comprehensive review of the literature. J Allergy Clin Immunol 2012;**129**:628–34.

23 Van der Heijden J, Geissler J, van Mirre E et al. A novel splice variant of FcγRIIa: a risk factor for anaphylaxis in patients with hypogammaglobulinaemia. J Allergy Clin Immunol 2013;**131**:1408–16.

24 Bentley P, Rosso M, Sadnicka A et al. Intravenous immunoglobulin increases plasma viscosity without parallel rise in blood pressure. J Clin Pharm Ther 2012;**37**:286–90.

25 Desborough M, Miller J, Thorpe SJ et al. Intravenous immunoglobulin-induced haemolysis: a case report and review of the literature. Transfus Med 2014;**24**:219–26.

26 Misbah SA. Rituximab-induced accelerated cryoprecipitation in HCV-associated mixed cryoglobulinaemia has parallels with intravenous immunoglobulin-induced immune complex deposition in mixed cryoglobulinaemia. Arthritis Rheum 2010;**62**:3122.

27 Schiff RI. Transmission of viral infections through intravenous immunoglobulin. N Engl J Med 1994;**15**:1649–50.

28 Misbah SA. Should therapeutic immunoglobulin be considered a generic product? An evidence-based approach. J Allergy Clin Immunol Pract 2013;**1**:567–72.

29 Chapel HM, Spickett GP, Ericson D, Engl W, Eibl MM, Bjorkander J. The comparison of the efficacy and safety of intravenous versus subcutaneous immunoglobulin replacement therapy. J Clin Immunol 2000;**20**:94–100.

30 Misbah SA, Baumann A, Fazio R et al. A smooth transition protocol for patients with multifocal motor neuropathy going from intravenous to subcutaneous immunoglobulin therapy: an open label proof-of-concept study. J Peripheral Nerv Syst 2011;**16**:92–7.

31 Rajabally YA. Subcutaneous immunoglobulin therapy for inflammatory neuropathy:current evidence base and future prospects. J Neurol Neurosurg Psychiatry 2014;**85**:631–7.

Further Reading

Castigli E, Geha RS. Molecular basis of common variable immunodeficiency. J Allergy Clin Immunol 2006;**117**:740–6.

Cavazzano-Calvo M, Fischer A. Gene therapy for severe combined immunodeficiency: are we there yet? J Clin Invest 2007;**117**:1456–65.

Eibel H, Salzer U, Warnatz K. Common variable immunodeficiency at the end of a prospering decade: towards novel gene defects and beyond. Curr Opin Allergy Clin Immunol 2010;**10**:526–33.

Jolles S, Sewell WAC, Misbah SA. Clinical uses of intravenous immunoglobulin. Clin Exp Immunol 2005;**142**:1–11.

Misbah S, Kuijpers T, van der Heijden J et al. Bringing immunoglobulin knowledge up to date: how should we treat today? Clin Exp Immunol 2011;**166**:16–25.

33 Transfusing Neonates and Infants

Ronald G. Strauss

Department of Pathology and Pediatrics, University of Iowa College of Medicine, Iowa City, USA; LifeSource/ITxM, Chicago, USA

Introduction

It is frequently stated that children are not small adults, when considering either normal physiology or the pathophysiology of disease. This concept can be extended to state that neonates and infants are not small children, particularly when considering the physiology of very low-birthweight (VLBW), premature infants and the pathological mechanisms of the diseases/disorders they experience (especially during the neonatal period).

The majority of preterm neonates and/or infants, particularly those with birthweight below 1.0 kg (VLBW) receive transfusions; red cells most frequently, followed closely by platelets and then plasma and cryoprecipitate, with the last two being given only occasionally. Because of the high frequency of transfusions to these tiny patients (>80% of VLBW infants in most studies) and the many controversial/variable aspects of neonatal/infant transfusion management, this chapter will focus on neonates and infants. Contrary to the adage that children are not small adults, when transfusions of red cells, platelets or plasma are indicated by clinical circumstances, children beyond the age of infancy are transfused according to guidelines that are similar to those for adults, although doses/quantities of blood components transfused must be adjusted to body size.

For the reasons discussed above, plus limitations of space, transfusions of red cells and platelets, but not plasma or cryoprecipitate, given to neonates and infants will be critically reviewed in this chapter. Transfusions prescribed for children older than infants will not be discussed further in this chapter.

Many aspects of haematopoietic physiology are unique to fetuses and, consequently, are unique in preterm infants, who in some respects, are 'fetuses *ex utero*' with physiological switches/adaptations to 'extrauterine life' that cannot occur at the moment of birth. As discussed in later sections of this chapter, one of the consequences is a diminished capacity of the neonate to produce red cells, platelets and neutrophils when stressed with life-threatening illnesses encountered after preterm birth such as sepsis, severe pulmonary dysfunction, necrotising enterocolitis and immune cytopenias. Similarly, hepatic function is immature, resulting in low levels of both procoagulant and anticoagulant plasma proteins. Transfusions play a major role in the management of many medical and surgical problems complicating prematurity that are associated with phlebotomy blood losses, bleeding, haemolysis and consumptive coagulopathy.

In summary, preterm infants begin life with quantities of blood cells and haemostatic proteins that are barely adequate. Additionally, these infants have a diminished ability to increase production adequately to compensate for the haematological problems they encounter and to fulfil physiological needs posed by rapid

Practical Transfusion Medicine, Fifth Edition. Edited by Michael F. Murphy, David J. Roberts and Mark H. Yazer.
© 2017 John Wiley & Sons Ltd. Published 2017 by John Wiley & Sons Ltd.

growth and expanding blood volume. These circumstances lead to the need for blood component transfusions which, although prescribed by guidelines that in some respects are quite controversial and vary among physicians, truly are life saving.

Red Cell Transfusions for the Anaemia of Prematurity

Physiology and Pathophysiology

Preterm infants, especially those with birthweight less than 1.0 kg and with respiratory distress, are often given numerous red cell transfusions early in life because of several interacting factors. Neonates delivered before 28 weeks of gestation (birthweight <1.0 kg) are born before the bulk of iron transport from mother to fetus has occurred via the placenta and before the onset of marked erythropoietic activity of fetal marrow during the third trimester. Hence, preterm infants of very low birthweight enter extrauterine life with low iron stores and a small circulating volume/mass of red cells. Severe respiratory disease can lead to repeated blood sampling for laboratory studies and, consequently, to replacement red cell transfusions. As a final factor, preterm infants rely primarily on hepatic production of erythropoietin (EPO), as the physiological 'switch' to renal EPO has not occurred, and they are unable to mount an effective EPO response to decreasing numbers of red cells, thus contributing to the diminished ability to compensate for anaemia and resulting in the need for red cell transfusions.

During the first weeks of life, all infants (term and preterm) experience a decline in the number of circulating red cells caused by normal physiological factors. In sick preterm infants, phlebotomy blood losses also contribute to this decline. In healthy term infants, the nadir blood haemoglobin (Hb) concentration rarely decreases below 9 g/dL (mean 11–12 g/dL) at an age of approximately 10–12 weeks. Because this postnatal decrease in Hb is universal and is well

tolerated by term infants, it is commonly called the *physiological anaemia of infancy*. In preterm infants, this decline occurs at an earlier age and is more pronounced in severity. The mean Hb decreases to approximately 8 g/dL in infants of 1.0–1.5 kg birthweight and to 7 g/dL in infants weighing less than 1.0 kg. In preterm infants, this marked decline in Hb frequently is exacerbated by phlebotomy blood losses and may be associated with symptomatic anaemia that necessitates red cell transfusions, making the *anaemia of prematurity* unacceptable as a 'purely physiological' condition.

Physiological factors that influence erythropoiesis and the biological characteristics of EPO are critical in the pathogenesis of the anaemia of prematurity. Growth is extremely rapid during the first weeks of life, and red cell production by neonatal marrow must increase commensurately to avoid a decreasing haematocrit caused by an insufficient number of circulating red cells being diluted within the expanding blood volume. It is widely accepted that the circulating life span of neonatal red cells in the bloodstream is shorter than that of adult red cells. This shorter survival of neonatal red cells, likely, is an artefact because studies of transfused autologous red cells labelled with biotin or radioactive chromium underestimate red cell survival in the infant's bloodstream for technical reasons. However, in healthy adults – when body size is stable so that blood and red cell volumes are constant (i.e. not increasing with growing body size and commensurate increase in erythropoiesis), when no transfusions are given and when large volumes of blood are not being taken for laboratory studies – the gradual disappearance of transfused labelled red cells, caused by the expected dilution with red cells produced endogenously by the marrow, accurately reflects red cell survival in the bloodstream. In contrast, the confounding factors of rapid growth, red cell transfusions and phlebotomy blood losses present in infants introduce error into the calculations performed when red cell survival is determined by the disappearance of labelled red cells.

A key clinical factor is the need for repeated blood sampling to monitor the condition of critically ill neonates. Small preterm infants are the most critically ill, require the most frequent blood sampling and suffer the greatest proportional loss of red cells because their circulating red cell volumes are smallest. In the past, the mean volume of blood removed for sampling has been reported to range from 0.8 to 3.1 mL/kg/day during the first few weeks of life for preterm infants requiring intensive care. Promising 'in-line' devices that withdraw blood, measure multiple analytes and then reinfuse the sampled blood have been reported [1] to decrease the need for red cell transfusions. However, until these devices are proven more extensively to be practical, effective and safe, replacement of blood losses from phlebotomy will remain a vital factor responsible for transfusions given to critically ill neonates during the first weeks of life.

A key reason why the nadir Hb concentrations of preterm infants are lower than those of term infants is that preterm infants have a relatively diminished EPO plasma level in response to anaemia. Although anaemia provokes EPO production in premature infants, the plasma levels achieved in anaemic infants, at any given haematocrit, are lower than those observed in comparably anaemic older persons. Erythroid progenitor cells of preterm infants are quite responsive to EPO *in vitro*, a finding suggesting that inadequate production of EPO (not marrow unresponsiveness) is the major cause of physiological anaemia.

The mechanisms responsible for the diminished EPO output by preterm neonates are only partially defined and, likely, are multiple. One mechanism is that the primary site of EPO production in preterm infants is in the liver, rather than kidneys [2]. This dependency on hepatic EPO is important because the liver is less sensitive to anaemia and tissue hypoxia, resulting in a relatively sluggish EPO response to the decreasing haematocrit. The timing of the switch from the liver to kidneys is set at conception and is not accelerated by preterm birth. Viewed from a teleological perspective,

decreased hepatic production of EPO under *in utero* conditions of tissue hypoxia may be an advantage for the fetus. If this were not the case, normal levels of fetal hypoxia *in utero* could trigger high levels of EPO and produce erythrocytosis and consequent hyperviscosity. Following birth, however, diminished EPO responsiveness to tissue hypoxia is disadvantageous and leads to anaemia because it impairs compensation for low haematocrit levels caused by rapid growth and red cell losses caused by phlebotomy, clinical bleeding, haemolysis, etc.

Diminished EPO production cannot entirely explain low plasma EPO levels in preterm infants, because extraordinarily high plasma levels of EPO have been reported in some fetuses and infants. Moreover, macrophages from human cord blood produce normal quantities of EPO messenger RNA and protein [3]. Thus, additional mechanisms contribute to diminished EPO plasma levels, such as metabolism (clearance) as well as production. Data in human infants [4] have demonstrated low plasma EPO levels resulting from increased plasma clearance, increased volume of distribution, more rapid fractional elimination and shorter mean plasma residence times than comparative values in adults. Thus, accelerated catabolism accentuates the problem of diminished EPO production, so that the low plasma EPO levels are a combined effect of decreased synthesis plus increased metabolism.

Red Cell Transfusion Practices

Red cell transfusions are given to maintain the haematocrit at a level judged best for the clinical condition of the infant [5]. General guidelines acceptable to most neonatologists are listed in Box 33.1, acknowledging that many aspects of neonatal red cell transfusion therapy are controversial and vary among physicians. This lack of consistency stems from incomplete knowledge of the cellular and molecular biology of erythropoiesis during the perinatal period, of the pathophysiological effects of neonatal anaemia and of the infant's physiological response to

---

Box 33.1   Guidelines for small-volume (15 mL/kg) red cell transfusions for neonates/infants.

- Maintain >34% haematocrit for *severe* cardiopulmonary disease
- Maintain >30% haematocrit for *moderate* cardiopulmonary disease
- Maintain >30% haematocrit during *major* surgery
- Maintain >22% haematocrit for infants with *symptomatic* anaemia, especially with:
  Unexplained breathing disorders
  Unexplained tachycardia
  Unexplained poor growth

Words in italics must be defined locally. For example, 'severe' pulmonary disease may be defined as requiring mechanical ventilation with >0.35 FiO_2 and 'moderate' as less intensive assisted ventilation.

---

red cell transfusions. In some instances, the value of red cell transfusions is clear (e.g. to manage anaemia that has caused congestive heart failure), but in others it is not (e.g. to correct irregular patterns of heart or respiratory rates).

An important controversy that is still unresolved is the wisdom – or lack thereof – of prescribing red cell transfusions for neonates using restrictive guidelines (i.e. low pre-transfusion haematocrit values) versus liberal guidelines (i.e. conventional, relatively high pre-transfusion haematocrit values). This issue is currently being addressed by an ongoing multicentre randomised clinical trial (Transfusion of Prematures (TOP) Trial sponsored by the National Institutes of Health NHLBI and NICHD) which was prompted by two earlier randomised controlled trials with seemingly contrary results [6,7].

In both trials, preterm infants were randomly assigned to receive small-volume red cell transfusions per either restrictive or liberal guidelines, based on a combination of the pre-transfusion haematocrit or Hb, age of the neonate and clinical condition at the time each transfusion was given. Both studies found that neonates in the restrictive transfusion group received fewer transfusions, without an increase in mortality or in morbidity based on several clinical outcomes. However, one critical discrepancy was present. Bell et al [6] found increases in apnoea, intra-ventricular bleeding and brain leukomalacia in infants transfused per restrictive guidelines, whereas Kirpalani et al [7] found no differences

between infants in the restrictive versus liberal groups. However, rates of serious outcomes were fairly high in both groups of the Kirpalani study, perhaps a result of the extreme prematurity of the study infants. Because neonates in the liberal transfusion group in the Bell et al study had substantially higher haematocrit/Hb levels than neonates in the liberal group of Kirpalani et al (average haematocrit of 6% or Hb of 2 g/dL higher), the initial speculation was that the higher haematocrit levels in some way protected the brain of liberally transfused infants in the Bell et al study.

However, the initial conclusions were contradicted by long-term observations. Neurological follow-up studies for the Bell et al trial (done years later when the subjects were approximately 11 years old) surprisingly revealed that intracranial volumes were substantially smaller in the transfused infants in the liberal arm than in those in the restrictive arm. In addition, the children in the liberal arm were found to perform more poorly than those in the restrictive arm on measures of fluency, visual memory and reading [8]. In the multicentre Kirpalani et al study, long-term follow-up at age approximately 18 months revealed no statistically significant difference in combined death or severe adverse neurodevelopmental outcomes, supporting their initial conclusions. However, to add to the confusion, in a *post hoc* analysis there was a significant difference favouring the liberal transfusion strategy. Thus, it is unclear whether a relatively high pre-transfusion Hb is 'neuro-protective' or 'neurodamaging'. To this end, the TOP Trial commenced in 2013 and will randomly assign 1824 VLBW (<1000 g) infants to a liberal or restrictive red cell transfusion protocol. The pre-transfusion Hb thresholds will be based on the presence of respiratory support and postnatal age, with the primary outcome of death or significant neurodevelopmental impairment in survivors.

Until more definitive data are available, the rationale underlying the recommendations for red cell transfusions given to neonates/infants in Box 33.1 are as follows.

Maintain Haematocrit >34% for Severe Cardiopulmonary Disease

In neonates with severe respiratory disease, such as those requiring high volumes of oxygen with ventilator support, it is customary to maintain the haematocrit at normal levels of approximately 35% (Hb at 12–13 g/dL), particularly when blood is being drawn frequently for testing. This practice is based on the belief that transfused donor red cells, containing adult Hb with its superior interaction with 2,3-diphosphoglycerate (2,3-DPG), will provide optimal oxygen delivery throughout the period of diminished pulmonary function. Consistent with this rationale for ensuring optimal oxygen delivery in neonates with pulmonary failure, it seems logical to maintain a similar haematocrit in infants with congenital heart disease that is severe enough to cause cyanosis and/or congestive heart failure.

Maintain Haematocrit >30% for Moderate Cardiopulmonary Disease

Following similar logic, it seems reasonable to maintain the haematocrit above 30% for moderate cardiopulmonary disease in neonates/infants.

Maintain Haematocrit >30% During Major Surgery

Definitive studies are not available to establish the optimal haematocrit for neonates during major surgery. However, it seems reasonable to maintain the haematocrit >30% because of the limited ability of the neonate's heart, lungs and vasculature to compensate for anaemia. Additional factors include the inferior off-loading of oxygen to tissues by the infant's own red cells because of the diminished interaction between fetal Hb and 2,3-DPG plus the developmental impairment of neonatal pulmonary, renal, hepatic and neurological function. Because this transfusion guideline is simply a recommendation – not a firm indication – it should be applied with flexibility to individual infants facing surgical procedures of varying complexity (i.e. minor surgery may be judged not to require a haematocrit >30%). The amount of anticipated blood loss must be strongly considered in preoperative transfusion decisions; with a likelihood of large blood loss, some physicians might prefer the preoperative haematocrit to be relatively high. Following surgery, red cell transfusions are needed only if significant bleeding and/or symptomatic anaemia occurs.

Maintain Haematocrit >22% for Infants with Symptomatic Anaemia

Clinical recommendations for red cell transfusions in preterm infants who are not critically ill but, nonetheless, develop moderate anaemia (haematocrit <22% or Hb <7.5 g/dL) are extremely variable. In general, infants who are clinically stable with modest anaemia do not require red cell transfusions, unless they exhibit significant clinical problems that are ascribed to the presence of anaemia or are predicted to be corrected by donor red cells. As an example, proponents of red cell transfusions to treat disturbances of cardiopulmonary rhythms believe that a low blood level of red cells contributes to tachypnoea, dyspnoea, apnoea and tachycardia or bradycardia because of decreased oxygen delivery to the respiratory centre of the brain. If true, it follows that red cell transfusions might decrease the number of apnoeic spells by improving oxygen delivery to the central nervous system. However, results of clinical studies have been contradictory.

Another controversial clinical indication for red cell transfusions is to maintain a reasonable haematocrit level as treatment for unexplained growth failure. Some neonatologists consider poor weight gain to be an indication for transfusion, particularly if the haematocrit is <22% and if other signs of distress are evident (e.g. tachycardia, respiratory difficulty, weak suck and cry and diminished activity). In this setting, growth failure has been ascribed to the increase in metabolic expenditure required to support the work of laboured breathing. However, results of clinical studies have not documented efficacy of red cell transfusions for this purpose. Similarly, there are no data to justify maintaining any predetermined haematocrit level by prophylactic, small-volume red cell transfusions in stable, growing infants who seem to be otherwise healthy.

In practice, the decision of whether to transfuse is based on the desire to maintain the haematocrit concentration at a level judged to be most beneficial for the infant's clinical condition. Investigators who believe this 'clinical' approach is too imprecise have suggested the use of 'physiological' criteria such as red cell mass, available oxygen, mixed venous oxygen saturation, measurements of oxygen delivery and utilisation, blood/red cell flow through the microcirculation and levels of tissue oxygenation to develop guidelines for transfusion decisions. These promising but technically demanding methods have been useful in research settings, but at present are too difficult to apply in the day-to-day practice of neonatology.

Red Cell Products to Transfuse

Most transfusions are given to preterm infants as small-volume transfusions (10–15 mL/kg body-weight) of red cells in extended-storage media (additive solution AS-1, AS-3, AS-5) at a haematocrit of approximately 55–60% (Table 33.1), with aliquots often taken from a single dedicated unit throughout the 42 days of storage. Unfortunately, some neonatologists persist in preferring red cells stored for shorter periods of time in citrate-phosphate-dextrose-adenine (CPDA) solution at a haematocrit of approximately

Table 33.1 Formulation of red blood cell anticoagulant-preservative solutions.

Constituent	CPDA	AS-1	AS-3	AS-5
Volume (mL)	63*	100[†]	100[†]	100[†]
Sodium chloride (mg)	None	900	410	877
Dextrose (mg)	2010	2200	1100	900
Adenine (mg)	17.3	27	30	30
Mannitol (mg)	None	750	None	525
Trisodium citrate (mg)	1660	None	588	None
Citric acid (mg)	206	None	42	None
Sodium phosphate (monobasic) (mg)	140	None	276	None

* Approximately 450 mL of donor blood is drawn into 63 mL of CPDA solution. One red cell unit (haematocrit ~70%) is prepared by means of centrifugation and removal of most plasma. Results of calculations will be slightly different if 500 mL of donor blood is drawn.

[†] When additive solution AS-1 or AS-5 is used, 450 mL of donor blood is first drawn into 63 mL of CPD, which is identical to CPDA except it contains 1610 mg dextrose per 63 mL and has no adenine. When AS-3 is used, donor blood is drawn into CP2D, which is identical to CPD except it contains double the amount of dextrose. After centrifugation and removal of nearly all plasma, the cells are resuspended in 100 mL of the additive solution (AS-1, AS-3 or AS-5) at a haematocrit of approximately 55–60%.

70%; in the author's view, this is a misguided practice for several reasons.

- The superiority of CPDA solution over extended-storage/additive solution has not been shown by clinical trials and, as discussed later in this chapter, randomised clinical trials report equivalence.
- Because the routine blood banking practice is to collect/store red cells in extended-storage/additive solutions, the insistence on transfusing CPDA red cell units to infants creates inventory management problems for both blood suppliers and hospital transfusion services.
- The need to transfuse one red cell product to some patients and another red cell product to others increases the chance of transfusion errors. Because of the small quantity of extracellular fluid (storage solution) infused very slowly with small-volume transfusions, the type of anticoagulant-preservative solution used and the duration of storage pose no risk for premature infants [9,10].

Acceptance of red cells stored for up to 42 days in extended-storage/additive solutions has changed transfusion practices for VLBW infants. The traditional use of relatively fresh red cells (<7 days of storage) has been replaced in many centres by transfusing aliquots of red cells from a dedicated unit of red cells stored for up to 42 days in an effort to diminish the high donor exposure rates among infants who undergo numerous transfusions. Neonatologists who object to prescribing stored red cells and insist on transfusing fresh red cells generally express the following four concerns:

- the increase in the level of potassium in the plasma (i.e. supernatant fluid)
- the decrease in the level of 2,3-DPG
- the possible risks of additives such as mannitol and the relatively large amounts of glucose (dextrose) and phosphate present in extended-storage/additive solutions
- the changes in red cell shape and deformability that may lead to poor flow through the microvasculature.

As recently reviewed [11], none of these concerns have, in fact, materialised in clinical practice for even the smallest infants, when assessed by laboratory (pre- versus post-transfusion changes in assay results) and clinical outcomes assessed by both short-term and long-term studies, including a multicentre randomised clinical trial involving 377 premature infants, in which transfusion of fresh red cell units stored for 5.1 ± 2.0 days (mean $\pm$ SD) did not improve multiple clinical outcomes when compared to red cell units stored for 14.6 ± 8.3 days.

In addition to the results of randomised clinical trials that established the short-term and relatively long-term efficacy and safety of stored red cells for small-volume transfusions given to neonates and infants, the post-transfusion intravascular circulating kinetics of transfused 'stored/aged' donor red cells has been reported to be nearly identical to 'fresh' donor red cells. The intravascular recovery was normal 24 hours after transfusion ('fresh' = 98.6% versus 'stored/aged' = 96.9%) and long-term survival (short storage = 81.2% versus long storage = 87.5%), measured in human infants using biotinylated red cells [11].

In conclusion, because the risks of multiple donor exposure can be eliminated by transfusing red cells from dedicated, stored red cell units and because increased risks of transfusing stored versus fresh red cells have not been demonstrated, it seems prudent to transfuse stored red cells for small-volume transfusions.

Prevention of Transfusion-Transmitted Cytomegalovirus (TTCMV)

Leucocyte reduction, when performed according to the manufacturer's instructions by the blood supplier, is the optimal way to prevent TTCMV. The combined 'belt-and-suspenders' approach (i.e. transfusing red cell units that are known to be both leucocyte-reduced and seronegative for antibody to CMV) likewise effectively prevents TTCMV, but has the disadvantage of delaying transfusions when sero/antibody-negative units are not readily available and significantly increases the costs, compared to using leucocyte reduction alone [12].

Irradiated Red Cell Units

Neonates, particularly those who are extremely preterm, are believed by many to be at risk of transfusion-associated graft-versus-host disease (TA-GVHD). Although the extent of this risk is controversial [12], in most hospitals caring for preterm neonates/infants, a blanket policy exists to transfuse irradiated cellular blood components to all infants to a specified age.

Platelet Transfusions for the Thrombocytopenia of Prematurity

Physiology and Pathophysiology

The physiology underlying fetal and neonatal thrombopoiesis and blood platelet counts, the pathophysiology/mechanisms of thrombocytopenia and the guidelines for platelet transfusion practices in neonates and infants differ in many respects from those present in older children, with older children resembling adults. Accordingly, neonates and infants will be discussed here, with infants being defined as up to age two years or a bodyweight of 15 kg or about 30 pounds.

As reviewed by Ferrer-Marin et al [13], substantial differences exist between fetal/neonatal thrombopoiesis and that of adults. Briefly, thrombopoietin (TPO) plasma levels are higher in healthy neonates versus healthy adults. Megakaryocyte progenitors of neonates are more sensitive to TPO, have higher proliferative potential and give rise to larger megakaryocyte colonies than do adult platelet progenitors, when cultured *in vitro*. Fetal/neonatal megakaryocytes are smaller in size and have lower ploidy than do their adult counterparts – an important factor because small megakaryocytes of low ploidy produce fewer platelets than larger megakaryocytes of higher ploidy. Presumably, this allows the expanding bone marrow of the growing fetus and neonate to generate sufficient numbers of megakaryocytes for growth, by the enhanced proliferation of megakaryocyte precursors, while avoiding thrombocytosis during proliferation because of the lower number of platelets produced by each proliferating megakaryocyte.

An important difference is that older children and adults respond to situations of increased platelet demand by first increasing megakaryocyte size and ploidy, which is followed in 3–5 days by increased megakaryocyte number, all driven by TPO. In contrast, thrombocytopenic neonates increase their megakaryocyte numbers but not the size of their megakaryocytes. Moreover, although cytoplasmic maturation is achieved in neonatal megakaryocytes per TPO stimulation, increases in ploidy are relatively diminished, and actually appear to be inhibited by TPO, resulting in large numbers of small megakaryocytes that are cytoplasmically mature but with low ploidy [13].

It is generally accepted that human neonates have blood platelet counts within the same normal range as older children and adults (i.e. $150–450 \times 10^9$/L). However, recent data suggest a lower normal limit of 120×10^9/L for VLBW neonates during the first days following birth. Using the conventional lower limit of 150×10^9/L for normal values, fewer than 1% of term neonates experience thrombocytopenia, whereas 20–35% of preterm neonates admitted to a neonatal intensive care unit (NICU) will have blood platelet counts less than 150×10^9/L. When only a subset of VLBW neonates (<1000 g at delivery) was considered, 73% had one or more platelet counts below 150×10^9/L and platelet transfusions were given to 62% of thrombocytopenic neonates [14]. Among all thrombocytopenic preterm neonates, 25–38% will have blood platelet counts less than 50×10^9/L (i.e. severe thrombocytopenia) and usually will receive platelet transfusions. Thus, between 2% and 8% of all preterm neonates admitted to an NICU will receive a platelet transfusion, with VLBW neonates given platelet transfusions much more frequently (45% overall, whether or not documented to be thrombocytopenic, and 62% when thrombocytopenic [14]).

Platelet Transfusion Practices

Platelet transfusion practices vary greatly. Although it has not been possible to precisely or consistently correlate major bleeding in neonates with either the severity of thrombocytopenia or the number of platelet transfusions given, in one study, blood platelet counts $<100 \times 10^9$/L posed significant clinical risks [15]. Neonates with birthweights less than 1.5 kg and platelet counts $<100 \times 10^9$/L were compared with neonates of similar size who did not have thrombocytopenia. The incidence of intracranial haemorrhage was 78% among thrombocytopenic neonates with birthweight less than 1.5 kg versus 48% for similar neonates without thrombocytopenia, and the extent of haemorrhage and neurological morbidity was greater with thrombocytopenia.

As discussed, one randomised clinical trial has been reported of prophylactic platelet transfusions to prevent intracranial bleeding in preterm neonates [16], and another multicentre trial is in progress in the UK, but to date, no randomised clinical trials of therapeutic platelet transfusions have been reported for bleeding thrombocytopenic neonates. Until more definitive data are published, it seems reasonable to transfuse thrombocytopenic neonates/infants per the guidelines presented in Box 33.2, based on the following rationale.

Maintain >50×10^9/L Platelets for Significant Bleeding

Virtually all clinicians agree with this recommendation, as a minimum threshold, when overt bleeding is present, with the post-transfusion goal being a platelet count >100×10^9/L. Although some may prefer a higher pre-transfusion threshold/'trigger', there are no definitive data to support this preference.

> **Box 33.2 Guidelines for platelet transfusions for neonates/infants to age two years.**
>
> - Maintain >50×10^9/L platelets for *significant* bleeding
> - Maintain >50×10^9/L platelets during *invasive* procedures, with >30×10^9/L post procedure until haemostasis stable
> - Maintain >20×10^9/L prophylactically for *clinically stable neonates/infants*
> - Maintain >30×10^9/L prophylactically for *clinically unstable* neonates/infants
>
> ---
>
> Words in *italics* must be defined locally. For example, consider bleeding site, extent and degree of prematurity and underlying medical condition.

Maintain >50×10^9/L During an Invasive Procedure, With >30×10^9/L Post Procedure Until Haemostasis is Stable

No disagreement exists over using a pre-transfusion platelet count of 50×10^9/L as a minimum transfusion trigger to prevent or treat bleeding immediately before and during an invasive procedure. No definitive data support a preference for a higher pre-transfusion threshold/trigger. There are no definitive data to support maintaining a platelet count of >50×10^9/L after the invasive procedure is completed, but physicians are reluctant to transfuse platelets per the usual prophylactic pre-transfusion count of 20×10^9/L. Accordingly, although definitive data do not support it, it seems reasonable to maintain the platelet count >30×10^9/L for a few days post procedure to help stabilise haemostasis/clotting

Maintain >20×10^9/L Platelets Prophylactically If Clinically Stable and >30×10^9/L If Clinically Unstable

The vast majority of platelet transfusions are given prophylactically to clinically stable neonates/infants per the traditional pre-transfusion threshold of 20×10^9/L. There are no definitive data to support the lower value of 10×10^9/L commonly used in adults. However, platelet transfusions are given to neonates at platelet counts >50×10^9/L or even >100×10^9/L by some physicians with the intent of reducing either the threat of, or the worsening of, intracranial haemorrhage in clinically unstable preterm neonates. No data exist to establish the efficacy of platelet transfusions at these relatively high platelet levels. Perhaps surprisingly, most preterm neonates with intracranial haemorrhages (for whom blood platelet counts are available) have normal platelet counts at the time actual bleeding occurs. Severe thrombocytopenia occurs most commonly among sick infants who, because of illness, may also receive medications (e.g. indomethacin, nitric oxide and antibiotics) that are well known to impair platelet function by *in vitro* tests and, by logical extension, can (at least theoretically) compromise the function of their already diminished number of platelets.

Because these factors are more pronounced in extremely preterm infants, who are clinically unstable and often receiving medications, some neonatologists favour prophylactic platelet transfusions whenever the platelet count decreases to <50×10^9/L, or even to <100×10 9/L, in critically ill infants rather than the 20×10^9/L threshold. However logical the rationale for these liberal transfusion practices, convincing data from definitive randomised clinical trials either do not exist or are inconsistent.

Platelet Products to Transfuse

When a platelet transfusion is prescribed for a thrombocytopenic neonate or infant, within the first two years of life, the usual goal is to increase the blood platelet count by 50 to 100×10^9/L above the pre-transfusion count (e.g. from 20×10^9/L before transfusion to between 70 and 120×10^9/L post-transfusion). This increment can be achieved by transfusing 10 mL/kg (infant bodyweight) of an *unmodified* platelet unit (i.e. either a platelet concentrate prepared from a whole blood unit or a platelet unit prepared by plateletpheresis collection that has not been

volume reduced by an additional centrifugation step) [17]. Routinely reducing the volume of platelet concentrates to increase the number of platelets per millilitre by means of additional centrifugation and resuspension steps is both unnecessary and unwise.

The volume of platelet concentrate to be transfused is withdrawn from the primary platelet unit into a syringe for infusion. As discussed in the red cell section, leucocyte reduction, as performed in the blood centre/transfusion laboratory to ensure adequate leucocyte removal, is all that is needed to prevent CMV transmission. Superior efficacy has never been shown for the well-intended 'belt-and-suspenders' approach of leucocyte reduction of units obtained from donors seronegative for antibodies against CMV. Leucocyte reduction is known not to prevent TA-GVHD and irradiation is required.

Both CMV and TA-GVHD are prevented by the FDA-approved INTERCEPT system for plasma and platelet preparations, and consideration can be given to omitting leucocyte reduction and irradiation done for these purposes. As with all blood products, filtration through a standard 150–180 micron blood filter is needed at the time of transfusion. The rate of infusion is as rapid as volume considerations and the infant's condition permit – preferably within one hour or so. Based on *in vitro* studies, the quality of platelets is maintained for at least six hours in syringes while awaiting and during transfusion.

In the selection of platelet units for transfusion, it is highly desirable that the neonate/infant and the platelet donor be ABO blood group identical (i.e. O to O, A to A etc.). A single 'out of group' platelet transfusion is only rarely problematic, but it is important to minimise repeated transfusions of group O platelets to group A, B or AB recipients because large quantities of passive anti-A or anti-B in the plasma can lead to haemolysis donation from ABO donors who are incompatible because of the presence of A or B antibodies.

KEY POINTS

1) Preterm infants with birthweight >2000 g and term infants who do not have an underlying haematological disease rarely need blood component transfusions. In contrast, the vast majority of VLBW preterm infants (<1000 g birthweight) are given red cells and/or platelet transfusions to treat the 'developmental disorders' of the anaemia of prematurity and the thrombocytopenia of prematurity.

2) The mechanisms underlying the anaemia of prematurity include phlebotomy blood losses for laboratory testing, deficiency of plasma EPO due to combined insufficient production and increased catabolism, and rapid growth and need for commensurate increase of red cell mass. Individual infants may have additional factors such as haemolysis and bleeding due to underlying disorders.

3) The mechanisms underlying the thrombocytopenia of prematurity are due to developmental factors in which the neonatal megakaryocytes proliferate rapidly to populate the expanding marrow of rapidly growing neonates, but do not increase their ploidy sufficiently to efficiently produce platelets. In a sense, the megakaryocytes are working at a very rapid rate under basal conditions and, accordingly, are incapable of further increasing their output when challenged by disorders in which blood platelets are lost or consumed.

4) Because neither the anaemia of prematurity nor the thrombocytopenia of prematurity is widely treated with growth factors (e.g. EPO, TPO or mimetic drugs), the major therapy is allogeneic red cell and platelet transfusions. Transfusion guidelines vary among hospitals/physicians, but the guidelines offered in Boxes 33.1 and 33.2 offer reasonable starting points that can be altered to fit local practices – practices based on conclusions reached via evidence-based discussions among local physicians.

5) Strong evidence supports using red cells stored in extended-storage/additive solutions throughout the 42 days of storage permitted, when prescribed as small-volume (15 mL/kg) transfusions for anaemia of prematurity. The superiority of 'fresh' red cells stored in alternative solutions has not been shown by clinical endpoints reported by randomised clinical trials.

6) Platelet transfusion practices are quite variable, and definitive data from randomised clinical trials are limited. However, considerable information from less definitive reports supports the guidelines offered in Box 33.2. Although there is a temptation to volume-reduce or concentrate platelet-aliquots before transfusion, strong evidence exists to discourage this practice as unnecessary.

7) Nothing has been shown to be superior to leucocyte reduction, as done effectively by the blood supplier, to prevent TTCMV. Leucocyte reduction is known not to completely prevent TA-GVHD, and irradiation is needed. However, the pathogen reduction INTERCEPT system, as approved for platelet preparations and plasma, is efficacious and offers the possibility to supplant leucocyte reduction and irradiation in plasma-rich components.

References

1 Widness JA, Madan A, Grindeanu LA et al. Reduction in red blood cell transfusions among preterm infants: results of a randomized trial with an in-line blood gas and chemistry monitor. Pediatrics 2005;**115**:1299–306.

2 Strauss RG. Controversies in the management of the anemia of prematurity using single-donor RBC transfusions and/or recombinant human erythropoietin. Transfus Med Rev 2006;**20**:34–44.

3 Ohls RK, Li Y, Trautman MS, Christensen RD. Erythropoietin production by macrophages from preterm infants: implications regarding the cause of the anemia in prematurity. Pediatr Res 1994;**35**:169–70.

4 Widness JA, Veng-Pedersen P, Peters C et al. Erythropoietin pharmacokinetics in premature infants: developmental, nonlinearity, and treatment effects. J Appl Physiol 1996;**80**:140–8.

5 Strauss RG. How I transfuse red blood cells and platelets to infants. Transfusion 2008;**48**:209–17.

6 Bell EF, Strauss RG, Widness JA et al. Randomized trial of liberal versus restrictive guidelines for red blood cell transfusions in preterm infants. Pediatrics 2005;**115**:1685–91.

7 Kirpalani H, Whyte RK, Andersen C et al. The Premature Infants in Need of Transfusion (PINT) study: a randomized, controlled trial of a restrictive (low) versus liberal (high) transfusion threshold for extremely low birth weight infants. J Pediatr 2006;**149**:301–7.

8 Nopoulos PC, Conrad AL, Bell EF et al. Long-term outcome of brain structure in premature infants: effects of liberal vs restricted red blood cell transfusions. Arch Pediatr Adolesc Med 2011;**165**:443–50.

9 Strauss RG. Data-driven blood banking practices for neonatal RBC transfusions. Transfusion 2000;**40**:1528–40.

10 Luban NLC, Strauss RG, Hume HA. Commentary on the safety of red blood cells preserved in extended storage media for neonatal transfusions. Transfusion 1991;**31**:229–35.

11 Strauss RG, Mock DM, Widness JA et al. Post-transfusion 24-hour recovery and subsequent survival of allogeneic red blood cells in the bloodstream of newborn infants. Transfusion 2004;**44**:871–6.

12 Wong ECC, Josephson CD, Punzalan RC et al (eds). Overview of special products, in Pediatric Transfusion: A Physician's Handbook, 4th edn. AABB Press, Bethesda, 2015, pp.185–212.

13 Ferrer-Marin F, Liu ZJ, Gutti R et al. Neonatal thrombocytopenia and megakaryocytopoiesis. Semin Hematol 2010;**47**:281–8.

14 Christensen RD, Wiedmeier HE, Stoddard RA et al. Thrombocytopenia among extremely low birth weight neonates: data from a multihospital healthcare system. J Perinatol 2006;**26**:348–53.

15 Andrew M, Castle V, Saigal S et al. Clinical impact of neonatal thrombocytopenia. J Pediatr 1987;**110**:457–64.

16 Andrew M, Vegh P, Caco C et al. A randomized, controlled trial of platelet transfusions in thrombocytopenic premature infants. J Pediatr 1993;**123**:285–91.

17 Strauss RG. Platelet transfusion volume reduction: it can be done, but why do it? Transfusion 2013;**30**:3029–31.

Further Reading

Strauss RG. Platelet transfusion in neonates and children, in Platelet Transfusion Therapy (eds J Sweeney, M Lozano M). AABB Press, Bethesda, 2013, pp.359–69.

Strauss RG. Blood components for infants, in Blood Components: From Bench to Bedside (eds M Blajchman, J Cid, M Lozano). AABB Press, Bethesda, 2011, pp.231–46.

Wong ECC, Josephson CD, Punzalan RC et al (eds). Blood components, in Pediatric Transfusion: A Physician's Handbook, 4th edn. AABB Press, Bethesda, 2015, pp.1–44.

Wong ECC, Josephson CD, Punzalan RC et al (eds). Hemostatis disorders, in Pediatric Transfusion: A Physician's Handbook, 4th edn. AABB Press, Bethesda, 2015, pp.81–134.

Wong ECC, Josephson CD, Punzalan RC et al (eds). Special patient populations, in Pediatric Transfusion: A Physician's Handbook, 4th edn. AABB Press, Bethesda, 2015, pp.213–54.

34 Development of a Patient Blood Management Programme

Jonathan H. Waters

Department of Anesthesiology, Magee Womens Hospital of UPMC, Pittsburgh, USA; Departments of Anesthesiology and Bioengineering, University of Pittsburgh, Pittsburgh, USA; Patient Blood Management program of UPMC; Acute Interventional Pain Program of UPMC

Introduction

The first bloodless medicine and surgery programmes were created in the 1980s to care for Jehovah's Witness patients. Over the next decade, it became apparent that outcomes for patients treated without allogeneic transfusion were equivalent and sometimes better than those of patients cared for with allogeneic transfusion. In conjunction with the creation of these bloodless programmes, studies associating allogeneic transfusion with a number of adverse outcomes were published. Recognising that bloodless medicine and surgery might be good for all patients, the domain of patient blood management (PBM) arose. In essence, a PBM programme recognises that allogeneic transfusion may be life saving but, like any medical therapy, is associated with risks. As such, it should be reserved for circumstances in which a clear benefit will result. This chapter describes a structure for how a hospital might implement a PBM programme. Box 34.1 outlines a six-step strategy for implementing such a programme. The following discussion highlights this strategy.

Step 1: Leverage Computerised Physician Order Entry (CPOE) Systems to Guide Evidence-Based Transfusions [1]

Over the last decade, multiple studies have suggested that more restrictive use of allogeneic blood results provides no difference in patient outcome compared to patients transfused more liberally, but leads to avoidance of certain complications associated with transfusion and does so at a reduced cost of care. These results have been demonstrated in a wide variety of patient populations, including critically ill intensive care [2], paediatric critical care, geriatric patients and patients with orthopaedic hip fracture [3], gastrointestinal bleeding, cardiac surgery [4], septic shock [5] and traumatic brain injury. Authors of a recent meta-analysis [6] concluded that a restrictive strategy significantly reduced cardiac events, re-bleeding, bacterial infections and mortality. Also, these studies suggest that little benefit is gained from transfusing patients with haemoglobin levels above the 7–8 g/dL range.

Practical Transfusion Medicine, Fifth Edition. Edited by Michael F. Murphy, David J. Roberts and Mark H. Yazer.
© 2017 John Wiley & Sons Ltd. Published 2017 by John Wiley & Sons Ltd.

Given that allogeneic transfusion is costly and provides no benefit to aggressive transfusion, a key component of a PBM programme is to drive clinicians to transfuse when evidence shows the

---

Box 34.1 Strategy for developing a PBM programme.

Step 1 Leverage computerised physician order entry (CPOE) systems to guide evidence-based transfusions

Step 2 Reduce all forms of waste related to blood transfusion practices

Step 3 Promote alternative blood transfusion methods and systems

Step 4 Promote anaemia management strategies

Step 5 Limit iatrogenic blood loss

Step 6 Provide blood management education, awareness and auditing for clinician

---

possibility of patient benefit. Another big opportunity to save money and improve outcomes is to reduce variability in transfusion behaviour, given the high variability in transfusion practice. To do this, transfusion review committees have historically retrospectively reviewed cases. Most would consider this retrospective auditing limited in changing behaviour. More recently, the introduction of electronic medical records and CPOE systems has facilitated compliance with accepted standards. These systems allow for prospective monitoring of transfusion orders, as well as facilitating a process for monitoring transfusions that do not meet an institutional standard.

Figure 34.1 shows an order page from an electronic ordering system produced by Cerner (Kansas City, MO) [7]. This page shows historical trends in the patient's haemoglobin levels and requires that a reason for the transfusion be chosen. If the transfusion order does not comply with institutional guidelines, an alert page is prompted, telling the clinician that they are

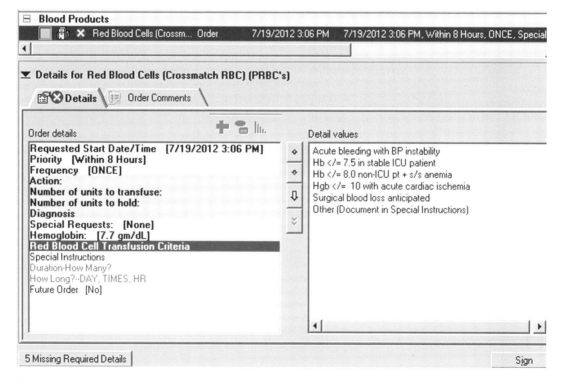

Figure 34.1 Computerised Physician Order Entry Page for Red Blood Cells. (*See insert for colour representation of the figure.*)

deviating from the institutional standard. While the clinician can proceed with the transfusion, it leaves an auditing trail, which allows for the transfusion review committee to generate transfusion variance reports. Figure 34.2 shows such a report. On this report, service lines that are least compliant are identified so that focused education can be performed. Though not shown in Figure 34.2, it also allows for the opportunity to drill down to the specific clinician who is deviating from the institutional guideline.

Step 2: Reduce All Forms of Waste Related to Blood Transfusion Practices

The second step in starting a PBM programme should focus on waste reduction associated with transfusion practice. Waste is rampant throughout healthcare and provides a significant opportunity for cost savings [8]. Blood and blood products are wasted in many ways. The practice of having a patient donate blood for

Facility	Total orders	Total alerts	Alerted orders not placed	Percent orders alerted	Percent alerts heeded
PUH	248	182	23	73.4%	12.6%
SHY	208	138	21	66.3%	15.2%
HAM	198	77	21	38.9%	27.3%
PAS	144	74	10	51.4%	13.5%
SMH	146	59	7	40.4%	11.9%
EAS	73	37	10	50.7%	27.0%
HZN	58	28	4	48.3%	14.3%
MER	275	27	4	9.8%	14.8%
NOR	39	23	0	59.0%	0.0%
MWH	103	20	2	19.4%	10.0%
MCK	62	12	3	19.4%	25.0%
BED	15	10	3	66.7%	30.0%

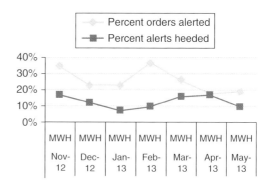

Total orders = Crossmatch Red blood cells, Red blood cells (Crossmatch RBC)
Percent orders alerted = Total alerts / Total orders
Percent alerts heeded = Alerted orders not placed / Total alerts

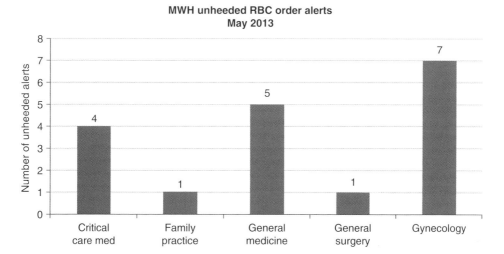

Figure 34.2 Transfusion variance report. (*See insert for colour representation of the figure.*)

themselves weeks prior to a surgical procedure, known as preoperative autologous donation (PAD), is one source of waste. Research using mathematical modelling and meta-analysis suggests that PAD increases instead of prevents transfusion; transfusion occurs at a higher rate than when no PAD has taken place [9]. In addition, at least 50% of these units are never used [10]. Thus, many major medical centres no longer coordinate PAD for surgical patients.

Crossmatch to transfusion (C:T) ratios are another source of waste. Here, crossmatching is performed at a rate significantly greater than actual transfusions. With every crossmatch, cost is incurred. A general standard is that the C:T ratio should be less than 2. Recently, the introduction of the computer crossmatching process for patients without antibodies allows crossmatched blood to be available for transfusion much more rapidly than if a serological crossmatch was necessary (also see Chapter 23). An electronic crossmatch can be performed in less than five minutes, which means that a unit of blood can be made available at the patient bedside sooner and is not delayed because of the crossmatching process. Education as to the availability and speed of the electronic crossmatch can drive down the C:T ratio.

The Maximum Surgical Blood Ordering Schedule (MSBOS) is another cause of elevated C:T ratios. The MSBOS was developed so that a patient would not arrive in the operating room (OR) without adequate blood being available. The original version of the MSBOS was derived by the consensus of surgeons performing the procedure. In many institutions, the MSBOS has not been updated to reflect changes in surgical procedures. As such, an attempt to generate a data-driven MSBOS should be made [11].

Excessive phlebotomy is another source of waste. An estimated 30% of transfusions that take place in an intensive care unit (ICU) compensate for excessive phlebotomy [12].Over the course of a hospitalisation, a patient can be subjected to draws of hundreds of millilitres of blood. This starts with the 'rainbow draw' at admission. Figure 34.3 illustrates the concept of

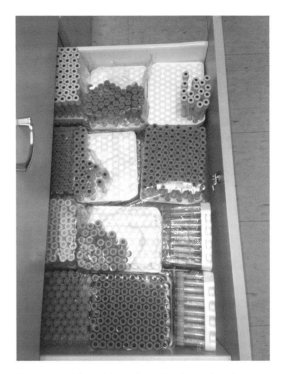

Figure 34.3 The rainbow draw. (*See insert for colour representation of the figure.*)

the 'rainbow draw', in which a well-intentioned nurse draws blood to fill vacutainer tubes of every colour in the hope that a patient will not have to be rephlebotomised when a fickle physician changes their mind about specific blood tests. In addition, the well-intentioned nurse may also draw double tubes of every colour just in case the laboratory rejects a specific sample. This excessive phlebotomy extends into the hospital stay, during which routine phlebotomy occurs every morning simply because the sun rises. As such, routine phlebotomy should not be allowed within a physician order entry system so that the clinician is forced to order testing only when there is a clinical question to be answered.

Blood mishandling also produces waste. This typically occurs when blood has been dispensed to a clinical area but is allowed to warm or sit unused for a prolonged period of time. Blood waste can be significantly reduced by educating clinicians in appropriate handling practices.

More importantly, the whole product ordering process needs to be reengineered. Typically, blood transfusion laboratories distribute blood to a clinical area based on a physician order but the nurse, who might be the one to administer the unit, may have multiple other patients to care for. In addition, the nurse may also need to administer premedication prior to the transfusion and ensure that a patient's intravenous line is available. One facility in which the blood bank distribution process was driven by a nurse demonstrated a 79% reduction in platelet wastage [13].

Lastly, waste arises from unnecessary ordering of blood to the OR. Having a cooler of blood at the patient bedside provides comfort to the anaesthesiologist and surgeon, but the vast majority of blood delivered to the OR in this fashion goes unused [14]. Not only is this blood wasted, but also the blood transfusion laboratory needs to carry a larger inventory to keep these products sitting at the foot of an OR table.

Step 3: Promote Alternative Blood Transfusion Methods and Systems

In many surgical procedures such as multilevel spine fusion or open thoracoabdominal aneurysm repair, heavy blood loss is highly probable. In strategising intraoperative management, reducing red cell transfusion through intraoperative blood recovery and reinfusion (cell salvage) should be considered, as well as normovolaemic haemodilution or component sequestration to reduce plasma and platelet transfusion.

Intraoperative blood salvage, more commonly called cell salvage, involves the collection of shed blood from the surgical field. The shed blood is then concentrated, washed, filtered and readministered to the patient. A rate of return of 60% of the lost cells can optimally be achieved with this technique. With this technology, multiple complete blood volumes can be processed prior to needing allogeneic red blood cell supplementation [15].

Normovolaemic haemodilution entails the withdrawal of autologous blood prior to the start of the surgical procedure and replacing volume with asanguineous intravenous fluids [16]. The primary goal of this technique is to create a relative anaemia in the patient so that bloodshed during the operative procedure effectively contains a reduced number of red cells. Once the threat of blood loss is diminished, the harvested cells are returned to the patient. A significant disadvantage to normovolaemic haemodilution is that it does not work very well to prevent red cell transfusion. The savings attributable to normovolaemic haemodilution are estimated at 100–200 mL, hardly enough to significantly reduce allogeneic exposure [17]. The value of haemodilution relates to its ability to treat coagulopathy that might develop during a major blood loss procedure. Intraoperative blood salvage allows for allogeneic red blood cell avoidance up to 2–3 blood volumes, while sequestered plasma and platelets from normovolaemic haemodilution protect the patient when a dilutional or consumption coagulopathy occurs. In general, removal of a litre of whole blood through normovolaemic haemodilution, and then reinfusion, is adequate for platelet and plasma transfusion avoidance.

Step 4: Promote Anaemia Management Strategies

Attention should be paid to the future surgical patient's haemoglobin concentration in the preoperative period. The prevalence of preoperative anaemia is striking; it has been documented to range from 5% in female geriatric hip fracture patients to over 75% in colon cancer patients. Other studies have shown that anaemia exists in 34% of non-cardiac surgery patients and 35% of those undergoing total knee or hip replacement. Preoperative anaemia is the greatest risk factor for perioperative transfusion. In addition, it has been associated with higher mortality rates in surgical patients.

Optimisation of a patient's haemoglobin can take place through the use of iron, vitamins and occasionally through the use of erythropoietin (Figure 34.4).

In general, determining the reason for the patient's anaemia is the best strategy. For instance, many patients undergoing joint replacement surgery are at an age where they are at risk for colon cancer. A patient with an occult colon cancer would be far better served by having the mechanism for their anaemia evaluated prior to a joint replacement because they might more greatly benefit from a colon resection.

How anaemia management is structured should be tailored to the hospital or health system. Many hospitals use a nurse manager to individually manage patients, while larger hospitals might find this strategy cost-prohibitive.

Step 5: Limit Iatrogenic Blood Loss

Limiting blood loss from phlebotomy is achieved through point-of-care testing devices. A wide variety of laboratory tests are available through these devices, including blood gas, electrolyte, glucose level, haemoglobin concentration and coagulation function tests. Testing devices measuring these factors require microlitres of blood rather than the standard 3–4 mL necessary with standardised laboratory testing. Point-of-care testing allows for the treating clinician to make decisions based on quantitative data at the point of care. This is most valuable in the operating room or ICU where transfusion needs are traditionally guessed. In cardiac surgery, where point-of-care testing has been implemented, blood use has been reduced by up to 70% [18].

In addition to point-of-care testing devices, hospitals can use paediatric vacutainer tubes for routine laboratory testing. These tubes aspirate 0.5–1 mL of blood, which further reduces routine phlebotomy losses. While resistance to this practice is frequently encountered from laboratory staff, patient safety should be the focus and not the convenience of the laboratory.

Another system which can reduce phlebotomy loss exists in conjunction with invasive lines. Routinely, 10 mL of blood is drawn through these lines prior to drawing the laboratory sample. The first 10 mL is then discarded. Systems in which this drawn blood is sterilely aspirated and then reinjected following sampling have been implemented.

Step 6: Provide Blood Management Education, Awareness and Auditing for Clinicians

The last step in the PBM implementation strategy is to benchmark blood use for commonly performed surgical procedures. Figure 34.5 shows a report on blood use for primary total hip replacement procedures. On the left side of the figure, the variability seen among a group of hospitals is demonstrated. On the right of the figure, variability by surgeon is demonstrated. This variability relates to multiple factors, including surgeon differences in tolerability of anaemia, surgical approach, deep venous thrombosis prevention practices and use of antifibrinolytics. By developing such reports and publicly sharing them, surgeons will self-regulate their transfusion behaviour.

Cost of Blood

While the risks of allogeneic transfusion are controversial, the cost of providing blood for patients is significant. When developing a PBM programme, it is important to understand the costs associated with transfusion in order to convince hospital administrators to support such a programme. The cost per red cell unit for an individual patient has been estimated to range from $726 to $1183 (£484 to

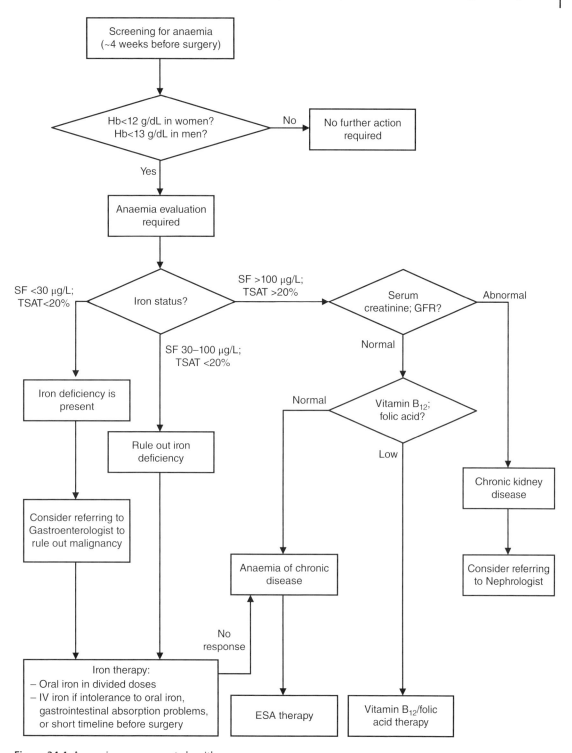

Figure 34.4 Anaemia management algorithm.

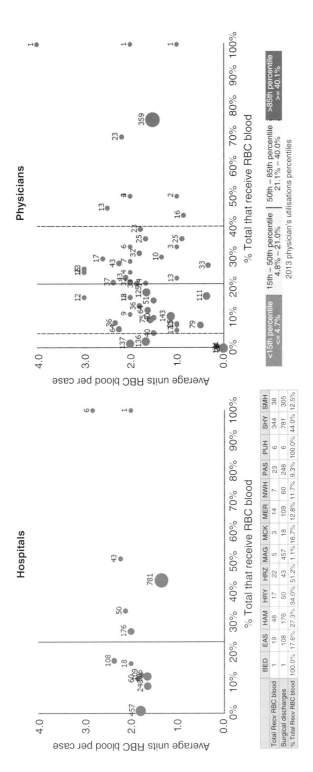

Hospitals

Physicians

	BED	EAS	HAM	HRY	HRZ	MAG	MCK	MER	NWH	PAS	PUH	SHY	SMH
Total Recv RBC blood	1	19	48	17	22	5	3	14	7	23	6	344	38
Surgical discharges	1	108	176	50	43	457	18	109	60	248	6	781	305
% Total Recv RBC blood	100.0%	17.6%	27.3%	34.0%	51.2%	1.1%	16.7%	12.8%	11.7%	9.3%	100.0%	44.0%	12.5%

<15th percentile <= 4.7%	15th – 50th percentile 4.8% – 21.0%	50th – 85th percentile 21.1% – 40.0%	>85th percentile >= 40.1%

2013 physician's utilisations percentiles

	2013/Apr	2013/May	2013/Jun	2013/Jul	2013/Aug	2013/Sep	2013/Oct	2013/Nov	2013/Dec	2014/Jan	2014/Feb	2014/Mar
Surgical discharges	192	182	206	155	197	189	222	224	179	208	193	215
Total receiving RBC blood	58	48	51	39	34	52	53	50	34	39	48	41
% Total that receive RBC blood	30.2%	26.4%	24.8%	25.2%	17.3%	27.5%	23.9%	22.3%	19.0%	18.8%	24.9%	19.1%
Avg units RBC blood per transfused case	1.83	1.77	1.59	1.41	1.91	1.27	1.79	1.66	1.50	1.33	1.31	1.54
Total receiving TXA	103	98	106	79	95	100	126	130	112	132	137	143
% Total that receive TXA	53.6%	53.8%	51.5%	51.0%	48.2%	52.9%	56.8%	58.0%	62.6%	63.5%	71.0%	66.5%
Avg units TXA per transfused case	1.07	1.07	1.07	1.08	1.17	1.07	1.08	1.08	1.14	1.21	1.26	1.24
ALOS w blood	3.4	3.3	3.1	3.2	3.6	2.8	3.0	2.6	2.5	2.3	2.9	3.0
ALOS w/o blood	2.9	2.8	3.0	2.8	2.9	3.0	2.8	2.7	2.7	3.0	2.7	2.8
% Autologous	0.0%	0.0%	3.9%	2.6%	2.9%	0.0%	1.9%	0.0%	0.0%	0.0%	0.0%	0.0%

Figure 34.5 Benchmarking report. (*See insert for colour representation of the figure.*)

£789) [19]. The national healthcare costs related to blood products are even more staggering. The United States currently spends $1.8 billion (£1.2 billion) of direct costs for blood products. Management of the blood supply and associated costs drive the overall price tag to between two and four times, or $3.6 to $7.2 billion (£2.4 to £4.8 billion).

KEY POINTS	
1) The easiest method to reduce exposure to donor blood is to use a restrictive transfusion trigger for all blood products.	4) Safe and appropriate blood use is facilitated by the use of information technology throughout the transfusion process.
2) Consider red cell transfusion only if the haemoglobin concentration is 80 g/L or less in haemodynamically stable patients, including asymptomatic patients with stable cardiovascular disease.	5) Computerised physician order entry (CPOE) systems can be leveraged to guide evidence-based transfusions.
3) Measures for patient blood management, e.g. for treating anaemia, minimising iatrogenic blood loss and intraoperative blood salvage, should be considered as alternatives to transfusion with donor blood.	6) All forms of waste related to blood transfusion practices should be addressed.
	7) Education in patient blood management should be provided for clinicians and patients.

References

1 Murphy MF, Waters JH, Wood EM, Yazer MH. Transfusing blood safely and appropriately. BMJ 2013;**347**:f4303.

2 Hebert PC, Wells G, Blajchman MA et al. A multicenter, randomized, controlled clinical trial of transfusion requirements in critical care. N Engl J Med 1999;**340**:409–17.

3 Carson JL, Terrin ML, Noveck H et al, for the FOCUS Investigators. Liberal or restrictive transfusion in high risk patients after hip surgery. N Engl J Med 2011;**365**:2453–62.

4 Hajjar LA, Vincent JL, Galas FRBG et al. Transfusion requirements after cardiac surgery: the TRACS randomized controlled trial. JAMA 2010;**304**:1559–67.

5 Holst LB, Haase N, Wetterslev J et al, for the TRISS Trial Group and Scandinavian Critical Care Trials Group. Lower versus higher hemoglobin threshold for transfusion in septic shock. N Engl J Med 2014;**371**:1381–91.

6 Salpeter SR, Buckley JS, Chatterjee S. Impact of more restrictive blood transfusion strategies on clinical outcomes: a meta-analysis and systematic review. Am J Med 2014;**127**:124–31.

7 McWilliams B, Triulzi DJ, Waters JH, Alarcon LH, Reddy V, Yazer MH. Trends in RBC ordering and use after implementing adaptive alerts in the electronic computerised physician order entry system. Am J Clin Pathol 2014;**141**(4):534–41.

8 Berwick DM, Hackbarth AD. Eliminating waste in US healthcare. JAMA 2012;**307**:1513–16.

9 Cohen JA, Brecher ME. Preoperative autologous blood donation: benefit or detriment? A mathematical analysis. Transfusion 1995;**35**:640–4.

10 Renner SW, Howanitz PJ, Bachner P. Preoperative autologous blood donation in 612 hospitals: a College of American Pathologists' Q-probes study of quality issues in transfusion practice. Arch Pathol Lab Med 1992;**116**:613–19.

11 Frank SM, Rothschild JA, Masear CG et al. Optimizing preoperative blood ordering with data acquired from an anesthesia information management system. Anesthesiology 2013;**118**:1286–97.

12 Corwin HL, Parsonnet KC, Gettinger A. RBC transfusion in the ICU. Is there a reason? Chest 1995;**108**:767–71.

13 Collins RA, Wisniewski MK, Waters JH, Triulzi DJ, Yazer MH. The effectiveness of multiple initiatives to reduce blood component wastage. Am J Clin Pathol 2014;**141**:78–84.

14 Staves J, Davies A, Kay J, Pearson O, Johnson T, Murphy MF. Electronic remote blood issue: a combination of remote blood issue with a system for end-to-end electronic control of transfusion to provide a "total solution" for a safe and timely hospital blood transfusion service. Transfusion 2008;**48**:415–24.

15 Waters JH, Shin Jung Lee J, Karafa MT. A mathematical model of cell salvage compared and combined with normovolemic hemodilution. Transfusion 2004;**44**:1412–16.

16 Olsfanger D, Fredman B, Goldstein B, Shapiro A, Jedeikin R. Acute normovolemic hemodilution decreases postoperative allogenic blood transfusion after total knee replacement. Br J Anesth 1997;**79**:317–21.

17 Matot I, Scheinin O, Jurim O, Eid A. Effectiveness of acute normovolemic hemodilution to minimize allogeneic blood transfusion in major liver resections. Anesthesiology 2002;**97**:794–800.

18 Nuttall GA, Oliver WC, Santrach PJ et al. Efficacy of a simple intraoperative transfusion algorithm for nonerythrocyte component utilization after cardiopulmonary bypass. Anesthesiology 2001;**94**:773–81.

19 Hofmann A, Ozawa S, Farrugia A, Farmer SL, Shander A. Economic considerations on transfusion medicine and patient blood management. Best Pract Res Clin Anaesthesiol 2013;**27**:59–68.

Further Reading

Boisen ML, Collins RA, Yazer MH, Waters JH. Pretransfusion testing and transfusion of uncrossmatched erythrocytes. Anesthesiology 2015;**122**:191–5.

Konig G, Hamlin BR, Waters JH. Topical tranexamic acid reduces blood loss and transfusion rates in total hip and total knee arthroplasty. J Arthroplast 2013;**28**:1473–6.

Seeber P, Shander A (eds). Basics of Blood Management, 2nd edn. Chichester: Wiley-Blackwell, 2013.

Spiess BD, Spence RK, Shander A (eds). Perioperative Transfusion Medicine, 2nd edn. Philadelphia: Lippincott, Williams and Wilkins, 2005.

Waters JH. Blood Management: Options for Better Patient Care. Bethesda: AABB Press, 2008.

Waters JH. Patient blood management, in Technical Manual, 17th edn (eds Roback JD, Grossman BJ, Harris T, Hillyer CD. Bethesda: AABB Press, 2011, pp. 671–85.

Yazer MH, Waters JH. How do I implement a hospital-based blood management programme? Transfusion 2012;**52**:1640–5.

35 Perioperative Patient Blood Management

Martin Rooms[1], Ravishankar Rao Baikady[1] and Toby Richards[2]

[1] *The Royal Marsden NHS Foundation Trust, London, UK*
[2] *University College London, London, UK*

Introduction

Patient blood management (PBM) is a programme of care that focuses on a patient-centred approach to the management and utilisation of blood transfusion. The three pillars of PBM are ideally applicable to a patient's journey through surgery from preoperative preparation to intraoperative techniques and post-operative restrictive practice (Figure 35.1). In the UK, there has been a considerable reduction in the use of blood transfusion in surgery [1], mirrored by increased development of laparoscopic surgery and minimally invasive interventions. However, PBM could not be more relevant in surgical practice where anaemia and transfusion use are both common and have both, independently, been associated with increased perioperative risk and poor outcomes [2]. Therefore, surgical practice is the ideal role model for PBM as part of a quality improvement programme in transfusion practice.

Patient blood management has been endorsed by the WHO [3] and in the UK, as a Department of Health initiative promoted by NHS Blood and Transplant (NHSBT) [4]. As a strategy, the benefits of PBM were demonstrated by the Western Australia (WA) Department of Health. In 2008, a five-year jurisdictional change in practice implemented a comprehensive PBM programme across the healthcare system. Overall, despite an increase in hospital admissions of 10%,

there was a stepwise reduction in blood usage in WA from 31.8 units to 27.9 units per 1000 population, with the greatest reduction seen in surgery (27%). Specifically in surgery, fewer patients (3% to 2.5%) received less blood (average 3.5 units to 3.0 units transfused). No notable impact on patient care or readmission was seen; indeed, in orthopaedic surgery where PBM had significant impact, there was a reduction in complications and length of hospital stay. Financially, the direct cost savings were AUD 4.7 million and indirectly considerably more, AUD 21 million [5] (around £9 million, October 2015). In Europe, there has been variable development of PBM [6], although recently the PREPARE trial reported, through a study of elective orthopaedic surgery, that transfusion rates and patient outcomes were improved in those hospitals with established PBM pathways [7].

Anaemia and Major Surgery

Preoperative anaemia affects about a third of all patients undergoing non-day-case surgery, rising to 40–60% of those undergoing major cardiac and non-cardiac operations [2]. Despite this, the investigation and management of anaemia before surgery are frequently overlooked [2]. Preoperative anaemia is strongly predictive of perioperative morbidity and mortality – even mild anaemia is associated with increased risk

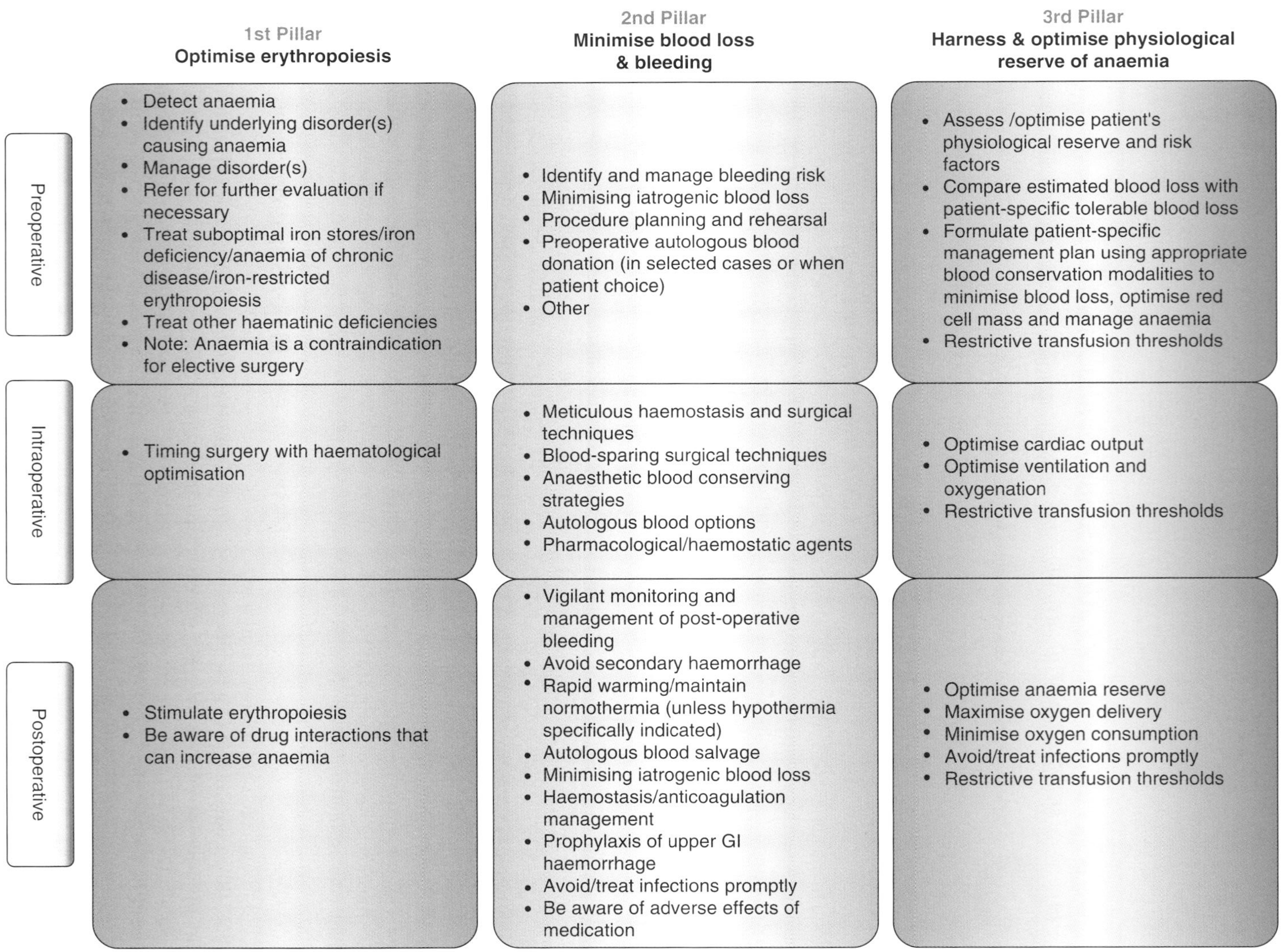

Figure 35.1 The three-pillar, nine-field matrix of perioperative patient blood management. This matrix, designed for the Western Australia Patient Blood Management Program, highlights the multiple patient blood management strategies that may be considered in the perioperative period in a patient/ procedure-specific context. GI, gastrointestinal. *Source: Adapted from Hofmann A, Friedman D, Farmer S. Western Australian patient blood management project 2008–2012: analysis, strategy, implementation and financial projections. Western Australia Department of Health, Canberra, 2007. (See insert for colour representation of the figure.)*

in the perioperative period of 30–40%, with a further relationship of more severe anaemia with worse outcome [8]. The EuSOS survey demonstrated that moderate or severe anaemia was associated with increased in-hospital mortality (odds ratio (OR) 1.99 and 2.28 respectively) [9]. Although a causal link between anaemia and adverse outcomes is not proven, the association has been repeatedly shown across most surgical specialties [2].

A recent NHSBT audit looked at PBM in surgical practice [1]. Fourteen elective procedures likely to be associated with high transfusion use were reviewed, including orthopaedic, cardiac, colorectal, urological, gynaecological and vascular surgery. Approximately 8500 units of red cells were transfused in 3897 patients from 190 sites over a three-month period in 2015. Preoperative anaemia was common, present in half of patients. However, anaemia was identified late in the preoperative pathway, with only a third of patients having an Hb level tested at least 14 days preoperatively. This was despite an average 42 days between listing for elective surgery and the operation itself. Even in colorectal surgery, where many cases may have been urgent for cancer, there was a median 18 days between listing and operation [1]. Consequently, time does exist in the normal pathways of care and there is a need to address and manage anaemia appropriately before operation, as anaemia is a potentially correctable risk factor for patients undergoing an operation [2,8,10].

Just Give Blood?

Transfusion of packed red cells has been the standard solution for anaemia in the perioperative period. However, replacing red cells does not address the underlying cause of anaemia, so in this regard blood transfusion should not be regarded as a treatment [2]. Aside from the fact that blood is a precious resource, it is not without risk. The risk of infection is small but well known, and other risks such as febrile reaction and fluid overload occur far more frequently

than the transmission of viruses by transfusion. Indeed, in the NHSBT audit described above, 0.6% of all transfusions were stopped due to some form of adverse event.

More recently, the current practices of blood transfusion in surgery have been brought into question. In two large database analyses (1 million and 1.6 million patients) [11,12], blood transfusion was found to be associated with increased morbidity and mortality in surgical patients. Data were retrospective and, importantly, do not address either the indication for blood transfusion or any causal link between transfusion and outcome. Consequently, these data cannot reliably comment on the blood product itself. However, they do link the current practice of the intervention (blood transfusion) and poor outcomes in surgical patients. Consequently, these data analyses suggest that blood transfusion may not be the most appropriate solution for anaemia in the surgical patients and if used, consideration should be given to appropriateness of the 'therapy' and potential impact of the intervention.

Patient Blood Management in Surgical Practice

Preoperative Optimisation

Two key aspects are important: the management of anticoagulant/antiplatelet therapy and the identification and management of preoperative anaemia. Preoperative PBM management also includes identification of the high-risk patient and therefore should trigger appropriate planning of further intraoperative and postoperative PBM strategies.

Management of antiplatelet/anticoagulant agents is an important step in the planning for surgery. Stopping agents for a period of time to allow clotting ability to return to normal can aid in reducing intraoperative blood loss [13]. Agents often need to be stopped for a period of five days or several weeks to allow new platelets or clotting factors to be generated, depending on the agent involved. Despite this, in the NHSBT audit, nearly a third of patients on warfarin underwent an operation with an international normalised ratio (INR) >1.4. This was frequently associated with late (poor) planning and discontinuation of warfarin in an appropriate manner [1]. Continuing treatment for underlying conditions may be needed, and bridging this gap with low molecular weight heparin (LMWH) can be undertaken, with treatment stopped the day before surgery.

To assess for preoperative anaemia, the recommended tests prior to major elective surgical procedures should preferably be undertaken 30 days beforehand and should include full blood count (FBC), iron studies, a marker of inflammation and B12 and folic acid levels (if a cause other than iron deficiency is suspected) [10]. The main causes of anaemia in the general population – iron, folate and vitamin B12 deficiency, gastrointestinal disease, renal failure or haemoglobinopathy – are rarely newly diagnosed at preoperative assessment. Surgical patients may indeed have an established or treated cause of anaemia, but are likely to also suffer from anaemia due to the condition for which they are undergoing surgery. This could either be directly related, for example due to gastrointestinal blood loss in colorectal cancer, or indirectly as a consequence of chronic disease. The latter has traditionally been regarded as *anaemia of chronic disease* (ACD), which is the most common type of anaemia seen in hospitalised patients.

This diagnosis of ACD has evolved with the understanding of iron metabolism in disease. The traditional definition of iron deficiency anaemia refers to depletion of the body's iron stores due to dietary deficiency or chronic blood loss, resulting in an *absolute iron deficiency* (AID), diagnosed by a blood ferritin <16 ng/mL. It is now recognised that disease states, in particular inflammation, have a direct effect on the iron regulatory protein, hepcidin. Hepcidin mediates the pathway of iron absorption and metabolism and activation of this can lead to a state of iron deficiency and anaemia [2]. Consequently, those patients previously diagnosed with ACD are now recognised to have *functional iron deficiency* (FID), where despite the presence of normal, or even increased, iron stores, there is inability to utilise these stores (Figure 35.2). The exact definition of FID in the perioperative setting as yet is not clear. However, clinical trials frequently use criteria of ferritin

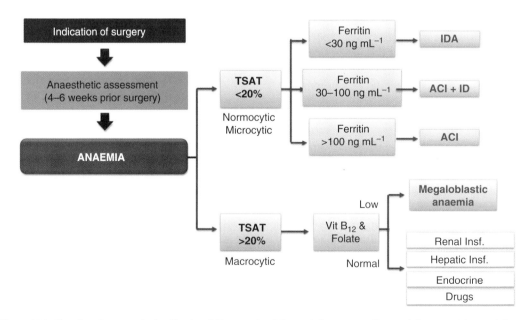

Figure 35.2 Flowchart for anaemia classification. ACI, anaemia of chronic inflammation; ID, iron deficiency; IDA, iron deficiency anaemia; TSAT, transferrin saturation. *Source:* Munoz et al. 2015 [10]. Reproduced with permission of Oxford University Press. (*See insert for colour representation of the figure.*)

<100 ng/mL or transferrin saturations <20% to define FID.

Patients treated for iron deficiency anaemia may benefit from oral iron therapy, provided that a minimum of 4–6 weeks is available prior to surgery. Oral iron is often effective, although can be poorly tolerated due to gastrointestinal side effects in about a quarter of patients, and has relatively poor bioavailability of 10–15% in the ferrous form, and less than this in the ferric form [2]. This bio-absorption is further impacted by inflammation, so its role in patients with FID is limited. Nevertheless, oral iron preparations are cheap and readily available, so consideration should be given to using oral iron as the first-line treatment for iron deficiency anaemia in patients undergoing elective non-urgent surgery, such as orthopaedic joint replacement.

An intravenous iron infusion provides an alternative to oral iron therapy in the perioperative setting. This route of administration bypasses the effects of hepcidin on GI absorption and macrophage sequestration. Complete restoration of iron reserves can be achieved in a single infusion and modern preparations enable a full treatment dose of 1000 mg or more as a short infusion without significant problems or side effects (Table 35.1). With current IV iron compounds, a rate of serious adverse events is estimated as <1:200 000, which is comparable to the risk associated with blood transfusion [10].

A period of at least five days should be available to see an effect before surgery and peak response is seen at three weeks post infusion. As yet, IV iron has not been formally tested in a randomised controlled trial (RCT) in perioperative patients and some concerns do exist around the impact of iron on infection rates. Again, these risks must be balanced against the risk of anaemia, the speed with which the haemoglobin concentration must be increased, and also blood transfusion [10].

Recombinant human erythropoietin (rHuEPO) is approved in Europe for decreasing allogeneic blood transfusion rates in patients with Hb of 100–130 g/L with adequate iron stores in orthopaedic surgery with expected moderate blood loss. Dosing regimens have been proposed from 10–21 days prior to surgery up to four days afterwards [10]. rHuEPO and IV iron have been used effectively together in the perioperative setting to improve Hb levels preoperatively. There is some concern around increased risk of thromboembolic events with perioperative rHuEPO use, although evidence is mixed and ABT carries its own thromboembolic risk [10]. Concerns have also been raised around promoting tumour growth through promotion of angiogenesis [14] and research into this area is ongoing, with a mixed evidence base at present. This treatment is, however, expensive and the cost-effectiveness in the perioperative period

Table 35.1 Intravenous iron formulations.

Formulation	Iron dextran	Iron sucrose	Ferric carboxymaltose	Iron isomaltoside
Maximum single dose	20 mg/kg	200 mg	20 mg/ 1000 mg per dose	20 mg/kg
Dosage	Single dose infusion	Repeated doses 3 × week	Single dose infusion	Single dose infusion
Adverse events	5% non-serious Anaphylactoid reactions 1:100–1:1000 Serious anaphylactic/ anaphylactoid reactions <1:10 000	0.5–1.5% non-serious Anaphylactoid reactions 1:1000–1:10 000 Serious anaphylactic/ anaphylactoid reactions <1:10 000	3% non-serious Anaphylactoid reactions 1:100–1:1000 Serious anaphylactic/ anaphylactoid reactions <1:10 000	>1% non-serious Anaphylactoid reactions 1:100–1:1000 Serious anaphylactic/ anaphylactoid reactions <1:10 000
Duration of infusion	4–6 hours	8 minutes (to 50 mg) 15 minutes (to 100 mg) 30 minutes (to 200 mg)	15 minutes	15 minutes (<1000 mg) 30 minutes (>1000 mg)

needs investigation. Nevertheless, the use of a one-size-fits-all approach (IV iron + EPO for anaemia) has been promoted and is currently being tested in a RCT in preoperative anaemia before cardiac surgery.

In an elective situation, preoperative anaemia should be considered to be a contraindication to surgery and cancellation or postponement of a procedure must be contemplated if more time is required to effectively investigate and manage an anaemic patient.

Intraoperative Management

Intraoperative management as part of PBM focuses on surgical and anaesthetic techniques for the prevention and management of blood loss, by pharmacological methods and surgical techniques. Transfusion, when required, should preferably be guided by access to near-patient testing.

At the start of surgery, anticipation, and therefore preparation, is key. Several PBM measures should be initiated. Avoidance of hypothermia is advocated, as it can adversely affect platelet function and also create an increased metabolic demand post-operatively as the body attempts to rewarm itself. Fluid warmers, forced air blankets and heated mattresses should be employed routinely to combat falling body temperature that otherwise occurs intraoperatively.

Inhibitors of clot lysis (antifibrinolytics), specifically tranexamic acid (TXA), are well known and highlighted by the CRASH-2 trial [15]. TXA is cheap and readily available. The action of TXA is to prevent clot breakdown. TXA does not 'cause clotting', as is often misinterpreted. The effect of TXA is to reduce blood loss in the operative and immediate post-operative period, often reported in clinical trials by endpoints of reduced output in surgical drains. TXA is safe and well used in cardiac and orthopaedic surgery, where it should be routine standard therapy for all cases, with TXA 1 g IV at induction. In the setting of general surgery, it is similarly highly recommended.

Surgical techniques to minimise blood loss are vital, including meticulous surgical haemostasis and minimally invasive/laparoscopic/robotic surgery where possible. Preoperative embolisation of highly vascular lesions can be considered, and tourniquets used in limb surgery can provide a bloodless field in which to operate. The use of electrical diathermy, laser cautery, topical haemostatic agents (sealants, glues, even topical TXA) and local anaesthetic with adrenaline as a vasoconstrictor all contribute to reducing intraoperative blood losses. Close collaboration with anaesthesia is vital in all major surgery to anticipate and respond to any problems. Fluid optimisation, through the use of goal-directed fluid therapy and cardiac output monitors, helps optimise cardiac output and therefore oxygen delivery. In specific cases, hypotension induced in a controlled manner can be used to minimise blood loss and allow a clear surgical field for faster completion of a procedure.

Where blood losses do occur, these can be collected, processed and returned to the patient through the use of cell salvage machines or wound drain collection/filtration devices. Concerns around reintroduction of unwanted material or cells have been mitigated in many scenarios through the use of leucocyte reduction filters. Orthopaedics, obstetrics, cardiac and cancer surgery have all found cell salvage techniques to be a useful part of a PBM strategy in suitable cases. Cell salvage is recommended in all operations with an estimated blood loss >500 mL [16].

Transfusion, when employed, should be guided by near-patient testing. This incorporates simple Hb testing (Hemocue®) to more advanced haemostasis testing such as thromboelastography, ROTEM® or platelet mapping. Near-patient testing enables rapid diagnosis of evolving abnormalities in correctly targeted cases as major haemorrhage. This can be useful in guiding decisions around blood products or appropriate use of other pharmacological agents including promotors of clot strength and stability (fibrinogen concentrate, factor XIII concentrate) and promotors of clot formation (prothrombin complex concentrate) and also in cases of major haemorrhage or correctly targeted cases.

The ideal haemoglobin value to aim for is an ongoing controversy, although it is becoming increasingly clear that one number does not benefit all patient groups [17,18]. Current practice in the perioperative setting has moved towards a restrictive transfusion trigger at an Hb of 70 g/L for most patients or 90–100 g/L in patients with unstable cardiac disease [19,20].

Major Haemorrhage

Major haemorrhage can create a rapidly changing situation, and in these instances a pre-prepared management plan in the form of a hospital-based guideline is essential to provide structure to management efforts [10]. The design of this plan should weave in appropriate PBM techniques to maximise efficacy of efforts to conserve blood and manage bleeding as well as provide information on the use of blood products to replace lost blood volume (Figure 35.3) (see also Chapter 26).

When undertaking transfusion in a patient suffering a major haemorrhage, the concept of a balanced ratio of plasma, platelets and red blood cells has been developed from military and civilian trauma research. The benefits of using a fixed ratio transfusion technique was proposed following an observational study (the PROMMTT trial [21]) and has been widely taken up by trauma centres and increasingly in the operating theatre. The PROPRR trial [22] attempted to refine the ideal ratio further, and examined patients suffering from severe trauma and major bleeding. The authors compared early administration of plasma, platelets and red blood cells in a 1:1:1 ratio compared with a 1:1:2 ratio, but did not demonstrate significant differences in mortality at either 24 hours or 30 days. Nevertheless, fixed ratio regimens have become the *de facto* standard of care for trauma patients, but an actual RCT proving that point is still lacking.

Post-operative Patient Blood Management

There are several areas post-operatively that can be addressed in a PBM strategy. Most research in this setting has focused on the need (or lack thereof) for a 'top up' or liberal transfusion.

A restrictive transfusion trigger is recommended through the post-operative period (Hb 70–80 g/L), although following cardiac surgery a more liberal target of 90 g/L versus 75 g/L was not inferior in terms of outcome [17]. As previously mentioned, anaemia should prompt the consideration of what is appropriate for the physiology of the patient at the time. In a patient with anaemia following blood loss, simple replacement of the blood may correct the Hb number but the patient may not have the reserves to manufacture and further recover their own blood count. Early establishment of nutrition with vitamin supplementation is vital, and in cases where intake is insufficient to meet demand for haematopoiesis, then iron replacement can be undertaken [23]. Post-operative oral iron is ineffective due to the inflammatory mediated hepcidin activation preventing iron absorption from the gut and macrophage sequestration. Intravenous iron replacement and management of functional iron deficiency are likely to be of increasing interest in the future.

Blood sampling is an essential aspect of monitoring and guiding patient treatment post-operatively, but hidden blood losses via this route can be significant and contribute to the overall burden. Reduction of post-operative sampling to only essential tests is advisable, and an effort should be made to instil this into a hospital's culture as part of an overarching PBM programme [10].

In the setting of critical illness, oxygen delivery is of primary importance and facilitating this in the context of anaemia is essential to allow recovery after surgery. This may be achieved through optimisation of cardiac output and ventilation in a critical care setting if required. Equally important is to actively seek and treat those things which raise metabolic oxygen demand, and so treating infections quickly and managing pain effectively are essential.

Finally, and most importantly, the use of blood transfusion in surgery is an intervention. It is a very good intervention and good treatment for blood loss. However, it is not necessarily the best treatment for all patients with anaemia. Knee-jerk prescriptions of two or more units to achieve an Hb >10 g/L need to be avoided. A structured programme of PBM includes appropriate transfusion

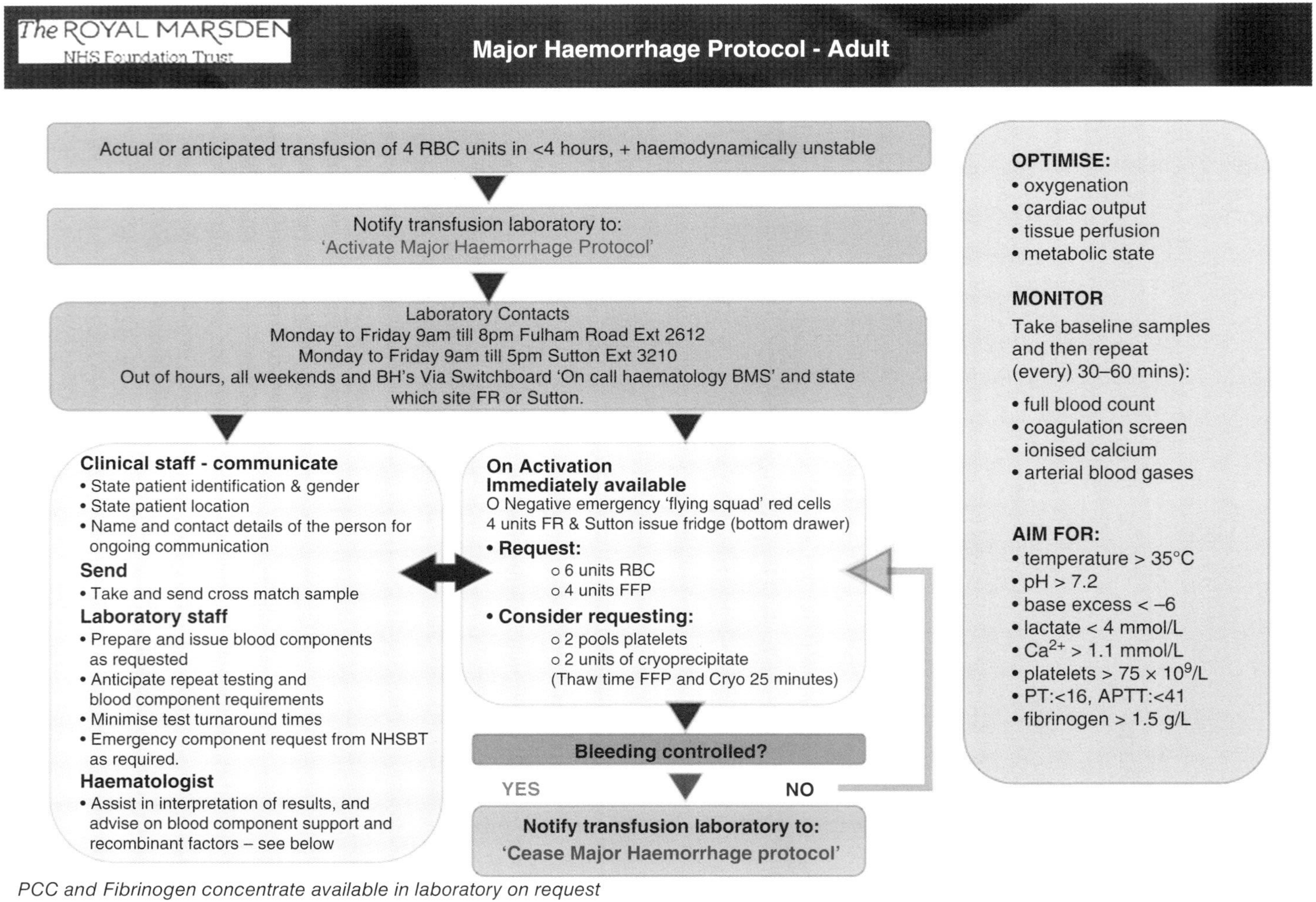

The ROYAL MARSDEN
NHS Foundation Trust

Major Haemorrhage Protocol - Adult

Actual or anticipated transfusion of 4 RBC units in <4 hours, + haemodynamically unstable

Notify transfusion laboratory to:
'Activate Major Haemorrhage Protocol'

Laboratory Contacts
Monday to Friday 9am till 8pm Fulham Road Ext 2612
Monday to Friday 9am till 5pm Sutton Ext 3210
Out of hours, all weekends and BH's Via Switchboard 'On call haematology BMS' and state which site FR or Sutton.

Clinical staff - communicate
- State patient identification & gender
- State patient location
- Name and contact details of the person for ongoing communication

Send
- Take and send cross match sample

Laboratory staff
- Prepare and issue blood components as requested
- Anticipate repeat testing and blood component requirements
- Minimise test turnaround times
- Emergency component request from NHSBT as required.

Haematologist
- Assist in interpretation of results, and advise on blood component support and recombinant factors – see below

On Activation
Immediately available
○ Negative emergency 'flying squad' red cells
4 units FR & Sutton issue fridge (bottom drawer)
- **Request:**
  ○ 6 units RBC
  ○ 4 units FFP
- **Consider requesting:**
  ○ 2 pools platelets
  ○ 2 units of cryoprecipitate
  (Thaw time FFP and Cryo 25 minutes)

Bleeding controlled?

YES

NO

Notify transfusion laboratory to:
'Cease Major Haemorrhage protocol'

OPTIMISE:
- oxygenation
- cardiac output
- tissue perfusion
- metabolic state

MONITOR
Take baseline samples and then repeat (every) 30–60 mins):
- full blood count
- coagulation screen
- ionised calcium
- arterial blood gases

AIM FOR:
- temperature > 35°C
- pH > 7.2
- base excess < –6
- lactate < 4 mmol/L
- Ca^{2+} > 1.1 mmol/L
- platelets > 75×10^9/L
- PT:<16, APTT:<41
- fibrinogen > 1.5 g/L

PCC and Fibrinogen concentrate available in laboratory on request

Figure 35.3 Major haemorrhage protocol (Royal Marsden NHS Foundation Trust). *Source:* Dougherty 2015. Reproduced with permission of John Wiley and Sons. (*See insert for colour representation of the figure.*)

practice, where Hb levels are taken and the patient clinically reassessed, before and after blood transfusion and the intervention is only repeated if necessary. This, a single unit transfusion policy, should be standard of care and blood transfusion practice in all stable patients.

Conclusion

Patient blood management is an individualised, evidence-based perioperative strategy used to reduce risks associated with anaemia and blood transfusion in an effort to improve patient outcome. Over 100 PBM measures have now been described [24]. These measures are largely not new, but require education and alteration to the pathways patients take through to surgery and beyond, in order to make these interventions and assessments a routine part of care.

Understanding the impact of preoperative anaemia is vital to appropriate management before surgery to reduce surgical risk (Figure 35.4). Haemorrhage management is proactive, and the use of TXA, cell salvage and organised major haemorrhage protocols is essential.

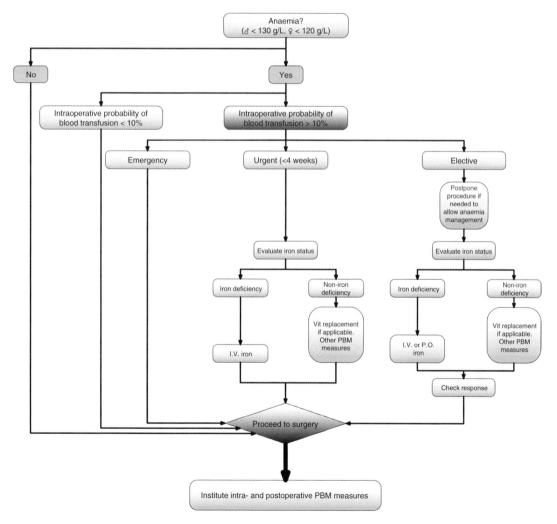

Figure 35.4 Pathways to surgery for patients with preoperative anaemia. IV, intravenous; PBM, patient blood management; PO, per os. (*See insert for colour representation of the figure.*)

Where required, the intervention of a blood transfusion should be stepwise, a single unit at a time.

Patient blood management requires a multi-disciplinary team to contribute to this effort through the perioperative period and a strong leader/champion of PBM is required to embed the concepts and processes of PBM into the culture of the hospital.

KEY POINTS

1) Hospitals should establish PBM multidisciplinary teams with PBM pathways of patient care integrated into anaesthetic and surgical pathways.
2) Hospitals should have a preoperative management pathway/protocol with clear stated arrangements for the following.
   - Timely identification and treatment of anaemia before elective surgery.
   - Preoperative haemostasis assessment with review and management of anticoagulant and antiplatelet therapy.
   - An individualised PBM strategy incorporating key interventions as below, proportionate to the anticipated blood loss.
   - Discussion with patients together with explanation of risks, benefits and transfusion alternatives available.
3) Hospitals should have protocols for the routine use of tranexamic acid in surgery.
4) Use of cell salvage and near-patient haemostasis testing should be considered in all cases where blood loss is anticipated to be >500 mL.
5) Hospitals should have protocols agreed between surgical, anaesthetic and transfusion teams for the management of major bleeding in surgery.
6) In the patient without active bleeding, a restrictive transfusion threshold should be used.
7) A single unit transfusion policy, followed by laboratory and clinical reassessment, should be adopted as the standard practice for blood transfusion.

References

1 Murphy MF, Gerrard R, Babra P, Grant-Casey J. 2013 National Patient Blood Management Survey. National Health Service Blood And Transplant. Available at: (http://hospital.blood.co.uk/media/27840/generic-pbm-survey-2013-report.pdf (accessed 16 November 2016).

2 Clevenger B, Richards T. Pre-operative anaemia. Anaesthesia 2014;**70**:20–8.

3 Availability, Safety and Quality of Blood Products. Presented at the Sixty-Third World Health Assembly, Geneva, 17–21 May 2010. Available at: http://apps.who.int/gb/ebwha/pdf_files/WHA63-REC1/WHA63_REC1-en.pdf (accessed 16 November 2016).

4 Department of Health. Health Service Circular HSC 2007/001: Better Blood Transfusion – Safe and Appropriate Use of Blood. Available at: file:///C:/Users/Owner/Downloads/nbtc_bbt_hsc_07.pdf (accessed 16 November 2016).

5 Farmer SL. Drivers for change: Western Australia Patient Blood Management Program (WA PBMP), World Health Assembly (WHA) and Advisory Committee on Blood Safety and Availability (ACBSA). Best Pract Res Clin Anaesthesiol 2013;**27**(1):43–58.

6 Shander A, van Aken H, Colomina MJ et al. Patient blood management in Europe. Br J Anaesth 2012;**109**(1):55–68.

7 Lasocki S, Krauspe R, Mezzacasa A, von Heymann C, Spahn DR. Postoperative anaemia and the need for effective patient blood management (PBM) are major concerns in

elective orthopaedic surgery– a multicentre observational study (PREPARE). Eur J Anaesthesiol 2012;**29**:97–8.

8   Musallam KM, Tamim HM, Richards T et al. Preoperative anaemia and postoperative outcomes in non-cardiac surgery: a retrospective cohort study. Lancet 2011;**378**:1396–407.

9   Baron DM, Hochrieser H, Posch M et al. Preoperative anaemia is associated with poor clinical outcome in non-cardiac surgery patients. Br J Anaesth 2014;**113**:416–23.

10 Munoz M, Gomez-Ramirez S, Kozek-Langeneker S et al. "Fit to fly": overcoming barriers to preoperative haemoglobin optimization in surgical patients. Br J Anaesth 2015;**115**(1):15–24.

11 Ferraris VA, Davenport DL, Saha SP et al. Surgical outcomes and transfusion of minimal amounts of blood in the operating room. Arch Surg 2012;**147**:49–55.

12 Whitlock EL, Kim H, Auerbach AD. Harms associated with single unit perioperative transfusion: retrospective population based analysis. BMJ 2015;**350**:3037–7.

13 Myles PS, Smith J, Knight J et al. Aspirin and Tranexamic Acid for Coronary Artery Surgery (ATACAS) Trial: rationale and design. Am Heart J 2008;**155**(2):224–30.

14 Okazaki T, Ebihara S, Asada M, Yamanda S, Niu K, Arai H. Erythropoietin promotes the growth of tumors lacking its receptor and decreases survival of tumor-bearing mice by enhancing angiogenesis. Neoplasia 2008;**10**(9):932–9.

15 CRASH-2 Trial Collaborators. Effects of tranexamic acid on death, vascular occlusive events, and blood transfusion in trauma patients with significant haemorrhage (CRASH-2): a randomised, placebo-controlled trial. Lancet 2010;**376**(9734):23–32.

16 Waters JH, Dyga RM, Waters JF, Yazer MH. The volume of returned red blood cells in a large blood salvage program: where does it all go? Transfusion 2011;**51**(10):2126–32.

17 Murphy GJ, Pike K, Rogers CA et al. Liberal or restrictive transfusion after cardiac surgery. N Engl J Med 2015;**372**(11):997–1008.

18 Goodnough LT, Levy JH, Murphy MF. Concepts of blood transfusion in adults. Lancet 2013;**381**(9880):1845–54.

19 Holst LB, Haase N, Wetterslev J et al. Lower versus higher hemoglobin threshold for transfusion in septic shock. N Engl J Med 2014;**371**(15):1381–91.

20 Carson JL, Carless PA, Hebert PC. Transfusion thresholds and other strategies for guiding allogeneic red blood cell transfusion. Cochrane Database Syst Rev 2012;**4**:CD002042.

21 Holcomb JB, del Junco DJ, Fox EE et al. The Prospective, Observational, Multicenter, Major Trauma Transfusion (PROMMTT) Study. JAMA Surg 2013;**148**(2):127–21.

22 Holcomb JB, Tilley BC, Baraniuk S et al. Transfusion of plasma, platelets, and red blood cells in a 1:1:1 vs a 1:1:2 ratio and mortality in patients with severe trauma. JAMA 2015;**313**(5):471–12.

23 Wallis JP, Wells AW, Whitehead S, Brewster N. Recovery from post-operative anaemia. Transfus Med 2005;**15**:413–18.

24 NHSBT. Patient Blood Management. Available at: www.transfusionguidelines.org.uk/uk-transfusion-committees/national-blood-transfusion-committee/patient-blood-management (accessed 16 November 2016).

Further Reading

National Blood Authority Australia. Patient Blood Management Guidelines. Available at: www.blood.gov.au/pbm-guidelines (accessed 16 November 2016).

Network for Advancement of Patient Blood Management, Haemostasis and Thrombosis (NATA). Provides detailed summaries of all PBM techniques with up to date reports of key articles. Available at: www.nataonline.com (accessed 16 November 2016).

NHSBT. Patient Blood Management. Available at: www.transfusionguidelines.org.uk/uk-transfusion-committees/national-blood-transfusion-committee/patient-blood-management (accessed 16 November 2016).

NHSBT. Patient Blood Management Toolkit. Available at: www.transfusionguidelines.org.uk/index.asp?Publication=NTC&Section=27&pageid=814 (accessed 16 November 2016).

Society for the Advancement of Blood Management (SABM). Provides education and research on transfusion medicine. Available at: www.sabm.org/(accessed 16 November 2016).

36 Restrictive Transfusion Practice and How to Implement It

Lawrence Tim Goodnough[1,2] and Neil Shah[1]

[1] *Department of Pathology, Stanford University, Stanford, USA*
[2] *Department of Medicine, Stanford University, Stanford, USA*

Introduction

Blood transfusion was the most frequently performed therapeutic procedure in 2010 [1] and a significant percentage of transfusions have been identified as inappropriate [2]. Allogeneic blood transfusions carry inherent risk, and studies have linked transfusions with adverse clinical patient outcomes, including morbidity and mortality [3], although this link was not present in several recent randomised controlled trials (RCTs) [4]. Differences in outcomes caused by the storage age of blood have also gained increased interest, despite randomised trials finding no differences in clinical patient outcomes for patients who received fresher (7–10 days) versus older (more than 21 days) red cell transfusions. Two additional trials are pending [5,6].

Accreditation agencies including the AABB and the Joint Commission (TJC) have initiated patient blood management (PBM) programmes, in order to promote restrictive transfusion practices [7]. The Choosing Wisely campaign by the American Board of Internal Medicine (ABIM) has identified blood transfusion as the most overused therapy in the United States [8]. Recently, seven key RCTs have provided level 1 evidence in adults that supports a restrictive red cell transfusion practice; however, there remains a heterogeneity of guidelines for blood transfusion by various medical societies, reflecting a lack of consensus on specific criteria for managing hospitalised, anaemic patients to guide blood transfusion therapy [9].

Clinical decision support (CDS) has been demonstrated to be effective in improving blood utilisation. This tool uses a haemoglobin concentration (Hb) threshold number in a smart Best Practices Alert (BPA) at physician order entry (POE), in order to trigger concurrent self-review for whether blood transfusion therapy is appropriate. However, it is poorly understood how physician behaviour is changed based on such a recommendation, or even whether such a recommendation is valid for complex patients who have with multiple comorbidities. The effectiveness of the BPA alone also has to be measured against other CDS tools such as accompanying educational activities, any targeted use of dashboards and benchmarking given to clinical services or providers or a combination of these interventions.

This chapter summarises level 1 evidence that supports restrictive transfusion practices. Traditional educational approaches to improving blood utilisation will also be reviewed, along with newer strategies made possible by CDS via electronic health records (EHR), that more recently have demonstrated value in improving blood utilisation by promoting restrictive transfusion practices.

Practical Transfusion Medicine, Fifth Edition. Edited by Michael F. Murphy, David J. Roberts and Mark H. Yazer.
© 2017 John Wiley & Sons Ltd. Published 2017 by John Wiley & Sons Ltd.

Level 1 Evidence Supports Restrictive Red Cell Transfusion Practices

Key Clinical Trials

There are a number of randomised trials providing level 1 evidence for restrictive blood transfusion practices, reviewed recently [9]. A systematic review prior to 2000 had identified 10 such trials, concluding that existing evidence supported the use of restrictive transfusion triggers in patients who were free of serious cardiac disease. A Cochrane systematic review of prospective, randomised trials up to 2012 compared 'higher' versus 'lower' Hb thresholds for blood transfusion in 19 trials involving 6264 patients. The authors found that lower Hb thresholds were as well tolerated as higher Hb levels. Blood transfusions could be reduced by 34%, with a mean reduction of 1.2 red cell units in cohorts using a lower Hb threshold for transfusion. A subsequent meta-analysis of trials with 2364 participants found that a restrictive red cell transfusion strategy targeting a Hb transfusion trigger <70 g/L was accompanied by reduced cardiac events, re-bleeding, bacterial infections and mortality. When 19 trials for restrictive transfusion strategies were pooled together with a total of 6936 patients, the restrictive strategy was still associated with a significant reduction in hospital mortality, 30-day mortality, pulmonary oedema, bacterial infections and re-bleeding.

There are seven key RCTs in adult patients that have compared 'restrictive' versus 'liberal' red cell transfusion strategies in various clinical settings (Table 36.1) [9]. The Transfusion Requirements in Critical Care (TRICC) trial in critical care patients found that randomisation to a restrictive transfusion strategy (Hb range 70–90 g/L, 82 g/L on average) had no difference in 30-day mortality rate, when compared to patients transfused more liberally (Hb range 100–120 g/L, 105 g/L on average). The Transfusion Requirements after Cardiac Surgery (TRACS) trial in cardiothoracic (CT) surgery patients was a large, single-centre study with randomisation to

Table 36.1 Seven key clinical trials of blood transfusion in adults.

Clinical setting	Haemoglobin threshold (g/L)	Age (years)	(%) Patients transfused	(%) Deviation from protocol	Mean haemoglobin (g/L)	% of screened patients enrolled in study
Intensive care	70	57.1	67	1.4	8.5	41
	100	58.1	99	4.3	10.7	
CT surgery	80	58.6	47	1.6	9.1	75
	100	60.7	78	0.0	10.5	
Hip fracture repair	80	81.5	41	9.0	7.9	56
	100	81.8	97	5.6	9.2	
Acute upper GI bleeding	70	NA	49	9.0	7.3	93
	90	NA	86	3.0	8.0	
Symptomatic CAD	80	74.3	28.3	1.8	7.9	12.2
	100	67.3	NA	9.1	9.3	
Septic shock trial	70	67	64	5.9	7.7	82
	90	67	99	2.2	9.3	
Cardiac surgery	75	69.9	53.4	30	8–9	98
	90	70.8	92.2	45	9.2–9.8	

CAD, coronary artery surgery; CT, cardiothoracic; GI, gastrointestinal; NA, not available.
Source: Goodnough & Shah [9].

receive either restrictive (haematocrit >24%) or liberal (haematocrit >30%) red cell transfusions post-operatively. Thirty-day all-cause mortality was not different (10% versus 11%, respectively) between the two cohorts. The FOCUS trial in patients undergoing repair of hip fracture found that elderly (mean >80 years of age) patients were able to tolerate post-operative blood transfusion to a Hb threshold of 80 g/L. It is noteworthy that symptomatic patients in this trial could be transfused at higher Hb levels. A prospective study of patients with upper gastrointestinal (UGI) bleeding has demonstrated that patients randomised to a restrictive (Hb <70 g/L) versus a liberal (Hb <90 g/L) Hb threshold for blood transfusions actually had statistically significantly improved clinical patient outcomes, including 45-day mortality and re-bleeding rates. However, significantly more protocol violations occurred in the restrictive group. Thus, if patients in the restrictive group should have died but were rescued by being transfused outside the protocol, the small difference in mortality between the two groups (that turned out to be significant) could have been eliminated. Still, the overall finding of the study, that restrictive threshold for these patients does not lead to worse outcomes, should stand.

The MINT trial was a pilot study of liberal (Hb ≥100 g/L) versus restrictive (Hb <80 g/L) transfusion thresholds in patients with symptomatic coronary artery disease (acute coronary syndrome or stable angina undergoing cardiac catheterisation), which was terminated after enrolment of only 110 of 200 planned patients. Of the screened patients who were eligible, only 12% were enroled (see Table 36.1). The primary composite outcome (death, myocardial infarction or revascularisation) occurred in only 11% of the liberal transfusion cohort, compared to 26% of the restrictive cohort (P = 0.054), and mortality occurred in 1.8% and 13.0%, respectively (P = 0.032). This trial provided evidence that a more liberal transfusion practice to maintain Hb thresholds above 100 g/L may represent prudent transfusion management for high-risk patients who

have coronary artery disease, but this conclusion awaits confirmation in a larger study.

A trial in patients with septic shock of lower (<70 g/L) versus higher (<90 g/L) Hb thresholds for red cell transfusion found equivalent 90-day mortalities (43% versus 45%, respectively) in the two patient cohorts. Finally, the TITRe2 trial studied elective cardiac surgery patients randomised to single unit blood transfusions at a restrictive Hb threshold of 75 g/L or liberal Hb threshold of 90 g/L. There was no significant difference in the primary composite outcome of serious infectious (sepsis or wound infections) or ischemic events (stroke, myocardial infarction, ischemic bowel and acute renal injury) between these two groups. While only 53% versus 92% of patients received blood transfusions in the restrictive and liberal cohorts, there was no difference in the primary outcome (35.1% and 33.0%), respectively, nor was 30-day mortality different. However, the average daily Hb levels were not that far apart (80–90 g/L versus 92–98 g/L); moreover, deviations from the protocol occurred in 30% and 45%, respectively, of the restrictive versus liberal threshold cohorts, perhaps accounting for the inability to demonstrate a predicted difference in the primary outcome. The authors conducted a *post hoc* analysis of 90-day mortality that was higher in the restrictive group, compared to the liberal group (4.2% versus 2.6%, P = 0.045).

Attempts to interpret a Hb threshold level as a 'transfusion trigger' from the results in these studies is problematic. For example, the mean pretransfusion Hb for patients in the 'restrictive' red cell transfusion arm of the TRACS trial was 91 g/L (see Table 36.1), compared to the 'target' Hb threshold of 80 g/L. Similarly, the mean Hb for patients in the 'restrictive' arm of the TRICC trial was 85 g/L; it is commonly interpreted from this study that a Hb of 70 g/L is the appropriate threshold to be used for blood transfusion in critical care patients [10]. Finally, and most importantly, since Hb is a concentration and not an absolute value, it is not only affected by changes in plasma volume, but also poorly reflects the degree of anaemia (reduced red cell mass) in dynamic situations such as acute blood loss.

Clinical Practice Guidelines

The number of published clinical practice guidelines for blood transfusion attests to the concerns of medical societies that some blood transfusions are administered inappropriately (Table 36.2) [11]. The identification of a discrete Hb as a 'trigger' for red cell transfusion has been controversial. For example, guidelines from the American College of Physicians (ACP) chose not to identify a single Hb number as a threshold for transfusions but rather, recommended that only one blood unit be transfused per transfusion event [12]. The guidelines do acknowledge the necessity of considering patient morbidities or other patient-specific criteria in making a transfusion decision. It is generally agreed that transfusion is not of benefit when the Hb is greater than 100 g/L for most patients, but may be beneficial when the Hb is less than 60–80 g/L.

However, some editorials have identified a 'new normal' Hb level of 70 g/L [13] or questioned how low we can go [14] for Hb thresholds used for transfusion decisions, and that 'it is no longer acceptable to recommend that we transfuse using vague approaches such as clinical judgement or in the hope of alleviating symptoms' [10].

Table 36.2 Clinical practice guidelines for blood transfusion.

Year	Society	Recommendations	Reference
1988	NIH Consensus Conference	<70 g/L (acute)	JAMA 1988;260:2700
1992	American College of Physicians	No number	Ann Intern Med 1992;116:393–402
1996/2006	American Society of Anaesthesiologists	<60 g/L (acute) No number	Anaesthesia 1996;84:732–47 Anaesthesia 2006;105:198–208
1997/1998	Canadian Medical Association	No number 60 g/L*	Can Med Assoc J 1997;156: S1–24 J Emerg Med 1998;16:129–31
1998	College of American Pathologists	60 g/L (acute)	Arch Pathol Lab Med 1998;122:130–8
2001 2012	British Committee for Standards in Haematology	70–80 g/L No number	Br J Haematol 2001;113:24–31 www.bcshguidelines.com/documents/BCSH_Blood_Admin_-_addendum_August_2012.pdf
2001	Australasian Society for Blood Transfusion	70 g/L	www.nhmrc.gov.au/_files_nhmrc/publications/attachments/cp78_cp_blood_components.pdf
2007/2011	Society of Thoracic Surgeons Society of Cardiovascular Anaesthesiologists	70 g/L or 80 g/L*	Ann Thorac Surg 2007;83:S27–86 Ann Thorac Surg 2011;91:944–82
2009	ACCM SCCM	70 g/L 70 g/L	Crit Care Med 2009;37:3124–57 J Trauma 2009;67:1439–42
2011	SABM	80 g/L	Trans Med Rev 2011;25:232–46
2012	National Blood Authority, Australia	No number	www.blood.gov.au/system/files/documents/pbm-module-1-qrg.pdf
2016	AABB	70–80 g/L or 80 g/L**	Transfusion 2016;56:2627–30.
2012	KDIGO	No number	Kid Int 2012;2:311–16
2012	National Cancer Centre Network	70–90 g/L	JNCCN 2012;10:628–53

* For patients with acute blood loss.
** For patients with symptoms of end-organ ischemia.
KDIGO, Kidney Dialysis Improvement Global Outcomes.
Source: Goodnough 2013 [11]. Reproduced with permission of Elsevier.

This approach advocates treating a laboratory number, rather than patient co-variables, and risks underestimating the heterogeneity of anaemias (e.g. acute versus chronic) and the heterogeneity of patients (e.g. cardiovascular comorbidities or age). Thus, the search for a transfusion threshold that combines clinical judgement, familiarity with the patient's unique circumstances and medical history, and objective laboratory guidance, continues.

Given the increasing evidence that blood transfusions are poorly effective and possibly harmful when used inappropriately, the guiding principle for transfusion therapy should be that 'less is more'. In the ABIM Choosing Wisely campaign, the AABB and American Society of Hematology (ASH) recently recommended that single unit red cell transfusions be administered for nonbleeding hospitalised patients, echoing guidelines published over 20 years ago by the ACP [15]. Additional blood units should be prescribed only after reassessment of the patient between transfusion events. This best practices framework is supported by the recent meta-analysis by Holst et al., which concluded that liberal transfusion strategies have not been shown to improve clinical outcomes [16].

Strategies for Improving Blood Utilisation

Educational Interventions

Historically, retrospective review of blood transfusions has been initiated by the laboratory-based transfusion service, with results reported to a hospital-based transfusion committee for peer review. Despite the resource-intensive nature of retrospective utilisation review, this model has been ineffective in improving transfusion practices, since only a fraction of cases are sampled (e.g. 5%) and retrospective review does little to modify future behaviour in the absence of continuous follow-up and feedback.

Review strategies concurrent with physician ordering have been described for red cell as well as for plasma and platelet products, through a combination of education and audits. While concurrent review of each product upon request can be successful, it is very labour intensive, difficult to sustain long term and can delay delivery of blood products. In traditional blood utilisation review, quality indicators have generally compared inventory management metrics, such as blood outdate and wastage rates, as well as crossmatch to transfusion (CT) ratios, against national benchmarks. However, while this focus on laboratory-based metrics is important, it does not consider quality metrics that link blood transfusion therapy to clinical patient outcomes.

Clinical Decision Support

Historical Approaches

A computerised method was shown to be effective in altering transfusion triggers for ordering red cells more than 25 years ago. Recent efforts using laboratory databases and patient EHRs, coupled with automated and manual reports to medical directors, have reported some success. Others have used education coupled with computerised provider order entry (CPOE) to reduce inappropriate red cell transfusions, as well as improving utilisation of plasma, cryoprecipitate and platelets [17,18]. Some limitations have been defined: teams (not individuals) frequently make transfusion decisions; trainees may overestimate required laboratory results/interventions, to avoid rounding delay; level 1 evidence may not be fully developed to support best practice recommendations; patient populations may be too heterogeneous for a one-size-fits-all BPA; and improved patient outcomes may not be demonstrably linked to the CDS intervention.

How Effective is CDS?

The financial impetus provided by the HITECH Act of 2009 increased the use of EHRs in office-based practices from 48% to 78% between 2009 and 2013. The implementation of EHRs implicitly promised advanced data analytics to improve patient care and prevent unnecessary treatment. The use of EHR systems has enabled tailored feedback to the provider at the critical time of order entry to promote appropriate use [19]. While several studies have shown beneficial impacts of CDS, large meta-analyses have failed to show a mortality benefit or meaningful impacts in reducing length of stay, adverse events or costs. The potential benefits of CDS can be maximised using intelligent design; taking a targeted approach that encompasses education and user awareness; continuous audit and feedback with dashboards and benchmarking; and dealing with acknowledged barriers to acceptance such as lack of time, relevance and alert fatigue [20].

Design elements leading to effective CDS have been published. A review of CDS found that 68% improved clinical practice and in 32 systems that possessed four key features, 94% significantly improved clinical practices. These four key features can be summarised as computer-based decision support that provides recommendations (rather than assessments) automatically at time of POE, through normal workflow. Subsequent analyses highlighted some unique aspects contributing to success: presenting CDS to both providers and patients, involving local users in the development process and not requiring additional data entry by providers. A required override or acknowledgment reason from providers increases adherence to CDS recommendations.

Overall, there is not generalisability in CDS. A recommendation with low or no dependencies would benefit from automated, provider-input free action (e.g. flu vaccine order for appropriate individuals) whereas complex CDS such as those used in sepsis care or preventing readmission would benefit from increased provider input at time of recommendation. CDS parameters should be designed appropriately to meet the clinical and business needs along with the right exclusions to avoid alert fatigue and false-positive alerting. These parameters include the audience (provider versus pharmacists versus nurse), the setting (inpatient, outpatient,

operating areas) and mode of alerting such as passive (information pulled by users), semi-active (knowledge representation and call to action) or active (automatic action without user intervention or knowledge).

A separate review took a more holistic approach to CDS by examining how different factors in healthcare affect user acceptance based on the Unified Theory of Acceptance and Use of Technology (UTAUT) model. This analysis found facilitators and barriers to CDS in three broad categories: user performance expectancy of system, user effort expectancy and social/cultural factors. Key themes within barriers included provider lack of time/competing clinical duties, poor design (complex or unfriendly interface, lack of agreement with system, lack of awareness of content) and cultural factors (reluctance to use CDS in front of patients, poor computer skills, financial constraints and low social acceptance of CDS). This analysis provides a road map for the future design and redesign of CDS to better engage end users to achieve more meaningful clinical impact. We must acknowledge that provider engagement is important for both the build and acceptance of these systems, but the resources supplied to physicians to meet these demands or financial incentives to drive these recommendations are absent. It is a pivotal time for hospitals and healthcare systems to restructure provider salary to be based on quality instead of work relative value units (RVUs). Otherwise, the discrepancy between national and systemic financial models versus local/provider ones will make the new healthcare framework untenable in the United States.

Improving Blood Utilisation: The Stanford Experience

At Stanford Health Care (SHC), we implemented a CDS system (Figure 36.1) for ordering blood transfusion in which a smart BPA is triggered when a provider orders blood for patients whose pretransfusion Hb is above a threshold (70 g/L, or 80 g/L for patients with acute coronary

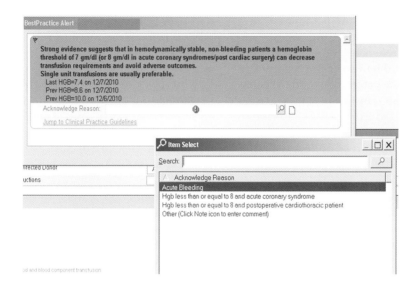

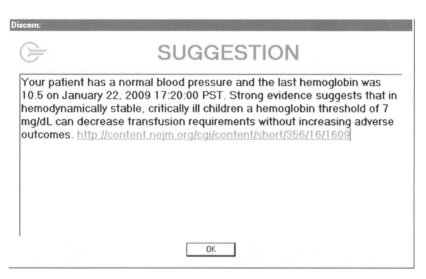

Figure 36.1 Best practices alert (BPA) screenshots at Stanford University Medical Centrr (SUMC). Screenshot from an electronic physician order entry (POE) for blood transfusion in adult patients at Stanford Hospital and Clinics (SHC) illustrates an 'interruptive alert' as a reminder for the merits of a restrictive transfusion practice versus liberal transfusion practice. An acknowledgment/exception field allows the physician to provide the indication for transfusion (acute bleeding, haemoglobin <80 g/L in the acute coronary syndrome or postcardiothoracic surgery patient, other clinical scenario) if such clinical scenarios were not updated in the problem list. The BPA for paediatric patients at Lucille Packard's Children's Hospital (LPCH) triggers only for children ages 1–18 years with haemoglobin >70 g/L who are normotensive in the last six hours. The alert did not trigger in patients from cardiac, haematology-oncology and neonatal ICU wards. *Source:* Goodnough and Shah 2014 [21]. Reproduced with permission of Oxford University Press.

syndrome or postcardiothoracic procedure) [21,22]. The purpose of the Hb level is to serve as a threshold for triggering concurrent, utilisation self-review (by the ordering medical team) and provide links to published medical literature. The BPA does not identify a 'correct' Hb level as even the most intelligent design (inclusion and exclusion factors in BPA triggering) cannot capture all relevant parameters in a dynamic patient with charting delays and availability of discrete data. Nevertheless, since implementation of the BPA for red cell transfusion in July 2010, the percentage of transfusions in patients whose pretransfusion Hb was greater than 80 g/L decreased from 60% beforehand to 35% in the six months after implementation, with a continued downtrend to less than 30% through 2013 (P < 0.001) [23].

Overall, CDS reduced red cell transfusions at SHC by 42%, from 2009 through 2015 (see Figure 36.2), despite increases in patient days at risk and case mix complexity over this time period. Hospital-wide patient clinical outcomes, as demonstrated by mortality showed statistically significant improvement, while length of stay and 30-day readmission rates remained stable. Outcomes in the subcohort of transfused patients before and after implementation of CDS showed pronounced improvement (P < 0.01 for all three outcomes) [23]. While the improvement in patient outcomes concurrent with reduction in red cell transfusions cannot be proven to be causal, it is reassuring that there was no deleterious effect on patient outcomes after hospital-wide adoption of restrictive transfusion practices, particularly in view of lower discharge Hb levels [25]. A study monitoring for inappropriate undertransfusion found no evidence that cases of nonadministration of blood were unjustified [26].

Additional benefits of our restrictive transfusion strategy included a significant improvement in the laboratory budget, with net savings of $1.6 million (£1.3 million) annually [22]. Purchase acquisition costs represent a fraction of total costs of blood transfusion that additionally include laboratory testing, reagent costs, nursing time dedicated to transfusion and monitoring. An activity-based cost summary of blood transfusions estimates that total costs related to transfusion are 3.2–4.8 times the purchase costs. Hence, the total transfusion-related saving potentially surpasses $30 million, over a four-year period. We recently implemented a smart BPA for plasma, triggered when the last

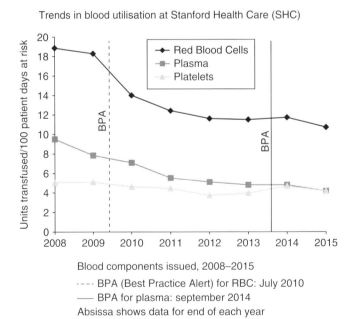

Trends in blood utilisation at Stanford Health Care (SHC)

Blood components issued, 2008–2015
---- BPA (Best Practice Alert) for RBC: July 2010
—— BPA for plasma: september 2014
Absissa shows data for end of each year

Figure 36.2 Trends in blood utilisation. Blood components issued to patients at Stanford Health Care. Transfusion of red cells decreased by 24% from 2009 through 2014. *Source:* From, Goodnough LT, Panigrahi A. Med Clin N Amer 2017 [24]. Reproduced with permission of Oxford University Press.

recorded INR is less than or equal to 1.7, to guide more appropriate plasma transfusion; preliminary analysis indicates a 17% reduction in plasma utilisation.

This model of concurrent real-time utilisation review can be supplemented by benchmarking between service lines and between providers in a service line for appropriateness of transfusion. Since up to 30% of red cell transfusions continue to occur in patients whose Hb was greater than 80 g/L at our institution, benchmarking can increase stakeholder acceptance, help reduce variability between providers and/or help modify the CDS triggers for known clinical exceptions. This process serves as continuous education and feedback, which is seen as vital in the success of utilisation programmes by augmenting improvements through CDS.

Other programmes have been able to utilise EHRs to improve blood utilisation in a different manner. One approach is to reconfigure the CPOE system for nonbleeding (excluding procedural units such as operating rooms, cardiac catheterisation labs) patients to remove single-click ordering for two-unit red cell transfusions; the provider must select from a drop-down menu if additional red cell units are desired. The proportion of two-unit red cell transfusions at one centre decreased from 47% before to 15% after this intervention. Similarly, reductions in two-unit red cell orders (48% to 33%) and an increase in one-unit red cell transfusions (22% to 48%) had been found after a comprehensive education and audit programme promoting restrictive transfusion practices. While CDS can improve red cell usage, further data are needed to assess whether CDS can improve plasma and platelet utilisation.

Future Directions

According to the Institute of Medicine, in 2009 $2.5 trillion (£2.0 trillion) was spent on healthcare, consuming 17.6% of GDP. Almost a third of this healthcare expenditure is estimated to be wasteful. Reducing this waste not only helps to improve patient outcomes by reducing exposure to unnecessary treatments/tests, but also addresses patient concerns over the ability to pay for the high cost of healthcare. Blood transfusion has been targeted among five key overuse measures by the American Board of Internal Medicine. The increased adoption of EHRs and features such as alerting allows the practice of prospective, real-time monitoring of transfusion therapy in an automated fashion at the critical time of physician order entry.

While alerting can help conform clinical practice towards published guidelines, this electronic tool may often be ignored if it is implemented in a vacuum without concurrent education. The contributions of the individual elements of the CDS (the alert, link to relevant literature, acknowledgment/exception) need to be further analysed to understand components affecting end-user action. Frequent and ill-designed CDS exacerbates 'alert/click fatigue', where users begin to mechanistically cancel pop-ups without reading the message, particularly when these occur at the time of order signing. Future measures include providing the prescriber with evidence-based and practical red cell ordering options; limiting low-impact CDS; moving the decision making and support downstream to pharmacy, radiology or pathology; and distributing the CDS burden to personnel with the highest knowledge base to make a decision. Displaying recommendations alongside user search items at order entry, instead of at the time of signing, would prevent disruptions in workflow and may lead to higher acceptance of CDS. An additional item missing from many CDS is follow-up of users and groups/services that commonly disregard best practices. Long term, these groups will have to be engaged for further education or refinement of CDS for continuous quality improvement.

Conclusion

Inappropriate blood transfusions and related costs can be substantially addressed through real-time CDS. Clinical patient outcomes improve after implementation; these observations provide assurance that a restrictive transfusion strategy can be successfully implemented institution-wide, improve patient safety and avoid patient harm. CDS design will require continued maturation to optimise user engagement and end-action while minimising 'alert fatigue'. In deriving increased value out of healthcare, CDS also can be applied to other overuse measures in laboratory testing, radiology and other therapies such as antibiotics, as outlined by the ABIM Choosing Wisely Campaign [8].

KEY POINTS

1) Blood transfusions are one of the most common inappropriately ordered therapies.
2) Clinical decision support is effective at improving blood utilisation.
3) Restrictive transfusion practices are associated with improved clinical outcomes.

References

1 Pfuntner A, Wier LM, Stocks C. Most frequent procedures performed in U.S. hospitals, 2010. HCUP Statistical Brief #149. Agency for Healthcare Research and Quality, Rockville. Available at: www.hcup-us.ahrq.gov/reports/statbriefs/sb149.pdf (accessed 16 November 2016).

2 Spahn DR, Goodnough LT. Alternatives to blood transfusion. Lancet 2013;**381**(9880):1855–65.

3 Goodnough LT. Blood management: transfusion medicine comes of age. Lancet 2013;**381**(9880):1791–2.

4 Yazer MH, Triulzi DJ. Things aren't always as they seem: what the randomized trials of red blood cell transfusion tell us about adverse outcomes. Transfusion 2014;**54**(12):3243–6; quiz 2.

5 Heddle NM. Informing fresh versus standard issue red cell management –International Standard Randomized Controlled Trial Number Register (ISRCTN). Available at: www.isrctn.com/ISRCTN08118744 (accessed 16 November 2016).

6 Cooper DJ. Standard Issue Transfusion versus Fresher Red Blood Cell Use in Intensive Care – A Randomized Controlled Trial – International Standard Randomized Controlled Trial Number Register (ISRCTN). Available at: https://clinicaltrials.gov/ct2/show/NCT01638416 (accessed 16 November 2016).

7 Goodnough LT, Shander A. Patient blood management. Anaesthesiology 2012;**116**(6):1367–76.

8 ABIM Foundation. Five things physicians and patients should question. Choosing Wisely. Available at: www.choosingwisely.org (accessed 16 November 2016).

9 Goodnough LT, Shah NK. Is there a 'magic' hemoglobin number? Clinical decision support promoting restrictive transfusion practices. Am J Hematol 2015;**90**(10):927–33.

10 Carson JL, Hebert PC. Should we universally adopt a restrictive approach to blood transfusion? It's all about the number. Am J Med 2014;**127**(2):103–4.

11 Goodnough LT, Levy JH, Murphy MF. Concepts of blood transfusion in adults. Lancet 2013;**381**(9880):1845–54.

12 Welch HG, Meehan KR, Goodnough LT. Prudent strategies for elective red blood cell transfusion. Ann Intern Med 1992;**116**(5):393–402.

13 Hebert PC, Carson JL. Transfusion threshold of 7 g per deciliter – the new normal. N Engl J Med 2014;**371**(15):1459–61.

14 Waters JH, Yazer MH. Patient blood management: where's the bottom? Transfusion 2015;**55**(4):700–2.

15 Audet AM, Goodnough LT. American College of Physicians Position Paper: Strategies for elective red blood cell transfusion. Ann Intern Med 1992;**116**:403–6.

16 Holst LB, Petersen MW, Haase N, Perner A, Wetterslev J. Restrictive versus liberal transfusion strategy for red blood cell transfusion: systematic review of randomised trials with meta-analysis and trial sequential analysis. BMJ 2015;**350**:h1354.

17 Yazer MH, Triulzi DJ, Reddy V, Waters JH. Effectiveness of a real-time clinical decision support system for computerized physician order entry of plasma orders. Transfusion 2013;**53**(12):3120–7.

18 Collins RA, Triulzi DJ, Waters JH, Reddy V, Yazer MH. Evaluation of real-time clinical decision support systems for platelet and cryoprecipitate orders. Am J Clin Pathol 2014;**141**(1):78–84.

19 Yazer MH, Waters JH. How do I implement a hospital-based blood management program? Transfusion 2012;**52**(8):1640–5.

20 Kawamoto K, Houlihan CA, Balas EA, Lobach DF. Improving clinical practice using clinical decision support systems: a systematic review of trials to identify features critical to success. BMJ 2005;**330**(7494):765.

21 Goodnough LT, Shah N. The next chapter in patient blood management: real-time clinical decision support. Am J Clin Pathol 2014;**142**(6):741–7.

22 Goodnough LT, Shieh L, Hadhazy E, Cheng N, Khari P, Maggio P. Improved blood utilization using real-time clinical decision support. Transfusion 2014;**54**(5):1358–65.

23 Goodnough LT, Maggio P, Hadhazy E et al. Restrictive blood transfusion practices are associated with improved patient outcomes. Transfusion 2014;**54**:2753–9.

24 Goodnough LT, Panigrahi AK. Blood Transfusion Therapy. Med Clin North Am 2017;**101**(2):431–447.

25 Goodnough LT, Murphy MF. Do liberal blood transfusions cause more harm than good? BMJ 2014;**349**:g6897.

26 Hibbs S, Miles D, Staves J, Murphy MF. Is undertransfusion a problem in modern clinical practice? Transfusion 2015;**55**(4):906–10.

Further Reading

Goodnough LT, Baker S, Shah N. How do I use clinical decision support to improve red blood cell utilization? Transfusion 2016;**56**(10):2406–2411.

Goodnough LT, Levy JH, Murphy MF. Concepts of blood transfusion in adults. Lancet 2013;**381**(9880):1845–54.

Goodnough LT, Maggio P, Hadhazy E et al. Restrictive blood transfusion practices are associated with improved patient outcomes. Transfusion 2014;**54**:2753–9.

Goodnough LT, Murphy MF. Do liberal blood transfusions cause more harm than good? BMJ 2014;**349**:g6897.

Goodnough LT, Murphy MF. How I train specialists in transfusion medicine. Transfusion 2016;**56**(12):2923–2933.

Goodnough LT, Shieh L, Hadhazy E, Cheng N, Khari P, Maggio P. Improved blood utilization using real-time clinical decision support. Transfusion 2014;**54**(5):1358–65.

Hibbs S, Miles D, Staves J, Murphy MF. Is undertransfusion a problem in modern clinical practice? Transfusion 2015;**55**(4):906–10.

37 Using Data to Support Patient Blood Management

Steven M. Frank and Jack O. Wasey

Department of Anesthesiology/Critical Care Medicine, Johns Hopkins Medical Institutions, Baltimore, USA

> *It is entirely possible that fast food chains and auto parts stores have better automated data collection than hospitals.*
>
> (Steven M. Frank MD)

Introduction

Patient blood management (PBM) is a relatively recent development in medicine that, in simple terms, has been described as giving the right product, at the right dose, at the right time, to the right patient, for the right reason. Although a strong PBM programme is multifaceted in its approach, all aspects of running a PBM programme are data intensive. Until very recently, we were living in the dark ages for data collection in the medical field. In the year 2013, it was determined that more than half of all US hospitals were still using paper anaesthesia records [1]. Given the difficulty in analysing data from paper records, the electronic medical record (EMR) is a big step forward. One problem with EMRs is that they are primarily designed for putting data in and not for getting data out, and their focus is often billing. Once a process is developed for data extraction, the EMR will be a gold mine of data that can be used to improve clinical practice.

Although the kinds of data in the EMR are numerous, the most important variables used to support a PBM programme are listed in Table 37.1. Data for the entire hospital can show changes in overall blood utilisation, which can then be narrowed down to the department level (specialty service), and then down to the individual provider level. Provider-level data can be challenging to interpret owing to problems with attribution. For example, in the operating room, the decision to transfuse may come from either the surgeon or the anaesthesiologist, and likewise in the intensive care unit (ICU), the decision may come from either the intensivist or the primary surgeon. Each facility should come to an agreement over how to handle these attribution challenges. Some institutions have mandated that an authorising physician be indicated in the electronic order set for each transfusion order, to address the attribution problem.

Transfusion Triggers and Targets

Because end-organ oxygen delivery is difficult or impossible to measure, the indication for transfusion is most often based on laboratory test results. The haemoglobin (Hb) trigger, for example, is defined as the lowest Hb concentration that will be tolerated before transfusion therapy is initiated. This method of determining the need for red blood cell transfusion is very useful, as long as the patient has adequate intravascular volume and is not actively bleeding.

Practical Transfusion Medicine, Fifth Edition. Edited by Michael F. Murphy, David J. Roberts and Mark H. Yazer.
© 2017 John Wiley & Sons Ltd. Published 2017 by John Wiley & Sons Ltd.

Table 37.1 Data variables used to support patient blood management.

Parameter measured	Data variable	Units of measure	Implications
Blood utilisation	Average number of units/hospital inpatient	Mean units/patient	Best method to measure success of a PBM programme Has direct implications for cost savings Is inherently adjusted by patient volume
	Percentage of inpatients transfused	Percentage of patients	Useful information on trends for transfusion avoidance
	Total units transfused	Units per month or year	Useful to assess overall blood use and costs, but is not patient volume adjusted Can be used to include outpatient transfusions
Transfusion guideline compliance	Transfusion triggers	Percentage of transfusion orders placed outside evidence-based guidelines assessed by laboratory tests	Can be assessed by 'true trigger' (the most recent lab value before transfusion) or by nadir Hb during the hospital stay
	Transfusion targets	Percentage of transfused patients with discharge laboratory values outside evidence-based range, as assessed by laboratory tests	Can be assessed by posttransfusion laboratory values, but is more easily assessed by last laboratory value before discharge
Clinical outcomes	Incidence of morbid events	Percentage of patients with morbid event (e.g. ischaemic, thrombotic, infection, renal or respiratory) (see Table 37.2)	Useful to determine whether PBM efforts affect quality of care
	Incidence of mortality	Percentage of patients not surviving the hospital stay	Useful to determine whether PBM efforts affect mortality
	Length of stay (LOS)	Days – best analysed as median (IQR) because LOS is not normally distributed	Has direct implications on cost of care; transfusion is associated with increased LOS
Costs	Hospital costs	$/hospitalisation Can be subdivided into direct and indirect costs	Useful because costs of blood and overall patient care are both included
	Hospital charges	$/hospitalisation	Less useful because hospitals aren't always paid what they charge
Risk-adjustment variables	Case Mix Index APR-DRG Wt MS-DRG Wt	0–30-point scale 0–30-point scale	Takes into account both severity of illness and complexity of procedures; used for Medicare billing and reimbursement; is directly related to transfusion requirements
	Charlson Comorbidity Index	0, 1–2, 3–4 and ≥5 scores are directly related to 1-year and 10-year mortality	A weighted index that takes into account comorbidities; may correlate with transfusion requirements

APR-DRG Wt, weighted all-patient refined diagnosis-related group; IQR, interquartile range; LOS, length of stay; MS-DRG Wt, weighted Medicare severity diagnosis-related group; PBM, patient blood management.

Over the past decade, eight large randomised trials have compared a restrictive transfusion strategy (Hb trigger of 70–80 g/L) to a liberal strategy (Hb trigger of 90–100 g/L) to determine differences in clinical outcomes. In general, the findings support the use of a restrictive strategy, with a trigger of 70 g/L in most patients and 80 g/L in those with cardiovascular disease. The first of these studies, the Transfusion Requirements in Critical Care (TRICC) trial [2], showed that even the sickest patients in the hospital (ICU patients with a 25% overall mortality rate) did no better with a 100 g/L trigger than with a 70 g/L trigger. What has been largely ignored in these large trials, however, is the average daily Hb concentration in the restrictive and liberal groups after the triggers are put into practice. If the trigger represents the Hb threshold for transfusion, the 'Hb target' is the desired Hb value after the transfusion [3].

The Hb target is also a means to assess the dose of blood given. Even with a perfect evidence-based, restrictive Hb transfusion trigger, if a large dose of blood is administered, the Hb target will exceed the evidence-based range. By encouraging single-unit red cell transfusions, practitioners can avoid exceeding the Hb target and conserve blood. The problem is that one must read the large randomised trial publications carefully to determine what Hb target was actually achieved in the liberal and restrictive groups. Figure 37.1 illustrates these findings and clearly shows that the average target Hb in these trials is often 10–15 g/L higher than the Hb trigger that defines the transfusion strategy. The FOCUS trial, for example, compared Hb triggers of 80 and 100 g/L, but the two groups ended up with Hb target concentrations of 95 and 110 g/L, respectively [4]. The results provided in the abstract of the publication can be

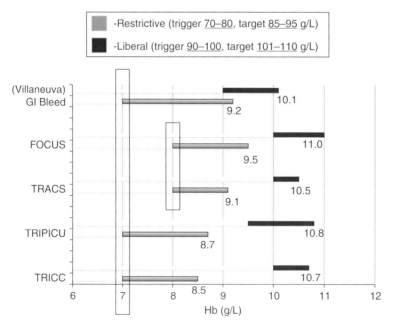

Figure 37.1 Haemoglobin (Hb) triggers (the Hb before transfusion) and Hb targets (the Hb after transfusion) are shown from the five large randomised trials [2,4,19–21] that compared restrictive and liberal transfusion strategies. Although the trial results advocate for the use of a restrictive transfusion strategy, with Hb triggers of 70–80 g/L for most patients, the Hb target concentration in the restrictive group was 85–95 g/L. When this finding is considered in the Functional Outcomes in Cardiovascular Patients Undergoing Surgical Hip Fracture Repair (FOCUS) trial, for example, the two groups compared (Hb trigger 80 versus 100 g/L) had actual daily average Hb concentrations that were 95 in the restrictive group and 110 g/L in the liberal group. (*See insert for colour representation of the figure.*)

deceiving because only the triggers are mentioned. In reality, we treat patients not numbers, so other factors like symptoms of anaemia, active bleeding and intravascular volume should be part of the transfusion decision process. One notable gap in the evidence base is data showing the ideal transfusion trigger for ischaemic heart syndromes. To date, for myocardial infarction patients, there have not been randomised trials, other than small feasibility pilot studies.

Because it is often difficult to collect accurate data on pre- and posttransfusion Hb levels, especially when patients receive multiple transfusions, some have advocated using trigger and target surrogate values that are easier to collect and analyse. The nadir Hb level for an entire hospital stay has been used as a surrogate for the Hb trigger, and the last Hb measured before discharge can be used as a surrogate for the Hb target. In reality, both the real trigger (Hb measured before transfusion) and the surrogate trigger could be misleading if the laboratory tests were not ordered, for example, during a bleeding episode. The same methods can be used for the international normalised ratio (INR) and plasma transfusions, or for platelet counts and platelet transfusions. However, this approach is limited because evidence is scant for bleeding outcomes and triggers based on laboratory tests alone for these blood components.

Blood Utilisation Metrics

Besides triggers and targets, other metrics commonly used to assess blood utilisation include the following (see Table 37.1).

1) *Average number of units transfused per patient*: this measure is calculated by dividing all transfused units by all patients. This measure has been used as the classic definition of 'blood utilisation' [5], perhaps because it correlates most closely with overall transfusion costs when adjusted for a facility's patient volume. This metric is probably the most useful method of tracking the success of a PBM programme. However, when used to compare providers to their peers, it is only useful if all providers are performing similar procedures on similar patients [6].

2) *Average number of units per transfused patient*: this measure is calculated by dividing the number of all transfused units by the number of all transfused patients. Although this metric is used in some PBM programmes, it is less useful than #1 above because it ignores all patients who avoid transfusion, often as a result of successful blood conservation measures.

3) *Percentage of patients transfused*: this measure is calculated by dividing the number of patients transfused by the total number of patients. As with # 1 above, this metric is most useful for comparing providers to their peers when they are all performing similar procedures in similar patients. However, it is less useful than #1 because, regardless of whether a given patient receives one or 10 units, he/she counts as only one transfused patient.

Sources of Data

Although it is possible to collect data from paper medical records, this process is arduous and useful only for random sampling of transfusion guideline compliance. With the increasing use of EMRs, data are plentiful but extraction can be challenging. A dedicated data manager with expertise in relational database management is ideal for extracting, analysing and preparing dashboards and reports to support PBM. The cost of putting in place an automated system for reporting blood utilisation can be substantial, and the data manager must continually monitor the system to keep pace with changes in the underlying databases and security requirements. Therefore, some institutions outsource this process. Specific EMRs offer their own reporting tools, which require additional training, but often an institution has multiple different computer systems and databases. Consequently, the reporting tool for one EMR is likely not adequate.

Another data source is the anaesthesia information management system [7], which is the term for the electronic anaesthesia records. The limitation of this data source is that only the intraoperative period is covered. We were surprised to learn that only about one-sixth of all transfused units are administered in the operating room at our institution (Johns Hopkins Hospital, Maryland, USA). In addition, transfusion triggers are often different during surgery, when many patients are actively bleeding.

For institutions that lack expertise, commercially available packages are available that are designed specifically for PBM programmes. The web-based blood management intelligence portal called IMPACT Online (Haemonetics Corp., Braintree, MA) is one such application, which outsources a large part of the data processing and reporting for PBM. The data are kept on a server at the company's headquarters, which receives hospital data monthly, packaged as text files derived from the hospital's blood transfusion laboratory and billing record databases. The reports and dashboards are then made available via a web portal. Most of the variables listed in Table 37.1 are included in IMPACT Online, and raw data can be exported in spreadsheet format, allowing the use of any chosen software package. Figure 37.2a was taken directly from the portal to illustrate the changes in Hb trigger compliance over a five-year time period. Figure 37.2b was created in Microsoft Excel from downloaded data. It shows the corresponding changes in blood utilisation (in red cell units per patient) for the 10 surgical services at Johns Hopkins Hospital [8]. Although red cell transfusions ordered with a preceding Hb level above 80 g/L (i.e. outside guidelines) decreased

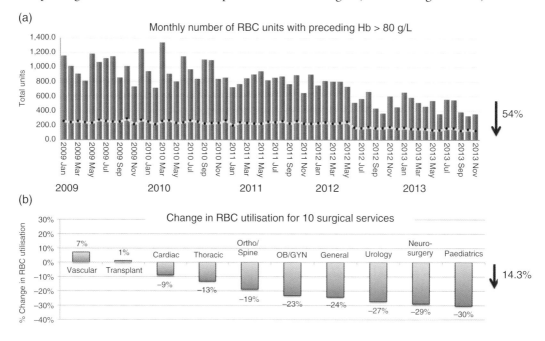

Figure 37.2 Effect of a patient blood management programme (PBM) on red blood cell utilisation. (a) The number of red cell units/month that were ordered with a preceding haemoglobin (Hb) >80 g/L is shown over a five-year period. With a multifaceted PBM programme that includes education, and computerised provider order entry with clinician decision support and a best practice alert, we achieved a 54% decrease in out-of-guideline red cell transfusions between the months of January 2009 and November 2013. (b) We also saw an overall decrease in red cell utilisation for eight out of 10 surgical services and an overall decrease in surgical blood utilisation of 14.3% over the same time period. *Source*: Modified from Zuckerberg et al. 2015 [8]. Reproduced with permission of John Wiley and Sons. (*See insert for colour representation of the figure.*)

by 54% over time, the change in overall blood utilisation (units per patient, averaging all 10 surgical services) was 14.3%. This discrepancy in rate of change is likely explained by timing and the dose of transfusions.

Data Extraction, Analysis and Presentation to Improve Practice

Extracting data from the EMR is often the hardest task. The data may be scattered across databases and across units within an institution. This lack of centrality introduces administrative and technical barriers. Extracting and merging these data require specialised skills, such as structured query language (SQL) programming. The simplest form of extracted data is a 'flat file', with one row per item of interest (e.g. patient admission). This format entails loss or aggregation of information, such as multiple surgical events per admission. For a typical analysis, the extracted data is imported into an application, which may be a spreadsheet programme, but more sophisticated tools may be needed, such as those provided by SAS or JMP (SAS Institute, Cary, NC), or Stata (StataCorp LP, College Station, TX). One useful application now is 'R' (www.r-project.org), a versatile statistical programming language that dates back to 1984 and is free to download. It has a steeper learning curve than other choices, but it has thousands of contributed add-on libraries for any imaginable data analysis or presentation task.

In our experience, the most effective method of showing data to providers is the rank order bar graph (Figure 37.3). When providers are compared directly to their peers [7], usually within their own specialty service, the individuals transfusing more blood, or to higher Hb values outside the evidence-based range, will want to change their practice to be closer to the mid range on the graph. It is debated whether to present such data with physician codes or with their names but the most impact occurs when names accompany the data. One lesson we have learned is that comparing surgeons by average Hb triggers and targets is better received than comparing surgeons to their peers by percentage of patients transfused, or by average number of units transfused per patient. To give an example, surgeon #44 (in Figure 37.3), with the highest average Hb trigger and target, had no idea where he stood on the Hb curve until we showed him the data. Afterward, his blood utilisation in average units per patient decreased by more than 60%.

Another effective method of presenting transfusion data is shown in Figure 37.4. We obtained the most recent measured pretransfusion Hb level (Hb trigger) by comparing the EMR timestamps of the laboratory tests and the transfusion orders. If no Hb test had been ordered within 24 hours before transfusion, then the trigger was considered to be missing. The various attending physicians in Figure 37.4 are shown in rank order by the number of red cell orders placed over the selected time period. The proportion of red cell orders is shown according to the Hb trigger levels: green shows the percentage of orders with a trigger <70 g/L; yellow, a trigger of 70–79 g/L; and red, a trigger ≥80 g/L. This method has been used in our institution for the past three years with great success. The same graphic presentation can be used to show the percentages of red cell orders that were placed for one unit or ≥2 unit units of red cells. Given that recent guidelines have emphasised a restrictive transfusion strategy and single-unit red cell transfusions in nonbleeding, haemodynamically stable patients [9], this rank order bar graph method with evidence-based, colour-coded depiction of guideline compliance is easy to interpret and can make a difference in improving practice.

Clinical Outcome Data

Nothing matters more than clinical outcomes, but these can be hard to capture. Morbid events, which are commonly assessed in PBM

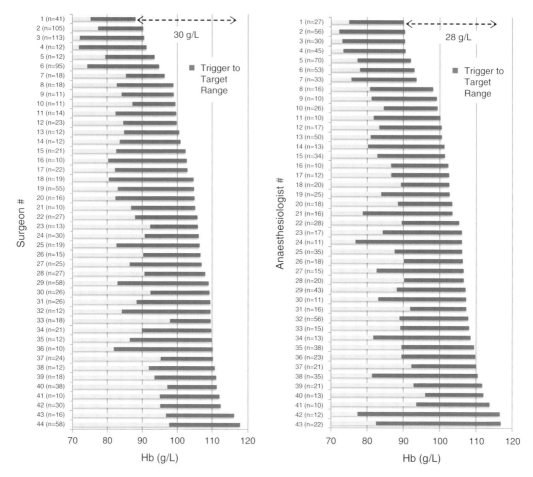

Figure 37.3 Comparison of mean transfusion haemoglobin (Hb) triggers and targets for all surgeons and anaesthesiologists who had 10 or more patients in the anaesthesia information management system (AIMS) database. The mean Hb triggers are designated by the left edge of the red bars and the mean Hb targets by the right edge of the red bars. The span between the lowest and highest Hb triggers was 26 g/L for surgeons and 24 g/L for anaesthesiologists. The span between lowest and highest Hb targets was 30 g/L for surgeons and 28 g/L for anaesthesiologists. *Source*: Modified from Frank et al. 2012 [7]. Reproduced with permission of Wolters Kluwer Health Inc. (*See insert for colour representation of the figure*.)

programmes, include those listed in Table 37.2. These 21 morbid events can be grouped into six major categories to ease interpretation and presentation of outcome data. If further simplification is needed, one can use a composite morbid event rate, which is a dichotomous outcome that includes the occurrence of any one of the individual morbid events.

In-hospital mortality is an important clinical outcome, and, unlike 30-day or one-year mortality, is obtainable from the EMR. It is clearly recognised that compared to nontransfused patients, transfused patients have a threefold higher composite morbid event rate and a ninefold higher in-hospital mortality rate (unpublished data from Johns Hopkins, 2009–15). Although morbidity and mortality are clearly *associated* with transfusion, it quickly becomes apparent that the transfused patients have more comorbidities and undergo more complex procedures [10].

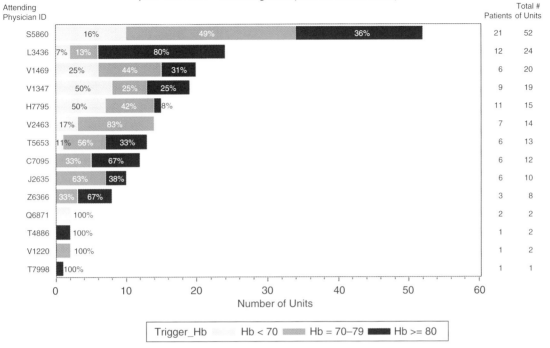

Department of Orthopaedics – Number and % of RBCs Given by Hb Trigger
(Oct–Dec 2014 – Excluding Intraoperative Transfusions)

Attending Physician ID	Total # Patients	# of Units
S5860	21	52
L3436	12	24
V1469	6	20
V1347	9	19
H7795	11	15
V2463	7	14
T5653	6	13
C7095	6	12
J2635	6	10
Z6366	3	8
Q6871	2	2
T4886	1	2
V1220	1	2
T7998	1	1

Trigger_Hb: Hb < 70 | Hb = 70–79 | Hb >= 80

Figure 37.4 These data were taken from the computerised provider order entry system. Individual physicians (y-axis) were compared by the number of red blood cell orders placed (x-axis) over a three-month time period, along with the percentage of orders placed by haemoglobin (Hb) trigger. The proportion of orders for which the most recent Hb preceding the order was <70 g/L is shown in green, 70–79 g/L in yellow and ≥80 g/L in red. An accompanying table for each department is provided showing the five-digit codes on the y-axis correspond to the names of attending physicians. (*See insert for colour representation of the figure.*)

Table 37.2 Clinical outcomes to assess in a PBM programme.

Morbid event category	Individual morbid events
Infections	Surgical site infection Drug-resistant infections Sepsis *C. difficile* infection
Thrombotic	Venous thrombotic event Pulmonary embolus Disseminated intravascular coagulation
Ischaemic	Myocardial infarction Transient ischaemic attack Cerebral vascular accident
Respiratory	Ventilator-associated pneumonia Acute respiratory distress syndrome
Renal	Renal insufficiency Renal failure – requiring renal replacement therapy
Transfusion-related morbidity	Transfusion-related acute lung injury Transfusion-associated cardiac overload Allergic reactions Haemolytic reactions Febrile nonhaemolytic reactions Bacterial contamination Hyperkalaemia

This phenomenon has been referred to as 'confounding by indication'. Thus, it becomes important to risk-adjust transfusion data.

Clinical outcome data may be collected and analysed from International Classification of Disease (ICD-9 or ICD-10) codes, which are determined by professional medical coders after patient discharge and entered into billing databases. Hospital-acquired morbid events of each type can be found by searching for a particular set of ICD-9 codes in the discharge data. Other sources of data that are prospectively collected include registry data, when hospitals participate in these programmes. The National Surgical Quality Improvement Program (NSQIP) and the Society for Thoracic Surgery (STS) registries are national examples that include outcome data. These registries take steps to ensure completeness and accuracy of data, whereas billing databases follow complicated rules that reflect reimbursement and regulatory obligations.

Risk Adjustment

Risk adjustment is critical when considering PBM data. Sicker patients and those who undergo more invasive procedures receive more transfusions, and they are also at risk for worse outcomes, hence the need to adjust any such outcomes with the patient-specific risk variables. In the 1980s, early attempts at risk adjustment included the Charlson Comorbidity Index [11]. ICD-9 codes can be converted to Charlson scores using statistical software packages (e.g. 'icd9' for R [Jack O. Wasey (2014). icd9: Tools for Working with ICD-9 Codes, and Finding Comorbidities. http://cran.r-project.org/web/packages/icd9/index.html]). This weighted score for patient comorbidities was shown to predict mortality over both a one-year and a 10-year time frame, and has also been shown to correlate with transfusion requirements.

A recent method of risk adjustment is the Case Mix Index (CMI). Created by the company 3M (Oakdale, MN), this diagnosis-related group (DRG)-based scoring system has evolved over the past two decades into the CMI values currently used to determine Medicare reimbursement – the All Patient Refined (APR)-DRG weighted score and the Medicare Severity (MS)-DRG weighted score [12,13]. These scores take into account both severity of illness and complexity of procedure, ultimately by using ICD-9 codes and patient characteristics. Our group has shown a strong relationship between these CMI numbers and utilisation of red cells, plasma and platelets (Figure 37.5) [5]. Thus, it is helpful to track CMI changes over time as a PBM data variable. The CMI also helps with benchmarking one institution's blood utilisation data against that of others, as this type of risk adjustment can account for differences in blood use caused by case mix alone.

Crossmatch-to-Transfusion Ratio

Since the concept of a maximum surgical blood order schedule (MSBOS) was first described in the mid-1970s, efforts have been made to optimise the process of ordering blood before surgery. The original MSBOS was created using data from 300 hospitals to determine the ideal blood orders for 50 common surgical procedures [14]. Using electronic anaesthesia records that accurately record transfusion data, we have described methods for creating an institution-specific MSBOS with 135 unique categories of surgical procedures [15]. We have since shown that updating the MSBOS in this fashion can reduce unnecessary preoperative blood ordering and result in substantial cost savings, especially for cases that are never or rarely transfused [16]. Ideally, the methods we describe will allow other facilities to create their own institution-specific MSBOS using data from their anaesthesia information management systems.

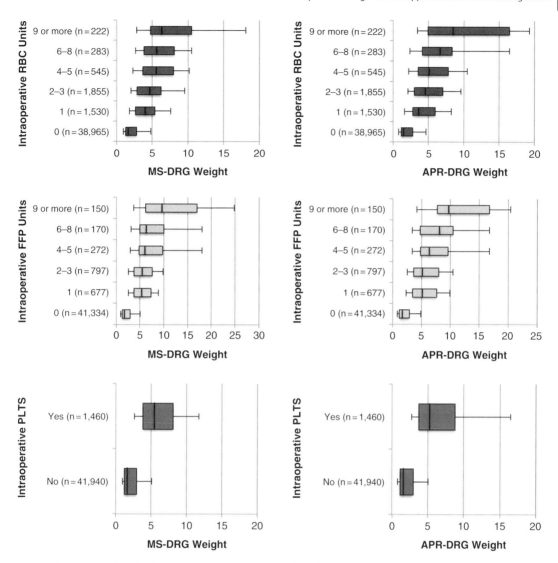

Figure 37.5 Intraoperative blood component requirements are plotted as a function of Case Mix Index (CMI). Left side: CMI is represented by the weighted Medicare Severity Diagnosis-Related Group (MS-DRG Weight). Right side: CMI is represented by the weighted All Patient Refined Diagnosis-Related Group (APR-DRG Weight). The data show a clear relationship between a higher CMI value and greater intraoperative transfusion requirements for red blood cells, fresh frozen plasma (FFP) and platelets (PLTS). Differences in CMI values among transfusion requirement groups are significant for all six analyses shown (P < 0.0001). *Source*: Modified from Stonemetz et al. 2014 [5]. Reproduced with permission of John Wiley and Sons. (*See insert for colour representation of the figure.*)

Preoperative Anaemia Screening and Management

Various performance measures designed to diagnose and treat preoperative anaemia before elective surgical procedures have been proposed. For example, the Joint Commission (the hospital-accrediting body in the United States) has proposed, but not yet mandated, that patients who are scheduled for elective surgery and have a high probability of requiring a blood transfusion have their Hb level tested between 45 and 14 days before the procedure. The data typically collected to satisfy such performance measures include a numerator (number of patients with anaemia screening) and a denominator (number of patients scheduled for surgery). Recently, this measure has been proposed, along with other PBM performance measures, with the aim of collecting such data from electronic health records. Because of the electronic data source for these performance measures, they have been termed 'electronic PBM (ePBM) performance measures'.

Conclusion

The variety and volume of data that can be collected to support a PBM programme are almost limitless. The challenge is to extract these data and focus on variables that will have the greatest ability to promote evidence-based practice. The methods of presenting data to providers are critical. Because blood transfusion is the most common procedure performed in US hospitals [17], and has also been named one of the five most overused procedures [18], managing its use has great potential to reduce risks, improve outcomes and reduce cost. Because quality/cost = value, a successful PBM programme will be an asset to any hospital or health system.

KEY POINTS

1) When assessing compliance with transfusion guidelines, the Hb target (after the transfusion) is equally as important as the Hb trigger (prior to transfusion). The Hb target is usually 10–15 g/L higher than the trigger in the randomised clinical trials that support a restrictive transfusion strategy.

2) The most useful blood utilisation metric to determine the impact of a PBM programme is the average number of units/patient, as this parameter inherently adjusts for changes in case load or hospital inpatient case volume.

3) Comparing providers to peers within their specialty service for haemoglobin transfusion triggers and targets is an effective method of presenting data to improve practice.

4) Clinical outcomes that should be assessed in a PBM programme include mortality, length of stay and morbid events. Morbid events can be obtained from ICD-9 or ICD-10 codes in the hospital's billing database.

5) Variables used to risk-adjust blood utilisation data include the Charlson Comorbidity Index and the Case Mix Index. CASE MIX INDEX adjusts for both complexity of procedure and severity of illness.

References

1 Stonemetz JL. 2013 AIMS Market Update. American Society of Anesthesiologists Newsletter 2013;77.

2 Hebert PC, Wells G, Blajchman MA et al. A multicenter, randomized, controlled clinical trial of transfusion requirements in critical care. Transfusion Requirements in Critical Care Investigators, Canadian Critical Care Trials Group. N Engl J Med 1999;**340**:409–17.

3 Frank SM, Resar LM, Rothschild JA, Dackiw EA, Savage WJ, Ness PM. A novel method of data analysis for utilization of red blood cell transfusion. Transfusion 2013;**53**:3052–9.

4 Carson JL, Terrin ML, Noveck H et al. Liberal or restrictive transfusion in high-risk patients after hip surgery. N Engl J Med 2011;**365**:2453–62.

5 Stonemetz JL, Allen PX, Wasey J, Rivers RJ, Ness PM, Frank SM. Development of a risk-adjusted blood utilization metric. Transfusion 2014;**54**:2716–23.

6 Yazer MH, Waters JH. How do I implement a hospital-based blood management program? Transfusion 2012;**52**:1640–5.

7 Frank SM, Savage WJ, Rothschild JA et al. Variability in blood and blood component utilization as assessed by an anesthesia information management system. Anesthesiology 2012;**117**:99–106.

8 Zuckerberg GS, Scott AV, Wasey JO et al. Efficacy of education followed by computerized provider order entry with clinician decision support to reduce red blood cell utilization. Transfusion 2015;**55**(7):1628–36.

9 Choosing Wisely. Available at: www.aabb.org/pbm/Documents/Choosing-Wisely-Five-Things-Physicians-and-Patients-Should-Question.pdf (accessed 17 November 2016).

10 Carson JL, Hebert PC. Here we go again – blood transfusion kills patients? Comment on "Association of blood transfusion with increased mortality in myocardial infarction: a meta-analysis and diversity-adjusted study sequential analysis". JAMA Intern Med 2013;**173**:139–41.

11 Charlson ME, Pompei P, Ales KL, MacKenzie CR. A new method of classifying prognostic comorbidity in longitudinal studies: development and validation. J Chronic Dis 1987;**40**:373–83.

12 Baram D, Daroowalla F, Garcia R et al. Use of the All Patient Refined-Diagnosis Related Group (APR-DRG) Risk of Mortality Score as a severity adjustor in the medical ICU. Clin Med Circ Respirat Pulm Med 2008;**2**:19–25.

13 Bush H. How hospitals can prepare for the new MS-DRGs. Hosp Health Netw 2008;**82**:5 p following 44.

14 Friedman BA. An analysis of surgical blood use in United States hospitals with application to the maximum surgical blood order schedule. Transfusion 1979;**19**:268–78.

15 Frank SM, Rothschild JA, Masear CG et al. Optimizing preoperative blood ordering with data acquired from an anesthesia information management system. Anesthesiology 2013;**118**:1286–97.

16 Frank SM, Oleyar MJ, Ness PM, Tobian AA. Reducing unnecessary preoperative blood orders and costs by implementing an updated institution-specific maximum surgical blood order schedule and a remote electronic blood release system. Anesthesiology 2014;**121**:501–9.

17 Healthcare Cost and Utilization Project. Available at: www.hcup-us.ahrq.gov/reports/statbriefs/sb149.pdf

18 Joint Commission. National Summit on Overuse, 2012. Available at: www.jointcommission.org/assets/transcripts/Overuse_Summit_Chassin_transcript.pdf (accessed 17 November 2016).

19 Hajjar LA, Vincent JL, Galas FR et al. Transfusion requirements after cardiac surgery: the TRACS randomized controlled trial. JAMA 2010;**304**:1559–67.

20 Lacroix J, Hebert PC, Hutchison JS et al. Transfusion strategies for patients in pediatric intensive care units. N Engl J Med 2007;**356**:1609–19.

21 Villanueva C, Colomo A, Bosch A et al. Transfusion strategies for acute upper gastrointestinal bleeding. N Engl J Med 2013;**368**:11–21.

Further Reading

Choosing Wisely. Available at: www.aabb.org/pbm/Documents/Choosing-Wisely-Five-Things-Physicians-and-Patients-Should-Question.pdf (accessed 17 November 2016).

Carson JL, Guyatt G, Heddle NM, et al. Clinical Practice Guidelines From the AABB: Red Blood Cell Transfusion Thresholds and Storage. JAMA 2016;**316**:2025–35.

Carson JL, Carless PA, Hebert PC. Outcomes using lower vs higher hemoglobin thresholds for red blood cell transfusion. JAMA 2013;**309**:83–4.

Gammon HM, Waters JH, Watt A, Loeb JM, Donini-Lenhoff A. Developing performance measures for patient blood management. Transfusion 2011;**51**:2500–9.

Goodnough LT, Shander A. Patient blood management. Anesthesiology 2012;**116**:1367–76.

Joint Commission. Electronic Patient Blood Management Performance Measures. Available at: www.jointcommission.org/electronic_clinical_quality_measures_for_patient_blood_management/(accessed 17 November 2016).

Kaufman RM, Djulbegovic B, Gernsheimer T et al. Platelet transfusion: a clinical practice guideline from the AABB. Ann Intern Med 2015;**162**:205–13.

Roback JD, Caldwell S, Carson J et al. Evidence-based practice guidelines for plasma transfusion. Transfusion 2010;**50**:1227–39.

Shander A, Fink A, Javidroozi M et al. Appropriateness of allogeneic red blood cell transfusion: the international consensus conference on transfusion outcomes. Transfus Med Rev 2011;**25**:232–46, e53.

Waters JH, Ness PM. Patient blood management: a growing challenge and opportunity. Transfusion 2011;**51**:902–3.

38

Regulation and Accreditation in Cellular Therapy

Zbigniew (Ziggy) M. Szczepiorkowski[1] and Daniel Hollyman[2]

[1] *Transfusion Medicine Service, Cellular Therapy Center, Dartmouth-Hitchcock Medical Center and Geisel School of Medicine at Dartmouth, Hanover, USA*
[2] *Diagnostics Development and Reference Services, NHS Blood and Transplant, Bristol, UK*

Introduction

In recent years there have been considerable advances in cellular therapies. The most widely used type of cellular therapy has been haematopoietic stem cell transplantation (HSCT) from its inception in 1968. In many cases, patients with haematological and nonhaematological diseases are cured after HSCT. There have also been considerable advances in the immunotherapy of cancer and viral infections and in the use of cellular therapy for tissue regeneration and repair.

A number of different agencies and professional bodies are involved in the regulation and accreditation of cellular therapy in the US and Europe. The regulations and standards depend on the source of the cell to be transplanted, the way it is used and the nature of any manipulations carried out. As a result of this, the last two decades have seen a seemingly bewildering growth in regulatory and accreditation requirements and these have put pressure on both clinical and laboratory services.

The drivers for these are:

- traceability of products from donor to recipient
- microbiological safety (related to donor/patient as well as collection/processing)
- enhanced product quality
- consistent measures of product function.

There are multiple organisations involved in the process of accreditation and standard setting of HSCT programmes. Figure 38.1 illustrates the timeline of this involvement by different organisations.

Haematopoietic Stem Cell Transplant Activity

The numbers of transplants have increased considerably in recent years so that between 50 000 and 70 000 are performed each year. The majority are autologous and related (usually sibling) donor procedures, although the number of transplants using unrelated donor stem cells increased from 3237 in 1997 to over 12 000 in 2015. The overall number of unrelated donors available on international registries increased from 4.8 to over 26 million during that time period [1]. In the last 10–15 years, there has been a switch to the use of peripheral blood progenitor cells (PBPC), which are now regarded as the source of choice in 98% of autografts and 74% of allografts in Europe, as well as a great increase in the use of cord blood (CB) units so that, in patients under the age of 16, they now account for 30% of transplants and their use has stabilised in adults.

In 1990, 4200 HSCTs were reported to the European Blood and Marrow Transplant Group

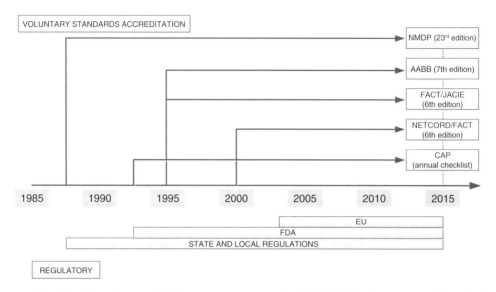

Figure 38.1 Timeline of involvement of different organisations in the field of cellular therapy. AABB (formerly the American Association of Blood Banks); CAP, College of American Pathologists; FACT, Foundation for the Accreditation of Cellular Therapy; EU, European Union; FDA, US Food and Drug Administration; JACIE, Joint Accreditation Committee (ISCT and EBMT); NMDP, National Marrow Donor Program.

(EBMT), a number that had risen by 2013 to 39 209. Autologous transplants comprised 57% of these and 43% were allografts; 37% of first-time allografts are now from identical siblings and 53% from unrelated donors. HSCT has increased in all diseases reported to the EBMT and Center for International Blood and Marrow Transplant Research (CIBMTR), with the exception of chronic myeloid leukaemia (CML), where the advent of the tyrosine kinase inhibitor imatinib has reduced numbers (see Chapter 41). Furthermore, there is a continuing increase in haploidentical transplants, both in Europe and in the US (Figure 38.2).

The Structure of SCT Programmes

Figure 38.3 shows the journey of an allogeneic stem cell product from a registry or sibling donor or CB unit where a blood sample is typed in the histocompatibility and immunogenetics (H&I) laboratory to determine the HLA type,

via the marrow, peripheral blood or CB collection facility and the cell processing laboratory to the clinical transplant unit. The many relevant accreditation and regulatory bodies and their areas of involvement in HSCT are shown.

European Union Directives and Legislation

Documents published in Europe in 1978 and 1994 stressed the need for international standardisation of tissue and cell collection practices and the harmonisation of legislation relating to the collection and transplantation of substances of human origin. It was recommended that there should be functional definitions of tissue banks and that such banks should be non-profit-making and licenced by national health authorities; the cells collected should be tested for infectious disease markers (IDMs); appropriate records should be kept and there should be consent for removal or collection of cells and tissues.

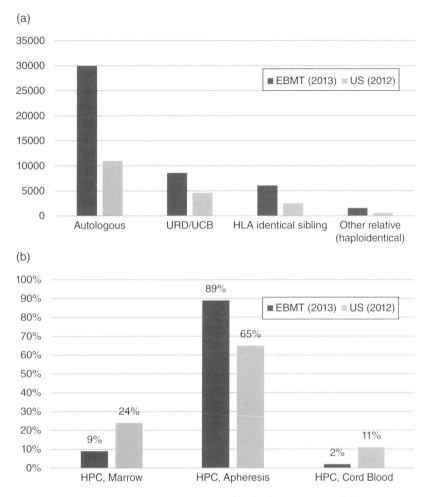

Figure 38.2 Comparison of the types of HSCT (a) and source of grafts (b) in Europe and the US in 2013 and 2012, respectively. HPC, haematopoietic progenitor cells; UCB, umbilical cord blood unit; URD, unrelated donor. *Source:* Adapted from Pasquini and Zhu 2014 [23] and Passweg et al. 2015 [24].

In 2004, the European Union (EU) Directive on Tissues and Cells was published as Directive 2004/23/EC [2]. In 2006, two technical annexes supplying more detailed information were published as Commission Directives 2006/17/EC (donation, procurement and testing) and 2006/86/EC (coding, processing, preservation, storage and distribution) [3,4]. The Directives are legally binding with a requirement that they are transposed into European law.

In 2005, Competent Authorities (CA) were appointed or established in the UK and other European Member States and these subsequently became responsible for the licencing of facilities storing tissues or cells. In the UK, the Human Tissue (Quality and Safety for Human Application) Regulations, which translate the EU Directive into UK law, were published in 2006 and 2007; all three directives were fully implemented. Of relevance to HSC transplantation and immunotherapy, the following cells and tissues are included within the scope of the Directive:

- haematopoietic stem cells from peripheral blood, bone marrow and CB
- donor leucocytes and other cellular therapies
- adult and embryonic stem cells.

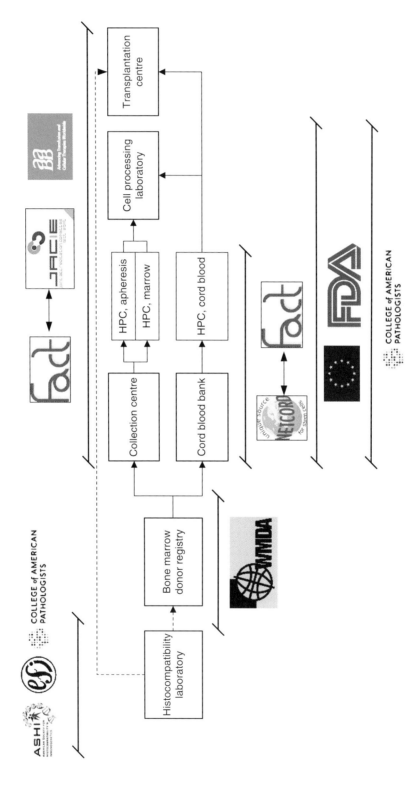

Figure 38.3 Regulatory environment for haematopoietic stem cell transplantation. Note that this figure does not reflect all potential regulatory reporting requirements for transplantation centres. (*See insert for colour representation of the figure.*)

The various sections of the Directive describe:

- the requirements for the person in charge of a cellular therapy or tissue facility (the responsible person or designated individual)
- the arrangements for the facility itself and its staffing
- the role of the CA and the need for twice-yearly inspections
- the requirements for consent
- traceability with retention of key records for a period of 30 years
- the reporting of adverse events and reactions to the CA
- conditions to be met when stem cells are imported or exported.

The Human Tissue (HT) Act 2004

This key piece of legislation serves as a good example of how national legislation for cell and tissue collection and processing operates [5,6]. It was introduced in the UK in 2006, repealing and replacing the HT Act of 1961 as well as the Anatomy Act (1989) and Human Organ Transplants Act (1989). It established the Human Tissue Authority (HTA) as the CA for the UK. Its aim is to regulate the collection, testing, storage, use and disposal of human bodies, body parts, organs and tissues.

The HT Act ensured that consent became the fundamental principle underpinning the lawful storage and use of organs and tissues. In addition, the Act also applies to the removal of transplantable material from the deceased. Consent is required when tissue is removed from the living or deceased for the purposes of:

- anatomical examination
- determining the cause of death
- obtaining scientific or medical information about a person relevant to another
- public display
- research in connection with disorders or functioning of the human body (unless the material is made anonymous and for specific, ethically-approved research)
- transplantation.

The HT Act is supported by two governmental regulations (Statutory Instruments 2006 no. 1659 (37) and 2006 no. 1260 (38)), directions issued by the HTA to help explain and interpret the Act and also a number of Codes of Practice, of which three are particularly relevant to cell and tissue therapies [7]:

- Code 1: Consent
- Code 5: Disposal of human tissue
- Code 6: Donation of allogeneic bone marrow and peripheral blood stem cells for transplantation.

Obtaining legally valid consent is extremely important and the HT Act states that it is a positive act, that it is voluntary and may be withdrawn at any time (other than where a tissue has already been used). Appropriate information should be provided and the person giving consent must have the capacity to do so. Children may consent if they are competent to do so. Consent prior to death is sufficient for organ and tissue donation and relatives have no legal right to overrule such consent. From December 2015, the Human Transplantation (Wales) Act 2013 allows the use of deemed consent for deceased organ and tissue donation in Wales (where no record of a person's decision on organ donation is held, they will be deemed to have given their consent, with some notable exemptions as detailed in the Code of Practice on the Human Transplantation (Wales) Act) [8].

United States Food and Drug Administration

The Food and Drug Administration (FDA) of the Department of Health and Human Services of the USA has been involved in the area of cellular therapy since the early 1990s [9]. The FDA recognised the need for regulatory oversight in the area of cell, gene and tissue therapies and products. Initial guidance documents were issued based on the Public Health Service Act, Section 361 (42 USC 264).

FDA Good Tissue Practice (GTP) Regulations for human cells, tissues and tissue-based products (HCT/Ps) require institutions shipping

HPC, Cord Blood; HPC, Apheresis; and TC, Apheresis, but not HPC, Marrow, to be registered with the FDA as manufacturers. There are specific requirements for donors who may be eligible/ineligible based on a suitability determination and defined in final guidance documents (see below). An annual update is required.

The regulatory approach implemented by the FDA based on the 1997 proposal for regulation included cellular therapy products (named HCT/P – human cells, tissues and tissue-based products) with gene therapy and tissues rather than with blood components. This different approach had significant implications for the field by defining minimal requirements for establishments involved in manufacturing of HCT/P. The FDA also introduced a concept of risk assessment which includes: (1) the relationship between the donor and the recipient (i.e. autologous, allogeneic related, allogeneic unrelated); (2) the amount of processing and manipulation (non-manipulated, minimally-manipulated and more than minimally-manipulated); and (3) the purpose for which the tissues are used (homologous and non-homologous use, where homologous use is defined as repair, replacement or supplementation of a recipient's cells or tissues with an HCT/P that performs the same basic functions in the recipient as in the donor).

The last of the aspects of risk assessment has been debated by the cellular therapy community as one that potentially assigns a different level of regulatory scrutiny based on the intended use despite equivalent risk in the first two areas, such as donor and the level of manipulation.

For very practical reasons, it is common amongst cellular therapy practitioners in the US to discuss products as '351' and '361' products. This nomenclature relates to two different sections of the Public Health Service Act. The 361 products are covered in 21 Code of Federal Regulations (CFR) 1271 A, B, C, D, E, F (i.e. Good Tissue Practice), whilst the 351 products are covered in multiple regulations including 21 CFR 1271 C, D; 21 CFR 207.20 (f); 21 CFR 210–211; 21 CFR 807.20 (d); 21 CFR 820.1 (a); 21 CFR 312 (investigational new drug regulations (IND)) and others. The 361 products are defined as (1) minimally manipulated; (2) intended for homologous use; (3) not involving combination with a drug or a device, except for a sterilising, preserving or storage agent, if the agent does not raise new clinical safety concerns and (4) not having a systemic effect and not dependent upon the metabolic activity of living cells for its primary function, or has a systemic effect and is for autologous use, or for allogeneic use in a first-degree and second-degree blood relative or for reproductive use. All products that do not fulfil these requirements are considered 351 products.

Based on the assignment of 351 and 361 products, there are different requirements for biological product deviation reporting.

It is important to note that there are tissues excluded from 21 CFR 1271 that include vascularied organs; whole blood and blood components; human milk and minimally-manipulated bone marrow. Thus, HPC, Marrow (minimally-manipulated) is regulated by a different set of regulations, which are under the authority of the Health Resources and Services Administration (HRSA).

For a thorough discussion of FDA regulatory activities and current guidance documents, the reader is referred to the agency website: www.fda.gov/BiologicsBloodVaccines/default.htm.

The ultimate goal of the FDA regulatory structure is to bring cellular therapy products to the licenced status. In October 2009, the FDA issued the guidance document regarding the biological licenced application for HPC, Cord Blood. The regulations required that after October 2011, all CB units would be either licenced by the CB banks or issued based on the IND [10] (see the guidance document for more information). These requirements led to a significant effort by the CB banks to submit a biological licenced application (BLA) to the FDA for approval. At the time of writing (November 2015), only five products (Hemacord (New York Blood Center); HPC Cord Blood (University of Colorado Medical School), Duracord (Duke University School of Medicine), Allocord (SSM Cardinal Glennon Children's Medical Center) and HPC, Cord Blood (LifeSouth Community Blood Centers, Inc.)) have been licenced. Only two new CB products were licenced in the period November 2012 to November 2015. There is growing concern that many CB banks would not be able to meet the heavy burden of BLA and the licencing process.

The CB units that are not licenced are issued under IND protocol (e.g. NMDP is a holder of one of the INDs).

Non-governmental (Voluntary) Accreditation

Many programmes elect to be accredited by one of the voluntary accrediting organisations, in addition to observing governmental regulations.

There are multiple reasons for voluntary accreditation, ranging from recognition by healthcare insurance providers for reimbursement purposes, through to improved quality of care to fulfilling requirements by some of the local governmental regulations (e.g. Commonwealth of Massachusetts requires FACT accreditation from all transplantation centres). The NHS England Clinical Commissioning Policy for Haematopoietic Stem Cell Transplantation now requires HSCT providers to be JACIE accredited [11].

All accrediting organisations require adherence to local and governmental laws and regulations in addition to individual standards established by each of them. The published standards, which are typically updated in defined time intervals, describe a minimum level of expectations. Table 38.1 summarises major differences

Table 38.1 Overview of voluntary accreditation/registry organisations (see individual websites to identify accredited centres, laboratories and registries as these data change often).

	FACT	JACIE	NetCord/FACT	AABB	CAP	NMDP	WMDA
Membership	No	No	No	No	No	Yes	Yes
Accreditation	Yes	Yes	Yes	Yes	Yes	No	Yes
Scope							
Registries	na	na	na	na	na	na	++
Recruitment	na	na	na	na	na	++	+
Donor	+	+	++	+	+	++	++
Collection	++	++	++	++	++	++	+
Processing	++	++	++	++	++	++	na
Transplantation	++	++	na	+	na	++	na
Products							
HPC, Apheresis	Yes	Yes	No	Yes	Yes	Yes	Yes
HPC, Marrow	Yes	Yes	No	Yes	Yes	Yes	Yes
HPC, Cord Blood	No	No	Yes	Yes	Yes	Yes	Yes
TC, Lymphocytes	Yes	Yes	No	Yes	Yes	Yes	No
Other CTCs	Yes	Yes	No	Yes	No	No	No
Standards structure	Checklist	Checklist	Checklist	ISO based	Checklist	Checklist	Checklist
Current edition/version	6th	6th	6th	7th	2015	23rd	2014

AABB, formerly American Association for Blood Banks; CAP, College of American Pathologists; CTC, cellular therapy products; FACT, Foundation for the Accreditation of Cellular Therapy; JACIE, Joint Accreditation Committee (ISCT and EBMT); NMDP, National Marrow Donor Program; WMDA, World Marrow Donor Association.

(and similarities) between different accrediting organisations.

Standards are prepared by a group of experts within the organisation, typically called the Standards Committee, which established minimum expectations for the facilities willing to participate in the accrediting programme. Once the final version of the standards is approved, a tool is created, which is used during the inspection process.

The accreditation process generally consists of three phases: phase I – the application step, when the applicant facility submits necessary documentation to the accrediting body and certifies that it is compliant with the standards; phase II – the confirmation step, when the accrediting body using on-site inspection confirms that the applicant facility truly follows the standards and phase III – the recognition step, when a certificate of accreditation is issued based on the documentation submitted and the results of on-site inspection and, if necessary, satisfying responses to identified shortcomings in the applicant facility. The accreditation certificate has an expiry date and stipulates that if there are any significant changes in the programme structure and/or performance, these will be promptly reported to the accrediting body. Each of the accrediting organisations may have additional requirements.

FACT and JACIE

In 1994, the Foundation for Accreditation of Cell Therapy (FACT) in the US initiated a voluntary inspection and accreditation scheme for cell therapy facilities. Five years later, its European counterpart, the Joint Accreditation Committee of the ISCT (International Society for Cell Therapy) and EBMT (JACIE), was founded. FACT–JACIE is a voluntary system that accredits clinical transplant programmes as well as the cell collection, processing and banking elements that are covered by current EU legislation [12,13]. Whilst FACT–JACIE accreditation is not compulsory, there are pressures for the clinical, collection and laboratory parts of HSCT programmes to comply with

their requirements in some countries. These include purchasing agreements with healthcare funders. The primary aim of FACT and JACIE is to improve the quality of HSCT through external inspection of facilities to ensure compliance with the FACT–JACIE standards. A further aim is to ensure consistency between these standards and other national and international standards, including the EU Tissues and Cells Directive (Directive 2004/23/EC) and the related Commission Directives 2006/17/EC and 2006/86/EC (see above).

FACT–JACIE accreditation is voluntary, but provides a means whereby transplant facilities can demonstrate that they are working within a quality system that covers all aspects of the transplantation process. Accreditation of HPC transplant facilities is through online submission of documentation and centres may apply for accreditation as complete programmes comprising a clinical programme, collection facility and processing laboratory or, for example, as a single collection or processing facility that may serve a number of clinical programmes.

FACT–JACIE Standards

The 6th edition of the standards was published in 2015 and covers all aspects of clinical transplant programmes, bone marrow and peripheral blood stem cell collection facilities, as well as processing laboratories. The standards also apply to the use of therapeutic cells (TC) derived from the peripheral blood or bone marrow, including donor lymphocytes and mesenchymal stem cells. The standards cover the clinical use of HPC(CB) by clinical programmes, but not the collection or banking of CB, which is covered by the related NetCord–FACT standards and inspected and accredited by NetCord–FACT (see below). The standards are available on the FACT and JACIE websites, and contain essential principles that apply throughout.

- Establishment and maintenance of a quality management programme.
- Requirement for documentation of policies, procedures, actions and requests, which extends

to all aspects of transplant activity. Personnel must not only be appropriately qualified, they must be trained in the procedures they regularly perform and their competency to perform the task after training must be assessed and documented.

- Validation of all equipment and procedures. Validation is a term used to describe the activity required to prove that any procedure, process, equipment, material, activity or system actually leads to the expected results. For example, a new apheresis machine must be shown to produce the expected results in terms of cell yields. The most recent version added stronger requirements for outcome analysis and donor follow-up, amongst other changes (see FACT and JACIE website for details).

Quality Management

An active quality management programme (QMP) is essential to the FACT–JACIE standards. A QMP is a mechanism to ensure that procedures are being carried out by all staff members in line with agreed standards and to maintain this standard of practice. In a transplant programme, this ensures that the clinical, collection and laboratory units are all working together to achieve good communication, effective common work practices and increased guarantees for patients. It is a means of rapidly identifying errors or accidents and resolving them so that the possibility of repetition is minimised. It assists in training and clearly identifies the roles and responsibilities of all staff. The culture and systems for quality management are well established in laboratories but are relatively new in clinical units and it is recommended that HSCT programmes have dedicated quality managers.

Experience of Centres Implementing FACT and JACIE

It was anticipated that implementation of the FACT–JACIE standards would pose some difficulties for applicant centres, particularly in relation to establishing a quality management system (QMS). To assess this in Europe, a survey was designed to assess the difficulties experienced by centres in preparing for JACIE accreditation. The results showed that the most difficult part of preparation was implementing the quality management (QM) system, adverse event reporting system and other documentation. All centres felt that accreditation was worth the effort invested. In addition, with the implementation of the EU Directive on Safety of Tissues and Cells (2004/23/EC), it is likely that collection and processing facilities will increasingly view compliance with JACIE standards as important in providing evidence that they are complying with the requirements of the Directive.

A detailed analysis of transplant outcome in 107 000 European patients transplanted between 1999 and 2007 showed that acquisition of JACIE accreditation was associated with improvement in overall patient survival. However, two recent studies interestingly showed different results as to the value of accreditation. It remains unclear whether accreditation status translates into better patient outcomes, but it is quite well established that accredited centres have a higher level of organisational prowess and better preparation of external inspections [14,15].

NetCord–FACT

In the same way that FACT and JACIE cooperate to produce a globally agreed set of standards and a guidance manual for accreditation of HSCT programmes, FACT collaborates with NetCord, which is an international organisation for CB banking [16]. Their combined international standards, first issued in 2000, are the gold standard for CB banks worldwide. The most recent standards (6th edition) were published in 2016.

American Association of Blood Banks (AABB)

Established in 1947, the AABB is an international, not-for-profit association dedicated to the advancement of science and the practice of transfusion medicine and related biological therapies. The AABB approach to the field of cellular therapies has aimed to balance flexibility in an outcome-based approach with the need for rigorous evidence-based standards. The standards are written using an ISO-based template. The 10 chapter headings are based on the AABB Quality System Essentials (QSEs), published in 1997 as AABB Association Bulletin 97-4. The 10 QSEs correlate directly with ISO. The AABB Standards for Cellular Therapy Services (7th edition published in 2015) [17], which are revised and updated every 24 months, cover all cellular therapy products and cell sources including autologous, allogeneic and cadaveric donors, including, for the first time, clinical services. AABB also coordinates the production of a cell therapy product Circular of Information (COI) [18].

Under a QM system approach, each chapter progresses from general policies to specific procedures. The chapters are:

- Organisation
- Resources
- Equipment
- Agreements
- Process Control
- Documents and Records
- Deviations and Nonconforming Products or Services
- Internal and External Assessments
- Process Improvement
- Safety and Facilities.

The AABB accreditation is valid for two years and each accredited institution is assessed every 24 months. Recently, the AABB, following other accrediting organisations, introduced unannounced assessments. These occur on any day within 90 days of the accreditation expiry date.

College of American Pathologists

The College of American Pathologists (CAP) is a medical society serving nearly 16 000 physician members and the laboratory community throughout the world [19]. It is the world's largest association composed exclusively of pathologists and is widely considered the leader in laboratory quality assurance. More than 6000 laboratories are accredited by the CAP and approximately 23 000 laboratories are enrolled in the College's proficiency testing programmes. There are two proficiency tests currently offered for cellular therapy products: Stem Cell Test and Cord Blood Test.

The CAP primarily accredits laboratories in clinical and anatomical pathology, but the accreditation process also includes other entities such as cellular therapy laboratories, HLA laboratories and reproductive laboratories.

The accreditation process, called the Laboratory Accreditation Program, is based on fulfilling the CAP checklist (self-assessment and on-site inspection), which consists of three major parts: the discipline-specific checklist(s), the laboratory general checklist and the all common checklists. Each checklist component consists of subject header, declarative statement and evidence of compliance. The questions on tissue banking were added to the transfusion medicine checklist in 1993. There were five questions covering (1) the authority, responsibility and accountability of the programme; (2) processing and infectious disease testing for each tissue stored; (3) procedures defining storage conditions of the different tissues handled and retention of records; (4) records showing proper storage conditions and (5) records allowing for identification of the donor and recipient for each tissue handled. In 2004, the CAP expanded the tissues and the haematopoietic progenitor cells sections of the checklist. In general, new editions of CAP checklists are released once a year, however, some important updates can be issued more frequently.

The CAP inspection is performed every other year and generally lasts two days. The accredited facilities are also required to perform self-evaluation in the year when there is no on-site inspection.

World Marrow Donor Association

The World Marrow Donor Association (WMDA) is an international organisation that publishes standards to which HSCT donor registries wishing to achieve accreditation for their activities must adhere [20]. These standards are available on the WMDA website (www.worldmarrow.org). Important areas described by the standards include general organisation of the donor registry, donor recruitment, assessment, counselling, histocompatibility and immunogenetic characterisation of donors, other testing, including an infectious disease marker, IT requirements, donor searches, collection and transport of cells. At the present time, accreditation is given after a detailed review of documentation submitted by the registry by independent reviewers, but site visits are not done, although a pilot scheme to introduce them is under way. Accreditation is valid for five years.

Histocompatibility Accreditation [21,22]

The American Society for Histocompatibility and Immunogenetics (ASHI) and its European counterpart, the European Federation of Immunogenetics (EFI), accredit H&I laboratories after reviewing documentation and conducting a site visit. The College of American Pathologists also accredits histocompatibility laboratories. The accreditation by CAP fulfils requirements of the National Marrow Donor Program 23rd edition of standards (October 2015), but at the time of writing has not been accepted by the FACT–JACIE standards. This creates an unfortunate situation where the transplant programmes cannot utilise CAP-accredited histocompatibility laboratories for HLA testing.

Conclusion: How Do HSCT Programmes Respond to the Challenge?

The requirements of regulatory and accreditation bodies place huge demands on transplant programmes. In some cases, they may need to construct new and improved facilities for HSC collection, processing and storage. A key feature is the need to develop robust quality management programmes as described above, which will include detailed policies and procedures to cover all their activities. Initial staff training and ensuring ongoing competency are crucial. HSCT programmes should remember that deficiencies commonly found at inspection involve the QMP, policies and procedures, donor assessment and testing and the labelling of cell therapy products. The interaction between the different component parts of programmes should work seamlessly and where, for example, cell processing or laboratory testing is performed outside the programme by external agencies, then service-level agreements will need to be in place. Most units that achieve compliance with regulatory and accreditation standards feel that the exercise has been worthwhile and that the quality of the services they offer has been improved.

KEY POINTS

1) There have been considerable advances in cellular therapy in the last 20 years and newer developments include the use of cell therapy products for regenerative medicine and immunotherapy.
2) The accreditation and regulatory environment has become increasingly complex and its aim is to enhance product quality and safety.
3) The development of robust quality systems is central to achieving compliance with these new requirements.
4) Some regulations are mandatory, e.g. the EU Directive and FDA requirements, whilst others, such as FACT–JACIE or AABB accreditation, are voluntary.
5) Increased resource is required to successfully implement the changes needed to achieve compliance.

References

1 World Marrow Donor Association Annual Report. 2015. Available at: www.worldmarrow. org/(accessed 17 November 2016).

2 Directive 2004/23/EC on setting standards of quality and safety for the donation, procurement, testing, processing, preservation, storage and distribution of human tissues and cells.

3 Implementing Directive 2004/23/EC of the European Parliament and Council as regards traceability requirements, notification of severe adverse reactions and events and certain technical requirements for the coding, processing, preservation, storage and distribution of human tissues and cells, C.D. 2006/86/EC.

4 Implementing Directive 2004/23/EC of the European Parliament and Council as regards certain technical requirements for the donation, procurement and testing of human tissues and cells, C.D. 2006/17/EC.

5 Human Tissue Act 2006 (Scotland) 2006.

6 Human Tissue Act 2004 (except Scotland) 2004.

7 Human Tissue Authority (HTA): Codes of Practice for Consent (Code 1), for Donation of Solid Organs for Transplantation (Code 2), for Disposal of Human Tissue (Code 5), for Donation of Allogeneic Bone Marrow and Peripheral Blood Stem Cells (Code 6) and for Import and Export of Human Bodies, Body Parts and Tissues (Code 8). Available at: www. hta.gov.uk (accessed 17 November 2016).

8 Code of Practice on the Human Transplantation (Wales) Act 2013. Available at: www.hta.gov.uk (accessed 17 November 2016).

9 FDA documents. Available at: www.fda.gov/ cber/tiss.htm and www.fda.gov/cber/gene.htm (accessed 17 November 2016).

10 Guidance for Industry Minimally Manipulated, Unrelated Allogeneic Placental/Umbilical CB Intended for Hematopoietic Reconstitution for Specified Indications; October 2009. Available at: http://www.fda.gov/cber/guidelines.htm (accessed 17 November 2016).

11 NHS England Clinical Commissioning Policy: Haematopoietic Stem Cell Transplantation. Available at: www.england.nhs.uk/ commissioning/wp-content/uploads/sites/ 12/2015/01/b04-haematp-stem-cll-transplt. pdf (accessed 17 November 2016).

12 FACT-JACIE International Standards for Hematopoietic Cellular Therapy Product Collection, Processing and Administration from the Foundation for the Accreditation of Cell Therapy (FACT) and the Joint Accreditation Committee of ISCT–Europe and EBMT (JACIE), 6th edn. Available at: www.jacie.org and www. factwebsite.org (accessed 17 November 2016).

13 FACT Common Standards for Cellular Therapies 2015. Available at: www.factwebsite. org (accessed 17 November 2016).

14 Marmor S, Begun J, Abraham J, et al. The impact of center accreditation on hematopoietic cell transplantation (HCT). Bone Marrow Transplant 2015;**50**(1):87–94.

15 Purtill D, Smith K, Devlin S et al. Dominant unit CD34+ cell dose predicts engraftment after double-unit cord blood transplantation and is influenced by bank practice. Blood 2014;**124**(19):2905–12.

16 NetCord–FACT International Standards for CB Collection, Processing, Testing, Banking, Selection and Release, 6th edn. Available at: www. factwebsite.org (accessed 17 November 2016).

17 Standards for Cellular Therapy Services, 7th edn. AABB, Bethesda, 2015.

18 Circular of Information for the Use of Cellular Therapy Products. Available at: http://www. aabb.org/aabbcct/coi/Documents/ CT-Circular-of-Information.pdf (accessed 17 November 2016).

19 CAP Checklist. Available at: www.cap.org under Accreditation and Laboratory Improvement (accessed 17 November 2016).

20 World Marrow Donor Association. International Standards for Unrelated Hematopoietic Progenitor Cell Donor Registries. Available at: https://www.wmda. info/(accessed 17 November 2016).

21 American Society for Histocompatibility and Immunogenetics (ASHI) Standards. Available at http://www.ashi-hla.org/(accessed 17 November 2016).

22 European Federation for Immunogenetics (EFI) Standards. Available at: www.efiweb.org (accessed 17 November 2016).

23 Pasquini MC, Zhu X. Current uses and outcomes of hematopoietic stem cell transplantation: 2014 CIBMTR Summary Slides. Available at: http://www.cibmtr.org (accessed 17 November 2016).

24 Passweg JR, Baldomero H, Bader P et al. Hematopoietic SCT in Europe 2013: recent trends in the use of alternative donors showing more haploidentical donors but fewer cord blood transplants. Bone Marrow Transplant 2015;**50**(4):476–82.

Further Reading

Cornish JM. JACIE accreditation in paediatric haemopoietic SCT. Bone Marrow Transplant 2008;**42** (Suppl. 2):S82–6.

Gratwohl A, Brand R, Niederwieser D et al. Introduction of a quality management system and outcome after hematopoietic stem-cell transplantation. J Clin Oncol 2011;**29**(15):1980–6.

Hurley CK, Foeken L, Horowitz M et al., for the WMDA Accreditation and Regulatory Committees. Standards, regulations and accreditation for registries involved in the worldwide exchange of hematopoietic stem cell donors and products. Bone Marrow Transplant 2010;**45**(5):819–24.

Pamphilon D, Apperley JF, Samson D, Slaper-Cortenbach I, McGrath E. JACIE accreditation in 2008: demonstrating excellence in stem cell transplantation. Hematol Oncol Stem Cell Ther 2009;**2**(2):311–19.

Wall DA. Regulatory issues in cord blood banking and transplantation. Best Pract Res Clin Haematol 2010;**23**(2):171–7.

Stem Cell Collection and Therapeutic Apheresis

Khaled El-Ghariani[1] *and Zbigniew (Ziggy) M. Szczepiorkowski*[2]

[1] *NHS Blood and Transplant and Sheffield Teaching Hospitals NHS Trust and University of Sheffield, Sheffield, UK*
[2] *Transfusion Medicine Service, Cellular Therapy Center, Dartmouth-Hitchcock Medical Centre and Geisel School of Medicine at Dartmouth, Hanover, USA*

Introduction

The word *apheresis* is derived from the Greek meaning 'a withdrawal' Therapeutic apheresis is the process of using apheresis technology to manipulate a patient's circulatory contents through removal or exchange, to achieve a therapeutic goal. The rationale for this is that it will remove or reduce a substance or substances implicated in the pathology of the disease being treated. Plasma exchange is the process of exchanging part of the patient's plasma with suitable replacement fluid. Different cellular components can be removed with high precision. Red cells can be exchanged, circulating stem cells and lymphocytes can be collected for transplantation and the excess white cells or platelets that are present in myeloproliferative disorders can be removed. Molecules such as low-density lipoproteins and immunoglobulins can be specifically removed through the use of adsorption columns.

A decision to offer these treatments to patients should be based on factors such as temporary benefits of apheresis, potential adverse effects and the availability and efficacy of other treatment modalities.

Cell Separators

Efficient cell separators are currently available. These machines are equipped with sophisticated software and safety alarm systems to detect air and changes in access or inflow pressure. Apheresis technology is based on either filtration or centrifugal systems. Filtration systems use permeable membranes to separate blood into its cellular and noncellular components by subjecting it to sieving through a membrane with suitably sized pores. An example of a filtration system is the Infomed HF440 (Plate 39.1 in the plate section). Centrifugal systems use the forces generated by rotation (usually quantified as multiples of the force of gravity or 'g forces') to separate blood into different components. Centrifugation of blood within apheresis machines results in sedimentation of its components into distinct layers. Based on increasing density, these layers are plasma, platelets, monocytes, lymphocytes and haematopoietic progenitor cells (HPCs), granulocytes and red cells.

Apheresis machines use either continuous- or intermittent-flow technology. In the continuous-flow machines, blood is continuously pumped into a spinning disposable harness

Practical Transfusion Medicine, Fifth Edition. Edited by Michael F. Murphy, David J. Roberts and Mark H. Yazer.

where separation takes place and components are either diverted to a collection bag or returned to the patient as required. These machines often require two points of access to the circulation, one for withdrawal and another for return blood to the subject. Examples of continuous-flow systems are Spectra Optia (TerumoBCT) (Plate 39.2 in the plate section), Amicus (Fenwal) and Com.Tec (Fresenius Kabi). Intermittent-flow machines collect blood into a bowl during the draw cycle and then centrifuge it down to separate plasma and cellular components. Different components are diverted to the collection bag or returned to the patient along with replacement fluid during the return cycle. This process could be achieved by a single point of access to the circulation. An example of a current intermittent-flow system is the UVAR XTS (Therakos Inc.). Apheresis systems are primed with normal saline to displace air from the harness and also to ensure isovolemia, an important prerequisite for patients with haemodynamic instability or sickle cell disease. In children and small adults, the extracorporeal volume may be relatively high and the system will need to be primed by a mixture of packed red blood cells and normal saline or albumin [1].

Cell separators must be qualified and maintained according to the manufacturer's recommendations and must be operated by trained personnel.

Patient Assessment and Treatment Planning

A physician experienced in the use of cell separators should undertake clinical assessment, to weigh the patient's current health status and expected benefit against potential risks and inconvenience. Plasma exchange often provides relief of the patient's symptoms for variable lengths of time and it is usually only part of the patient's treatment plan. Valid consent must be obtained from all patients and donors according to national practice. Laboratory evaluations before the first procedure should be tailored to the patient's clinical

status; these may include a full blood count, coagulation screen and biochemistry. These tests are repeated thereafter as required. Apheresis treatment plans will include the type of vascular access, volume to be exchanged, type of replacement fluid, frequency of procedures and monitoring of response to therapy.

Adequate vascular access is crucial. Peripheral veins, usually located in the antecubital fossa, should be evaluated by apheresis staff early in planning and should be used wherever possible, especially for patients requiring a limited number of procedures. Central venous catheterisation is required for patients who have inadequate peripheral veins or who require frequent procedures. A rigid double-lumen catheter should be used. Trained staff must undertake central vein cannulation and postinsertion catheter care [2]. Maximum effort should be exerted to avoid failure of vascular access during the procedure as this is associated with disappointment to patients and delays and difficulties for the staff.

Haematopoietic Progenitor Cell Mobilisation

Currently, haematopoietic cell transplantation in adults is more commonly undertaken using mobilised peripheral blood rather than bone marrow as a source of stem cells (see also Chapter 36). This is because HPC, Apheresis engrafts faster than marrow and can be harvested without the need for hospital admission or general anaesthesia [3]. In the steady state, HPCs circulate in the peripheral blood, albeit in very low numbers, of less than 0.1% of the total white blood cell count. To ensure adequate graft, mobilisation of such cells from the marrow into the peripheral circulation is necessary. Granulocyte colony-stimulating factor (G-CSF) is used to mobilise healthy donors, whereas mobilisation of cells from patients undergoing autologous HSCT can be achieved by G-CSF and/or the administration of chemotherapy such as cyclophosphamide or disease-specific combination chemotherapy.

The dissection of the mechanism of HPC mobilisation has revealed a number of different molecular pathways. One of them involves CXCR4, expressed by HPCs among other cells, and its ligand, stromal-derived factor 1 (SDF-1; CXCL12), which is produced by marrow stromal cells. The association of CXCR4 with its ligand mediates stem cell homing, trafficking and retention. Proteolytic enzymes, such as elastase, cathepsin G and matrix metalloproteinase-g, released from neutrophils following administration of chemotherapy and/or G-CSF, are thought to degrade molecules such as CXCR4 and SDF-1, which are important for anchoring stem cells to marrow stroma and inducing mobilisation. Also, G-CSF may have an inhibitory effect on expression of CXCR4 mRNA and the reduced expression of CXCR4 receptors enhances mobilisation.

Most healthy donors are mobilised by G-CSF at a dose of 10 µg/kg/day. Progenitor cells usually peak after the fourth injection when harvesting starts and the procedure may be repeated until the target number of stem cells is achieved. Donor age, steady-state CD34 levels and the dose of G-CSF may impact on the CD34+ cell mobilisation. G-CSF used in healthy donors has proven to be both effective and reasonably safe [4]. The most common side effects of G-CSF are bone pain, headaches, fatigue and nausea. Reduction in arterial oxygenation has also been noted. Rare but serious effects of G-CSF have been reported. Splenic enlargement is common and there are a few case reports of splenic rupture, either spontaneously or precipitated by minor trauma or viral infection. Donors are encouraged to report any pain or discomfort that they may experience over the splenic region. G-CSF has a procoagulant effect and may increase the risk of myocardial infarction or ischemic strokes in susceptible individuals. Current data do not suggest adverse effects of G-CSF on genomic stability or possible long-term leukaemogenesis. However, donor registries regularly monitor volunteer donors for

these and accumulated long-term follow-up data should rule out such complications [5]. Recently, four cases among allogeneic unrelated donors of intracerebral bleeding were identified. These complications generated additional questions to evaluate potential donors for the risk of intracerebral bleeding.

Pegylation of G-CSF is a process in which a polyethylene glycol (PEG) moiety is conjugated to a G-CSF molecule. This increases its molecular mass, reduces its renal excretion and prolongs its half-life in excess of 30 hours. One or two injections of pegfilgrastim have been used to mobilise stem cells but data are limited and gave mixed outcomes [6]. Two branded forms of G-CSF (Granocyte and Neupogen®) have been available since the early 1990s. Extensive data are available concerning their safety. Recently, G-CSF biosimilar agents have become available. These are alternative biological versions of G-CSF with significantly lower cost. Reviews have shown no difference between biosimilar and reference products in biological mode of action or side effects [5]. However, most volunteer donor registries only use original products while the safety of biosimilars is being evaluated in a long-term follow-up study [7].

The response of individuals to mobilisation regimens is variable and some donors fail to mobilise enough HPCs into the circulation to allow collection of an adequate graft. Such poor mobilisation is more common in autologous than allogeneic donors. The mechanism of poor mobilisation in healthy donors is unclear. However, experiments in mice have suggested a genetic control of the vigour and timing of mobilisation.

In the autologous settings, the average mobilisation failure rate in myeloma and lymphoma patients is 20% but can be as high as 40% in certain patient groups. Mobilisation failure is defined as the inability to collect the minimum recommended stem cell dose for autologous transplant, which is 2×10^6 CD34+ cells/kg recipient body weight [6]. Factors associated with poor mobilisation include stem cell damage due to old age, previous exposure to chemotherapy and radiotherapy, disease involvement of bone marrow, the use of stem cell-toxic agents such as melphalan, carmustine, fludarabine, alkylating agents or lenalidomide, the diagnosis of non-Hodgkin's lymphoma and coexisting diabetes [6].

Patterns of donors' responses to mobilisation treatment are likely to continue to change in the future, depending on changes in types of diseases treated, the patients' age profiles and comorbidities, as well as the use of novel cancer treatments and their effects on stem cells. A few reports suggested that therapies such as rituximab and bortezomib may not adversely affect mobilisation. The management of mobilisation failure has improved with better understanding of the biology of stem cells and the availability of new therapeutic agents such as plerixafor. Box 39.1 lists the options available to predict and manage poor mobilisation.

Plerixafor (Mozobil) is a CXCR4 antagonist that blocks this receptor reversibly and inhibits its interaction with SDF-1. This leads to HPC release into the circulation. Plerixafor synergises with G-CSF and is usually administered the night before the planned first day of collection, at $240\,\mu g/m^2$ subcutaneous injection. The introduction of plerixafor has provided clinical practice with a safe and effective new mobilising agent [8,9]. Although current use of plerixafor is limited by increased drug cost, its judicious use in an appropriately selected patient population has been proven to be cost-effective [10] and the drug has been approved by the US Food and Drug Administration (FDA) and the European Medicine Evaluation Agency (EMEA) for autologous HPC donations for patients with myeloma and non-Hodgkin's lymphoma. Because most patients are good mobilisers, the universal use of plerixafor is not justified.

Plerixafor can be used in combination with G-CSF in patients who have previously failed mobilisation with a success rate of up to 70% [11]. This is known as the rescue approach. However, plerixafor could be used preemptively to prevent mobilisation failure in the first place. Use of plerixafor during the first mobilisation of selected high-risk patients could be more helpful by eliminating the need for a second mobilisation, reducing the number of apheresis sessions required and avoiding delays in transplantation. This could be achieved by adopting the preemptive course otherwise known as a 'just-in-time' approach where patients' blood CD34+ cell counts on the predicted day of harvest are monitored. Those with low CD34+ cell count (fewer than 15 per microlitre) would be identified as potential mobilisation failures and given plerixafor during their first mobilisation attempt [10,12].

Box 39.1   Options to predict and manage mobilisation failure.

- Patients should be considered for stem cell mobilisation and harvesting, if required, early in the course of their treatment and before stem cell toxic agents are used. High-risk patients should be carefully monitored during the mobilisation process.
- Plerixafor is used preemptively in patients with low circulating CD34+ cells on the predicated day of harvest to prevent mobilisation failure.
- Patients who have failed a mobilisation attempt could be rescued by further mobilisation attempts using G-CSF and plerixafor (± chemotherapy).
- The use of large-volume apheresis, new mobilising agents (within clinical trials) and marginally low numbers of stem cells for transplantation are options that clinicians could consider on an individual basis.
- Bone marrow is harvested instead. However, bone marrow from poor mobilisers may not be of good enough quality and delayed engraftment may follow.

Peripheral Blood HPC Collection (Leucocytapheresis)

Leucocytapheresis, following chemotherapy and G-CSF mobilisation, could commence when leucocyte counts are rising ($\geq 1 \times 10^9$/L). However, currently, most centres use surface expression of CD34 on peripheral blood mononuclear cells (PBMCs), measured by flow cytometry, to predict the optimal time to start HPC collection, to predict the success of collection and to enumerate HPC in the collected product [13]. CD34 is a heavily glycosylated phosphoglycoprotein expressed on progenitor cells of all lineages within the lymphohaemopoietic system, but not on mature cells. Endothelial progenitors, marrow stromal cells and osteoclasts also express CD34. Approximately 1.5% of aspirated normal marrow mononuclear cells, less than 0.1% of nonmobilised PBMCs and approximately 0.5% of cord blood cells are CD34+. The function of CD34 molecules remains elusive but analysis of its structure indicates that these molecules may have a role in cellular signal transduction and/or cell adhesion. CD34 is a surrogate marker for stem cells. Purified autologous CD34+ cells mediate haemopoietic engraftment whereas CD34– cells do not engraft. There is a clear correlation between the number of CD34+ cells infused and the rate of subsequent recovery of both neutrophils and platelets post transplant [14]. Compared with marrow harvests, G-CSF mobilised grafts contain three- to fourfold higher CD34+ cells and about a 10–20-fold increase in CD3+ T-cells.

The optimal number of infused HPC, Apheresis required for transplantation is not fully defined. However, to ensure timely engraftment and graft survival, there is a consensus to infuse at least 2.0×10^6/kg recipient body weight of CD34+ cells for autologous transplant and 4×10^6/kg of recipient body weight for allogeneic transplant [13]. The required number of CD34+ cells for allogeneic transplants is increased with increased HLA disparity between donor and recipient. In addition, a higher number of cells should be collected if tandem transplant or graft manipulation is contemplated. The maximum number of cells to be infused is not defined. However, in the autologous setting, the inconvenience and cost of harvesting of much higher cell numbers are not justified by improvement of clinical outcome. In some studies, infusion of very high numbers of allogeneic cells was found to be associated with a higher risk of extensive chronic graft-versus-host disease (GVHD) [14].

Administration of G-CSF just before leucocytapheresis should be avoided. G-CSF injections are usually followed by temporary reduction of circulating stem cells lasting for about four hours. The optimal harvesting time is between four and 12 hours after subcutaneous injection of G-CSF. Serial measurement of peripheral blood CD34+ cell count in autologous donors is usually obtained as soon as their total leucocyte count approaches 1×10^9/L. Collection, started at a level of 20 CD34+ cells/μL, gives the best yield. Healthy donors usually follow a more predicted course and their peak mobilisation is usually reached at day 5, after four G-CSF injections. Some donors require further injections either because of delayed mobilisation or because not enough cells were collected at the first collection.

Collection of HPC, Apheresis is a technically challenging procedure and different machines collect cells with different efficiency and selectivity. Machine efficiency is measured by the percentage of CD34+ cells that can be collected at a specific peripheral CD34+ cell count. The collected yield can be enhanced by the machine's ability to process more volumes of donor blood within a reasonable period of time and without inconvenience to the donor. Selective machines manage to target HPC, Apheresis with less contamination by other unwanted blood cells. This reduces platelet and red cell contamination of the harvest, which is important in two respects: first, such contamination affects stem cell cryopreservation and may increase infusion complications and, second, collection of other cells such as platelets may lead to thrombocytopenia in the donor.

Apheresis units should observe good manufacturing practice (GMP) and qualify new machines against published data, as well as against existing equipment, to ensure that new technologies are safe and convenient to the donors, as well as being able to meet required product specifications. This is particularly important in cases where the unit deals with special donor groups such as children or heavily pretreated autologous patients, who tend to mobilise poorly. International standards for practice are widely available [15].

There are other important operational features of apheresis machines that should be taken into consideration. A low volume of the endproduct is an advantage as smaller volumes are easy to cryo-preserve, require a smaller storage space and are associated with less dimethylsulfoxide (DMSO) infusion toxicity. Also, the contamination of the final product with granulocytes should be mini-mised, as they have been shown to be a cause of infusion-related adverse reactions. Machines that have smaller extracorporeal volumes are less likely to cause transient anaemia and hypovolae-mia in small subjects and children and so avert the need to prime with blood. Machines that are using a single point of access (i.e. single needle) to the circulation are usually associated with an ability to process a smaller volume of blood and so may give a lower yield of CD34+ cells.

Several machines, such as COBE Spectra Optia (TerumoBCT), Amicus (Fenwal) and Com.Tec (Fresenius Kabi), are able to collect stem cells with different efficiencies and selec-tivity. Spectra Optia is automated and has small end-harvest and extracorporeal volumes and is commonly used in the UK.

A total of 2–3 patient blood volumes are usually processed by the apheresis machine at each leucocytapheresis procedure. Large-volume leu-cocytapheresis (processing of 3–6 blood volumes over a longer period of time or by increasing the blood flow into the apheresis machine) has been tried and was shown to collect significantly higher CD34+ yields. This may reduce the number of leucocytapheresis procedures required and also limit exposure to G-CSF [16]. Although this practice is associated with donor inconvenience, citrate toxicity and platelet loss, it has been used successfully, particularly for allogeneic donors.

Plasma Exchange

Plasma exchange is an effective treatment for many conditions, mainly immune in nature. Exchanging a patient's plasma can remove or substantially reduce the concentration of a patho-logical substance or substances; an example is immunoglobulin in situations of hyperviscosity or autoimmune disorders such as myasthenia gravis. However, the response of diseases such as multiple sclerosis, not primarily mediated by autoantibodies, to plasma exchange has suggested other possible mechanisms of actions of this treatment [17]. These are summarised in Box 39.2.

Box 39.2 Possible mechanisms of action of plasma exchange.

- Removal of pathogenic antibodies.
- Sensitisation of antibodies-producing cells to immunosuppressant and chemotherapeutic agents.
- Removal of pathogenic immune complexes which could prevent splenic blockade and hence improve monocyte/macrophage functions.
- Removal of cytokines and adhesion molecules.
- Replacement of missing plasma component (eg TTP).
- Alteration of the cellular immune system. Observed alterations include:
  - changes in lymphocyte numbers and distribution (decline in B-cells and increase in T-cells)
  - changes in NK cell numbers and activity
  - increased in Tsuppressor or Tregulatory cell function
  - shift from Th2 to Th1 predominant pattern.

Source: Adapted from Reeves and Winters [17].

The removed plasma is most commonly replaced with human albumin solution (HAS) of 4.5%. (In the USA, it is called human serum albumin and is usually 5%.) Up to one-third of the exchange volume can be replaced by normal saline if the patient's starting albumin level is normal; otherwise hypotension and/or peripheral oedema may follow. HAS is used because it provides the necessary oncotic pressure with fewer allergic reactions and an impressive safety record with regard to infection transmission. In other clinical scenarios, the exchange process is required not only to remove factors implicated in the disease pathogenesis but also to replace necessary plasma constituents. In thrombotic thrombocytopenic purpura (TTP), for example, plasma exchange removes autoantibodies to the von Willebrand factor-cleaving protease, an important enzyme otherwise known as ADAMTS13, and the associated ultra-large von Willebrand factor multimers. Plasma exchange is also required to replace the missing ADAMTS13; hence fresh frozen plasma (FFP) is used as a replacement fluid for TTP. Solvent detergent plasma is the recommended replacement fluid for TTP in the UK, while in the USA this product, though approved for use, is not currently widely available. Clotting factors may also require replacement during the course of plasma exchange. A therapeutic dose of FFP (10–15 mL/kg) may be included as the last replacement fluid to be infused in cases where repeated exchange with albumin has depleted clotting factors in patients at high risk of bleeding.

Plasma exchange treatment plans include determination of the amount of plasma to be exchanged in relation to the patient's estimated plasma volume and how to space the procedures to ensure efficiency. An exchange of 1.0–1.5 of the patient's plasma volume will exchange between 63% and 78% of their plasma and is therapeutically effective in most situations. Larger volume exchange is associated with inconvenience and use of larger amounts of replacement fluid, and brings little extra benefit (Figure 39.1) [18]. The frequency and total number of exchanges depend on the disease being treated and on the patient's response. Hyperviscosity, TTP and Goodpasture's syndrome require daily exchanges; other conditions may respond to a less intensive course of treatment, such as five exchanges over 7–10 days.

The response to treatment varies between patients. Criteria to monitor response to treatment should be agreed early in the treatment plan to avoid undertreatment, overtreatment or the continuation of ineffective treatment. TTP is monitored by measuring the platelet

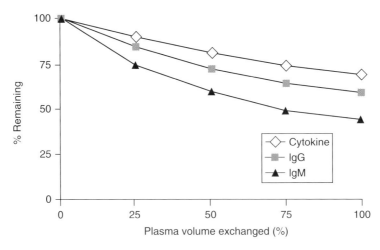

Figure 39.1 Kinetics of plasma exchange. *Source*: Reproduced from El-Ghariani and Unsworth 2006 [18], with permission from the Royal College of Physicians.

count and other parameters of haemolysis while Guillain–Barré syndrome and myasthenia gravis are assessed by clinical neurological improvement. Evidence is accumulating regarding the effectiveness, or otherwise, of different apheresis procedures to treat various disease processes (Box 39.3). The American Society for Apheresis (ASFA) regularly publishes a guideline document with assignment of ASFA category (I to IV) and recommendation grade for different diseases [19].

Although large randomised trials support the use of plasma exchange in the treatment of Guillain–Barré syndrome, intravenous immunoglobulin (IVIg) is equally effective. Given the ease of administration, IVIg is usually a first-choice therapy. However, either of the two treatment modalities can be used if the other fails. Chronic inflammatory demyelinating polyneuropathy also responds to both plasma exchange and IVIg and the former can be used for maintenance treatment.

In myasthenia gravis, plasma exchange has a clear therapeutic effect but the disease control is temporary and may be followed by a rebound.

Plasma exchange is used to treat emergencies such as respiratory failure or swallowing difficulties and to prepare patients for thymectomy. Plasma exchange must be accompanied by an appropriate immunosuppressive regime if it is to be of long-term benefit in myasthenia gravis.

Paraproteinaemia causing clinically evident and progressive hyperviscosity syndrome is a medical emergency requiring urgent plasma exchange to lower the concentration of the responsible paraprotein. IgM, the largest immunoglobulin and mostly intravascular, is most likely to cause hyperviscosity. IgA and IgG3 tend to aggregate and, after IgM, are more likely than other isotypes or subclasses to be associated with hyperviscosity. One to three treatments will usually alleviate symptoms long enough for chemotherapy to take effect. These patients are often severely anaemic. They should not be transfused until the viscosity has been lowered as a rise in haematocrit can precipitate a serious worsening of their symptoms. Plasma exchange can also be life saving in cryoglobulinaemia associated with a fulminant clinical picture.

Box 39.3 Disorders for which apheresis is accepted as first-line therapy, either as a stand-alone treatment or in conjunction with other modes of treatment (ASFA Category I® indications).

Plasma exchange

Thrombotic thrombocytopenic purpura
Severe hyperviscosity in monoclonal gammopathies
Antiglomerular basement membrane disease (Goodpasture's syndrome)
ANCA-associated rapidly progressive glomerulonephritis (Wegener's syndrome)
Severe myasthenia gravis
Paraproteinemic polyneuropathies (IgG/IgA)
Guillain–Barré syndrome
Chronic inflammatory demyelinating polyradiculoneuropathy
ABO-incompatible kidney and liver transplantation (certain indications)

Red cell exchange

Acute stroke in sickle cell disease
Severe malaria (certain indications)

Photopheresis

Erythrodermic cutaneous T-cell lymphoma

Selective lipid removal

Usually by adsorption column, for homozygote familial hypercholesterolemia

Leucocytapheresis

Hyperleucocytosis causing leukostasis

Source: Adapted from the American Society for Apheresis guidelines [19].

Replacement fluids should always be warmed. At the same time, the cause of the cryoglobulinaemia must be determined and definitive chemotherapy instituted if appropriate.

Plasma exchange plays a limited role in the treatment of autoimmune cytopenia; however, it is the treatment of choice for TTP and should be started as soon as the diagnosis is suspected. Daily plasma exchange is needed for at least two days after the platelet count has returned to normal (i.e. over 150×10^9/L) and lactate dehydrogenase (LDH) is within the normal range. Plasma infusion can also be used to treat TTP if plasma exchange is not immediately available.

Plasma exchange is required as an adjuvant therapy in antiglomerular basement membrane disease (Goodpasture's syndrome). In the presence of pulmonary haemorrhage, it is important not to overload the patient with replacement fluids as this may provoke further bleeding. Plasma exchange may be used in certain cases of pauci-immune rapidly progressive glomerulonephritis and systemic vasculitis. Such cases need to be discussed with a specialist. Plasma exchange has no proven role in the management of systemic lupus erythematosus nephritis or uncomplicated rheumatoid arthritis.

Red Cell Exchange

Red cell exchange involves the removal of a patient's red cells and concomitant infusion of allogeneic donor cells. This procedure, evolved as a manual procedure, can be performed by apheresis machines and is most commonly used to treat sickle cell disease and some parasitic infections such as malaria or babesiosis. A major advantage of this automated procedure is the isovolaemic nature of the exchange, which is important in preventing further complications. A single red cell volume exchange removes approximately 60% of the red cells originally present in the patient's circulation. The patient's haematocrit, the fraction of the patient's red cells to be left in circulation after the exchange, the desirable final haematocrit and the haematocrit of the replacement fluid can be entered into the apheresis device's software, which then calculates the volume of red cells to be removed and estimates the volume of red cells to be used as replacement.

Exchange using normal red cells as a replacement fluid is beneficial in the treatment and prevention of certain sickle cell crises. Exchange should aim at raising the haemoglobin A to 70–80% to avoid further vasoocclusive crises and treat the ongoing one. However, the final haematocrit following exchange should not exceed 30%. Hyperviscosity, associated with a higher haematocrit, is associated with a reduction in oxygen delivery. Neurological events after partial exchange, usually for priapism, have been observed and are thought to be due to high end haemoglobin levels, a situation also known as ASPEN syndrome (Association of Sickle cell disease, Priapism, Exchange transfusion and Neurological events) [20]. Red cell exchange may not shorten an uncomplicated painful sickle cell crisis but may be considered in severe and frequent debilitating crises. A patient who survives an acute ischemic stroke could be maintained on a regular exchange programme to prevent recurrence. For acute chest syndrome, life- or organ-threatening complications, red cell exchange can provide rapid reduction of sickle haemoglobin and is less likely to cause iron accumulation. Red cell exchange in sickle cell disease is associated with concerns such as increased requirement of allogeneic blood, which is associated with the risk of red cell alloimmunisation.

Red cell exchange is an adjuvant therapy that should be considered for severely ill patients with malaria if parasitaemia is more than 10% or if the patient has severe malaria manifested by altered mental status, nonvolume overload pulmonary oedema or renal complications. Treatment is discontinued after achieving ≤5% residual parasitaemia. Absolute erythrocytosis causing hyperviscosity, thromboembolism or bleeding should be treated by tackling its primary cause and possibly by phlebotomy to maintain a normal haematocrit. However, erythrocytapheresis is also used to treat certain patients with polycythemia, where removed red cells are replaced with albumin or saline to maintain isovolemia. This procedure is particularly useful in patients with polycythemia rubra vera, complicated by acute thromboembolism, severe microvascular complications or bleeding, especially if the patient is haemodynamically unstable.

Extracorporeal Photochemotherapy (Photopheresis)

Extracorporeal photochemotherapy (ECP) is a process in which the patient's mononuclear cells (MNC) are collected and exposed to ultraviolet A light (UVA) in the presence of photoactivating agents such as 8-methoxypsoralen (8-MOP). This process brings about immunomodulation, which can be therapeutically beneficial to patients with advanced cutaneous T-cell lymphoma (CTCL), GVHD and cardiac transplant rejection as well as other indications [21,22]. The mechanism of action of ECP is not fully understood but it induces lymphocyte apoptosis, which leads to changes in cytokine secretion patterns, more tolerant antigen-presenting cells (APCs), induction of Tregulatory (Treg) cells and suppression of CD8+ effector cells. Interestingly, ECP does not lead to an increased incidence of opportunistic infection, a feature that is particularly useful in patients with extensive skin lesions.

Extracorporeal photochemotherapy can be best achieved by collecting MNC using a specialised cell separator such as the THERAKOS^{TM} CELLEX^{TM} system (most commonly used in the UK and USA). This machine delivers a calculated UVA radiation dose into the MNC suspension pretreated with 8-MOP, before returning the cells to the patient's circulation. Heparin and, less commonly, ACD-A are used as anticoagulants. Alternatively, ECP can be completed using a combination of a cell separator to collect leucocytes, 8-MOP is added to the apheresis product

and the suspension is then exposed to UVA using an irradiation source (UV light box), such as the UV-matic irradiator, and then reinfused. This practice is commonly used in Europe, but strict adherence to GMP regulations for reinfused products is required. ECP is contraindicated in the presence of psoralen hypersensitivity.

There is some evidence for the use of ECP in erythrodermic CTCL and steroid-refractory GVHD, but randomised controlled studies are needed. There is evidence supporting the use of ECP in preventing cardiac and lung rejection following transplantation. Randomised controlled trials have also shown a therapeutic benefit in type 1 diabetes mellitus, but the inconvenience associated with the procedure outweighs the clinical benefit. Patients with advanced CTCL (stage III/IV) typically receive ECP on two consecutive days once per month. For the management of chronic GVHD, an accelerated regime has been used to gain rapid control of the disease, with two consecutive treatments administered initially every two weeks. In the USA, often a higher frequency of two procedures per week for 12 weeks is used. ECP is a treatment option for patients with steroid-refractory acute GVHD [23].

Complications of Therapeutic Apheresis

Complications occur in up to 10% of procedures; most are mild but rarely, serious complications, including deaths, have been reported. Given the advances in technology, machine-related problems are unusual. Failure of the machine that will prevent red cell return can result in red cell loss of up to 200 mL of blood in newer instruments and up to 350 mL in older instruments. Central catheter-related complications, such as pneumothorax, internal bleeding, thrombosis and infections, are more common and can be serious. Allergic reactions to replacement fluids are uncommon but can be significant. These include anaphylactic reactions, hypotension and urticarial rashes. Reactions to

HAS are now rare as the preparations contain lower amounts of significant contaminants than previously, especially of vasoactive kinins. HAS essentially carries no risk of infection and does not increase the citrate return. Dilution of coagulation factors can occur following repeated plasma exchanges and may require the addition of FFP to the replacement fluid. FFP poses the risk of blood-borne infection (although virally inactivated products are now available) and allergic reactions, and also contributes to the citrate load as it contains approximately 14% citrate anticoagulant by volume. Side effects of the citrate anticoagulant, almost universally used, are particularly common. These result from hypocalcaemia and include paraesthesia (digital and perioral), abdominal cramps and, rarely, cardiac dysrhythmias and seizures. Citrate toxicity usually responds to simple measures such as slowing the rate of return and providing extra calcium orally. Intravenous calcium may be required. Patients with renal failure who are receiving large amounts of citrate during plasma exchange may develop a profound metabolic alkalosis. Patients receiving repeated treatments over a long period of time can lose significant quantities of calcium.

Complications during therapeutic apheresis may arise from underlying pathology or comorbidity. It is important that the clinical status is assessed prior to exchange. Where risks are increased but benefit is likely, a suitable location for the procedure such as a high-dependency unit may be required.

KEY POINTS

1) A physician experienced in the use of cell separators should assess the patient's need to have a therapeutic apheresis procedure, taking into consideration potential risks and inconvenience.
2) Adequate vascular access is crucial. Central venous catheterisation needs to be undertaken by trained staff to minimise risks to patients.
3) G-CSF with or without chemotherapy is currently the gold standard for HPC mobilisation. Donors who prove to be hard to mobilise may respond favourably to the addition of a CXCR4 antagonist (Plerixafor™) to the G-CSF mobilisation protocol.

4) Human albumin solution (4.5%) is the most commonly used replacement fluid for plasma exchange. Occasionally, plasma, possibly solvent detergent product, is needed.
5) Plasma exchange causes several changes to the immune system and the mechanisms of action that mediate these changes require further research.
6) Photopheresis induces immunomodulation without systemic immunosuppression and is indicated for treatment of specific indications of cutaneous T-cell lymphoma, GVHD and solid organ transplant rejection.

References

1 Kim HC. Therapeutic apheresis in pediatric patients, in Apheresis Principles and Practice, 3rd edn (eds BC Mcleod, ZM Szczepiorkowski, R Weinstein et al). AABB Press, Bethesda, 2010.
2 National Institute for Clinical Excellence. Guidance on the Use of Ultrasound Locating Devices for Placing Central Venous Catheters. Available at: www.nice.org.uk/guidance/ta49 (accessed 17 November 2016).
3 To LB, Roberts MM, Haylock DN et al. Comparison of haematological recovery times and supportive care requirements of autologous recovery phase peripheral blood stem cell transplants, autologous bone marrow transplants

and allogeneic bone marrow transplants. Bone Marrow Transplant 1992;**9**(4):277–84.

4 Pulsipher MA, Chitphakdithai P, Miller JP et al. Adverse events among 2408 unrelated donors of peripheral blood stem cells: results of a prospective trial from the National Marrow Donor Program. Blood 2009;**113**: 3604–11.

5 Boing H, Becker PS, Schwebig A, Turner M. Biosimilar granulocyte-colony-stimulating factor for health donor stem cell mobilization: need we be afraid? Transfusion 2015;**55**:430–9.

6 Giralt S, Costa L, Schriber J, DiPersio J et al. Optimizing autologous stem cell mobilization strategies to improve patient outcomes: consensus guidelines and recommendations. Biol Blood Marrow Transplant 2014;**20**:259–308.

7 Becker P, Brauninger S, Bialleck H et al. Biosimilar filgrastim mobilizes haematopoietic stem cells in health volunteer donors with expected efficiency and typical acute adverse effects: interim results of a post-authorization safety study. Bone Marrow Transplant 2013;**48**(2):S28 (0177).

8 Di Persio JF, Micallef IN, Stiff PJ et al. Phase III prospective randomized double-blind placebo-controlled trial of plerixafor plus granulocyte colony-stimulating factor compared with placebo plus granulocyte colony-stimulating factor for autologous stem-cell mobilization and transplantation for patients with non-Hodgkin's lymphoma. J Clin Oncol 2009;**27**(28):4767–73.

9 Di Persio JF, Stadtmauer EA, Nademanee A et al. Plerixafor and G-CSF versus placebo and G-CSF to mobilize hematopoietic stem cells for autologous stem cell transplantation in patients with multiple myeloma. Blood 2009;**113**(23):5720–6.

10 NHS England. Clinical Commissioning Policy: Use of Plerixafor for Stem Cell Mobilization (Update). Available at: www.england.nhs.uk/commissioning/wp-content/uploads/sites/12/2015/01/b04-use-plerixfr-stemcll-moblstn-fin.pdf (accessed 17 November 2016).

11 Durate RF, Shaw BE, Marin P et al. Plerixafor plus granulocyte CSF can mobilize hematopoietic stem cells from multiple myeloma and lymphoma patients failing previous mobilization attempts: EU compassionate use data. Bone Marrow Transplant 2011;**46**:52–8.

12 Li J, Hamilton E, Vaughn L et al. Effective and cost analysis of 'just-in-time' salvage plerixafor administration in autologous transplant patients with poor stem cell mobilization kinetics. Transfusion 2011;**51**: 2175–82.

13 Gutensohn K, Magens MM, Kuehnl P et al. Increasing the economic efficacy of peripheral blood progenitor cell collections by monitoring peripheral blood CD34+ concentrations. Transfusion 2010;**50**(3):656–62.

14 Heimfeld S. HLA-identical stem cell transplantation: is there an optimal CD34 cell dose? Bone Marrow Transplant 2003;**31**:839–45.

15 FACT-JACIE. International Standards for Hematopoietic Cellular Therapy Product Collection, Processing, and Administration, 6th edn. Available at: www.jacie.org/standards/6th-edition-2015 (accessed 17 November 2016).

16 Abrahamsen JF, Stamnesfet S, Liseth K. Large-volume leukopheresis yields more viable CD34+ cells and colony-forming units than normal-volume leukopheresis, especially in patients who mobilize low numbers of CD34+ cells. Transfusion 2005;**45**:248–53.

17 Reeves HM, Winters JL. The mechanisms of action of plasma exchange. Br J Haematol 2014;**164**:342–51.

18 El-Ghariani K, Unsworth DJ. Therapeutic apheresis – plasmapheresis. Clin Med 2006;**4**: 343–7.

19 Schwartz J, Padmanabhan A, Aqui N, Balogun RA, Connelly-Smith L, Delaney M, Dunbar NM, Witt V, Wu Y, Shaz BH Guidelines on the Use of Therapeutic Apheresis in Clinical Practice-Evidence-Based Approach from the Writing Committee of the American Society for Apheresis: The Seventh Special Issue J Clin Apheresis, 2016, **31**: 149–162.

20 Siegel JF, Rich MA, Brock WA. Association of sickle cell disease, priapism, exchange transfusion and neurological events: ASPEN syndrome. J Urol 1993;**150**(5 Pt 1):1480–2.

21 Scarisbrick JJ, Taylor P, Holtick U et al. UK consensus statement on the use of extracorporeal photopheresis for treatment of cutaneous T-cell lymphoma and chronic graft versus-host disease. Br J Dermatol 2008;**158**(4):659–78.

22 Knobler R, Berlin G, Calzavara-Pinton P et al. Guidelines on the use of extracorporeal photopheresis. J Eur Acad Dermatol Venereol 2014;**28**(Suppl. 1):1–36.

23 Perfetti P, Carlier P, Strada P et al. Extracorporal photopheresis for the treatment of steroid refractory acute GVHD. Bone Marrow Transplant 2008;**42**:609–17.

Further Reading

George JN. How I treat patients with thrombotic thrombocytopenic purpura. Blood 2010;**116**:4060–9.

Gertz MA. Current status of stem cell mobilization. Br J Haematol 2010;**150**:647–62.

Howell C, Douglas K, Cho G et al. Guidelines on the clinical use of apheresis procedures for the treatment of patients and collection of cellular therapy products. Transfus Med 2015;**25**(2):57–78.

Kim H. Red cell exchange: special focus on sickle cell disease. Hematology Am Soc Hematol Educ Program 2014;**2014**(1):450–6.

Scully M, Hunt B, Benjamin S et al. Guidelines on the diagnosis and management of thrombotic thrombocytopenic purpura and other thrombotic microangiopathies. Br J Haematol 2012;**158**(3):323–35.

Shaz BH, Schwartz J, Winters JL et al. ASFA guidelines support use of red cell exchange for severe malaria with high parasitemia. Clin Infect Dis 2014;**58**(2):302–3.

Siddiq S, Pamphilon D, Brunskill S et al. Bone marrow harvest versus peripheral stem cell collection for haemopoietic stem cell donation in healthy donors. Cochrane Database Syst Rev 2009;**1**:CD006406.

40 Haemopoietic Stem Cell Processing and Storage

Hira Mian[1] Ronan Foley[2] and Pamela O'Hoski[2]

[1] Department of Oncology, McMaster University, Hamilton, Ontario
[2] Department of Pathology and Molecular Medicine, McMaster University, Hamilton, Canada

Introduction

Once exclusively obtained from the posterior pelvis of a suitable donor under general anaesthesia, haemopoietic progenitor cells (HPCs) are now routinely collected from peripheral blood as well as from the umbilical cord and placenta post delivery. Recognition that haemopoietic growth factors (i.e. granulocyte-colony stimulating factor (G-CSF)), administered alone or following chemotherapy, result in mobilisation of HPCs into peripheral blood has had a profound impact on stem cell collection both for autologous transplantation and for healthy allogeneic stem cell donors. Identification of HPCs correlates with expression of the CD34+ antigen. Functional evaluation of colony-forming units (CFUs) of myeloid, erythroid, megakaryocytic and long-term culture initiating cells may be useful to complement immunophenotypic analysis.

Terminology to describe HPC and other cell-based human products derived from a bone marrow harvest (HPC, Marrow), from mobilised apheresis peripheral blood (HPC, Apheresis), from umbilical cord (HPC, Cord Blood) or from steady-state apheresis for donor lymphocyte infusion (DLI) (Mononuclear cells, Apheresis) (Table 40.1) has been proposed by the International Society for Blood Transfusion (ISBT 128 nomenclature). Each source exhibits different biological properties and graft composition which offer advantages and disadvantages for specific types of clinical transplant procedures. Cytokine mobilised apheresis products contain a higher number of CD34+ progenitors which may be ideal for reduced-intensity allogeneic and autologous transplants. Apheresis also harvests more T-lymphocytes which may increase chronic graft-versus-host disease (GVHD) [1]. Cord blood may have fewer progenitor cells, but compensates with a higher proliferative potential and a lower risk of GVHD [2].

Transplant Procedures

Autologous Stem Cell Transplant

Expanding indications support the use of autologous stem cell transplant (SCT) in a variety of clinical settings, including multiple myeloma (single or tandem) and relapsed non-Hodgkin's and Hodgkin's lymphoma (B and T aggressive histology lymphoma, mantle cell lymphoma, Burkitt's and follicular lymphoma). Autologous SCT is also a therapeutic option for patients with gonadal or retroperitoneal germ cell tumours refractory to cisplatin-based chemotherapy. At present, autologous progenitor cells are obtained by leucapheresis. Use of HPC, Apheresis reduces the time to engraftment with shorter hospitalisation, reduced transfusional support and reduced the use of antimicrobials [3], all leading to cost reductions.

Practical Transfusion Medicine, Fifth Edition. Edited by Michael F. Murphy, David J. Roberts and Mark H. Yazer.
© 2017 John Wiley & Sons Ltd. Published 2017 by John Wiley & Sons Ltd.

Table 40.1 Human haemopoietic progenitor cells (HPCs).

Name	Donor	Options	Storage
HPC, Marrow Collect 10–15 mL/kg recipient weight with maximum 20 mL/kg donor weight Dose $3–5 \times 10^8$/kg recipient weight	Matched related donor Matched unrelated donor Autologous (rare)	Standard intraoperative marrow harvest adults or children	Usually infused liquid within 6 hours following collection Cryopreservation post buffy coat concentration
HPC, Apheresis Process 12–20 litres of donor blood	Autologous patient (common)	Apheresis product collected following a stem cell mobilisation agent (G-CSF, pegylated G-CSF, GM-CSF, SCF, plerixafor) ± chemotherapy	Auto SCT – cryopreserved
	Matched related donor	Mobilise with 5–10 µg/kg G-CSF	Allo SCT – infused following collection or cryopreserved
	Matched unrelated donor	Mobilise with 5–10 µg/kg G-CSF	
	Haploidentical donor	Mobilise with 16 µg/kg G-CSF	CD34+ selection, T-cell depletion and cryopreservation
MNC-apheresis or T-cell apheresis Donor lymphocyte infusion	Matched related donor Matched unrelated donor	Same donor as original HPC product – steady state Dose = CD3+/lymphocyte/kg recipient weight	Graduated doses, first dose following collection, later doses cryopreserved
HPC, Cord	Cord blood approximately 100 mL Matched unrelated donor	Consenting parent(s) $>3.0 \times 10^7$/kg recipient weight *In utero* *Ex utero*	Red cell depleted cryopreserved

G-CSF, granulocyte-colony stimulating factor; GM-CSF, granulocyte macrophage-colony stimulating factor; MNC, mononuclear cell; SCF, stem cell factor; SCT, stem cell transplant.

Allogeneic Stem Cell Transplant

Allogeneic SCT involves replacement of a diseased bone marrow with haemopoietic elements from a healthy donor. Engraftment of both HPCs as well as donor immune T-lymphocytes are essential for long-term haemopoiesis and disease control. Donor lymphocytes contribute to both graft-versus-leukaemia (GVL) as well as GVHD. Shifting the balance of therapeutic efficacy solely from stem cell replacement to maintenance of a transplanted donor immune system has led to reduced intensity conditioning (RIC) allogeneic transplants.

Allogeneic donors may be a sibling or obtained from a bone marrow registry. Matches are based on the human leucocyte antigen (HLA) system composed of genes on chromosome 6. The major histocompatibility complex (MHC) is made up of two basic classes involved in antigen presentation and immune activation. MHC class I includes HLA-A, HLA-B and HLA-C, whereas MHC class II includes HLA-DR, HLA-DQ and HLA DP. Proteins encoded by HLA define self and directly instruct the immune system to recognise self versus non-self. HLA typing previously employed simple serological testing (antibody based) to provide low-resolution (LR) typing. Although useful in the related setting, there have been concerns regarding use of LR typing in unrelated donors. Many HLA laboratories now routinely perform high-resolution (HR) molecular typing.

If an unrelated match cannot be found, remaining options include haploidentical transplantation or allogeneic transplant using cryopreserved cord blood. Haploidentical SCT involves a family member with only a partial HLA match (4/8). Due to significant HLA barriers, large-volume CD34+ product must be rigorously purified (T-depleted). This may result in lasting immune deficiency with a high risk of fulminant infection (viral, cytomegalovirus (CMV), Epstein–Barr virus (EBV)) or relapse. Recently, clinical evidence has suggested that administration of cyclophosphamide following stem cell infusion may be an effective *in vivo* T-cell purge [4].

Donor Lymphocyte Infusions

Apheresis from an original HPC donor in an unstimulated state is called MNC-apheresis and T-cell apheresis (CD3+ content known). These DLI products may be used to boost a mixed chimerism to full donor chimerism after allogeneic HPC transplant or as preemptive therapy for treatment of an early relapse via a direct GVL effect. Given the risk of severe GVHD, graduated doses of donor T-cells are often administered over time. Lymphocyte content is calculated using automated or manual differential as well as flow cytometry (CD3+). The laboratory will aliquot doses (defined by institution or protocol) based on CD3+ $\times 10^6$/kg of recipient weight, often giving the first dose fresh and cryopreserving other doses.

Haemopoietic Progenitor Cell Products

Bone Marrow

Use of bone marrow (HPC, Marrow) remains a mainstay of treatment for paediatric or patients with aplastic anaemia. Collecting bone marrow involves placing a suitable donor under general anaesthesia and aspirating 10–15 mL/kg recipient weight (maximum 20 mL/kg donor weight) from both posterior iliac crests. Collected fresh product (mixed with ACD/heparin) is passed through 500 and 200 µm filters to remove bone and other debris prior to infusion or further processing. The target nucleated cell dose (automated counter) is $3–5 \times 10^8$/kg recipient weight. Use of marrow CD34+ enumeration suggests that a CD34+ cell dose $>3.0 \times 10^6$/kg correlates with improved recovery and five-year survival while $<1.2 \times 10^6$/kg correlates with inferior recovery [5,6].

Peripheral Blood

Mobilisation of CD34+ progenitor cells into blood with collection by leucapheresis (HPC, Apheresis) is the method of choice for autologous SCT. This procedure is based on obtaining sufficient CD34+ progenitor cells (defined as a minimum of 2.0×10^6 CD34+ cells/kg recipient weight and an optimal of 5.0×10^6 CD34+ cells/kg recipient weight). Lower doses of infused CD34+ cells can result in delayed or failed platelet engraftment. Case-by-case decisions are made based on the clinical situation and stability of the underlying disease, to proceed with autologous SCT when fewer than 2.0×10^6/kg CD34+ cells are available. For patients undergoing autologous SCT, two mobilisation strategies can be employed: either growth factor(s) alone or growth factors that follow administration of chemotherapy (chemo-mobilisation).

In some patients, G-CSF and chemotherapy still result in suboptimal stem cell yields. Plerixafor (AMD3100) can antagonise the binding of the chemokine stromal cell-derived factor-1 (SDF-1) to its cognate receptor CXCR4, and so rapid and reversibly mobilises haemopoietic stem cells into the peripheral circulation. It synergises with G-CSF and using this CXCR4 antagonist with G-CSF can salvage those who fail G-CSF mobilisation alone.

Healthy allogeneic donors may also be asked to provide mobilised peripheral blood progenitors collected by leucapheresis. Administration of G-CSF alone is the currently accepted strategy for mobilisation of normal healthy donors. Use of HPC, Apheresis as opposed to HPC,

Marrow appears to improve the time to haemopoietic recovery and offers a greater GVL effect [6], but carries a potentially higher risk of chronic extensive GVHD [7].

Umbilical Cord Blood

Characteristics of banked cord products include highly functional HPCs, less CMV contamination and a lower risk of GVHD. It is generally accepted that the kinetics of haemopoietic recovery are significantly slower. This may relate to fewer and less mature HPCs. A minimum target of approximately 3.0×10^7 nucleated cells per kg recipient weight per unit of cord blood is suggested. A higher dose may be considered depending on HLA disparity. Measurement of CD34+ cells/kg recipient weight may be more informative. The mean collection volume for a cord sample is approximately 100 mL (50–200 mL) including anticoagulant [8].

Several techniques for cord blood collection may be performed either before or after delivery of the placenta. Closed system collection techniques have improved rates of bacterial contamination. Cells can be stored in a smaller volume by immediately removing plasma and red blood cells. Characterisation of the cord unit includes volume, weight, total nucleated count, CD34+ cell count, colony-forming analysis, ABO/Rh and HLA typing, full panel transmissible disease testing and haemoglobin electrophoresis [9]. *In vitro* analysis has suggested reasonable viability to as long as 15 years, perhaps longer [10]. In an effort to hasten time to reconstitution in larger adult recipients, double UCB is now being considered [11].

Haemopoietic Progenitor Cell Product Assessment and Specialised Procedures

CD34 Enumeration

Flow cytometry on a fresh HPC product provides CD34+ enumeration in a timely manner (one hour). Given the importance of accurate CD34+ enumeration, the procedure should follow a standardised and validated methodology (i.e. ISHAGE guidelines) [12]. A CD34+ enumeration kit includes CD45-FITC/CD34-PE, isotype control PE, stem cell microbeads (known concentration/µL), lysing solution (ammonium chloride) and a viability dye 7-aminoactinomycin D (7-AAD). HPC samples stored at 18–20 °C should be processed within a few hours and samples kept overnight should be stored at 2–6 °C. Total viable CD34, apoptotic and necrotic cells can be measured with calculations based on product volume.

Peripheral blood CD34+ (expressed per microlitre) enumeration prior to collection may be instructive and predictive.

Viability Assays

Trypan blue (TB) is a simple exclusion dye test indicating viability. Cells that fail to exclude dye are considered nonviable. Use of fluorescent stains with dark-field microscopy may reduce background staining. 7-Aminoactinomycin (7-AAD) is a fluorescent chemical with affinity for GC-rich DNA. Nonviable cells lack membrane integrity and will take up 7-AAD, which can be measured by flow cytometry. When performing viability for cryopreserved HPC product, it is important to keep in mind that small aliquots will have different cooling properties that may diminish viability. Thus, viability results from a cryovial are simply an estimate of viability for an actual product contained in a bag.

In Vitro HPC Assays

Functional analysis of HPCs can be performed using cells grown in semi-solid methylcellulose (MC) to identify CFU. Resultant CFU-erythroid, CFU-granulocyte, CFU-mixed (CFU-GEMM) and CFU-megakaryocyte colonies help to characterise the short-term multipotency of a given HPC product. These assays are time consuming (two weeks) and do not provide real-time information for products that are administered shortly after collection. Facilities managing HPC, Cord products that are stored frozen over long periods may offer colony assay results together with CD34 content. These assays are useful in the evaluation of long-term storage and for validation of newer cryopreservation strategies.

Sterility Testing

Sterility testing suitable for detecting clinically significant bacteria and fungal contamination of an HPC product must be performed at a minimum post processing. It is our preference to collect cultures when the product arrives in the laboratory and after each step of processing. Paediatric bottles can be used to minimise the volume of sample removed from the product. Cultures should be performed (i) at the end of HPC product collection and the end of processing for cryopreservation and (ii) after each reprocessing step (washing cells, manipulation on cell processor, post-CD34+ selection). Cultures may also be obtained from each bag at the time of reinfusion.

ABO Incompatibility

Human leucocyte antigen-matched HPC SCT can proceed even if the blood groups of donor and recipient do not match. There are two types of ABO mismatch, each with its own interventions, which may need to occur before the transplant product can be infused [13]. ABO major mismatch results when the recipient's plasma contains a potent ABO antibody directed against donor red cells. HPC, Apheresis products have a haematocrit of 5–10%, whereas the red cell content of HPC, Marrow haematocrit is much higher, ranging from 25% to 30%. Significant intravascular lysis of red cells will cause a haemolytic transfusion reaction if the product is infused without a reduction in the level of the ABO antibody. Recipients who have an ABO antibody titre against donor red cells greater than 1:16 may be prepared by performing several apheresis procedures to replace plasma with 5% albumin. The titre of antibody can be further reduced by infusing plasma containing a soluble ABO substance that matches

the problem antibody. These measures are generally sufficient to allow safe infusion of HPC, Apheresis, but significant residual antibody after other interventions may require processing of HPC, Marrow to remove most of the red cell content. Red cell depletion of marrow is most commonly performed using a blood processor such as the Cobe 2991 with or without the addition of a regimenting agent like hydroxethyl starch (HES). Red cell content at completion of processing should be as low as possible while minimising loss of progenitor cells.

An ABO minor mismatch results when the donor's plasma contains a potent antibody directed against recipient red cells. The need for intervention is less common in this setting as the ratio of antibody to red cell antigen is much lower, but it is wise to assess the level of donor antibody against the intended recipient's red cells. The presence of an antibody with a titre above 1:256 may necessitate group O red cell exchange of the recipient if the product is HPC, Apheresis. HPC, Marrow should undergo plasma depletion to remove at least 80% of antibody either through manual centrifugation or in semi-closed mode using a Cobe 2991 or similar blood processor.

CD34+ Enrichment

CD34+ enrichment of HPC products is performed for a variety of reasons: haploidentical transplant, reduction of potential tumour burden in autologous HPC products and providing a T-cell-depleted product to a recipient at high risk of GVHD. Both HPC, Apheresis and HPC, Marrow can be enriched for CD34+ cells but the marrow product must first be processed to derive a buffy coat concentrate by reducing the overall volume and the red cell content. Commercially available CD34+ enrichment devices using monoclonal antibodies have proven highly effective. The CliniMacs™ instrument from Miltenyi Biotec produces an extremely pure product (with an average 98% T-cell depletion) while recovering 65–75% of the initial CD34+ cell content.

T-Cell Depletion

Despite the use of potent immunosuppressive agents (i.e. methotrexate, ciclosporin), GVHD remains a common (up to 50%) complication for patients undergoing allogeneic SCT. GVHD is primarily mediated by T-lymphocytes, which can be successfully removed from the graft prior to administration. T-cell depletion can clearly reduce GVHD but also may hinder engraftment, increase the incidence of leukaemic relapse and the risk of infections, including posttransplant lymphoproliferative disorders. *Ex vivo* procedures to reduce T-cells include physical separation by density gradient (counterflow centrifugal elutriation), depletion with lectins, cytotoxic drugs and the use of anti-T-cell antibodies (examples are CD2, CD3, CD5, CD8, CD25 and CD52) alone or in combination (complement, conjugated to toxin). Despite an ability to significantly eliminate T-cells to as low as $<1 \times 10^5$ CD3+ cells/kg recipient weight and attenuate acute GVHD, no differences in chronic GVHD, transplant-related mortality and disease-free survival have been proven to date [14].

Storage of Haemopoietic Progenitor Cell Products

In many instances, the HPC product is stored for short periods of time (hours) in an unmanipulated liquid state. Reported temperatures suitable for short-term storage range from 4 °C to 27 °C (Table 40.2). Ambient temperature is often preferred for short-term storage of HPC, Marrow [15] but 'ambient' should be a specific temperature range, for example 18–22 °C. HPCs collected by apheresis can be held at room temperature for 1–2 hours if further processing is to occur imminently, but are most commonly stored at 4 °C when longer storage is required. There is a progressive loss of progenitor cells during nonfrozen storage, with the rate of loss influenced by cell concentration, quantity and type of other cells contained in the product, the storage bag and the storage temperature [16].

The leucocyte count should be diluted with donor plasma to $<2 \times 10^8$/mL if overnight storage is planned.

The length of time the product can be stored should also be established by in-house viability measurements and an expiry date and time set for each type of product handled. Storage requirements should include designating a location dedicated to HPC products and a separate, clearly labelled location for any product that must be quarantined. A mechanism for monitoring and documenting temperature that includes both local and remote alarms must be in place. If the product is stored at 'ambient temperature', the temperature of the location of storage must be documented. There should be a posted contingency plan that deals with temperature outside the designated range or mechanical failure of the designated storage equipment.

Cryopreservation

The majority of allogeneic products are not cryopreserved. However, cryopreservation of allogeneic products may allow increased flexibility in the timing of the transplant related to the donor collection. In other cases, donor availability or a change in the recipient's condition may dictate that the collected product be cryopreserved. Virtually all products to be used for autologous SCT are cryopreserved to allow time for conditioning and clearance of chemotherapy drugs from the circulation.

Preparation of Products for Freezing

Haemopoietic progenitor cell products to be cryopreserved must be transported to the processing laboratory in a designated transport cooler that has been validated for transport time and temperature. The receiving staff must document the minimum/maximum and actual temperatures of transport and inspect the product for colour, leakage and correct labelling. All materials to be used in the cryopreservation process should have lot number and expiry date

Table 40.2 Stem cell laboratory processing procedures.

Procedure	Methods	Indication
Red cell depletion of HPC, Marrow	Semi-automated – Cobe 2991 cell processor with or without HES Manual centrifugation	Major ABO/other antigens Cryopreservation of HPC, Cord Blood
Plasma depletion of HPC, Marrow	Semi-automated – Cobe 2991 cell processor Manual centrifugation	Minor ABO mismatch
Buffy coat concentration	Centrifugation Semi-automated – Cobe 2991 cell processor	Volume reduction Cryopreservation of HPC, Marrow
Sterility	Bacterial and fungal detection Investigational products (mycoplasma, adventitial virus, endotoxin)	HPC products before cryopreservation and after thaw Cryoprotectant solutions
Viability	Dye exclusion (TB), fluorescence microscopy 7-AAD – flow cytometry	Products used after more than 2 years of storage
CD34/CD3 enumeration	Flow cytometry (i.e. ISHAGE)	HPC, Apheresis HPC, Marrow HPC-C (optional) MNC-apheresis
Functional HPC assays	CFU assays, LTC-IC	Viability post long-term storage Viability post investigative procedure (purging) Validation of new procedure to document HPC loss Assess stored cryopreserved product post 'warming event'
CD34 enrichment	Immunomagnetic bead-based separation	Related haploidentical SCT 'purge' technique Selected cases (GVHD prophylaxis) Clinical trial
T-cell depletion	Antibody based ± toxin Elutriation	Investigational product Selected cases Clinical trial
Cryopreservation	DMSO, HES/DMSO controlled-rate freezing or freeze in −80° C Liquid nitrogen storage below −150 °C	Option for all HPC products

AAD, aminoactinomycin D; CFU, colony-forming unit; DMSO, dimethyl sulfoxide; GVHD, graft-versus-host disease; HES, hydroxyethyl starch; HPC, haemopoietic progenitor cell; LTC-IC, long-term culture-initiating cell; MNC, mononuclear cell; SCT, stem cell transplant.

recorded. The product must be manipulated in a fully maintained and inspected biohazard safety cabinet. HPC, Marrow and HPC, Cord products require processing to reduce mature red cell content and volume reduction before cryo-preservation processing can occur. In most instances, the haematocrit of HPC, Apheresis is between 5% and 10%, so these products can be cryopreserved without removal of mature red cells. Plasma collected from the donor (apher-esis) or retained from red cell depletion (referred to as concurrent plasma) should always accom-pany the product to the processing laboratory in case there is a need to dilute the product.

Sterility testing must be performed on the product on arrival and after the addition of the cryoprotectant solution. Once sterility samples are collected, samples are drawn for a nucleated cell count and CD34 assessment; products with a nucleated cell count higher than 4.5×10^8/mL can be diluted with concurrent donor plasma.

Techniques for cryopreservation are designed to interfere with mechanisms that cause cell damage or death during the freezing process [18]. HPCs need to be protected from dehydration and ice crystal formation within the cell. Dimethyl sulfoxide (DMSO) is a 'penetrating cryoprotectant' that acts not only by slowing water absorption by the ice crystals but also by rapid diffusion into the cell and so facilitating movement of water out of the cell without excessive osmotic stress and before intracellular ice crystal formation can occur.

Freezing Cellular Products

The cooling rate should minimise ice formation potential and complement the cryoprotectant's adjustment of the solution's rate of cooling. The optimum concentration of DMSO to achieve good penetration of cells and moderation of the freezing point of the extracellular water is 10% volume/volume. Reduced concentrations of DMSO (5%) can be used if DMSO is combined with a macromolecular cryoprotectant such as HES [18]. Cryoprotection can be accomplished by using macromolecules alone but a 'combined' cryoprotectant seems to afford better cell recoveries than the use of macromolecules alone. This type of cryoprotectant solution is a complex blend of salts, sugars, DMSO and plasma proteins and requires careful preparation. Plasma proteins also have cryoprotectant properties and the addition of serum proteins as donor plasma or 5% human serum albumin to a cryoprotectant solution appears to improve HPC survival.

Red Cell Removal

Processing of products to remove mature red cells should be performed prior to cryopreservation for HPC, Marrow and HPC, Cord Blood,

to limit infusion of free haemoglobin and renal toxicity. Large quantities of red cells can also cause clumping of the product during processing. Bone marrow product may be processed before cryopreservation, not only to remove red blood cells but also to eliminate fat and the majority of plasma volume and so allow cryopreservation at a desirable cell concentration to optimise cell recovery and reduce the volume of the final product. Centrifugation can be performed manually between 800 g and 1000 g or in a semi-automatic manner using a Cobe 2991 cell processor. Most laboratories freeze HPCs at concentrations between 1.0 and 5.0×10^8/mL but successful cryopreservation and recovery have been reported using concentrations as high as 8×10^8/mL and as low as 1×10^6/mL.

Most centres avoid the risk of large ice crystal formation by storing at or below −150 °C in mechanical freezers or in the vapour or liquid phase of nitrogen. Products and temperature monitoring devices should be placed well below the rim of liquid nitrogen freezers to minimise the increase of temperature caused by opening the lid. Products exposed to frequent temperature change are at risk of progressive damage to stored cells and this can be reduced by placing products well below the rim of liquid nitrogen freezers and by using aluminium storage canisters and frameworks to moderate thermal changes in the freezer. Products may be stored for at least seven years. Engraftment kinetics are identical to those seen after transplantation for the first half of the product stored for only 1−2 months [19].

Thawing of Cryopreserved Haemopoietic Progenitor Cells

Thawing can occur at the patient bedside or in the laboratory. Units should be transported in a liquid nitrogen dry shipper with continuous temperature monitoring to maintain the temperature below −120 °C. In most instances, thawing is performed in a water bath between 35 °C and 39 °C. If the cells are thawed too slowly, there is risk of injury from ice recrystallisation; if the temperature is too high, there is loss of viability or clumping of protein material within the bag.

Cryoprotectant can cause toxicity to the recipient but if the dose of DMSO is carefully controlled, it is not necessary to remove it prior to infusion. The DMSO dose should be limited to less than 1 g/kg of recipient weight in a 24-hour period. If the total amount of DMSO exceeds this limit, infusion should occur over two days. DMSO can be removed using serial dilutions of protein-based solution to avoid osmotic shock to cells. DMSO infusion can cause nausea, chills, cardiac arrhythmias, neurological symptoms and respiratory arrest but the majority of reactions are transient and few patients require clinical treatment.

Quality Assurance

A quality programme defines the policies and environment necessary to attain acceptable outcomes and meet safety standards consistently. The components include standard operating procedures (SOPs) that address all activities, standardised and controlled labelling, documentation/record keeping that ensures traceability, personnel qualifications and training, building, facilities and equipment validation, environmental monitoring, regular auditing and error and accident system/management. Regulatory authorities worldwide have placed major emphasis on the establishment of an effective quality programme along with strict compliance to best practices in clinical, collection and laboratory settings. At the processing laboratory, the quality programme is the means by which good manufacturing practices are instituted and followed throughout product manufacturing and manipulation.

KEY POINTS

1) Clinical indications for both autologous and allogeneic stem cell transplants are increasing.
2) HPCs can be obtained from three sources: bone marrow, peripheral blood and umbilical cord blood. Characteristics of these products differ in terms of HPCs and other mature cells.
3) Validated methods for cryopreservation are a key requirement to ensure optimal graft performance following administration to a transplant recipient.

4) Accurate nucleated cell counting, CD34+ enumeration and sterility analysis before and after cryopreservation are essential.
5) Quality assurance testing of products at multiple stages of processing is essential to assure the safety, composition and potency of the product and must form part of an established quality assurance and accreditation programme to guarantee high standards in HPC transplantation.

References

1 Stem Cell Trialists' Collaborative Group. Allogeneic peripheral blood stem-cell compared with bone marrow transplantation in the management of hematologic malignancies: an individual patient data meta-analysis of nine randomized trials. J Clin Oncol 2005;**23**:5074–87.

2 Wagner JE, Barker JN, Defor TE et al. Transplantation of unrelated donor umbilical cord blood in 102 patients with malignant and nonmalignant diseases: influence of CD34 cell dose and HLA disparity on treatment related mortality and survival. Blood 2002;**100**:1611–18.

3 Vellenga E, van Agthoven M, Coockewit AJ et al. Autologous peripheral blood stem cell transplantation in patients with relapsed lymphoma results in accelerated haemopoietic reconstitution, improved quality of life and cost reduction compared with bone marrow transplantation: the Hovon 22 study. Br J Haematol 2001;**114**:319–26.

4 Luznik L, O'Donnell PV, Symons HJ et al. HLA-haploidentical bone marrow transplantation for hematologic malignancies using non-myeloablative condition and high-dose, post-transplantation cyclophosphamide. Biol Blood Marrow Transplant 2008;**14**:641.

5 Zubair AC, Zahrieh D, Daley H et al. Engraftment of autologous and allogeneic marrow HPCs after myeloablative therapy. Transfusion 2004;**44**:253–61.

6 Couban S, Simpson DR, Barnett MJ et al. A randomized multicenter comparison of bone marrow and peripheral blood in recipients of matched sibling allogeneic transplants for myeloid malignancies. Blood 2002;**100**:1525–31.

7 Schrezenmeier H, Passweg JR, Marsh JC et al. Worse outcome and more chronic GVHD with peripheral blood progenitor cells than bone marrow in HLA-matched sibling donor transplants for young patients with severe acquired aplastic anemia. Blood 2007;**110**:1397–400.

8 Reed W, Smith R, Dekovic F et al. Comprehensive banking of sibling donor cord blood for children with malignant and nonmalignant disease. Blood 2003;**101**:351.

9 Eichler H, Meckies J, Schmut N et al. Aspects of donation and processing of stem cell transplants from umbilical cord blood. Z Geburtshilfe Neonatol 2001;**205**:218.

10 Broxmeyer HE, Srour EF, Hangoc G et al. High efficiency recovery of functional haemopoietic progenitor cells from human cord blood cryopreserved for 15 years. Proc Natl Acad Sci USA 2003;**100**:645.

11 Wall DA, Chan KW. Selection of cord unit(s) for transplantation. Bone Marrow Transplant 2008;**42**:1.

12 Sutherland DR, Anderson L, Keeney M, Nayar R, Chin-Yee I. The ISHAGE guidelines for CD34 + determination by flow cytometry. International Society of Hematotherapy and Graft Engineering. J Hematother 1996;**5**:213–26.

13 Rowley SD, Donato ML, Bhattacharyya P. Red blood cell incompatible allogeneic haemopoietic progenitor cell transplantation. Bone Marrow Transplant 2011;**46**:1167–85.

14 Hale G, Zhang MJ, Bunjes D et al. Improving the outcome of bone marrow transplantation by using CD52 monoclonal antibodies to prevent graft-versus host disease and graft rejection. Blood 1998;**92**:4581.

15 Antonenas V, Garvin F, Webb M et al. Fresh PBSC harvest, but not bone marrow show temperature related loss of CD34 viability during storage and transport. Cytotherapy 2006;**8**:158–65.

16 Peltengell R, Wall PJ, O'Connor D et al. Viability of haemopoietic progenitors from whole blood, bone marrow and leucapheresis product. Effects of storage media, temperature and time. Bone Marrow Transplant 1994;**14**(5):703–9.

17 Bakken AM. Cryopreserving human stem cells. Curr Stem Cell Res Ther 2006;**1**:47–54.

18 Rowley SD, Feng Z, Chen L et al. A randomized phase III trial of autologous blood stem cell transplantation comparing cryopreservation using dimethylsulfoxide versus dimethylsulfoxide with hydroxyethyl starch. Bone Marrow Transplant 2003;**31**:1043–51.

19 Cameron G, Tantiworawit A, Halpenny M et al. Cryopreserved mobilised autologous blood progenitors stored for more than two years successfully support blood count recovery after high dose chemotherapy. Cytotherapy 2011;**13**(7):856–63.

Further Reading

Martin-Henao GA, Torrico C, Azqueta C et al. Cryopreservation of HPC from apheresis at high cell concentrations does not impair the hematological recovery after transplantation. Transfusion 2005;**15**:1917–24.

Thomas ED, Appelbaum FR, Blume KG, Forman SJ, Negrin RS. Haemopoietic Cell Transplantation, 4th edn. Wiley-Blackwell, Chichester, 2009.

41 Haematopoietic Stem Cell Transplantation

Robert D. Danby[1], Rachel Protheroe[2] and David J. Roberts[3,4]

[1] Churchill Hospital, Oxford University Hospitals NHS Foundation Trust, Oxford, UK
[2] Bristol Adult Bone Marrow Transplant Unit, University Hospitals Bristol, Bristol, UK
[3] Radcliffe Department of Medicine, Oxford University Hospitals NHS Foundation Trust, Oxford, UK
[4] NHS Blood and Transplant, John Radcliffe Hospital, Oxford, UK

Introduction

Although the treatment of haematological malignancies has improved over the last 40 years, many patients still have diseases that remain incurable with conventional chemotherapy alone. Bone marrow cells are exquisitely sensitive to chemotherapy and radiotherapy. The recognition that radiation could permanently kill bone marrow function while other organs were largely unaffected or fully recovered suggested that bone marrow transplantation (BMT) (also known as haematopoietic stem cell transplantation – HSCT) might be feasible [1].

Initially, pretransplant conditioning chemoradiotherapy was thought to provide 'space' for the incoming cells to engraft, as well as killing residual cancer cells. Therefore, *autologous* (HSC from the patient) and *allogeneic* (HSC from another individual) transplants were perceived as intensification of treatment with haematopoietic 'rescue' only. However, it became apparent that allogeneic HSCT also produced an immune-mediated graft-versus-tumour (GvT) effect, since patients with chronic graft-versus-host disease (GvHD) had less relapse and improved disease-free survival [2]. Some patients with chronic myeloid leukaemia (CML), who relapsed after allogeneic HSCT, could also return to full molecular remission by infusion of additional lymphocytes from the original donor (a donor lymphocyte infusion – DLI), further evidence of a GvT response [3].

Allogeneic HSCT is therefore a combination of chemotherapy and/or radiotherapy with the donor-derived immune response, providing a major component in treating the original disease. As such, allogeneic HSCT has a lower relapse rate, compared to autologous HSCT, but is associated with a higher incidence of post-transplant infections and immune-mediated complications.

Principles of Haematopoietic Stem Cell Transplants

Haematopoietic stem cell transplantation is used to:

- enable intensification of chemotherapy and radiotherapy so that toxicity to the bone marrow is no longer the major limiting factor in determining outcome
- ensure complete engraftment of the donor marrow through immunosuppression of the host (patient), so permitting tolerance to develop
- promote a GvT effect.

Practical Transfusion Medicine, Fifth Edition. Edited by Michael F. Murphy, David J. Roberts and Mark H. Yazer.
© 2017 John Wiley & Sons Ltd. Published 2017 by John Wiley & Sons Ltd.

Indications for haematopoietic stem cell transplants

Haematopoietic stem cell therapy is used when conventional dose treatment has failed or is expected to have a high likelihood of failure. The failure of primary therapy when disease recurs is a clear endpoint. However, the perception that failure is likely is more subjective, although some objective evidence may be present. For example, the presence of the Philadelphia chromosome in acute lymphoblastic leukaemia (ALL) or the presence of high-risk cytogenetics (e.g. monosomy 7) or molecular abnormalities (FLT-3 mutation) in acute myeloid leukaemia (AML) are associated with a high risk of relapse with chemotherapy alone [4]. Prognostic scoring systems (e.g. IPSS-R for myelodysplastic syndrome – MDS) can also be used to help select patients who may benefit from transplantation [5]. Current indications for HSCT are regularly reviewed and updated by the British Society for Blood and Marrow Transplantation (BSBMT) and are summarised in Table 41.1.

Source of Stem Cells

Autologous Cells

Collected from the patient and cryopreserved prior to transplant. Allows haemopoietic rescue but does not demonstrate a GvT effect.

Table 41.1 Classification of indications for blood and marrow transplants (www.bsbmt.org).

Degree of consensus	Allogeneic HSCT	Autologous HSCT
Very high level of agreement	Poor/intermediate risk AML CR1 AML other than CR1 Adults with ALL CR1 (sibling donor) ALL other than CR1 CML in CP1 if TKI intolerant/refractory, T315I mutation CML in CP2, accelerated phase High risk myelodysplasia High risk myelofibrosis Severe aplastic anaemia	Multiple myeloma first response Relapsed Hodgkin's disease Relapsed aggressive non-Hodgkin's lymphoma Poor risk neuroblastoma Germ cell tumour CR > 1
Some variation in practice between BMT units/nations	Adults with poor risk ALL CR1 (unrelated donor) Multiple myeloma Chronic lymphocytic leukaemia Low-grade NHL Relapsed high-grade lymphoma Low risk myelodysplasia Low/intermediate risk myelofibrosis Relapsed Hodgkin's disease	Multiple myeloma (second autograft) Amyloid/POEMS Ewing's sarcoma Soft tissue sarcoma Autoimmune disease
Little evidence in support of transplant	CML in blast crisis Refractory ALL	CML AML ALL Myelodysplasia Myelofibrosis Chronic lymphocytic leukaemia

ALL, acute lymphocytic leukaemia; AML, acute myeloid leukaemia; BMT, bone marrow transplant; CML, chronic myeloid leukaemia; CP, chronic phase of CML; CR, complete remission; CR1, first complete remission; HSCT, haematopoietic stem cell transplant; NHL, non-Hodgkin's lymphoma; POEMS, polyneuropathy, organomegaly, endocrinopathy, monoclonal gammopathy, skin changes; TKI, tyrosine kinase inhibitor.

Syngeneic Cells

Collected from an identical twin and with similar attributes to autologous stem cells.

Allogeneic Cells

The preferred allogeneic donor of choice is a healthy HLA-matched sibling, although one is only available in around 30% of patients requiring an HSC transplant. However, improved testing of patient and recipient HLA-genes (Class I [HLA-A, -B, -C] and Class II [HLA-DRB1, -DQB1]) using molecular typing has improved transplant outcomes when using HLA-matched (10/10) unrelated donors from volunteer donor registries. If not available, alternative options include single antigen mismatched (9/10) unrelated donors, cord blood or haploidentical family donors, with the toxicity and results of these procedures steadily improving [6] (Table 41.2).

- *Cord blood*: umbilical cord blood from unrelated donor cord blood banks was initially used for individuals with low bodyweight (<50 kg) because of the small number of stem cells available. However, in adults and larger children, using two different cord blood units improves engraftment and has now become a realistic option [7]. Although two cord blood units are infused, only one unit will prevail to provide long-term engraftment. The advantage of cord blood is that it is obtained from an immune naive source with greater capacity for immunological tolerance, so that HLA and other mismatches are better tolerated with less GvHD.
- *Haploidentical donors*: initial results with haploidentical donors were poor due to the high level of immune suppression and T-cell depletion required to prevent life-threatening GvHD, causing high rates of relapse. However, with the development of new conditioning regimens using post-transplant cyclophosphamide, GvHD can be reduced without the high rates of relapse [8]. The use of haploidentical donors is now increasing since the majority of patients will have a haploidentical donor available (i.e. sibling, parent or child).

Donor Care and Selection

When more than one donor is available, other factors in addition to HLA-matching should be considered, including CMV serostatus of donor and recipient, donor age, gender and blood group. CMV matching between the donor and recipient is important to minimise the risk of CMV reactivation post-transplant. Young male donors are generally preferred, as multiparous female donors can increase the risk of chronic GvHD and usually have lower bodyweight [8]. If there is an HLA mismatch between recipient and donor, the recipient should also be screened for anti-HLA antibodies and a donor selected whose HLA type does not match the specificity to these antibodies. An ABO-compatible donor is also preferable, although not essential.

Donors must always be treated with respect and the patient must not be used to transmit information to a potential sibling donor. A physician separate from the transplant team should take responsibility for donor care. The Human Tissue Authority (HTA) and the Joint Accreditation Committee of EBMT and the International Society for Cytotherapy-Europe (JACIE) have recommendations regarding donor care and, where the donor is a child, an independent assessor is essential. Doctors involved in advising donors, whether family or unrelated, must be aware of current guidance and legislation [9].

Collecting Haematopoietic Stem Cells

Haematopoietic stem cells may be obtained directly from the bone marrow or by peripheral blood stem cell (PBSC) harvesting. Bone marrow harvesting involves direct aspiration from both posterior iliac crests under general anaesthesia (target total nucleated cell dose of $2–4 \times 10^8$/kg) and usually requires overnight hospital admission. PBSC mobilisation, now more commonly used, involves collecting stem cells using cytapheresis over one or two days as

Table 41.2 Comparison of sources of stem cells.

	Sibling	Family haploidentical donor	Unrelated adult volunteer	Umbilical cord blood
Availability	~30% patients have a sibling donor match (25% chance of any one sibling being matched)	Almost every patient will have a donor (sibling/parent/child)	>29 million donors worldwide; about 70% chance of finding a matched donor for those of Western European origin	700,000 banked worldwide; 99% chance of finding a 4/6 HLA A, B, DR match
Matching requirements	Increasingly molecular matching with 9/10 allele match acceptable	5/10	High-resolution molecular matching; 10/10 (HLA-A, B, C, DR, DQ); 9/10 allele match acceptable	Low resolution (serological) for Class 1 (HLA-A and B) and high resolution (molecular) for Class 2 (HLA-DR); 6/6 preferred but can use 4/6
Speed of availability	3–4 weeks, can be quicker	As per sibling	3–4 months, can be quicker but difficult	Potentially available in days from identifying the preferred cord blood(s)
Engraftment	PBSC ~14 days; BM ~21 days	As for sibling though higher risk of rejection	As for sibling	~20–30 days; platelets may be slower in adult size recipients
Acute GvHD (Grade II–IV)	25–50% (highest with multiparous female donors)	20–40%, though may be severe	30–70%	30–70%
Chronic GvHD	30–40% for BM; 40–70% for PBSC (highest with multiparous female donors)	10–20%	40–50% for BM; 50–70% for PBSC	20–50%
Second donations/ DLI availability	Availability dependent on donor	Yes, but high risk of GvHD	Availability dependent on donor	Unavailable
Risk to the donor	Small	Small	Small	None
Pretransplant testing complete (HLA and virology)	Once donor identified, takes a week or so	As per sibling	Once donor identified and requested, may take several weeks	At time of cryopreservation and unit available for issue

BM, bone marrow; DLI, donor lymphocyte infusion; GvHD, graft-versus-host disease; PBSC, peripheral blood stem cell.

an outpatient (target CD34$^+$ dose of 4×10^6/kg). In healthy donors, PBSCs are mobilised using growth factor (granulocyte-colony stimulating factor – G-CSF) injections while patients undergoing autologous procedures receive G-CSF alone or a combination of chemotherapy and G-CSF.

The choice of whether to use BM or PBSC is dependent on donor preference, although some donors may be unfit for one method or the other. PBSC allografts produce more chronic, but not acute, GvHD than bone marrow transplants in siblings. This may be associated with less relapse in patients at high risk of recurrent disease [10]. Comparative data in unrelated donor transplants also suggest that the use of PBSC is associated with more chronic GvHD, but no difference in long-term survival [11]. As a result, BM harvests are usually preferred for patients being treated for non-malignant conditions (e.g. aplastic anaemia), when a GvT response is less important, to minimise the risk of GvHD.

Complications of Transplantation

Patients who are being considered for any form of HSCT must be given full information about the procedure prior to giving consent. All HSCT procedures carry major risks of mortality, morbidity and long-term complications and careful assessment of all potential transplant candidates is mandatory [12].

Regimen-Related Toxicity

The radiotherapy and chemotherapy conditioning regimen used in HSCT can cause significant toxicity, including mucositis, gut toxicity and reversible alopecia. Less commonly, the liver, heart, lungs and kidneys may suffer transient or even permanent damage and careful pretransplant assessment of the major organ function (heart, lungs, liver and kidneys) is essential.

For older patients (>40 years) and/or those with significant comorbidities, reduced intensity conditioning (RIC) transplants have been developed to harness the immunological benefits of allogeneic transplants, while avoiding much of the acute toxicity associated with the conditioning regimen [13]. RIC cytotoxic therapy is insufficient to completely ablate the recipient's bone marrow cells. Instead, RIC allografts rely on the immune-mediated effects of immune tolerance to facilitate engraftment of the donor transplant and the subsequent GvT effect to eradicate the underlying disease. DLI may also be used after the transplant to convert mixed donor chimerism to full chimerism. Although RIC transplants are sometimes known as 'mini-transplants', they are still intensive procedures requiring great commitment from the patient. Use of validated pretransplant comorbidity scoring systems (e.g. the Sorror HCT comorbidity index) can estimate the transplant-related mortality (TRM) risk for individual patients and may aid decisions [14].

Rejection

Rejection is an immune-mediated event in which the pretransplant conditioning and immunosuppression are insufficient to prevent residual recipient immune cells rejecting the donor cells. It only occurs in allogeneic transplants, although graft failure due to inadequate numbers of HSC in the transplant and/or pre-existing damage to the marrow microenvironment can occur in autologous transplants. HLA incompatibility between the patient and donor, prior sensitisation of the patient to HLA or other cell antigens, T-cell depletion of the graft and low cell count are risk factors for rejection.

Graft-versus-Host Disease

Graft-versus-host disease is the clinical manifestation of the alloimmune response seen when immune-competent donor T-lymphocytes recognise recipient antigens as foreign. GvHD is stimulated by tissue damage caused by conditioning therapy producing a pro-inflammatory environment, in which clonal donor T-cell expansion and cytokine release are promoted [15]. The risk of GvHD is increased by HLA mismatches between donor and recipient and use of unrelated donors. Despite prophylactic immunosuppression, many of the patients receiving allogeneic transplants will develop acute GvHD within the first 100 days. Acute GvHD is characterised histologically by apoptosis of epithelial cells with infiltrating immune cells. Clinically, there is a spectrum of symptoms affecting three organs:

- *skin:* an erythematous sunburn-like rash which can progress to a blistering, exfoliative erythroderma
- *liver:* typically involves the bile ducts with features of obstructive jaundice, although an hepatitic variant may lead to isolated elevated transaminases
- *gastrointestinal tract:* lower gut involvement is characterised by profuse watery diarrhoea, bloody and accompanied by abdominal pain or ileus in the most severe cases. Upper gastrointestinal upset is not uncommon, with anorexia, nausea and vomiting.

Chronic GvHD usually occurs later and has been reported in up to 70% of allogeneic HSCT, depending on the type donor and conditioning/immunotherapy used. Chronic GvHD can involve any organ of the body with typical features of autoimmune disease, including dry eyes, scleroderma, hypo/hyperpigmentation of skin, lichen planus of mouth, bronchiolitis obliterans and fasciitis/myositis [16]. Treatment of GvHD is with systemic immunosuppression (corticosteroids +/- Ciclosporin), topical steroid therapy and supportive care [17].

Relapse

Despite the intensive preparation for transplant, a significant proportion of patients will suffer recurrent disease post-transplant. Patients most at risk are those not in remission at the time of transplant or patients with more advanced disease, i.e. already relapsed after chemotherapy.

Absence of GvT effect, as in autologous HSCT, or when no GvHD is seen, also increases relapse risk, as does the use of RIC allografts [2].

Infectious Complications

In allogeneic HSCT, the conditioning regimen causes profound immune suppression to prevent rejection of the graft and the myelotoxicity results in neutropenia. In addition, immunosuppression is given for the first few months after transplant to control the new donor-derived immune response and reduce the incidence of GvHD. While haematopoietic recovery usually occurs within 2–3 weeks, full immune reconstitution can take much longer (12–18 months), making the recipient vulnerable to infections. Immune deficiency is further compounded by the presence of active GvHD and/or continued immunotherapy.

HSCT-related immune problems may be divided into three phases.

Immediate Post-HSCT

Characterised by severe neutropenia, lymphopenia and hypogammaglobulinaemia. During this period the patient is managed with:

- protective isolation, clean diet and filtered air to reduce fungal infections
- routine prophylactic antifungal, antiviral and antibacterial therapy
- pre-emptive use of therapeutic antimicrobials, including broad-spectrum antibiotics at the first sign of fever (temperature >38 °C), followed by antifungal treatment in the absence of prompt resolution.

Early Post-Engraftment

Following neutrophil recovery, the patient will now have marrow function and may be able to leave hospital. Although autologous transplant recipients rarely have major problems after this time, vigilance is necessary. In contrast, allogeneic HSCT recipients remain at risk of the following:

- bacterial infections related to central lines
- fungal infection

- viral infections. Most units will monitor for CMV reactivation using a polymerase chain reaction (PCR)-based test and treat patients with positive results before there is evidence of disease. Pre-emptive strategies are very effective and CMV is becoming a less important cause of mortality after allogeneic HSCT [18]. Such monitoring may be applied to other viruses (EBV, adenovirus) and patients are clinically monitored for respiratory viruses and herpes viruses, e.g. herpes zoster
- toxoplasmosis and pneumocystis
- hepatitis E. In light of the recent epidemic, a new guideline from the Advisory Committee for the Safety of Blood, Tissue and Organs (SaBTO) advises PCR-based screening of patients before and after allogeneic HSCT, providing hepatitis E-negative blood products to all allograft recipients until at least six months post-transplant and practising good food hygiene to reduce dietary acquisition (predominantly from undercooked pork).

Late Problems

Patients who have active GvHD requiring immunosuppressive therapy will continue to have impaired immunity, and most patients who have received unrelated donor transplants will have detectable abnormalities of the immune system. However, by three years post-transplant, most patients off immunosuppressive drugs will have almost normal immunity. However, important points to consider are:

- revaccination against common pathogens (e.g. polio, tetanus, MMR) is required, although patients still on immunosuppression may not respond optimally. HSCT patients should not receive live vaccines (other than MMR) [19]
- allogeneic transplant recipients are functionally hyposplenic and should be vaccinated against *Pneumococcus*, *Meningococcus* and *Haemophilus influenzae B* (HIB), as well as receiving lifelong prophylaxis, e.g. penicillin V.

Late Effects

There is a growing population of HSCT survivors; 85% of patients alive two years after transplant will go on to become long-term survivors [20]. However, there are many other medical problems that can occur in the years following HSCT, including:

- cataracts
- endocrine disorders such as hypothyroidism, growth retardation in children (especially after TBI +/− steroids), metabolic syndrome
- sexual dysfunction and infertility
- second malignancies
- iron overload and liver dysfunction from red cell transfusions.

Haematopoietic stem cell transplant recipients therefore require long follow-up at a centre familiar with the range of late complications and with a sufficiently large practice to ensure that emerging problems are identified promptly. There are published recommendations for the follow-up of these patients [21].

Bone Marrow Transplant Outcome

A detailed discussion of the results of HSCT is beyond the scope of this chapter as the results are dependent upon many factors, including diagnosis (e.g. AML, ALL); remission status at transplant (CR1, CR2, PR); transplant type (autologous, allogeneic); donor type (sibling, unrelated); HLA matching (matched, mismatched); recipient age; and comorbidities. Current data and results from the EBMT and the Center for International Blood and Marrow Transplant Research (CIBMTR) are available on their websites and provide up-to-date, precise information.

Registry data are of great importance, but cannot replace the careful assessment of individual patients in the light of their specific prognostic factors, such as co-existent disease, toxic effects of prior chemotherapy or previous invasive fungal infection. Also, registries report only data from patients with a minimum of three years follow-up and so evaluation of more recent developments requires scrutiny of primary research publications and reports to specialist meetings.

Post-Bone Marrow Transplant Chimerism and Molecular Monitoring

It has been possible to monitor leukaemic clones using sensitive molecular techniques for nearly 20 years. More recently, molecular techniques have been applied to routine monitoring of donor and recipient chimerism post-transplant. RIC transplants often exhibit a period of mixed chimerism early post-transplant, when the presence of both residual host and donor haemopoiesis is detectable. Mixed chimerism is associated with a higher risk of graft rejection or relapse and optimal GvT responses are dependent upon full donor chimerism [22]. Donor lymphocyte infusions (DLI) of graded numbers of T-lymphocytes can be used to drive haemopoiesis from mixed to full donor chimerism. However, this carries a significant risk of GvHD, as the particular subset of T-cells that will generate GvT without GvHD has yet to be identified.

Cytotoxic T-Cell Therapy

Donor lymphocyte infusions targeted against Epstein-Barr virus (EBV) have been used to treat lymphoproliferative disorder (LPD) patients who have received an unrelated donor HSCT, with the strong immunosuppression leading to EBV reactivation. By isolating T-cells and exposing them to EBV *in vitro*, it is possible to generate clonal cytotoxic T-cells that recognise EBV antigens and kill the LPD cells. This treatment has been used in both the prophylactic and therapeutic management of EBV LPD [23]. In the past few years, significant progress has been made in developing strategies

for using cytotoxic T-cells against other viruses, particularly CMV.

Regulatory Aspects of Haemopoietic Stem Cell Transplantation

An awareness of current regulations regarding HSCT is essential for medical, nursing and scientific staff responsible for HSCT services. In the EU, competent authorities regulate tissue banks, which include processing and storage of HSC. In the UK, for example, the HTA is the competent authority to ensure that the EU Directive on Tissues and Cells is implemented, and has legal powers. A professional international organisation, JACIE, inspects and sets standards for the safety and quality management of clinical and laboratory HSCT process. Although not having legal force, JACIE compliance is seen as vital to a safe and active HSCT programme.

Conclusion

Haematopoietic stem cell transplants can save the lives of patients with incurable leukaemia and lymphomas in many cases. Patients who survive the first five years are likely to enjoy long-term survival, although life expectancy does not return to normal. RIC transplants extend the benefits to more patients who might have been unfit to undergo the rigours of a myeloablative procedure. Whether the use of RIC transplants in a wider range of malignant diseases is effective will become apparent in the next few years. Autologous transplants may decline in importance as improved chemotherapy, immunotherapy and allogeneic HSCT reduce the number of patients for which they are applicable. Additional approaches are still needed to deal with those patients whose primary disease is poorly responsive to current chemoradiotherapy and to further reduce transplant-related mortality.

KEY POINTS

1) HSC transplants provide a curative treatment for patients with haematological malignancies, although they are still associated with significant risks of morbidity and mortality.

2) The number of transplants (autologous and allogeneic) performed each year is increasing worldwide, although the indications, type of transplant and donor source have changed over time.

3) Although RIC transplants have less immediate toxicity than conventional myeloablative transplants, they remain arduous procedures with many short- and medium-term complications.

4) National and international volunteer unrelated donor registries continue to expand, with particular emphasis on recruiting young,

healthy, male donors and donors from black and other ethnic minorities.

5) It is important to treat donors of stem cells as individuals and not as a means to an end.

6) There is increasing use of alternative donors for those patients who do not have an HLA-matched sibling or unrelated donor.

7) Use of haploidentical donors has increased in recent years, with the corresponding use of cord blood units declining. However, further long-term results from haploidentical transplantation are required to determine if this trend will continue.

8) Randomised controlled clinical trials remain the best way to produce definitive data as to the relative merits of treatments in blood and lymphoid malignancies.

References

1 Thomas ED, Lochte HL Jr, Lu WC, Ferrebee JW. Intravenous infusion of bone marrow in patients receiving radiation and chemotherapy. N Engl J Med 1957;**257**(11):491–6.

2 Weiden PL, Sullivan KM, Flournoy N, Storb R, Thomas ED. Antileukemic effect of chronic graft-versus-host disease: contribution to improved survival after allogeneic marrow transplantation. N Engl J Med 1981;**304**(25):1529–33.

3 Kolb HJ, Mittermuller J, Clemm C et al. Donor leukocyte transfusions for treatment of recurrent chronic myelogenous leukemia in marrow transplant patients. Blood 1990;**76**(12):2462–5.

4 Kottaridis PD, Gale RE, Frew ME et al. The presence of a FLT3 internal tandem duplication in patients with acute myeloid leukemia (AML) adds important prognostic information to cytogenetic risk group and response to the first cycle of chemotherapy: analysis of 854 patients from the United

Kingdom Medical Research Council AML 10 and 12 trials. Blood 2001;**98**(6):1752–9.

5 Greenberg PL, Tuechler H, Schanz J et al. Revised international prognostic scoring system for myelodysplastic syndromes. Blood 2012;**120**(12):2454–65.

6 Hough R, Danby R, Russell N et al. Recommendations for a standard UK approach to incorporating umbilical cord blood into clinical transplantation practice: an update on cord blood unit selection, donor selection algorithms and conditioning protocols. Br J Haematol 2016;**172**:360–70.

7 Brunstein CG, Gutman JA, Weisdorf DJ et al. Allogeneic hematopoietic cell transplantation for hematologic malignancy: relative risks and benefits of double umbilical cord blood. Blood 2010;**116**(22):4693–9.

8 Bashey A, Zhang X, Sizemore CA et al. T-cell-replete HLA-haploidentical hematopoietic transplantation for hematologic malignancies using post-transplantation cyclophosphamide results in outcomes

equivalent to those of contemporaneous HLA-matched related and unrelated donor transplantation. J Clin Oncol 2013;**31**(10):1310–16.

9 Sacchi N, Costeas P, Hartwell L et al. Haematopoietic stem cell donor registries: World Marrow Donor Association recommendations for evaluation of donor health. Bone Marrow Transplant 2008;**42**(1):9–14.

10 Schmitz N, Eapen M, Horowitz MM et al. Long-term outcome of patients given transplants of mobilized blood or bone marrow: a report from the International Bone Marrow Transplant Registry and the European Group for Blood and Marrow Transplantation. Blood 2006;**108**(13):4288–90.

11 Eapen M, Logan BR, Confer DL et al. Peripheral blood grafts from unrelated donors are associated with increased acute and chronic graft-versus-host disease without improved survival. Biol Blood Marrow Transplant 2007;**13**(12):1461–8.

12 Deeg HJ, Sandmaier BM. Who is fit for allogeneic transplantation? Blood 2010;**116**(23):4762–70.

13 Giralt S, Estey E, Albitar M et al. Engraftment of allogeneic hematopoietic progenitor cells with purine analog-containing chemotherapy: harnessing graft-versus-leukemia without myeloablative therapy. Blood 1997;**89**(12):4531–6.

14 Sorror ML, Maris MB, Storb R et al. Hematopoietic cell transplantation (HCT)-specific comorbidity index: a new tool for risk assessment before allogeneic HCT. Blood 2005;**106**(8):2912–19.

15 Goker H, Haznedaroglu IC, Chao NJ. Acute graft-vs-host disease: pathobiology and management. Exp Hematol 2001;**29**(3):259–77.

16 Filipovich AH, Weisdorf D, Pavletic S et al. National Institutes of Health consensus development project on criteria for clinical trials in chronic graft-versus-host disease: I. Diagnosis and staging working group report. Biol Blood Marrow Transplant 2005;**11**(12):945–56.

17 Dignan FL, Amrolia P, Clark A et al. Diagnosis and management of chronic graft-versus-host disease. Br J Haematol 2012;**158**(1):46–61.

18 Ljungman P, Reusser P, de la Camara R et al. Management of CMV infections: recommendations from the Infectious Diseases Working Party of the EBMT. Bone Marrow Transplant 2004;**33**(11):1075–81.

19 Rubin LG, Levin MJ, Ljungman P et al. 2013 IDSA clinical practice guideline for vaccination of the immunocompromised host. Clin Infect Dis 2014;**58**(3):309–18.

20 Wingard JR, Majhail NS, Brazauskas R et al. Long-term survival and late deaths after allogeneic hematopoietic cell transplantation. J Clin Oncol 2011;**29**(16):2230–9.

21 Majhail NS, Rizzo JD, Lee SJ et al. Recommended screening and preventive practices for long-term survivors after hematopoietic cell transplantation. Hematol Oncol Stem Cell Ther 2012;**5**(1):1–30.

22 Liesveld JL, Rothberg PG. Mixed chimerism in SCT: conflict or peaceful coexistence? Bone Marrow Transplant 2008;**42**(5):297–310.

23 Comoli P, Basso S, Zecca M et al. Preemptive therapy of EBV-related lymphoproliferative disease after pediatric haploidentical stem cell transplantation. Am J Transplant 2007;**7**(6):1648–55.

Further Reading

Anasetti C. Use of alternative donors for allogeneic stem cell transplantation. Hematol Am Soc Hematol Educ Program 2015;**2015**(1):220–4.

British Society of Blood and Marrow Transplantation (BSBMT) site: http://bsbmt.org/.

Centre for International Blood and Marrow Transplant Research (CIBMTR) site: www. cibmtr.org.

European Group for Blood and Marrow Transplantation (EBMT) site: www.ebmt.org/. Particularly the EBMT-ESH Handbook: http:// ebmtonline.forumservice.net/.

Majhail NS, Farnia SH., Carpenter PA et al. Indications for autologous and allogeneic hematopoietic cell transplantation:

guidelines from the American Society for Blood and Marrow Transplantation. Biol Blood Marrow Transplant 2015;**21**(11):1863–9.

Savani BN, Labopin M, Blaise D et al. Peripheral blood stem cell graft compared to bone marrow after reduced intensity conditioning regimens for acute leukemia – a report from the ALWP of the EBMT. Haematologica 2016;**101**:256–62.

Cord Blood Transplantation

Rachael Hough[1] and Robert D. Danby[2]

[1] University College London Hospital's NHS Foundation Trust, London, UK
[2] Oxford University Hospitals NHS Foundation Trust, Oxford, UK

Introduction

Over the last 50 years, transplantation of haemopoietic stem cells (HSCs) from related or unrelated donors has provided curative therapy for thousands of patients with a wide range of malignant, metabolic and immunological disorders [1]. HSCs have conventionally been harvested from bone marrow or granulocyte-colony stimulating factor (G-CSF) mobilised peripheral blood, with the optimal donor being a human leucocyte antigen (HLA)-identical sibling. However, the chance of any one brother or sister being 'matched' is only 1 in 4 and, as a result, a sibling allograft is an option for only around 30% of patients.

In recent years, there has been considerable success in expanding international volunteer donor registry panels, with over 29 million donors currently registered. However, the likelihood of identifying a 'suitably matched' unrelated donor is dependent on the ethnicity of the recipient; whilst Caucasians may have at least a 50% chance of finding a donor, the likelihood falls to around 10% for certain ethnic or mixed race groups who are poorly represented on the registry panels. In addition, the time taken from commencing an unrelated donor search to the delivery of HSCs to the patient is an average of four months. For patients who are clinically unstable and require an urgent transplant, this can be too long and patients may succumb to their disease or toxicity of interim chemotherapy. Furthermore, the use of more stringent molecular HLA typing methods to optimise donor selection and improve transplant survival outcomes has prolonged the search process and reduced the likelihood of finding any HLA-matched volunteer donor [2].

The use of alternative HSC sources such as umbilical cord blood (UCB) arose because suitable HLA-matched donors could not be identified for a substantial proportion of patients and the time to acquisition of donor cells was too long for those requiring urgent transplantation.

The first UCB transplant (UCBT) was performed in 1988 in a boy with Fanconi anaemia, using cells collected from his sibling's umbilical cord blood [3]. This successful transplant was proof of the principle that UCB could be harvested, cryopreserved and thawed and still contain sufficient viable stem cells to successfully repopulate the recipient's bone marrow and immune system. Further successful related and unrelated donor UCBTs followed quickly and led to the establishment of public UCB banks, the first of which was the New York Cord Blood Bank in 1993. These banks have rapidly expanded internationally since, with

Practical Transfusion Medicine, Fifth Edition. Edited by Michael F. Murphy, David J. Roberts and Mark H. Yazer.
© 2017 John Wiley & Sons Ltd. Published 2017 by John Wiley & Sons Ltd.

a current worldwide repository in excess of 720 000 units, which have facilitated over 35 000 UCBTs so far.

Umbilical Cord Blood Banking

Cryopreserved UCB may be safely stored for many years without significant deleterious effect on the viability of stem cells, in either public or private cord banks. Large public banks store UCB that has been altruistically donated for transplantation into unrelated recipients. Some countries also have national, publicly-funded banks for directed donations, usually collected for siblings with known life-threatening disease. More recently, siblings have been specifically conceived using preimplantation genetic diagnosis to select HLA-matched and disease-unaffected embryos for implantation, from whom UCB can be harvested after delivery and used for transplantation of an existing sick child [4]. The practice of storing UCB, collected by either altruistic or directed donations, is now well established and has already saved thousands of lives. To ensure consistency, quality assurance for the collection (including maternal consent), processing and storage of UCB is provided by inspection against international standards (Netcord-FACT standards).

An increasing number of private UCB banks are also becoming available and offer cryopreservation of UCB for the specific use of the donating family as an 'insurance policy' and source of stem cells for either:

- conventional indications for an HSC transplant, or
- future use in the treatment of other diseases (regenerative medicine).

At the present time, the utility of private cord banking is unclear. The chances of using a privately stored unit for transplantation have been estimated to be between 1 in 1400 and 1 in 20 000 [5]. The issue is further complicated by the possibility of contamination of autologous cord blood by disease, which subsequently presents in childhood, such as acute leukaemia. There is considerable current scientific exploration into the potential of cord blood as a source of non-haemopoietic cells that could be utilised in the treatment of many different conditions, in particular degenerative diseases. Should this potential be realised, the utility of storing autologous cord blood for subsequent use may become clearer.

Box 42.1 lists the key elements involved in the recruitment of expectant women who may wish to altruistically donate their baby's UCB to public banks. As the potential role of UCB becomes more widely appreciated, an increasing number of women actively seek the opportunity to donate. For others, literature or verbal information may be provided at booking clinics or antenatal classes. A history is taken from mothers-to-be who are interested in donation, focusing on ethnicity and the risks of transmissible infection or genetic disease. The consent process ensures that the future mother is aware that her child's UCB may be used at any time for transplantation in an unknown recipient, the need for testing for transmissible infectious or genetic diseases and the potential for discard or use in research if the unit collected does not meet key criteria for clinical grade banking.

Box 42.2 lists the mandatory tests of both mother and UCB, performed at the time of banking and prior to issue. There is an increasing tendency for collection centres to appoint and train a team of UCB harvesters who collect the placenta from the delivery room following placental delivery. This obviates the need for midwives to be involved in UCB collection, which might otherwise distract them from nursing the new mother and baby.

The exact timing of collection remains controversial. Some centres harvest UCB whilst the placenta is still *in utero*. Although this approach optimises the volume and stem cell yield from the collection, it potentially

---

Box 42.1   Donor recruitment, selection and consent.

Donor recruitment

Need consent to collect before delivery (EU Directive)

Prenatal information to mothers

Leaflets, posters, videos

Antenatal/parents classes

Brief medical history for obvious exclusions

Maternal interview 24–48 h post-delivery

Informed written consent for use for cord blood transplant and research and development

Medical, genetic, family, lifestyle, ethnic and travel history

Maternal samples

Follow-up donor interview

Telephone at 12 weeks if indicated (concerns re health of baby or mother at 24–48 h)

Postnatal health of mother and baby

Consent

Collection and storage of cord blood (CB) for transplantation into unrelated individuals worldwide

Possible risks and benefits to mother and/or infant, including medical and ethical concerns

Permission for microbiological testing, including for HIV, and for the donor to be counselled in the event of results relevant to their health

Exchange of anonymised relevant information to registries and transplant centres

Contact with mother and relevant clinical professionals as required to confirm safety of CB donation for use

Storage of personal information

Storage of samples for future testing

Right of the mother to refuse without prejudice

Research and development use or discard if the donation is unsuitable for clinical use

Source: Rachel Pawson, Oxford University Hospitals. Reproduced with permission of Rachel Pawson.

---

distracts from the birthing process and may present a risk to both mother and newborn. In fact, some midwives and obstetricians advocate delaying the clamping of the umbilical cord even after placental delivery. This recommendation is based on the observation that delayed cord clamping leads to a higher ferritin level in the newborn child, which may impact favourably on their subsequent development [6]. Unfortunately, delaying cord clamping will have a significant impact on the volume and number of stem cells present in each UCB unit, which may considerably limit the usefulness of many collected.

Box 42.2 Testing.

At processing/cryopreservation

Maternal

HIV (Ab + PCR), HCV (Ab + PCR), HBV, (HBsAg + anti-Hbcore +PCR), HTLV 1 + 2 Ab, TPHA, CMV IgG, ± discretionary tests such as Malaria Ab, *T. cruzi*

Cord sample

ABO/Rh grouping

Bacterial and fungal culture

HLA-A, -B, -DR (DNA typing)

FBC pre- and post-process

CD34 count and CD34 cell viability

Total nucleated cell count (TNC) and nucleated red cell count

Haemoglobinopathy test results obtained

Medical review and quality checked

At reservation

Maternal

HLA type to confirm linkage between mother and CBU

Cord sample

Confirmatory HLA typing (high resolution)

HIV (Ab + PCR), HCV (Ab + PCR), HBV, (HBsAg + anti-Hbcore +PCR), HTLV 1 + 2 Ab, TPHA, CMV (IgG and PCR)

Blood film examination if indicated

Contiguous line segment – TNC, CD34 count + viability
– CFU assay
– STR analysis to confirm linkage between mother and CBU

Update on health of mother and child via family doctor

Medical and quality review and results checked

Source: Rachel Pawson, Oxford University Hospitals. Reproduced with permission of Rachel Pawson.
Ab, antibody; CBU, cord blood unit; CFU, colony-forming unit; CMV, cytomegalovirus; FBC, full blood count; Hb, haemoglobin; HBV, hepatitis B virus; HCV, hepatitis C virus; HIV, human immunodeficiency virus; HLA, human leucocyte antigen; HTLV, human T-lymphotrophic virus; PCR, polymerase chain reaction; STR, short tandem repeat; TPHA, *Treponema pallidum* particle agglutination assay.

Clinical Outcomes of Umbilical Cord Blood Transplantation

Malignant Disease

The efficacy of allogeneic HSC transplantation in haematological malignant diseases is achieved by the cytoreductive impact of the conditioning chemotherapy and/or radiotherapy and a later immune-mediated clearance of any residual malignant cells, called the graft-versus-malignancy (GVM) or graft-versus-leukaemia (GVL) effect.

Early experience of UCBT in malignant disease used single unit transplants from related and, subsequently, unrelated donors in children. Table 42.1 summarises these outcome data compared to other stem cell sources. The key observations, established over time, are that UCBTs are associated with equivalent survival and relapse rates (demonstrating a preserved GVM effect) compared to bone marrow or peripheral blood stem cell transplants. Interestingly, the incidence and severity of acute and chronic graft-versus-host disease (GVHD) are less than observed with conventional HSC sources, which allows for a more permissive 'matching system' between the recipient and donor. In general, unrelated donors are only used if they are matched at nine or 10 out of 10 HLA alleles, whilst unrelated donor UCB units can be used if matched at four or more out of six alleles (with less stringent matching at class I antigens).

The key limitation of using UCB as an alternative stem cell source is that the time to and probability of 'engraftment' or recovery of the neutrophil and platelet counts are both inferior when compared to bone marrow or peripheral blood stem cell transplants. The time to neutrophil recovery is around one week longer than using bone marrow, leading to a prolonged risk of early transplant mortality, predominantly due to infection.

One of the key determinants of engraftment, transplant-related mortality and survival is the cell dose (as measured by the total nucleated cell count or CD34+ cell count) infused into the recipient [9,10]. Outcome improves with increasing cell dose, with an apparent pre-thaw threshold of around $3-3.5 \times 10^7$ total nucleated cells (TNC)/kg or $1.5-2 \times 10^5$ CD34+/kg, below which toxicity is prohibitively high. Engraftment, transplant-related mortality and survival also improve with closer HLA matching, although the deleterious impact of each mismatch may be overcome to some extent by a higher cell dose [10,11].

Initial outcome data in adults showed a high risk of graft failure and transplant-related mortality, with UCBT tending to be restricted to patients with advanced-stage disease who were heavily pretreated. However, with modified conditioning regimens (including reduced-intensity regimens) and an increasing awareness of the key factors in optimising graft selection, adult UCBT outcomes have improved considerably (Table 42.2) and are now also considered to be standard of care, when a conventional donor is unavailable.

Metabolic Disorders

The metabolic disorders are a range of diseases that result from enzyme deficiencies or transport protein defects, which cause accumulation of toxic substrates in critical organs, leading to progressive and often fatal organ failure. Allogeneic haemopoietic stem cell transplantation (HSCT) has been shown to arrest disease progression in selected disorders. The mechanism of benefit is unclear, but may be due to production of continuous and sufficient enzyme by graft-derived cells and a concomitant reduction of central nervous system inflammation.

The largest experience of HSCT in a metabolic disorder is in Hurler's syndrome, an autosomal recessive deficiency of α-L-iduronidase. The key factors considered in HSC choice for this disorder are:

- the need for rapid transplant before neurological damage occurs
- the lack of necessity for GVM (thus GVHD is less tolerable than in the context of malignancy).

Umbilical cord blood has the advantage of being rapidly available for transplant and, in a series of 93 patients, the three-year overall survival was 77% with an incidence of grade II–IV acute GVHD of 31% – outcomes at least equivalent to those previously reported for other stem cell sources [12]. A shorter interval from diagnosis to transplant was an independent predictor of improved event-free survival, reinforcing the advantage of rapid availability of UCB for transplantation.

Primary Immunodeficiencies

The primary immunodeficiency syndromes are a rare group of inherited disorders in which there is a single or combined deficiency in key

Table 42.1 Summary of large studies comparing cord blood transplant with haemopoietic stem cell (HSC) sources in paediatric patients with malignant disease.

Author	Period	Diagnosis	HSC source	n	Median age (range)	TNC dose ×10⁷/kg (range)	Days to ANC >0.5×10⁹/L	aGVHD II–IV (%)	cGVHD (%)	Relapse (%)	TRM (%)	OS (%)
Rocha et al. [7]	1990–7	Malignant & nonmalignant	Sibling CB	113	5 (<1–15)	4.7 (<10–36)	26	14	6	–	14	64
			Sibling BM	2052	8 (<1–15)	35 (<10–410)	18	22	15	–	12	66
Rocha et al. [8]	1994–8	AML/ALL	UD (CB)	99	6 (2.5–10)	3.8 (2.4–36)	32 (11–56)	35	25 #2	38 #2	39 #100	35 #2
			UD (BM)	262	8 (5–12)	42 (14–56)	18 (10–40)	58	46 #2	39 #2	19 #100	49 #2
			T-depleted UD (BM)	180	8 (6–12)	38 (11–53)	16 (9–40)	20	12 #2	47 #2	14 #100	41 #2

Data given at three years post-HSCT unless otherwise indicated (#100, 100 days; #2, 2 years).

aGVHD, acute graft-versus-host disease; ALL, acute lymphocytic leukaemia; AML, acute myeloid leukaemia; ANC, absolute neutrophil count; BM, bone marrow; CB, cord blood; cGVHD, chronic graft-versus-host disease; HSC, haemopoietic stem cell; MUD, matched unrelated donor; OS, overall survival; PB, peripheral blood stem cell; TRM, transplant-related mortality; UD, unrelated donor.

Table 42.2 Summary of studies comparing cord blood transplant with haemopoietic stem cell (HSC) sources in adult patients.

Author	Period	Diagnosis	HSC source	n	Median age (range)	TNC dose ×10^7/kg (range)	Days to ANC >0.5×10^9/L	aGVHD II–IV (%)	cGVHD (%)	Relapse (%)	TRM (%)	OS (%)
Takahashi et al. [13]	1998–2001	Malignant	CB	68	36 (16–53)	2.5 (1.1–5.3)	22 (16–41)	66	74	16[#2]	9[#1]	74[DFS]
			MUD (BM)	45	26 (16–50)	33 (6.6–50)	18 (12–33)	50	78	25[#2]	29[#1]	44[DFS]
Rocha et al. [14]	1998–2002	AML/ALL	CB	98	25 (15–55)	2.3 (0.9–6.0)	26 (14–80)	26	30 (20–40)[#2]	23[#2]	44[#2]	36[#2]
			MUD (BM)	584	32 (15–59)	29 (<10–90)	19 (5–72)	39	46[#2]	23[#2]	38[#2]	42[#2]
Laughlin et al. [15]	1996–2001	Leukaemia	CB	150	(16–60)	2.2 (1.0–6.5)	27 (25–29)	41	51	17	63	26
			MUD (BM)	367	(16–60)	24 (0.2–170)	18 (18–19)	48	35	23	46	35
			mMUD (BM)	83	(16–60)	22 (0.1–58)	20 (18–22)	52	40	14	65	20
Chen et al. [16]	2000–4	Malignant	CB	64	53 (19–67)	4.4 (1.0–8.5)	22 (13–70)	14	22[#2]	43	27	46
			UD (BM/PB)	221	58 (19–73)	–	13 (2–181)	20	54[#2]	50	10	50
de Latour et al. [17]	200–10	AML	CB	80	59 (50–71)	4 (3–4)	[85% d+28]	39	23	43	24	45
			MUD (PB)	35	59 (50–74)	110 (70–120)	[94% d+28]	38	41	29	14	53
Rodrigues et al. [18]	2000–8	Lymphoid	CB	104	48 (18–67)	–	18 (7–59)	29	26	28	29	56
			MUD (PB)	541	50 (18–70)	–	14 (3–31)	32	52	35	28	49
Marks et al. [19]	2000–10	ALL	CB	116	25	–	[57% d+28]	27	39	22	42	44
			MUD (BM/PB)	546	32	–	[95% d+28]	47	42	25	31	44
			mMUD (BM/PB)	140	33	–	[96% d+28]	41	45	28	39	43
Warlick et al. [20]	2000–10	AML	CB	151	(18–74)	–	–	24[g3–4]	–	36[#2]	20[#1]	36[#6]
			MUD (BM/PB)	55	(18–74)	–	–	15[g3–4]	–	20[#2]	25[#1]	54[#6]
			mMUD (BM/PB)	21	(18–74)	–	–	24[g3–4]	–	33[#2]	14[#1]	51[#6]
Robin et al. [21]	2005–11	MDS	CB	129	57 (20–72)	4.6 (1.4–13)	20 (6–72)	31	23[#2]	30[#2]	42[#2]	30[#2]
			MUD (PB)	379	60 (24–76)	96 (15–332)	16 (3–60)	29	44[#2]	23[#2]	32[#2]	50[#2]
			mMUD (PB)	107	61 (20–74)	–	–		37[#2]	28[#2]	36[#2]	43[#2]
Malard et al. [22]	2002–10	AML	CB	205	49 (19–69)	3.1 (0.2–8.2)	19 (0–106)	32	6[#5]	51[#5]	21[#5]	36[#5]
			MUD (PB)	347	57 (19–70)	85 (0.5–192)	16 (0–52)	31	12[#5]	32[#5]	21[#5]	49[#5]
			mMUD (PB)	99	55 (19–68)	87 (25–182)	15 (0–31)	39	10[#5]	36[#5]	31[#5]	33[#5]

Data given at three years post-HSCT unless otherwise indicated (#1, 1 year; #2, 2 years; #5, 5 years; #6, 6 years).

aGVHD, acute graft-versus-host disease; ALL, acute lymphocytic leukaemia; AML, acute myeloid leukaemia; ANC, absolute neutrophil count; BM, bone marrow; CB, cord blood; cGVHD, chronic graft-versus-host disease; DFS, disease-free survival; g3–4, grade III–IV; HSC, haemopoietic stem cell; mMUD, mismatched unrelated donor; MUD, matched unrelated donor; OS, overall survival; PB, peripheral blood stem cell; TRM, transplant-related mortality; UD, unrelated donor.

elements of the innate and/or adaptive immune systems. Early death due to infection may be prevented by enzyme therapy in some children and gene therapy offers the promise of disease amelioration for others in the future. However, for many, replacement of the immune system by allogeneic HSCT provides the only curative therapeutic strategy at present.

The outcome of allogeneic HSCT has improved considerably over recent years with improvements in supportive care, better prevention of GVHD and the use of reduced-intensity conditioning regimens. The critical determinant of a successful transplant is for the procedure to be performed prior to the onset of significant infections or comorbidities, which may lead to death within the first year of life in some disorders such as severe combined immune deficiency syndrome (SCID). Whilst the donor of choice for such children is a sibling, with overall survival rates of 70–100%, the likelihood of having an HLA-matched sibling who is unaffected by the same inherited disease is only around 10% [1].

Umbilical cord blood is an attractive stem cell source for children with primary immunodeficiencies, given the rapid availability and low risk of GVHD. In a retrospective study comparing 74 UCB transplants to 175 mismatched related donor transplants for patients with primary immunodeficiencies (SCID or Omenn syndrome), the five-year overall survival rate was 57% and 62%, respectively [24]. Although the slower engraftment rate compared to conventional transplants may increase the risk of peri-transplant infections, UCBT is an acceptable alternative when no sibling or unrelated donor is available.

Advantages and Disadvantages of Umbilical Cord Blood

The wealth of experience of UCBT to date has demonstrated a number of advantages and disadvantages compared to other stem cell sources, which are summarised in Table 42.3. The reduced stringency required in 'HLA matching' between recipient and donor, due to a lower incidence of GVHD following UCBT, allows

patients access to a life-saving allogeneic HSCT, when previously they would not have had a 'suitable' donor. This access is increased further by targeting collection centres in areas where the population has a broader ethnic mix, which allows specific harvesting of units from a racially-diverse HLA background, currently underrepresented on international volunteer donor panels. UCB can be collected with no risk to either the donor or mother. Once stored, UCB units are available immediately, thus allowing rapid access when a transplant is urgently indicated and also easy rearrangement of the transplant date when necessary. Adult volunteer donors may also become unwell or be unavailable for donation when required; there is no such 'donor attrition' with UCB. There is also a very low risk of transmission of infectious agents with transplantation of HSCs collected from a newborn baby.

The principal limitation of UCB is that it is a 'one-off' collection of a finite number of HSCs. Furthermore, stem cells cannot be harvested in the event of graft failure and donor lymphocytes cannot be given as immunotherapy in the management of relapse, serious infection or mixed chimerism. The stem cell dose is a crucial determinant of outcome and a single UCB will generally have insufficient HSCs to transplant a larger adolescent or adult patient safely. The other potential disadvantage of UCB is that the stem cells may harbour transmissible genetic disease, not yet apparent in the baby from whom it came.

Future Developments

The focus of recent and ongoing research efforts has been on improving engraftment and shortening the duration of cytopenia post-transplant, with the aim of reducing early mortality and improving survival (Table 42.4) [25].

The most successful so far has been the co-infusion of two unrelated UCB units in larger children, adolescents and adults. Initial concerns that this could lead to graft failure due to an immunological reaction between the two units or to prohibitive GVHD have not been substantiated. This work, pioneered by

Table 42.3 Advantages and disadvantages of different stem cell sources.

	Autologous HSCT	HLA-identical related donor HSCT	Unrelated donor HSCT	Unrelated donor UCBT	Haploidentical related donor HSCT
Available donor pool	–	–	>29 million	>720 000	–
Estimation of likelihood of suitable donor	>90%	Approx. 30%	10/10 = 40% 9/10 = 70% Ethnic minority = 20%	≥5/6 = 40% ≥4/6 = 70%	>90%
Speed of access	Immediate	Immediate	3–4 months	3–4 weeks	Immediate
Cost of graft	Low	Low	High	High	Low
Ability to rearrange infusion date	Easy	Easy	May be difficult	Easy	Easy
Ability to reaccess	Impossible	Yes	Possible	No	Yes
Quality of product	Assured	Assured	Assured	Variable	Assured
Speed of engraftment	Fast	Moderate	Moderate	Slow	Fast
Risk of graft failure	Low	Low	Moderate	High	Moderate
Risk of transplant-related mortality	Very low	Low	High	High	High
Risk of GVHD	None	Moderate	High	Moderate	Low
Speed of immune reconstitution	Rapid	Moderate	Moderate	Moderate	Very slow
Risk of viral transmission	None	Yes	Yes	None	Yes
Risk of transmission of congenital disease	Yes	Yes	No	Yes	No

Source: Adapted from Warwick & Brubaker [23].
GVHD, graft-versus-host disease; HSCT, haemopoietic stem cell transplant; UCBT, umbilical cord blood transplant.

Table 42.4 Strategies to overcome the limitations of lower cell dose.

Mechanism	Approach
Increase cell dose infused	Improved collection, processing, freezing and thawing Double unit transplant Co-infusion of CD34 selected haploidentical cells *Ex vivo* expansion
Improved homing	Direct intraosseous infusion Increased stromal-derived factor-1 (SDF-1) (CXCL12)/CXCR4 interaction *Ex vivo* fucosylation of HSC
Improved selection of CB	Enhanced HLA matching Avoiding CB with specificity against donor-specific anti-HLA antibodies
Modification of transplant regimen	Reduced-intensity conditioning Use of granulocyte-colony stimulating factor, SCF and/or Eltrombopag
Infusion of accessory cells	Mesenchymal stem cells Regulatory T-cells

CB, cord blood; HLA, human leucocyte antigen; HSC, haemopoietic stem cell; SCF, stem cell factor.

researchers in Minneapolis, has shown that the duration of neutropenia is acceptable and the likelihood of engraftment increased, even in large adult patients [26]. Although there is an increase in GVHD compared to a single unit transplant, the impact of this on survival appears to be offset by a reduced incidence of relapse. This strategy has led to safe and efficacious UCBT in adults, with a consequent rapid increase in the number of these transplants performed internationally. Interestingly, although both infused units contribute to initial haemopoiesis, ultimately one unit will predominate and will usually eradicate the 'losing' unit by around three months post-transplant.

Another significant development has been the use of reduced-intensity conditioning regimens. It has been shown that UCB will engraft even in this setting and, importantly, the duration of neutropenia is considerably reduced to around 12 days, due to a temporary contribution of haemopoiesis from non-ablated recipient stem cells [27]. Again, the engrafting unit will subsequently eradicate host cells that have effectively 'bridged' the neutropenic phase. This approach has made it possible for older patients or those with significant comorbidities to safely proceed to transplant.

Other approaches, including the co-infusion of CD34-selected haploidentical stem cells, *ex vivo* expansion and direct intraosseous injection of UCB, are also showing promising results in ongoing international clinical trials.

Conclusion

Allogeneic HSCT provides a life-saving treatment option for patients with many malignant and genetic diseases. Over the last 30 years, UCB has emerged as a safe and effective alternative stem cell source for patients lacking an HLA-matched sibling or unrelated donor, available within the required time frame. Previously considered a waste product, UCB is abundantly and rapidly available, without risk to the donor or mother. UCB also has a lower incidence of GVHD and transmissible infection. The limitations of finite cell dose and slower engraftment are being overcome by novel approaches, thus expanding access to transplantation to older, larger recipients and those with comorbidities.

KEY POINTS

1) Over the last 30 years, UCB, previously a biological waste product of pregnancy, has been shown to be an effective and safe alternative source of HSCs for transplantation in patients with life-threatening diseases who otherwise would not have a suitable related or unrelated donor.

2) The lower stringency required for recipient and donor matching and the targeted collection of ethnic minority and mixed race UCB units have extended access to transplantation considerably, particularly for those of racial backgrounds poorly represented on volunteer donor panels.

3) UCB collection presents no risk to the mother or baby and provides a rapidly available HSC source when urgently required, with no risk of donor attrition.

4) The incidence and severity of acute and chronic GVHD are lower following a UCBT compared to bone marrow transplant, despite greater HLA disparity. Transplant-related mortality, relapse rate and overall survival are at least comparable with bone marrow.

5) A limited cell dose, resulting in a slower and reduced probability of engraftment, remains the biggest obstacle to the wider use of UCBT.

6) Double unit UCBT has been shown to be safe and efficacious in larger adolescents and adults, in whom a single unit transplant would result in an unacceptably high risk of graft failure and early mortality.

7) Other strategies, such as *ex vivo* expansion, intraosseous injection and co-infusion of haploidentical CD34-selected stem cells, all show promise and may yet expand the utility of UCBT further.

References

1 Hough R, Cooper N, Veys P. Allogeneic haemopoietic stem cell transplantation in children: what alternative donor should we choose when no matched sibling is available? Br J Haematol 2009;**147**(5):593–613.

2 Eapen M, Klein JP, Sanz GF et al. Effect of donor–recipient HLA matching at HLA A, B, C, and DRB1 on outcomes after umbilical-cord blood transplantation for leukaemia and myelodysplastic syndrome: a retrospective analysis. Lancet Oncol 2011;**12**(13):1214–21.

3 Gluckman E, Broxmeyer HA, Auerbach AD et al. Hematopoietic reconstitution in a patient with Fanconi's anemia by means of umbilical-cord blood from an HLA-identical sibling. N Engl J Med 1989;**321**(17):1174–8.

4 Gluckman E, Ruggeri A, Rocha V et al. Family-directed umbilical cord blood banking. Haematologica 2011;**96**(11):1700–7.

5 Fisk NM, Roberts IA, Markwald R, Mironov V. Can routine commercial cord blood banking be scientifically and ethically justified? PLoS Med 2005;**2**(2):e44.

6 Mercer JS, Erickson-Owens DA. Rethinking placental transfusion and cord clamping issues. J Perinat Neonatal Nurs 2012;**26**(3):202–17; quiz 18–19.

7 Rocha V, Wagner JE Jr, Sobocinski KA et al. Graft-versus-host disease in children who have received a cord-blood or bone marrow transplant from an HLA-identical sibling. Eurocord and International Bone Marrow Transplant Registry Working Committee on Alternative Donor and Stem Cell Sources. N Engl J Med 2000;**342**(25):1846–54.

8 Rocha V. Comparison of outcomes of unrelated bone marrow and umbilical cord blood transplants in children with acute leukemia. Blood 2001;**97**(10):2962–71.

9 Rocha V, Gluckman E, Eurocord-Netcord Registry, European Bone Marrow Transplant Group. Improving outcomes of cord blood transplantation: HLA matching, cell dose and other graft- and transplantation-related factors. Br J Haematol 2009;**147**(2):262–74.

10 Barker JN, Scaradavou A, Stevens CE. Combined effect of total nucleated cell dose and HLA match on transplantation outcome in 1061 cord blood recipients with hematologic malignancies. Blood 2010;**115**(9):1843–9.

11 Eapen M, Klein JP, Ruggeri A et al. Impact of allele-level HLA matching on outcomes after myeloablative single unit umbilical cord blood transplantation for hematologic malignancy. Blood 2014;**123**(1):133–40.

12 Boelens JJ, Rocha V, Aldenhoven M et al. Risk factor analysis of outcomes after unrelated cord blood transplantation in patients with hurler syndrome. Biol Blood Marrow Transplant 2009;**15**(5):618–25.

13 Takahashi S, Iseki T, Ooi J et al. Single-institute comparative analysis of unrelated bone marrow transplantation and cord blood transplantation for adult patients with hematologic malignancies. Blood 2004;**104**(12):3813–20.

14 Rocha V, Labopin M, Sanz G et al. Transplants of umbilical-cord blood or bone marrow from unrelated donors in adults with acute leukemia. N Engl J Med 2004;**351**:2276–85.

15 Laughlin MJ, Eapen M, Rubinstein P et al. Outcomes after transplantation of cord blood or bone marrow from unrelated donors in adults with leukemia. N Engl J Med 2004;**351**(22):2265–75.

16 Chen YB, Aldridge J, Kim HT et al. Reduced-intensity conditioning stem cell transplantation: comparison of double umbilical cord blood and unrelated donor grafts. Biol Blood Marrow Transplant 2012;**18**(5):805–12.

17 Peffault de Latour R, Brunstein CG, Porcher R et al. Similar overall survival using sibling, unrelated donor, and cord blood grafts after reduced-intensity conditioning for older patients with acute myelogenous leukemia. Biol Blood Marrow Transplant 2013;**19**(9):1355–60.

18 Rodrigues CA, Rocha V, Dreger P et al. Alternative donor hematopoietic stem cell transplantation for mature lymphoid malignancies after reduced-intensity conditioning regimen: similar outcomes with umbilical cord blood and unrelated donor peripheral blood. Haematologica 2014;**99**(2):370–7.

19 Marks DI, Woo KA, Zhong X et al. Unrelated umbilical cord blood transplant for adult acute lymphoblastic leukemia in first and second complete remission: a comparison with allografts from adult unrelated donors. Haematologica 2014;**99**(2):322–8.

20 Warlick ED, Peffault de Latour R, Shanley R et al. Allogeneic hematopoietic cell transplantation outcomes in acute myeloid leukemia: similar outcomes regardless of donor type. Biol Blood Marrow Transplant2015;**21**(2):357–63.

21 Robin M, Ruggeri A, Labopin M et al. Comparison of unrelated cord blood and peripheral blood stem cell transplantation in adults with myelodysplastic syndrome after reduced-intensity conditioning regimen: a collaborative study from Eurocord (Cord blood Committee of Cellular Therapy & Immunobiology Working Party of EBMT) and Chronic Malignancies Working Party. Biol Blood Marrow Transplant 2015;**21**(3):489–95.

22 Malard F, Milpied N, Blaise D et al. Effect of graft source on unrelated donor hemopoietic stem cell transplantation in adults with acute myeloid leukemia after reduced-intensity or nonmyeloablative conditioning: a study from the societe francaise de greffe de moelle et de therapie cellulaire. Biol Blood Marrow Transplant 2015;**21**(6):1059–67.

23 Warwick R, Brubaker S. Tissue and Cell Clinical Use: An Essential Guide. Wiley-Blackwell Pubishing, Oxford, 2012.

24 Fernandes JF, Rocha V, Labopin M et al. Transplantation in patients with SCID: mismatched related stem cells or unrelated cord blood? Blood 2012;**119**(12):2949–55.

25 Danby R, Rocha V. Improving engraftment and immune reconstitution in umbilical cord blood transplantation. Front Immunol 2014;**5**:68.

26 Barker JN, Weisdorf DJ, DeFor TE et al. Transplantation of 2 partially HLA-matched umbilical cord blood units to enhance engraftment in adults with hematologic malignancy. Blood 2005;**105**(3):1343–7.

27 Barker JN, Weisdorf DJ, DeFor TE, Blazar BR, Miller JS, Wagner JE. Rapid and complete donor chimerism in adult recipients of unrelated donor umbilical cord blood transplantation after reduced-intensity conditioning. Blood 2003;**102**(5):1915–19.

Further Reading

Aldenhoven M, Kurtzberg J. Cord blood is the optimal graft source for the treatment of pediatric patients with lysosomal storage diseases: clinical outcomes and future directions. Cytotherapy 2015;**17**(6):765–74.

Ballen KK, Gluckman E, Broxmeyer HE. Umbilical cord blood transplantation: the first 25 years and beyond. Blood 2013;**122**:491–8.

Barker JN, Fei M, Karanes C et al. Results of a prospective multicentre myeloablative double-unit cord blood transplantation trial in adult patients with acute leukaemia and myelodysplasia. Br J Haematol 2015;**168**:405–12.

Brunstein CG Umbilical cord blood transplantation for the treatment of hematologic malignancies. Cancer Control 2011;**18**:222–36.

Brunstein CG, Setubal DC, Wagner JE. Expanding the role of umbilical cord blood transplantation. Br J Haematol 2007;**137**:20–35.

Munoz J, Shah N, Rezvani K et al. Concise review: umbilical cord blood transplantation:

past, present, and future. Stem Cells Transl Med 2014;**3**:1435–43.

Shah N, Boelens JJ. Umbilical cord blood: advances and opportunities. Cytotherapy 2015;**17**(6):693–4.

Shaw BE, Veys P, Pagliuca A et al. Recommendations for a standard UK approach to incorporating umbilical cord blood into clinical transplantation practice: conditioning protocols and donor selection algorithms. Bone Marrow Transplant 2009;**44**:7–12.

Stavropoulos-Giokas C, Charron D, Navarrete C. Cord Blood Stem Cells Medicine. Elsevier, London, 2014.

Wagner JE, Eapen M, Carter S et al. One-unit versus two-unit cord-blood transplantation for hematologic cancers. N Engl J Med 2014;**371**:1685–94.

43 Recent Advances in Clinical Cellular Immunotherapy

Mark W. Lowdell[1] and Emma Morris[2]

[1] Cell and Tissue Therapy, University College London; Cellular Therapy, Honorary Consultant Scientist, Royal Free London NHS Foundation Trust, London, UK
[2] UCL Institute of Immunity and Transplantation, London, UK

Introduction

Immunotherapy in the form of vaccination has been part of medical practice since Jenner in the eighteenth century. This so-called 'active' immunisation requires that the recipient has the capacity to mount an immune response against the antigens within the vaccine. In contrast, the infusion of antibodies or immune cells raised in other animals or individuals, in response to deliberate vaccination or prior antigen exposure, into patients at risk of infection ('passive' immunisation) allows treatment of immunodeficient or immunocompromised patients.

Until recently, infusion of pathogen-specific antisera was the only routine form of passive immunotherapy, equine anti-tetanus antisera being a well-known example. Successful passive (or adoptive) cellular immunotherapy requires precise matching of donor/recipient histocompatibility antigens and thus advances in human leucocyte antigen (HLA) typing over the past 40 years have underpinned these approaches. The infusion of donor-derived T-cells (donor lymphocyte infusion (DLI)) is now common practice following allogeneic haemopoietic stem cell transplantation (HSCT), but only in the last five years have advances in genetic engineering made possible the redirection of patient-derived (autologous) T-cells towards specific cancer or viral antigens. Cellular immunotherapy is now the focus of much attention, with many early-phase trials demonstrating impressive clinical responses.

Cellular Immunotherapy in Haemopoietic Progenitor Cell Transplantation

The antileukaemic activity of allogeneic bone marrow transplantation was first described, in murine experiments, more than 40 years ago, but was appreciated in the clinic only in the late 1970s when attempts at preventing graft-versus-host disease (GVHD) by T-cell depletion were sometimes frustrated by an increase in the risk of leukaemia recurrence. The clinical antileukaemic effect of GVHD was first reported in 1979 and confirmed later by registry data from the International Bone Marrow Transplant Registry (IBMTR) [1]. The observed benefit of GVHD was particularly evident in patients transplanted for chronic myeloid leukaemia and led to the trial of post-transplant DLI. The first peer-reviewed report of DLI therapy included a single patient who achieved molecular remission with no evidence of clinical GVHD, supporting the hypothesis that graft-versus-leukaemia (GVL) could be directed at leukaemia-specific, leukaemia-restricted target antigens or recipient haematopoiesis [2]. DLI utilises unmanipulated donor-derived T-cells, which mediate their effect in the recipient through the recognition of alloantigens, minor histocompatibility antigens or tumour-specific/associated antigens.

Currently, most allogeneic HSCT regimens incorporating T-cell depletion at the time of transplant (for the prevention of GVHD) include post-transplant DLI to boost immune reconstitution or to treat mixed chimerism and/or disease relapse/progression. The risk of GVHD after DLI has been somewhat reduced by the use of incremental doses of DLI but the search for the 'holy grail' of leukaemia-specific GVL in the complete absence of GVHD continues to be an active research theme.

Nonspecific T-Cell Immunotherapy

In the autologous setting, there is clear evidence that T-cell immunity can not only eradicate viral infection, but can protect against cancer. Immune checkpoint inhibitors, blocking inhibitory pathways such as CTLA4 and PD1, have shown impressive clinical benefits in cancer patients who had failed all conventional therapy options [3,4]. Immune checkpoint inhibition enables the activation of endogenous T-cell immunity [5,6].

In the allogeneic setting, dissecting GVHD from GVL has been attempted by the removal of alloreactive T-cells from donor grafts while retaining nonalloreactive cells which could mediate GVL and antiviral responses. These approaches were all based upon *ex vivo* stimulation of allogeneic donor T-cells with normal haemopoietic cells from the recipient to provoke a clinical-scale mixed lymphocyte response. Reacting T-cells were identified by the expression of activation antigens (e.g. CD25, CD69) and depleted by immunotoxin or immunomagnetic selection. While possibly successful in the reduction of GVHD, the clinical trials of this approach showed no evidence of a GVL effect, although antiviral immune responses have been enhanced in some cases. The principal criticism of these studies was that too few allo-depleted

T-cells were infused to definitively test the hypothesis that GVHD was prevented. Subsequent studies demonstrated that alloreactive T-cell activation *in vitro* generated random oligoclonal responses and was unpredictable from day to day. As such, not all alloreactive T-cell clones will activate in a single mixed cell reaction and thus clinically relevant minor alloreactive T-cells are likely to remain and induce GVHD *in vivo* after infusion.

Another nonspecific approach has been the selective depletion of CD8 T-cells from DLI [7]. Based upon the fact that the target cells of GVHD mostly lack expression of HLA class II, it has been considered that infusions of allogeneic CD4 T-cells induce less GVHD. Many haematopoietic malignancies express HLA class II antigens and are potential targets for CD4 T-cells. Evidence of GVL, resolution of mixed T-cell chimerism and improved antiviral immunity in the absence of GVHD have all been reported in clinical trials of CD8-depleted DLI. Trials of this form of immunotherapy are continuing and are reporting encouraging results with respect to reversal of mixed chimerism and GVL [8].

Tumour-Specific or Tumour-Restricted T-Cell Immunotherapy

Unselected DLI is currently the mainstay of antitumour cellular immunotherapy following HSCT; however, tumour antigen-specific T-cell responses can be generated by vaccination or by the generation of tumour antigen-specific T-cells for adoptive transfer. T-cell-recognised tumour antigens can be divided into two main categories:

- the first category is known as tumour-specific antigens (TSAs), and the genes encoding TSAs are only present in tumour cells and not in normal tissues
- the second group, called tumour-associated antigens (TAAs), are expressed at elevated levels in tumour cells but are also present in normal cells.

The majority of T-cell-recognised tumour antigens in humans are TAAs. The significance of this is that a low level of antigen expression in normal cells can lead to the inactivation of high-avidity T-cells by immunological tolerance mechanisms. As a consequence, the antigen-specific T-cells that escape immune tolerance typically generate low-avidity responses and are often inadequate in providing tumour protection. Therefore, TSAs are theoretically the most desirable target antigens for cellular immuno-therapy (vaccination or adoptive transfer), as there is no pre-existing immunological self-tolerance and TSA-specific immune responses are unlikely to damage normal tissues. Unfortunately, TSAs with specific mutations are often invisible to cytotoxic T-lymphocytes (CTL) as a result of impaired antigen presentation due to competition with normal cellular antigens for proteasomal degradation, transportation by TAP molecules and binding to major histocompatibility complex (MHC). To date, most tumour antigens indentified as CTL targets are TAAs.

The majority of antitumour vaccination trials in humans have been against melanoma antigens, and not in the context of stem cell transplantation. In these situations, vaccination can lead to TAA or TSA-reactive CTL responses, but there has rarely been a corresponding sustained clinical benefit.

Recently, vaccination against the Wilms' tumour antigen 1 (WT1, a leukaemia-associated antigen) has been shown to induce WT1-specific T-cell responses in patients with myeloid malignancies [9]. Current studies are testing whether vaccination against WT1 epitopes early post-transplant can augment the reconstitution of WT1-specific CTL and act as maintenance immunotherapy.

Gene-Modified T-Cells for Immunotherapy

Chimeric antigen receptors (CARs) can redirect T-cell specificity to antibody-recognised target antigens, and T-cell receptors (TCRs) target HLA-presented peptide epitopes (Figure 43.1).

CARs target antigens on the cell surface of cancer cells, while TCRs can target intracellular and nuclear proteins, which are processed and presented on the cell surface by HLA molecules. CAR or TCR gene transfer is efficiently achieved using retroviral and lentiviral vectors, but the clinical-grade production of these vectors is costly, and there is a risk of insertional mutagenesis resulting in malignant transformation when retroviral vectors are used [10].

Chimeric Antigen Receptor Modified T-Cells

Chimeric antigen receptors are 'man-made' antigen receptors encoded by a single cDNA that combine antigen targeting, T-cell activation (such as CD3ζ) and the provision of a co-stimulation signal (such as CD28 or 4-1BB) in a single molecule.

Sustained clinical responses have been observed in poor-risk chronic lymphocytic leukaemia (CLL) and acute lymphocytic leukaemia (ALL) patients treated with engineered T-cells expressing CARs that target CD19 [11–13]. The CD19 protein is expressed on malignant and normal B-cells. As predicted, the CD19-CAR therapy also abolished normal B-cells, an anticipated on-target/off-tumour side effect that is managed by treating patients with regular immunoglobulin infusions. CD19-CAR T-cells are now being tested in a wide range of B-cell malignancies, including follicular lymphoma, diffuse large B-cell lymphoma and small cell lymphoma.

Current research is focused on optimising the design of the CAR molecule to enhance T-cell function and persistence *in vivo*.

T-Cell Receptor Gene Transfer

Advances in gene and cell therapy technologies have now made it possible to rapidly and reproducibly generate autologous (or allogeneic) T-cells equipped with a TCR specific for a given tumour antigen (antigen-specific T-cells) independent of precursor frequency [14]. Both the specificity and avidity of the TCR-transduced T-cells are similar to the parental CTL clone from which the TCR has been isolated. Tumour antigen-specific TCR-transduced T-cells

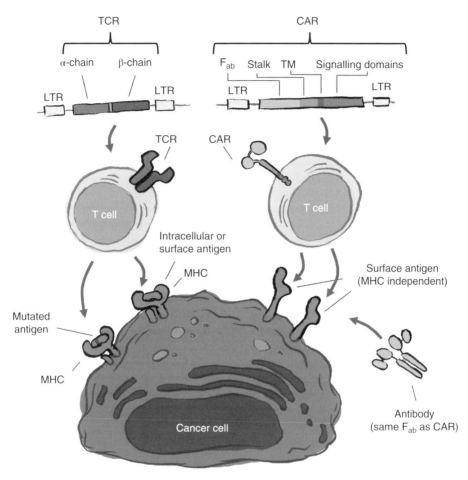

Figure 43.1 Generation of CAR or TCR gene-modified T-cells for cancer immunotherapy. Retroviral and lentiviral vectors encoding CAR or TCR molecules can be used to redirect the specificity of human T-cells. CAR molecules recognise proteins that are expressed on the surface of cancer cells. TCR molecules can recognise peptides that are derived from intracellular proteins, including mutated proteins. (*See insert for colour representation of the figure.*)

have been shown to provide tumour protection in murine models and result in recall responses up to three months post-adoptive transfer. A number of phase I/II clinical trials have now been reported which have demonstrated that TCR-transduced autologous T-cells can have antitumour effects, including TCRs specific for NY-ESO1, MART-1 and gp100 in synovial cell carcinoma and melanoma [15,16]. As MART-1 and gp100 are tissue-specific differentiation antigens expressed in the melanocyte linage, the on-target/off-tumour side effects include attack of melanocytes in the skin and the eye.

However, further modifications are required to the approach in order to maximise clinical benefit. These include:

- modifications of the TCR construct to enhance cell surface expression of the introduced TCR and reduce the incidence of mispairing with endogenous α and β chains (Figure 43.2)
- optimisation of the conditioning regimen used prior to adoptive transfer
- generation of functional TCR-transduced helper T-cells.

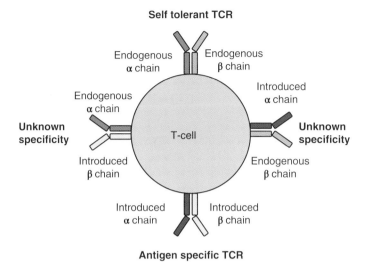

Figure 43.2 Schematic illustrating mispairing with endogenous TCR chains by the introduced TCR chains following retroviral TCR gene transfer. (*See insert for colour representation of the figure.*)

Tumour-Restricted Natural Killer Cell Immunotherapy

Some of the earliest trials of antitumour cellular immunotherapy were based upon infusion of NK cell activating cytokines or *ex vivo* activated NK cells. Most of the early trials were in the autologous setting and, with the notable exception of a single report of AML patients after autologous HSCT, were uniformly disappointing. However, these early trials were conducted before the complex mechanisms underlying NK cell function were understood.

Human NK cells are controlled by a variety of inhibitory and stimulatory signals through cell surface receptors which allow them to distinguish between normal and malignant or infected cells. These receptors fall into one of four families:

- killer immunoglobulin-like (KIR)
- C-type lectins
- immunoglobulin-like transcript (ILT)
- natural cytotoxicity receptors (NCR).

The first two families include both inhibitory and activating receptors while the ILT and NCR families contain only activating receptors. All human NK cells express multiple receptors from each family and it is now apparent that functional subsets of NK cells exist.

In the 1980s, Klaus Karre first demonstrated that murine NK cells preferentially lysed MHC class I negative tumours. This led him to construct his 'missing self' hypothesis in which he proposed that NK cells are inhibited from lysis of normal cells,which express MHC class I, but are capable of lysing MHC class I negative tumour cells. Murine NK cells express surface receptors for MHC class I molecules and their ligation transduces inhibitory signals which prevent NK-mediated lysis. As implied above, the human NK regulatory system is more complex. Killer immunoglobulin-like receptors (KIRs) bind to HLA class I molecules and the majority transduce inhibitory signals upon ligation by their specific HLA class I ligand. KIR molecules are classified on the basis of the number of extracellular domains and the length of the intracellular domain (Figure 43.3).

In a co-culture of NK cells, autologous normal cells and HLA class I deficient tumour cells, one can demonstrate the co-localisation of the KIR:HLA interaction between the NK and normal cell while the tumour cells show no such signalling (Figure 43.4).

Given the concept that NK cells are 'kept in check' by inhibitory signals initiated through

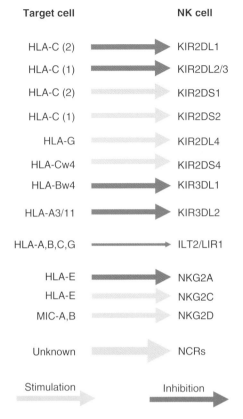

Line thickness indicates relative strength of signal

Figure 43.3 Ligands controlling NK cell activation and triggering. (*See insert for colour representation of the figure.*)

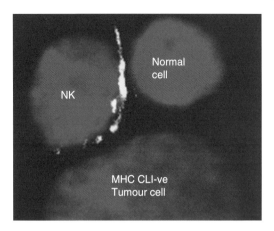

Figure 43.4 Capping of KIR molecules on NK cell. Anti-KIR antibody (*green*) shows co-localisation of KIR and MHC class I molecules at the synapse between the NK and autologous normal cell. In contrast, the MHC-negative tumour cell fails to initiate capping of the KIR molecules. (*See insert for colour representation of the figure.*)

binding HLA molecules on normal somatic cells, one might imagine that the KIR repertoire of any given individual is determined by their HLA type. This is not, however, the case and many healthy individuals will maintain NK cell clones which lack the appropriate inhibitory KIR molecules. However, the C-type lectin, NKG2A, which forms a heterodimer with CD94, appears to be universally expressed on human NK cells and presumably can provide the requisite inhibitory signals through its ligation to HLA-E. Most healthy individuals sustain a population of NK cells which lacks both KIR and NKG2A; these cells appear to be hyporesponsive to activating stimuli.

The clinical relevance of NK cell inhibition is evident in haploidentical HSCT where certain HLA class I mismatches generate a situation of HLA:KIR incompatibility. Highly significant reductions in relapse have been reported among AML patients receiving HLA:KIR incompatible haploidentical HPC grafts compared to patients receiving grafts in which the donor NK repertoire is matched to the HLA type of the patient.

The KIR effect seems to be limited to excessively T-cell-depleted haploidentical grafts and there is little or no role for CD94/NKG2A or for the activating receptors that appear so important in autologous NK cell function.

Natural killer activating signals may be provided via numerous receptors, although their ligands remain largely unknown. Recent published work has shown that, like T-cells, NK cells always require more than one signal to initiate cytokine secretion or lysis and that these signals may need to be provided sequentially to the cell [17].

Despite the lack of a complete understanding of human NK biology, clinical trials of allogeneic NK immunotherapy are already under way and some have been reported. The most notable clinical responses to NK cell therapy were reported as long ago as 1995 in a trial of *ex vivo* expanded and activated autologous NK cells. This remarkable trial from Seattle treated 16 patients with refractory lymphoma, of whom 12 were beyond second complete remission. These patients were treated with megadoses of autologous NK cells with additional *in vivo* low-dose interleukin (IL)-2 which was well tolerated. The five-year disease-free survival was 71% [18]. The complexity of delivery of megadoses of autologous NK cells and the increasing evidence of NK cell inhibition by MHC from murine studies meant that this approach was not pursued, but improved understanding of human NK cell biology in recent years is leading to a resurgence of interest in autologous NK cell therapies.

The clinical use of allogeneic NK cells remains an important area, the value of which was first reported from Minnesota, USA. In that study, minimally conditioned patients with AML, who received bolus infusions of partially-enriched IL-2-activated NK cells from HLA-mismatched donors without concomitant HPC transplant, showed engraftment of donor NK cells in the presence of recipient T-, B- and myeloid cells [19]. At the highest NK dose and the greatest level of preinfusion conditioning with cyclophosphamide and fludarabine, five of 19 patients achieved complete remission. Donor NK cells were detected in their peripheral blood and bone marrow. Despite the engraftment of haplomismatched NK cells, the patients maintained normal bone marrow function and normal levels of autologous T-cells, B-cells and granulocytes.

The antileukaemic effect was relatively short-lived in this trial but the data support the safety of such an approach. A similar trial design was used to treat AML patients with allogeneic NK cells primed with tumour ligands and reported similar success, even achieving disease clearance in one patient who had failed to achieve remission after conventional chemotherapy [20]. Most recently, allogeneic NK cells derived from cord blood CD34+ cells have shown the same clinical benefit in AML patients [21].

In all of these trials, the effects were transient, lasting a few months or up to two years. Although not tested yet, it is possible that such patients could receive multiple courses of NK cell infusions to maintain control of residual disease. The concept of repetitive passive cellular immunotherapy is novel and contrary to the design of most current approaches which have been conceived within a mindset of 'cure by vaccination'. However, most tumour antigens elicit relatively weak immune responses and the physiological immune response to tumours may be one of control rather than eradication.

Passive Cellular Immunotherapy of Infectious Disease

Possibly the most remarkable clinical results from cellular immunotherapies have been seen in the treatment of opportunistic viral infections in immunocompromised patients. Most of these trials have been in the post-transplant setting, particularly in recipients of allo-HSCT grafts.

- The earliest studies involved infusion of enormous numbers of cloned cytomegalovirus (CMV)-reactive CD8 T-cells which caused resolution of refractory CMV disease in patients post allo-HSCT.
- Subsequently, others elegantly demonstrated the specific resolution of post-transplant Epstein–Barr virus (EBV)-driven lymphoma following infusion of donor-derived anti-EBV CTLs.

Ex vivo generation of very large numbers of antiviral T-cells is complex and expensive. However, in 2003, a phase I trial of allogeneic donor-derived CMV-reactive T-cells grown for 21–28 days *ex vivo* on monocyte-derived dendritic cells, which were pulsed with fixed whole CMV, was reported. These expanded cells were infused into patients with molecular evidence of CMV reactivation post allo-HSCT and 8/16 patients resolved the reactivation without recourse to antiviral chemotherapy. No patient received a dose greater than 10^5 T-cells/kg bodyweight and the average dose of CMV-specific T-cells in each dose was no greater than 200–300 per kilogram. Despite this incredibly low dose of cells, virus-specific T-cells were detectable in the peripheral blood of responding recipients at levels equivalent to a 35 000-fold expansion. The small numbers of cells infused in this trial demonstrated that the production of donor-specific cell therapies could be cost-effective [22].

Despite the acknowledged clinical success of these trials, neither led to the wide-scale adoption of cellular therapy due to the extreme technical complexity of cell therapy production. However, with recent advances in the availability of clinical-grade reagents and disposables, the translation of laboratory-grade procedures to clinical application has advanced rapidly. For several years, immunologists have been able to immunomagnetically select specifically activated T-cells on the basis of the secretion of γ-interferon and its capture on the cell surface with a bispecific antibody complexed to a paramagnetic nanoparticle. This approach selects both CD4 and CD8 cells [23].

An alternative approach is the use of multimeric recombinant MHC class I complexes loaded with an immunodominant viral peptide antigen restricted to the specific class I antigen [24]. These HLA multimers can be complexed with the same sort of paramagnetic nanoparticles used in the γ-secretion process described above and directly select antiviral-specific CD8 T-cells from donor blood. These two patented technologies are now produced to clinical grade and are already central to a number of trials, including a phase III trial of allogeneic immunotherapy of CMV reactivation post HSCT, the first multicentre randomised clinical trial of directed donation cellular immunotherapy.

There is undoubted promise in the clinical application of cellular immunity and the field has advanced very substantially in the last five years. However, the true potential of adoptive cellular immunotherapy remains constrained by the perceived need for directed donations (autologous or HLA-matched allogeneic) and by confusion over the regulatory framework in which the therapies fall. The first issue is the greatest barrier, although some recent studies do support the feasibility of the ultimate goal of 'off-the-shelf' products. The haploidentical NK study, discussed above, used NK cells from HLA-mismatched donors and demonstrated transient engraftment. A group in Edinburgh, UK, recently used 'off-the-shelf' HLA-mismatched T-cell lines to treat post-transplant EBV lymphoma in recipients of renal transplants [25].

Technical Advances Facilitating Translational Research in Cellular Immunotherapy

In Europe, since the ratification of the EU Clinical Trials Directive in Member States in 2004, cellular immunotherapies have been regulated as investigational medicinal products (IMPs). Whether a specific cell therapy product constitutes an IMP is determined by the relevant authority in each Member State, but once a product is regulated as an IMP then production must meet Good Manufacturing Practice (GMP) and this has been difficult in the field of cellular immunotherapy. However, a number of European companies now manufacturer CE-marked reagents, consumables and devices for clinical-grade cell production. Closed and semi-closed systems are available for handling large-volume cell suspensions. Gas-permeable cell culture and expansion bags allowing closed-system culture are now widely available and the availability of clinical-grade cytokines is improving.

One of the most significant advances in the field has been the development of CE-marked clinical-grade immunomagnetic cell sorters. These are now widely used for the specific selection of subsets of haemopoietic progenitor cells and other leucocytes and can even select antigen-reactive cells on the basis of cytokine secretion, multimeric HLA peptide reagents or expression of activation markers.

As the regulatory position becomes clearer, more trials will be conducted to good clinical practice and the regulatory authorities will gather more evidence and experience of the field. In the not-too-distant future, the hospital blood bank may become more of a 'cell pharmacy' than ever before.

KEY POINTS

1) Allogeneic GVL by DLI is proof-of-principle of cellular immunotherapy.
2) Use of checkpoint inhibitors in a number of malignancies has demonstrated further the role of T-cell control of cancer.
3) Cellular immunotherapy of viral infections is becoming an alternative to antiviral chemotherapy.
4) Gene-modified autologous and allogeneic antigen-specific T-cells can be reliably generated using retroviral or lentiviral vectors.
5) CAR and TCR gene-modified T-cells have shown antitumour effects in a number of malignancies, with the most impressive clinical results observed using CD19-targeted CAR T-cells in ALL and CLL.
6) Technical and regulatory difficulties in production of cell therapies are being overcome.

References

1 Horowitz MM, Gale RP, Sondel PM et al. Graft-versus-leukemia reactions after bone marrow transplantation. Blood 1990;**75**:555–62.

2 Kolb HJ, Mittermueller J, Clemm C et al. Donor leukocyte transfusion for treatment of recurrent chronic myelogenous leukemia in marrow transplant patients. Blood 1990;**76**:2462–5.

3 Brahmer JR, Tykodi SS, Chow LQ et al. Safety and activity of anti-PD-L1 antibody in patients with advanced cancer. N Engl J Med 2012;**366**:2455–65.

4 Topalian SL, Hodi FS, Brahmer JR et al. Safety, activity, and immune correlates of anti-PD-1 antibody in cancer. N Engl J Med 2012;**366**:2443–54.

5 Gubin MM, Zhang X, Schuster H et al. Checkpoint blockade cancer immunotherapy targets tumour-specific mutant antigens. Nature 2014;**515**:577–81.

6 Powles T, Eder JP, Fine GD et al. MPDL3280A (anti-PD-L1) treatment leads to clinical activity in metastatic bladder cancer. Nature 2014;**515**:558–62.

7 Shimoni A, Gajewski JA, Donato M et al. Long-term follow up of recipients of CD8-depleted DLI for the treatment of CML relapsing after allogeneic progenitor cell transplantation. Biol Blood Marrow Transplant 2001;**7**:568–75.

8 Orti G, Lowdell M, Fielding A et al. Phase I study of high-stringency CD8 depletion of donor leukocyte infusions after allogeneic hematopoietic stem cell transplantation. Transplantation 2009;**88**:1312–18.

9 Uttenthal B, Martinez-Davila I, Ivey A et al. Wilms' tumour 1 (WT1) peptide vaccination in patients with acute myeloid leukaemia induces short-lived WT1-specific immune responses. Br J Haematol 2014;**164**(3):366–75.

10 Williams DA, Thrasher AJ. Concise review: lessons learned from clinical trials of gene therapy in monogenic immunodeficiency diseases. Stem Cells Transl Med 2014;**3**:636–42.

11 Brentjens RJ, Davila ML, Riviere I et al. CD19-targeted T-cells rapidly induce molecular remissions in adults with chemotherapy-refractory acute lymphoblastic leukemia. Sci Transl Med 2013;**5**:177ra138.

12 Maude SL, Frey N, Shaw PA et al. Chimeric antigen receptor T-cells for sustained remissions in leukemia. N Engl J Med 2014;**371**:1507–17.

13 Porter DL, Levine BL, Kalos M, Bagg A, June CH. Chimeric antigen receptor-modified T-cells in chronic lymphoid leukemia. N Engl J Med 2011;**365**:725–33.

14 Stauss HJ, Morris EC. Immunotherapy with gene-modified T-cells: limiting side effects provides new challenges. Gene Ther 2013;**20**(11):1029–32.

15 Morgan RA, Dudley ME, Wunderlich JR et al. Cancer regression in patients after transfer of genetically engineered lymphocytes. Science 2006;**314**:126–9.

16 Robbins PF, Morgan RA, Feldman SA et al. Tumor regression in patients with metastatic synovial cell sarcoma and melanoma using genetically engineered lymphocytes reactive with NY-ESO-1. J Clin Oncol 2011;**29**:917–24.

17 Sabry M, Lowdell MW. Tumor-primed NK cells: waiting for the green light. Front Immunol 2013;**4**:408.

18 Benyunes MC, Higuchi C, York A et al. Immunotherapy with interleukin 2 with or without lymphokine-activated killer cells after autologous bone marrow transplantation for malignant lymphoma: a feasibility trial. Bone Marrow Transplant 1995;**16**:283–8.

19 Miller JS, Soignier Y, Panoskaltis-Mortari A et al. Successful adoptive transfer and in vivo expansion of human haploidentical NK cells in patients with cancer. Blood 2005;**105**:3051–7.

20 Kottaridis PD, North, Tsirogianni M et al. Two-stage priming of allogeneic Natural Killer cells for the treatment of patients with acute myeloid leukemia; a phase I trial. PLoS One 2015;**10**(6):e0123416.

21 Dolstra H, Roeven MWH, Spanholtz J et al. A phase I study of allogeneic natural killer cell therapy generated from cord blood hematopoietic stem and progenitor cells in elderly acute myeloid leukemia patients. Blood 2015;**126**:1357.

22 Peggs KS, Verfuerth S, Pizzey A et al. Adoptive cellular therapy for early cytomegalovirus infection after allogeneic stem-cell transplantation with virus-specific T-cell lines. Lancet 2003;**362**(9393):1375–7.

23 Peggs K, Thomson K, Samuel E et al. Directly selected cytomegalovirus-reactive donor T-cells confer rapid and safe systemic reconstitution of virus-specific immunity following stem cell transplantation. Clin Infect Dis 2011;**52**:49–57.

24 Cobbold M, Khan N, Pourgheysari B et al. Adoptive transfer of CMV-specific CTL to stem cell transplant patients after selection by HLA-peptide tetramers. J Exp Med 2005;**202**:379–86.

25 Haque T, Wilkie GM, Jones MM et al. Allogeneic cytotoxic T-cell therapy for EBV-positive PTLD: results of a phase II multicentre clinical trial. Blood 2007;**110**:1123–31.

Further Reading

Stauss HJ, Morris EC, Abken H. Cancer gene therapy with T-cell receptors and chimeric antigen receptors. Curr Opin Pharmacol 2015;**24**:113–18.

44 Tissue Banking

Akila Chandrasekar, Paul Rooney and John N. Kearney

NHS Blood and Transplant, Tissue and Eye Services, Liverpool, UK

Introduction

Tissue banking has become an increasingly important area of activity for EU blood services, and allows expertise in donor and quality management to be applied to collect, process and store tissues in a carefully regulated environment. Consent for removal and use of all tissues must be obtained and recorded. Assessment of deceased donors must be thorough and retrieval of tissues rapid to reduce the potential for bacterial contamination. Processed heart valves, tendons, ligaments, bone and skin are used in a wide variety of surgical spheres. Decellularised tissues have the advantage of not inducing an immune response and of becoming repopulated by recipient cells and eventually being remodelled by the recipient, so the allograft becomes part of the host. New techniques have allowed transplantation of limbal stem cells in the eye or remodelling of large tissues such as the trachea using a donor scaffold and host stem cells. These novel technologies herald a new era of regenerative medicine.

Regulation

The European Union Tissue and Cells Directives (EUTCD) is made up of three Directives: the parent Directive (2004/23/EC), providing the framework legislation, and two technical directives (2006/17/EC and 2006/86/EC – amended in 2015/565), providing the detailed requirements of the EUTCD. The Human Tissue Act (2004) established the Human Tissue Authority (HTA) as the competent authority, with responsibility for regulating tissues and cells (other than gametes and embryos) for human application within England, Wales and Northern Ireland. There is separate legislation in Scotland – the Human Tissue (Scotland) Act 2006 – with a high degree of similarity between both acts. The EU Directives were fully implemented into UK law in 2007, via the Human Tissue (Quality and Safety for Human Application) Regulations 2007. Tissue banks in the USA are regulated by the Food and Drug Administration (FDA). The American Association of Tissue Banks (AATB) also provides a voluntary accreditation that tissue banks can apply for.

Consent

Consent is the fundamental principle of the Human Tissue Act and underpins the lawful removal, storage and use of donated tissue for any purpose. While provisions of the Human Tissue (Scotland) Act 2006 are based on authorisation rather than consent, these are essentially both expressions of the same principle. In Europe, the legal requirements for obtaining permission for retrieval of tissues after death vary from

Practical Transfusion Medicine, Fifth Edition. Edited by Michael F. Murphy, David J. Roberts and Mark H. Yazer.
© 2017 John Wiley & Sons Ltd. Published 2017 by John Wiley & Sons Ltd.

country-to-country [1]. However, even where 'opting out' or 'presumed consent' systems are operated, it is considered best professional practice to confirm that no relatives object to the donation proceeding.

Informed and valid consent must be obtained from an appropriate person, prior to tissue retrieval, to ensure that tissue donation for any purpose, such as clinical use or research/training, is lawful. With a living donor, the appropriate person is generally the donor themselves. For deceased donors, this can be the wishes of the deceased themselves expressed in life, for example through the organ donor register, or their nominated representative, a person who was appointed in life by the deceased to make these decisions. In the absence of either of these, the consent of a person in a 'qualifying relationship' with them immediately before they died must be sought. This may be (in order of priority) a spouse or partner, blood relation or friend.

Consent should be taken only by those trained to do so. It is important that the person giving consent is fully informed about all aspects of the donation process and, where appropriate, what the risks are. The duration of the consent must also be specified; the person giving consent may withdraw it at any point before or after donation, providing that the tissue has not already been used, and it is important that they are informed of this right. With the exception of anatomical examination or public display, where written consent is required, the Human Tissue Act does not specify the format in which consent should be recorded. Verbal consent, documented either by audio recording or in the patient's notes, is also valid.

Donor Selection and Testing

Tissue donors must be carefully selected to minimise the risk of transmitting diseases and to ensure suitable quality of grafts for transplantation. The major donor exclusion criteria described in the EU Directive (Box 44.1) are based on these two principles.

Box 44.1 Donor exclusion criteria.

History of disease of unknown aetiology

Presence or past history of malignancy (some exceptions)

Risk of transmission of prion disease(s)

Systemic infection or significant local infection uncontrolled at the time of donation

History or evidence of risk of transmissible viral infections such as HIV and hepatitis

History of chronic or systemic autoimmune disease that could have a detrimental effect on the tissues

Unknown cause of death for deceased donors

The donor selection process includes a structured interview with living donors to obtain a detailed medical and behavioural history. In the case of deceased donors, this interview is conducted with someone who knew the donor well – usually – but not always, a relative. The reliability of a family interview depends on how well the interviewee knew their deceased relative and additional sources of information can supplement the donor selection process. Information is sought from the general practitioner and, when necessary, from the referring hospital practitioner if the donor was admitted to hospital prior to death, to obtain as accurate a medical history as possible [2]. The result of postmortem examination is reviewed [2], if one was carried out.

Donor blood samples for testing must be obtained at the time of donation or within seven days post-donation for living donors. The sample from deceased donors must be obtained just prior to death or within 24 hours after death. Fluids administered in the 48 hours prior to death must be recorded to allow an estimation of any plasma dilution effect. Tissues from donors with plasma dilution of more than 50% can be accepted only if testing procedures used for screening are validated for such plasma dilution or if a pre-transfusion sample is available.

The minimum requirement for mandatory tests required by the EU Directive includes screening for hepatitis C (anti-HCV), hepatitis B (HBsAg and anti-HBc), HIV (anti-HIV I and II) and syphilis. Individual nations are permitted to set higher standards than the minimum requirements. There is a requirement in the EU Directive to quarantine living tissue donations to obtain a second blood sample from the donor after an interval of 180 days to repeat the mandatory tests; however, if the blood sample taken at the time of donation is additionally tested by the nucleic acid amplification method (NAT) for HIV, HCV and HBV, a retest is not required after 180 days. In UK Blood Services, all tissue donors are screened by NAT for HIV, hepatitis C and hepatitis B, in addition to the antibody and antigen tests mentioned above.

The interval between the time of infection to the onset of detectable infection on screening tests is known as the 'window period'. This window period for genome detection by NAT is much shorter than the window period for antibody detection. NAT thereby reduces the risk of transmission of infection during the early phase of the infection following exposure to a virus, before antibodies can be detected on screening. However, the serology screen may serve as an indicator of a past exposure and as an indicator of lifestyle risks. This combination of NAT and antibody test is especially important for testing of deceased tissue donors, where only a single blood sample can be taken at the time of donation. A negative NAT at the time of donation from a seronegative individual also removes the requirement for quarantining the donation from living donors, as explained above.

Tissue Procurement

Living donations are retrieved during surgery by the operating team. Clear, written instructions, staff training, and standard sterile kits are provided by the tissue bank for tissue collection. Regular auditing to ensure compliance with agreed procedures, detailed in a written agreement between the tissue bank and the hospital, is an integral part of a living donation program.

With deceased donors, it is important to ensure the quality of the tissues removed. Tissues can deteriorate postmortem due to microbial contamination and autolysis, or be contaminated during the retrieval process. The optimal time and place to procure tissues from deceased donors is in an operating theatre, immediately after death or post cessation of circulation. However, the availability of these facilities for tissue donation is limited, and is generally restricted to tissue grafts that can be obtained during routine organ procurement procedures, such as removal of the heart for valve donation. In the UK, the large majority of tissue donations are performed in hospital mortuaries or on rare occasions in funeral homes. In addition, National Health Service Blood and Transplant in England has a dedicated tissue donation facility in Liverpool, equipped with laminar air flow, for tissue retrieval; similar donation suites can be found in Europe and the USA.

Donor identification by means of a wristband or toe-tag is a crucial step before commencing the retrieval. A minimum of three points of identification, such as name, date of birth, hospital number and address, is required to positively identify the donor. Before tissue retrieval, a thorough external examination of the donor body appearance is conducted and recorded as part of donor assessment. This examination should include detection and recording of tattoos, jaundice, evidence of drug use, body piercing, open wounds or signs of infection, scars and bruises, intravenous cannula sites, operation incision sites and other significant abnormalities.

Reducing Bacterial Contamination

Following death, autodegradation of all tissues commences as cells die and release lytic enzymes into the tissue. The intestinal microflora begins to migrate throughout the body, contaminating other tissues. The rate of both these processes is critically dependent on temperature so it is crucial that warm ischaemia time is minimised and the body refrigerated as soon as possible after death. In general, tissues should be recovered within the shortest possible period from the time of death. Standards vary around the world, from 12 to 48 hours, depending on the tissue and the processing method to which it will be subjected.

Minimising bacterial contamination is further ensured by staff wearing sterile clothing and applying an aseptic technique during the tissue recovery process. This includes cleaning the donor using surgical detergents, alcohol wipes and sterile water; shaving the incision and skin retrieval areas; and draping the donor body before commencing the retrieval. Single-use equipment is employed where possible.

Generally, skin grafts (if consented for) will be retrieved first to prevent the skin becoming contaminated by internal body fluids following incisions to remove internal tissues. An important aspect of tissue recovery is the careful reconstruction of the donor body. Extendable plastic or wooden prostheses are used to replace large bones.

Tissue Processing

Tissue grafts are processed to improve safety and efficacy and for long-term storage of the donated material. There are multiple ways of processing, depending on the properties of the graft that need to be retained [3]. The core methodology by which viable tissues (skin, heart valve, cardiovascular and meniscus grafts) are processed comprises dissection, decontamination by antibiotic cocktail and cryopreservation. While it may be desirable to sterilise a graft to increase safety, this is not practical where retention of donor cell viability is required. For many types of tissue allograft, in particular musculoskeletal allografts, the presence of viable cells is not required and, in these cases, processing reduces the risk of disease transmission by

removal of blood and marrow and by reducing or eliminating contamination by chemical or physical means. Pooling of tissues from different donors during processing is not permitted by standards in Europe or the USA.

Each tissue bank should have a policy for acceptance or rejection of tissues if certain organisms are detected in bacterial screening during different stages of processing. The policy should be based on the pathogenicity of the organism and the validated effectiveness of any subsequent decontamination or sterilisation steps.

Femoral heads from living donors removed during surgery in an operating theatre can be frozen and transplanted without further processing in the absence of bacterial or fungal contamination in validated tests.

Supply and Traceability of Tissues

Directive 2006/86/EC requires the development of a European coding system, which will facilitate tracking of tissue from the donor to the recipient. Most tissue banks supply tissues direct to operating theatre departments and it is the responsibility of the receiving hospital to track from the receipt of the tissue to the graft's ultimate fate. Many tissue banks supply the hospital with a recipient record to be completed for each graft and returned to the bank. The users should always be advised to:

- keep a log of tissue received and used
- record any allograft unit numbers in the patient's notes
- inform the tissue bank immediately of any adverse reaction that might be attributable to the tissue graft.

In many cases, tissues are supplied for specific cases and stocks are not held locally, but some units prefer to keep stocks of tissue immediately at hand for use in emergency or unexpected cases. Depending on the type of tissue, the hospital may require a licence in the EU to store tissue grafts for more than 48 hours; tissues containing donor cells such as cryopreserved skin grafts require a licence for storage, whereas acellular tissues, such as processed freeze-dried bone grafts, do not.

Clinical Applications

Tissue allografts are used in a variety of clinical indications in orthopaedic, spinal, cardiac, vascular, ophthalmic and plastic and reconstructive surgical procedures. Some of them are listed in Table 44.1.

Serious Adverse Events and Reactions

Directive 2006/86/EC requires Member States to have systems for reporting adverse reactions and events related to the procurement, testing, processing, storage or distribution of the tissue, which might lead to the transmission of communicable disease, death or life-threatening, disabling or incapacitating conditions which might result in or prolong hospitalisation or morbidity in the recipient. In the UK, the HTA has developed an electronic reporting system for tissue and cell facilities, in line with the requirements of the Directive.

Advances in Tissue Processing and Regenerative Medicine

Regenerative medicine uses techniques of tissue engineering to remove donor cells without affecting the biological, biomechanical or biochemical parameters of the tissue [4].

Decellularised Tissues

Decellularised tissue, in particular decellularised dermis, has been available as an allograft

Table 44.1 Indications for tissue allografts.

Types of graft	Surgical specialty	Surgical procedure (examples)
Heart valves	Cardiac	Heart valve replacement
Tendons and ligaments	Knee surgery	Ligament reconstruction
Meniscus	Knee surgery	Replacement of damaged meniscus (in selected cases)
Frozen femoral head, morcellised bone grafts	Orthopaedic (hip and knee)	Impaction grafting at revision joint surgery
Massive bone allograft	Orthopaedics	Post trauma or tumour excision reconstruction
Demineralised bone	Spinal surgery, orthopaedic, oral and maxillofacial	Spinal fusion, nonunion or trauma defects, to fill cysts and tumour cavity defects
Cornea	Ophthalmology	Keratoconus, corneal ulcers, trauma, chemical burns
Skin	Burns	Burns, toxic epidermal necrolysis
Decellularised dermis	Plastic and reconstructive, breast surgery, abdominal surgery	Chronic wounds, breast reconstruction, abdominal wall repair
Blood vessels	Vascular	To replace infected prosthetic graft, lower limb ischaemia

since 1995 and several tissue banks now offer decellularised dermis and decellularised heart valves to surgeons. A major advantage of decellularised tissue becoming repopulated by recipient cells is that, over time, the grafted tissue becomes remodelled by the recipient cells, the donor extracellular matrix is replaced with recipient matrix and the allograft becomes part of the host. Two consequences of this are:

- a reduction in immune and/or inflammatory response
- the ability of the grafted/remodelled tissue to grow and be able to repair itself as part of the recipient.

Recent studies on implantation of decellularised heart valves indicate that the tissue does become repopulated with recipient cells and there is a reduction in complications and the need for further operations with time when compared to conventionally cryopreserved valves [5]. The use of decellularised heart valves opens up the possibility that when used in paediatric patients, only one heart valve transplant may be required during the lifetime of the patient and the implanted valve will increase in size when required as part of the recipient's natural growth.

Limbal Stem Cells

The ability to add cells to banked tissue allografts is a major step forward in regenerative medicine treatment. Amniotic membrane has been used as a conventional allograft to treat severe ocular surface diseases for several years owing to its ability to facilitate corneal re-epithelialisation and reduce scarring and inflammation; however, more recently, amniotic membrane has been used as a substrate on which epithelial stem cells can be expanded prior to transplant. The epithelial stem cells are derived from biopsies of the limbal region of the corneum; the stem cells can locate to stem cell niches when transplanted and thus provide a long-term solution to limbal stem cell deficiency. Limbal stem cells can be obtained either from the patient or from a donor.

Tracheal Transplants

Recent advances in regenerative medicine have involved adding recipient cells to a decellularised tissue, either in advance in the laboratory or at the point of transplant, making the procedure 'personalised' regenerative medicine. In 2008, a patient in Spain received a transplant of a portion of trachea that had been decellularised and then repopulated with her own cells, within a bioreactor [6]. Similar procedures were performed in the UK in 2010 using the entire trachea and adding stem cells 2–4 hours prior to transplant [7].

Regenerative medicine opens up the possibility of replacing almost every damaged or worn-out tissue with a new tissue capable of becoming part of the patient and returning normal functionality.

Conclusion

The banking of tissues is increasing within blood services, where expertise in donor selection, donor testing and quality management is being applied to the banking of tissues. For deceased donors, a thorough medical and behavioural history from a number of alternative sources is recorded to compensate for the lack of a direct donor interview. Tissues should be retrieved within the shortest possible time period after death to minimise the risk of bacterial contamination. Minimising bacterial cross-contamination is ensured by applying aseptic retrieval techniques. Tissue processing is necessarily open and usually involves decontamination or terminal sterilisation. Traceability is an essential aspect of the quality chain and should ideally be supported by machine-readable identification codes. Tissue banking and processing is a rapidly evolving field and is becoming more and more related to personalised regenerative medicine.

KEY POINTS

1) Tissue grafts are used in surgical procedures to replace damaged or lost tissues in patients. Most tissue allografts are donated by deceased donors and some by living donors undergoing surgery.
2) Selection criteria for donors are based on an analysis of risks and benefits related to application of specific tissues.
3) Processing tissue reduces the risk of disease transmission by removing blood and marrow and by reducing or eliminating contamination by chemical and physical means. Pooling of donations during processing is not permitted by standards in Europe or the USA.
4) Tissue allografts have been used in surgical procedures for many years with great success but with known limitations. Regenerative medicine using decellularised and tissue-engineered allografts may allow full incorporation of the graft into the patient such that it becomes part of the patient and is able to grow and repair itself.

References

1 Schulz-Baldes A, Biller-Andorno N, Capron AM. International perspectives on the ethics and regulation of human cell and tissue transplantation. Bull World Health Org 2007;**85**:941–8.
2 Chandrasekar A, Warwick RM, Clarkson A. Exclusion of deceased donors post-procurement of tissues. Cell Tissue Bank 2011;**12**:191–8.
3 Galea E (ed.). Essentials of Tissue Banking. Springer, New York, 2010.
4 Mirsadraee S, Wilcox H, Korossis S et al. Development and characterisation of an acellular human pericardial matrix for tissue engineering. Tissue Eng 2006;**12**:763–73.
5 Da Costa FD, Santos LR, Collatusso C et al. Thirteen years' experience of the Ross operation. J Heart Valve Dis 2009;**18**:84–94.
6 Macchiarini P, Jungebluth P, Go T et al. Clinical transplantation of a tissue-engineered airway. Lancet 2008;**372**:2023–30.
7 Baiguera S, Birchall MA, Macchiarini P. Tissue engineered tracheal transplantation. Transplantation 2010;**89**:485–91.

Further Reading

Barron DJ, Khan NE, Jones TJ, Willets RG, Brawn WJ. What tissue bankers should know about the use of allograft heart valves. Cell Tissue Bank 2010;**11**:47–55.

Eagle MJ, Rooney P, Lomas R, Kearney JN. Validation of radiation dose received by frozen unprocessed and processed bone during terminal sterilisation. Cell Tissue Bank 2005;**6**:221–30.

Getgood A, Bollen S. What tissue bankers should know about the use of allograft tendons and cartilage in orthopaedics. Cell Tissue Bank 2010;**11**:87–97.

Greaves NS, Benatar B, Baguneid M, Bayat A. Single stage application of a novel decellularised dermis for treatment resistant lower limb ulcers: positive outcomes assessed by SIAscopy, laser perfusion and 3D imaging, with sequential time histological analysis. Wound Repair Regen 2013;**21**:813–22.

Hogg P, Rooney P, Leow-Dyke S, Brown C, Ingham I, Kearney JN. Development of a terminally sterilised decellularised dermis. Cell Tissue Bank 2015;**16**:351–9.

Kearney JN. Guidelines on processing and clinical use of skin allografts. Clin Dermatol 2005;**23**:357–64.

McDermott ID. What tissue bankers should know about the use of allograft meniscus in orthopaedics. Cell Tissue Bank 2010;**11**:75–85.

45

Observational and Interventional Trials in Transfusion Medicine

Alan T. Tinmouth[1], Dean Fergusson[2] and Paul C. Hébert[3]

[1] *General Hematology and Transfusion Medicine, Division of Hematology, Department of Medicine, Ottawa Hospital, University of Ottawa Center for Transfusion Research, Clinical Epidemiology Program, Ottawa Health Research Institute, Ottawa, Canada*
[2] *University of Ottawa Center for Transfusion Research, Clinical Epidemiology Program, Ottawa Health Research Institute, Ottawa, Canada*
[3] *Department of Medicine, Centre Hospitalier de L'Université de Montreal, Centre Recherche de le Centre Hospitalier de Montreal, Montreal, Canada*

Introduction

Randomised controlled clinical trials (RCTs) are the 'gold standard' clinical research design used to distinguish the risks and benefits of therapeutic interventions. In 1948, for the first time a controlled clinical trial made use of random allocation, a control group and blinding. Additional principles guiding the design of RCTs were first elaborated by Sir Austin Bradford-Hill in the 1960s [1].

Many important questions regarding the use of blood products and alternatives such as blood conservation therapies have not been the subject of well-designed and executed RCTs. Clinicians frequently base decisions on suboptimal levels of clinical evidence. Their reasons for the relative paucity of large clinical trials in transfusion medicine include the following.

- Transfusion medicine has historically been a laboratory-based specialty with research focused on the product.
- Blood components are a supportive treatment for patients under the care of other physicians whose research focus is directed at the underlying disease.
- The impact of supportive therapy with blood components on important clinical outcomes may be difficult to measure.
- Difficulty in obtaining funding for research of a supportive, as opposed to a curative, therapy.
- Blood components have been part of standard care for years without good evidence to define the benefits or harms, or specific indications of use.
- Few industry partners are willing to invest in large clinical trials given that products are already in wide use.

In this chapter, we outline some of the methodological issues central to the development and conduct of observational and interventional trials, including RCTs, in transfusion medicine.

Types of Clinical Studies

To ascertain the effectiveness of an intervention, the RCT remains the preferred study design as it should minimise the most important biases if properly conceived and executed.

Despite being the 'gold standard', there are often practical, legal, financial and ethical limitations to the use of clinical trials. While many of these limitations have been well described, one unique obstacle in transfusion medicine is the conduct of a RCT when an intervention is universally implemented, such as a new processing method or testing procedure for the entire blood supply. By implementing an intervention such as universal prestorage leucocyte reduction, a RCT becomes impossible within that population. If a RCT is not possible, other study designs including quasi-experimental and observational designs should be considered.

Observational Studies

Two types of observational designs are often considered in clinical research: case–control studies and cohort or prognostic studies (Figure 45.1). In all observational studies, the first step is to define (a) the research hypothesis, (b) the population, (c) the exposure(s), (d) the outcome(s) and (e) the covariates (factors other than the exposure that may influence the occurrence of the outcomes). A case–control study is one which identifies a group of individuals with an outcome (cases) and another group of nonaffected individuals (controls) who would be

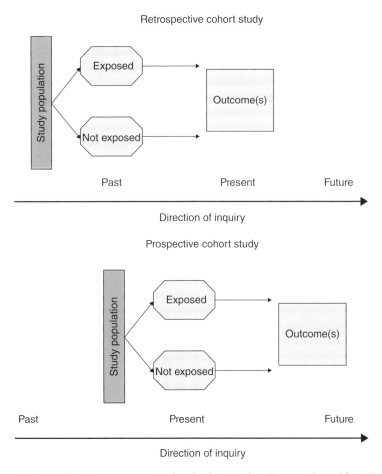

Figure 45.1 Observational study designs: case–control and cohort studies. *Source:* Adapted from Tay and Tinmouth 2007 [22]. Reproduced with permission of John Wiley & Sons. (*See insert for colour representation of the figure.*)

considered at risk of developing the outcome. The investigators then seek to identify potential risk factors in both groups. This classic epidemiological design is by definition a retrospective study and is ideally suited to the investigation of rare diseases and the identification of potential aetiological or risk factors, particularly if there is a long latency period [2]. In transfusion medicine, case–control studies would be ideally suited for the initial study of rare conditions such as transfusion-related acute lung injury (TRALI) or the association between blood transfusion and variant Creutzfeldt–Jakob disease (vCJD). For example, Silliman et al were able to identify that certain diagnoses (haematological malignancies and cardiac disease) and the age of the platelets were associated with TRALI using a case–control design [3]. Despite some of the potential advantages of this study design, it is difficult to do well, fraught with potential biases and, finally, does not allow causation to be determined.

The second observational design choice is a cohort study. Cohort studies follow patients forward in time and evaluate outcomes based on a known exposure, risk factor or treatment. In this type of study, individuals are identified well in advance of either developing a disease or the outcome of interest and followed forward in time. A cohort study may provide important clues to the aetiology of a disease or health state by comparing individuals who develop the disease and those who do not. It may also lead to a better understanding of the incidence of the disease or, in patients with an established disease, the course of the disease, the prognostic information or the effectiveness of treatments. If patients are identified and followed once a disease has developed, then this design may also provide invaluable prognostic information. This design is most powerful when all eligible individuals are identified early, followed prospectively throughout the course of the study and without any losses to follow-up.

The positive and negative attributes of cohort studies can be illustrated by some of the cohort studies that have examined the relationship between anaemia, red cell transfusion and mortality. A retrospective study of Jehovah's Witness patients conducted by Carson and colleagues demonstrated a clear association between increasing degrees of preoperative anaemia and mortality rates in the presence of ischaemic heart disease [4]. Ethically, a prospective RCT examining the question would not have been feasible. In contrast, multiple cohort studies, including a retrospective study of cardiac surgery patients, reported an association between prolonged red cell storage and adverse outcomes.

These observational studies all had major limitations, particularly interdependence of anaemia, comorbidities and transfusions. This is a classic example of a common bias affecting observational studies known as confounding by indication, which is the mixing or blurring of effects where an outcome is related to an exposure but effect is due to a third factor [5,6]. Subsequent large RCTs did not find an effect of prolonged red cell storage on mortality or other adverse outcomes, highlighting the potential biases and limitations of observational cohort studies and the inability of this study design to demonstrate causation or draw definitive conclusions.

The use of cohort studies can be of particular value in the evaluation of a universally implemented intervention such as prestorage leucocyte reduction. In such a case, subjects must either be sampled over a period of time prior to and after the implementation of the program (a 'before-and-after' or interrupted time-series study), or sampling must occur among subjects who received leucocyte-reduced blood products and another population that did not receive such products (standardised incidence study). In a before-and-after study design, the frequency of an outcome in a specified population is measured first during a period of time when the exposure is absent then in the same population during a period of time where exposure is present. Consecutive periods before and after the implementation of a treatment are often compared. When a single measurement in both the pre- and post-intervention periods is compared, there is the risk that changes occurring as a result of other ongoing factors may be attributed to the intervention. To limit this temporal bias, the changes in the experimental group may be compared to a control group not exposed to the intervention (controlled before-and-after study) or determinations of the outcome at multiple time points before and after the implementation of an intervention (interrupted time-series analysis) should ideally be used to account for temporal changes.

Well-executed case–control studies may provide clues about the aetiology or risk factors associated with the development of a disease or complication. A cohort study may provide the best estimate of incidence, prognosis and risks associated with the development of a disease or its complications. Both designs provide weak inferences regarding specific therapeutic interventions because many forms of bias and confounding remain even after complex multivariable analysis. Before-and-after studies and time-series analysis, both quasi-experimental designs, may provide some inferences regarding clinical consequences attributed to the implementation of a universal program when a RCT is not possible [7]. Inherent in both case–control and cohort studies is the inability to determine causality between a risk factor or treatment and a specific outcome.

Randomised Controlled Trials

Overall Design Approaches for RCTs

For therapeutic interventions, there is little debate that the highest quality of evidence is provided by a well-performed RCT. However, there should be an awareness that RCTs may be complex in terms of both their design and execution. In this section, a conceptual framework is provided for RCTs that should assist providers and consumers of clinical research.

The ideal RCT establishes whether therapeutic interventions work, and determines the overall benefits and risks of each alternative in predefined patient populations. In addition, the ideal RCT should attempt to fulfil its objectives with the fewest patients possible (often termed 'statistical efficiency'). Unfortunately, these objectives are often in direct conflict. More importantly, economic considerations often limit our ability to fulfil all these objectives. For instance, by maximising the efficiency of a study, investigators might sacrifice their ability to draw conclusions in clinically important subgroups because of inadequate sample size.

The most important consequence of these conflicting objectives is that choices made in the design of RCTs must focus on whether an intervention works or whether it results in more good than harm for patients [8]. Trials that attempt to determine therapeutic *efficacy* address the question 'Will the therapy work under ideal conditions?' Trials attempting to determine therapeutic *effectiveness* address the question 'Will the therapy do more good than harm under usual practice conditions in all patients who are offered the intervention?' Clearly, both questions will yield useful information. Efficacy is often established first (e.g. phase III pharmaceutical studies), then the intervention may be evaluated for its effectiveness, though this occurs more rarely.

As the characteristics of efficacy and effectiveness trials can differ considerably, the planning of a RCT should reflect the design that will best reflect the primary study question (Tables 45.1 and 45.2). Efficacy trials attempt to maximise internal validity, defined as the extent to which the experimental findings represent the true effect in study participants. This is often at the expense of external validity, defined as the extent to which the experimental findings in the study represent the true effect in the target population. For effectiveness studies, external validity is usually emphasised over internal validity.

An example of an efficacy trial is the Stroke Prevention in Sickle Cell Anaemia (STOP) trial which compared the efficacy of exchanges transfusions to prevent stroke in 130 paediatric sickle cell patients with abnormal transcranial Doppler studies [9]. In contrast, the Clinical Randomisation of an Antifibrinolytic in Significant Haemorrhage (CRASH-2) study was a large effectiveness trial

Table 45.1 Considerations in determining which design approach to implement in transfusion trials.

Criteria to consider	Choice of design	
	Favouring efficacy	**Favouring effectiveness**
Evidence	Limited evidence	Efficacy well documented
Importance of the question	Rare and less serious	Common and serious problem
Feasibility	Not demonstrated	Adequate accrual and confirmed feasibility
Risks	Unknown or significant consequences	Minimal or acceptable risks given benefits
Benefits	Limited or unknown benefits	Significant benefits anticipated.

Table 45.2 Comparison of study characteristics using either an efficacy or an effectiveness approach when designing a study.

Study characteristics	Efficacy trial	Effectiveness trial
Research question	Will the intervention work under ideal conditions?	Will the intervention result in more good than harm under usual practice conditions?
Setting	Restricted to specialised centres	Open to all institutions.
Patient selection	Selected, well-defined patients	A wider range of patients identified using broad eligibility criteria
Study design	Smaller RCT using stringent rules	Larger multicentre RCT using simpler rules
Baseline assessment	Elaborate and detailed	Simple and clinician friendly
Intervention	Tightly controlled Optimal therapy under optimal study conditions	Less controlled Therapy administered by investigators using accepted approaches
Treatment protocols	Rigorous and detailed	Very general
Compliance		Noncompliance tolerated
Endpoints	Disease-related Related to biological effect. Surrogate endpoints	Patient related such as all-cause mortality or quality of life
Analysis	By treatment received Noncompliers removed.	Intention-to-treat All patients included
Data management		
Data collection	Elaborate	Minimal and simple
Data monitoring*	Detailed and rigorous	Minimal

*Data monitoring refers to the review of source documents and adjudication/verification of outcomes.
RCT, randomised controlled trial.

that showed small but clinically important differences in all-cause mortality in 20000 trauma patients receiving tranexamic acid [10].

Many trials opt for a hybrid approach between large simple trials and tightly controlled clinical studies. The Transfusion Requirements in Critical Care (TRICC) trial [11], which allocated 838 critically ill patients to either a restrictive or liberal transfusion strategy, and the Platelet Dose (PLADO) trial [12], which randomised 1272 patients with hypoproliferative thrombocytopenia to low-, medium- or high-dose prophylactic platelet transfusions, provide examples.

RCT Design Alternatives

Parallel Group Design

Once investigators have chosen whether an efficacy, effectiveness or hybrid approach will best answer the research question, there are several design options that may be considered (see Table 45.2). A two-group parallel design is the most common of RCT design choices (Figure 45.2a). In this design, patients are randomly allocated to one of two therapeutic interventions and followed forward in time. It is the simplest to plan, implement, analyse and,

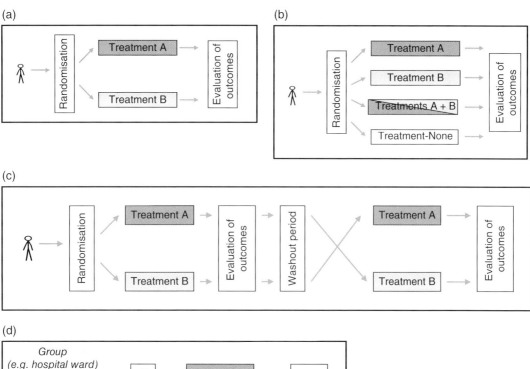

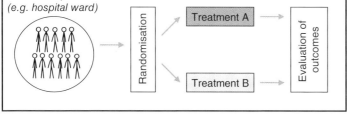

Figure 45.2 Design approaches for randomised controlled trials. (a) Randomised two-group parallel design: subjects randomly assigned to treatment A or B. (b) Factorial design: all subjects randomly assigned to treatment A, treatment B, treatment A + B or no treatment. (c) Randomised crossover design: subjects randomly assigned to treatment A followed by treatment B (after wash-out period) or treatment B followed by treatment A. (d) Randomised cluster design: all subjects in one group/area (e.g. by physician, by hospital, by ward) are assigned to treatment A or B. *Source:* Adapted from Tinmouth and Hebert 2007 [23]. (*See insert for colour representation of the figure.*)

most importantly, interpret. Therefore, a parallel group design is the most frequently adopted RCT design. Parallel group designs may also be used to independently compare three or more treatments [13].

Factorial Design

The use of factorial designs may also be considered when a number of therapies are being evaluated in combinations. For instance, in a 2×2 factorial design, two interventions are tested both alone and in combination, and compared with a control group (usually a placebo) (Figure 45.2b) [14]. This means that investigators can efficiently test two interventions with only marginal increases in sample size. In addition, the benefits of treatment combinations can be evaluated in a controlled manner. This design is most useful when interactions are either very strong or nonexistent [14]. Traditionally, the factorial design is used to answer two separate study questions. In a recent RCT using a factorial design, Robertson and colleagues randomised traumatic brain injury patients to (1) erythropoietin or placebo and (2) a restrictive or liberal transfusion threshold [15].

Crossover Design

Another RCT design option particularly amenable to an efficacy evaluation is a two-period crossover study in which patients are used as their own controls. In this trial, patients are randomised to one of two therapies for a fixed period of time and then proceed to receive the other therapy in a second comparable interval (Figure 45.2c). Minimising 'between-subject' variability in this manner makes significant gains in efficiency. Crossover studies are therefore best suited to relatively stable conditions (stability is required during the study), interventions with rapid onset of action and a very short half-life (the biological effect must disappear prior to the second treatment period), and rapidly modifiable endpoints [14]. MacLennan et al used a crossover design to compare the efficacy of platelets stored for 6–7 days versus 2–5 days on the proportion of days with clinically significant bleeding [16].

Cluster Design

All designs discussed so far have described the evaluation of interventions for individual patients. However, it is sometimes necessary to evaluate therapies, protocols, guidelines or treatment programs for groups of individuals. Using this design, groups or 'clusters' such as ICUs, wards, hospitals and physician practices are randomised to receive an intervention or control (Figure 45.2d). Cluster design may be the most appropriate for evaluating complex or multidimensional interventions such as the implementation of care paths, educational interventions, transfusion audits or other interventions to change transfusion practice. For these evaluations, the cluster is a more natural method of allocation than the individual [7]. Cluster trials are advantageous as there could be a risk of contamination such that the intervention will be implemented in all patients rather than only the patients assigned to receive the therapy, which would bias the results of the study. However, the allocation of interventions to groups rather than individuals will increase the sample size as a result of the nonindependence within the group and it is often difficult to infer what happened at an individual level. An additional concern in cluster trials is the possibility of large variations between clusters that may make it difficult to detect actual differences between therapies [17].

As an example of a cluster randomised trial, Murphy et al randomised wards at different hospitals to receive units of red cells with labels reminding nurses to check the patient and component identification[18]. The randomisation by wards was important to ensure that transfusions given without the reminder were not given by nurses who had been previously exposed to the reminder tags. In this study, the reminder tags did not result in an improvement in the bedside check for transfusion.

Selecting a Study Population

The choice of study population will invariably depend on the study question, the underlying hypothesis and a number of other factors. The choice of a hypothesis that will address either therapeutic efficacy or effectiveness will have a substantial impact on selection of the study population and the overall design of the study (Table 45.3) [8]. In choosing an efficacy approach, investigators usually perform the study in a well-defined patient population (using restrictive eligibility criteria and disease definitions) where the intervention has the highest probability of demonstrating an effect. This will decrease overall variability attributed to patient selection but may have adverse consequences on patient recruitment and jeopardise the generalisability of study results. When defining the eligibility criteria for an effectiveness trial, investigators should utilise more liberal criteria in a wide range of clinical settings. The study population may also be affected by other factors such as the spectrum of biological activity or the participation of specialised centres for recruitment.

Selecting Outcomes (Box 45.1)

In most clinical trials, the clinical investigative team should consider a number of potential outcomes, both fatal and nonfatal. An outcome is defined as a measurement (e.g. haematocrit) or an event (e.g. death) potentially modified following the implementation of an intervention. If all are given equal consideration, concerns arise about multiple comparisons and interpretation of a study with heterogeneous findings. Thus it is important to choose a primary outcome that will determine an intervention's therapeutic success or failure. Secondary outcomes will provide supportive

Table 45.3 Types of randomised clinical trial (RCT) designs.

Type of RCT	Description	Advantage	Disadvantage
Two-group parallel	Patients randomised to one of two groups	Simplest approach, widely used and accepted	Limited to simple comparisons
Factorial (2 × 2)	Patients randomised to one of four groups: therapy a, therapy b, therapy a + b or control	Combinations of therapy may be compared	Larger sample size required More complex design
Sequential study	Pairs of outcomes continuously compared in patients randomised to one of two therapies	Ongoing evaluations of therapy	Limited uses (efficacy only) Not a well-accepted approach Sample size unpredictable
Sequential study	Pairs of outcomes continuously compared in patients randomised to one of two therapies	Ongoing evaluations of therapy Sample size unpredictable	Limited uses (efficacy only) Not a well-accepted approach
Two-period cross-over	Patients allocated to one of two therapies then receive other therapy in second treatment period	Smaller sample required	Limited to reversible outcomes Major concern with carry-over effect
N of ... study	Single patient sequentially and repeatedly receives a therapy and a placebo	Optimal method of determining if a therapy is beneficial to a given patient	Results not generalisable Difficult in unstable patients Very labour intensive
Cluster design	Groups of patients are randomised	Ideal for program or guideline evaluation	Less well accepted in clinical practice Difficult to implement when large variability between clusters

Box 45.1 Guides to the choice of outcome measure in a randomised controlled trial.

- Is the outcome causally related to the consequences of the disease?
- Is the outcome clinically relevant to the healthcare providers and/or patients?
- Has the validity of the outcome (for complex outcomes such as scoring systems or composite outcomes) been established?
- Is the outcome easily and accurately determined?
- Is the outcome responsive to changes in a patient's condition?
- Is the outcome measure potentially able to discriminate between patients who benefit from a therapy and patients in the control group?

evidence in secondary analyses and assess potential adverse outcomes. The primary outcome is also essential in determining the sample size requirements in a clinical trial.

There are a number of factors that should be considered prior to selection of outcomes for a study. The primary outcomes should be considered clinically important and easily ascertained. By fulfilling these two criteria, the investigator will have a much greater chance of influencing clinical practice once a study has been completed and published. Outcomes should also measure what they are supposed to measure (validity), and be precise and reproducible. An outcome must be able to detect a clinically important true positive or negative change in the patient's condition following a therapy.

The sample size in a clinical trial comparing two therapies is based on the baseline event rate, the expected incremental benefit or difference, the level of significance (α) and the power to detect differences ($1 - \beta$). Establishing the incremental benefit of a new therapy is vitally important because of the enormous sample size repercussions. A sample size calculation for a RCT requires that the investigators establish the minimum therapeutic effect detectable within

the trial. This difference in outcomes between interventions is referred to as the minimally important difference (MID) or minimal clinically important difference (MCID) [8]. The MID is essentially establishing the level of discrimination in the study population who are exposed to the interventions given acceptable levels of type I (finding a difference when one does not truly exist) and type II (not finding a difference when one truly exists) errors and the baseline event rate. Too often, investigators calculate a sample size based on very large and unrealistic expected differences in outcomes.

To determine a plausible effect size, investigators should ask themselves the following questions.

- What difference or incremental benefit can be realistically expected of the experimental therapy? (Anticipated biological effect of therapy)
- Are the required number of patients available to participate in the clinical trial? (Feasibility)
- How much of a benefit, given the added costs and expected adverse effects of therapy, would be required for clinicians, patients and administrators to adopt a new therapy? (Overall benefit of therapy)

Investigators need to consider whether the absolute incremental benefit predicted is likely attainable using the experimental therapy. If not, another more discriminating outcome should be sought.

Frequently, the treatment effect or difference in the desired outcome is small. As a result, a surrogate or composite outcome may be chosen as the primary outcome for a trial to reduce the sample size. A surrogate outcome is defined as a laboratory or physical measure that accurately reflects a clinically meaningful outcome, and therefore can act as substitute outcome with the goal of reducing the sample size [19]. A composite outcome combines more than one individual outcome. The latter may increase statistical efficiency and can combine multiple endpoints that are equally important [20]. Both surrogate and composite outcomes must be used judiciously and results interpreted with caution [19,20]. Surrogate endpoints should clearly predict the clinical outcome, which may not be the case (e.g. corrected count increment and bleeding in platelet transfusion trials) [19,21]. Composite outcomes must be related and, equally important, biologically plausible, uniform in their anticipated direction of effect and clinically relevant [20,21].

Conclusion

Randomised controlled trials remain the 'gold standard' to evaluate therapeutic interventions, but many aspects of transfusion therapy have not been evaluated in well-designed and executed clinical trials. Given the expense and difficulty of performing RCTs, careful attention to the study design is required prior to enrolling any patients (Box 45.2). Different design alternatives, such as factorial designs or cluster randomisation, should be considered to ensure that the study design is optimal to address the research question. Decisions regarding the study population and outcomes must also consider the primary objective of the study question and feasibility.

Although RCTs provide the most unbiased and accurate assessment of the efficacy and effectiveness of therapeutic and preventive interventions, they remain challenging and expensive to conduct. As performing RCTs is not always feasible due to logistical and ethical constraints, observational studies including cohort and case–control studies can be useful study designs to evaluate specific outcomes but these studies are prone to bias. As more research groups form to address unanswered therapeutic questions in transfusion medicine, investigators will invariably better understand the strengths and limitations of different RCT and observational study design characteristics.

Acknowledgements

Alan Tinmouth is supported by an Ottawa Hospital Department of Medicine Research Award.

We wish to thank our students, teachers and colleagues who contributed many of the ideas outlined in this manuscript.

Box 45.2 Suggestions for planning a randomised controlled trial (RCT) in transfusion medicine.

- Explicitly determine whether you are primarily interested in establishing therapeutic efficacy or effectiveness.
- Whenever possible, undertake a RCT as part of a broader research program.
- If the study intervention is complex (or risky) or if other aspects of study feasibility are questionable, a pilot study should be considered.
- Whenever possible, investigators should use simple rather than complex designs (two-group parallel design vs factorial design).
- The study population should be tailored to the intervention.
- Ideally, the study intervention and treatment protocols should not aim to substantially modify or affect usual clinical practice.
- Given the complexity of RCTs, data collection should aim to clearly describe the study population, describe co-interventions and all major study outcomes.
- In choosing primary study endpoints, investigators should focus on patient-oriented outcomes rather than surrogate or biological markers.
- If you are planning a seminal RCT, you may only have one chance to get it right. When making compromises, always opt to answer questions that most clinicians consider most important.
- In establishing the minimally important difference, select a potentially achievable benefit.

KEY POINTS

1) Properly conducted RCTs are the best means to evaluate the risk and benefits of therapeutic interventions.
2) Observational studies can be useful when RCTs are not feasible: case–control studies are particularly useful to evaluate rare outcomes and cohort studies can examine outcomes following known exposures, risk factors or therapies. However, all observational studies are prone to bias and cannot show causation.

3) The design of a RCT depends on whether the investigators wish to evaluate the *efficacy* or the *effectiveness* of an intervention.
4) A two-group parallel group design is the simplest RCT to design, execute and evaluate, but alternative designs can be useful in specific circumstances.
5) Selecting the appropriate study population and the outcomes is critical to ensure both the feasibility of completing the RCT and the generalisability and clinical relevance of the study results.

References

1 Hill AB. The clinical trial. N Engl J Med 1952;**247**(4):113–19.

2 Kelsey RA, Whittemore AS, Evans AS, Thompson WD. Case control studies: I. Planning and execution, in Methods in Observational Epidemiology. Oxford: Oxford University Press, 1996, pp. 188–213.

3 Silliman CC, Boshkov LK, Mehdizadehkashi Z et al. Transfusion-related acute lung injury: epidemiology and a prospective analysis of etiologic factors. Blood 2003;**101**(2):454–62.

4 Carson JL, Duff A, Berlin JA et al. Perioperative blood transfusion and postoperative mortality. JAMA 1998;**279**(3):199–205.

5 Grimes DA, Schulz KF. Bias and causal associations in observational research. Lancet 2002;**359**(9302):248–52.

6 Van de Watering L. Pitfalls in the current published observational literature on the effects of red blood cell storage. Transfusion 2011;**51**(8):1847–54.

7 Grimshaw J, Campbell M, Eccles M, Steen N. Experimental and quasi-experimental designs for evaluating guideline implementation strategies. Fam Pract 2000;**17**(Suppl 1):S11–S16.

8 Sackett D. The principles behind the tactic of performing clinical trials, in Clinical Epidemiology: How To Do Clinical Practice Research (eds Haynes RB, Sackett D, Guyatt G et al). Philadelphia: Lippincott Williams and Wilkins, 2009, pp.173–243.

9 Adams RJ, McKie VC, Hsu L et al. Prevention of a first stroke by transfusions in children with sickle cell anemia and abnormal results on transcranial Doppler ultrasonography. N Engl J Med 1998;**339**(1):5–11.

10 Shakur H, Roberts I, Bautista R et al. Effects of tranexamic acid on death, vascular occlusive events, and blood transfusion in trauma patients with significant haemorrhage (CRASH-2): a randomised, placebo-controlled trial. Lancet 2010;**376**(9734):23–32.

11 Hebert PC, Wells G, Blajchman MA et al. A multicenter, randomized, controlled clinical trial of transfusion requirements in critical care. Transfusion Requirements in Critical Care Investigators, Canadian Critical Care Trials Group. N Engl J Med 1999;**340**(6):409–17.

12 Slichter SJ, Kaufman RM, Assmann SF et al. Dose of prophylactic platelet transfusions and prevention of hemorrhage. N Engl J Med 2010;**362**(7):600–13.

13 Fergusson DA, Hebert PC, Mazer CD et al. A comparison of aprotinin and lysine analogues in high-risk cardiac surgery. N Engl J Med 2008;**358**(22):2319–31.

14 Friedman LM, Furberg CD, DeMets DL. Fundamentals of Clinical Trials, 3rd edn. New York: Springer-Verlag, 1998.

15 Robertson CS, Hannay HJ, Yamal JM et al. Effect of erythropoietin and transfusion threshold on neurological recovery after traumatic brain injury: a randomized clinical trial. JAMA 2014;**312**(1):36–47.

16 MacLennan S, Harding K, Llewelyn C et al. A randomized noninferiority crossover trial of corrected count increments and bleeding in thrombocytopenic hematology patients receiving 2- to 5- versus 6- or 7-day-stored platelets. Transfusion 2015;**55**(8):1856–65.

17 Donner A, Klar N. Design and Analysis of Cluster Randomization Trials in Health Research. London: Arnold, 2000.

18 Murphy MF, Casbard AC, Ballard S et al. Prevention of bedside errors in transfusion medicine (PROBE-TM) study: a cluster-randomized, matched-paired clinical areas trial of a simple intervention to reduce errors in the pretransfusion bedside check. Transfusion 2007;**47**(5):771–80.

19 Arnold DM, Lim W. The use and abuse of surrogate endpoints in clinical research in transfusion medicine. Transfusion 2008;**48**(8):1547–9.

20 Heddle NM, Cook RJ. Composite outcomes in clinical trials: what are they and when should they be used? Transfusion 2011;**51**(1):11–13.

21 Heddle NM, Arnold DM, Webert KE. Time to rethink clinically important outcomes in platelet transfusion trials. Transfusion 2011;**51**(2):430–4.

22 Tay J, Tinmouth A. Observational studies: what is a cohort study? Transfusion 2007;**47**(7):1115–17.

23 Tinmouth A, Hebert P. Interventional trials: an overview of design alternatives. Transfusion 2007;**47**(4):565–7.

Further Reading

Campbell DT, Stanley JC. Experimental and Quasi-experimental Designs for Research. Chicago: Rand McNally College Publishing Company, 1966.

Friedman LM, Furberg CD, DeMets DL. Fundamentals of Clinical Trials, 3rd edn. New York: Springer-Verlag, 1998.

Grimes DA, Schulz KF. Bias and causal associations in observational research. Lancet 2002;**359**(9302):248–52.

Guyatt GH, Sackett DL, Cook DJ. Users' guides to the medical literature II. How to use an article about therapy or prevention. A. Are the results of the study valid? JAMA 1993;**270**: 2598–601.

Haynes RB, Sackett DL, Guyatt GH, Tugwell P. Clinical Epidemiology: A Basic Science for Clinical Medicine, 3rd edn. Philadelphia: Lippincott Williams and Wilkins, 2006.

Heddle NM. Clinical Research: Understanding the Methodology Toolbox. Bethesda: AABB Press, 2013.

Sackett DL. Bias in analytic research. J Chron Dis 1979;**32**:51–63.

Sackett DL. The competing objectives of randomized trials. N Engl J Med 1980;**303**:1059–60.

Sackett DL, Gent M. Controversy in counting and attributing events in clinical trials. N Engl J Med 1979;**301**:1410–12.

Weijer C, Grimshaw JM, Eccles MP et al, for the Ottawa Ethics of Cluster Randomized Trials Consensus Group. The Ottawa Statement on the Ethical Design and Conduct of Cluster Randomized Trials. PLoS Med 2012;**9**(11):e1001346.

46 Getting the Most Out of the Evidence for Transfusion Medicine

Simon J. Stanworth[1], Susan J. Brunskill[2], Carolyn Dorée[2] and Sally Hopewell[3]

[1] *NHS Blood and Transplant and Department of Haematology, Oxford University Hospitals, Oxford, UK;*
Radcliffe Department of Medicine, University of Oxford, Oxford, UK
[2] *NHS Blood and Transplant, Systematic Review Initiative, Oxford, UK*
[3] *Oxford Clinical Trials Research Unit, University of Oxford, Oxford, UK*

What is Meant by Evidence-Based Medicine?

Evidence-based medicine (EBM) has been described by Sackett as 'the integration of best research evidence with clinical expertise and patient values' [1]. Proponents of EBM have particularly highlighted the nature of the evidence that is used to make clinical decisions, i.e. where is it from, how believable is it, how relevant is it to my patient and can it be supported by other data? However, evidence is only one of the factors driving clinical decision making, and clinicians will also need to consider the available resources and opportunities, individual patients' values and needs (physical, psychological and social), local clinical expertise and cost. In some situations, clinical judgement will determine that the available evidence for a specific problem is not applicable.

Evidence-based medicine is not just about obtaining and evaluating clinical research evidence; it is also a means by which effective strategies for self-learning can be applied, aimed at continuously improving clinical performance. The focus of this chapter will be to discuss core elements of EBM with particular reference to clinical research in transfusion medicine and to provide a practical approach to critical appraisal and study design.

Hierarchies of Clinical Evidence

Health research studies are designed to ultimately show evidence of causality. While causality is extremely difficult (or impossible) to prove, hierarchical levels of evidence provide increasing support for such association. Optimal evidence is the best evidence available to answer a question. Data derived from randomised controlled trials (RCTs) have generally been regarded as the strongest support for evidence of efficacy or effectiveness.

In 1948, the first modern RCT in medicine was published comparing streptomycin and bed rest for patients with pulmonary tuberculosis [2]. The authors chose to perform a controlled trial because 'the natural course of pulmonary tuberculosis is in fact so variable and unpredictable that evidence of improvement or cure following the use of a new drug in a few cases cannot be accepted as proof of the effect of that drug'. In that trial, assignment of patients to streptomycin or bed rest was done by 'reference to a statistical series based on random sampling numbers drawn up for each sex at each centre'. There were fewer deaths in the patients assigned to streptomycin (four out of 55 patients) compared to bed rest alone (14 out of 52 patients) [2]. If the process of randomisation is done correctly, differences in outcome(s) between groups should be attributable to the intervention and not to other confounding factors related to the patient's demography, study setting or quality of care.

The most common (and simple) design for an RCT is a parallel design, in which participants are randomly allocated to one of two groups. However, the RCT design comes with inherent challenges.

- RCTs are costly and logistical problems can arise if these studies are conducted at multiple centres (which is necessary for large trials).
- Small RCTs may overestimate the effect of the intervention and may place too much emphasis on those outcomes with more striking results.
- Small RCTs may be designed to detect unreasonably large treatment effects (which they will never be able to show because of their small size).
- RCTs with non-significant results may never be fully reported or only found in abstract form – a phenomenon known as publication bias.
- Effects of interventions may be overgeneralised and inappropriately applied to different patient populations.
- RCTs are not suited to investigating low-frequency rare adverse effects, prevalence rates or diagnostic criteria.

In contrast to RCTs, observational studies, such as cohort or case–control studies, whether prospective or retrospective, may demonstrate an association between intervention and outcome; however, it is often difficult to be sure that this association does not reflect the effects of unknown confounding factors. The influence of confounding factors and biased participant selection can dramatically distort the accuracy of the study findings in observational studies. This does not mean that findings from well-designed observational studies should be disregarded; such study designs can be very effective in establishing or confirming effects of large size. Interpretation is more difficult when the observed effects are small. Clinical questions addressing possible aetiology or monitoring adverse effects may be more suited to observational studies.

In order to identify any limitations in a study and understand the possible impact of these on the study findings and their overall interpretation, it is important for readers, and investigators gearing up to design their own studies, to know how to critically appraise the methodological quality of the research. Critical appraisal and evaluation will be discussed next.

Appraisal of Primary Research Evidence for Its Validity and Usefulness

One component of EBM is the critical appraisal of evidence generated from a study. Published RCTs should report sufficient detail pertaining to the study design, population, condition, intervention and outcome to allow the reader to make an independent assessment of the trial by examining its methodological quality. Guidelines and checklists have been designed to help with the reporting [3–5]. As shown in Box 46.1, key components of the critical appraisal process for clinical trials relate to the methodology of the study (the participants, interventions and comparators, the outcomes, the sample size, the methods used for the randomisation process and whether research staff were blinded to treatment allocation) and the reporting of the results (the numbers randomised and the numbers analysed/evaluated, the numbers not available for analysis with reasons and the role of chance, i.e. confidence intervals). Inadequate methodology and poor reporting of the study methods and its findings do not provide the needed reassurance to readers that patient selection, study group assignment and outcome detection were not prone to bias, which may result in inaccurate inferences drawn from the data. Critical appraisal guidelines are also useful for authors of primary research because they define the information that should be included in their published reports.

One aspect of trial appraisal concerns the understanding of chance variation and sample size calculation. One needs to distinguish

---

Box 46.1   Key components of the critical appraisal process for clinical trials.

Did the trial address a clearly focused issue?

Was the assignment of patients to treatments randomised?

Were patients, health workers and study personnel blinded to treatment allocation?

Were all the participants who entered the study accounted for within the results?

Were all the participants followed up and data collected in the same way?

Aside from the experimental intervention, were the groups treated equally?

How are the results presented and how large was the treatment effect?

How precise was the estimate of the treatment effect?

Were all the important outcomes for this patient population considered?

Can the results be applied to practice/different populations?

Source: Adapted from the Critical Appraisal Skills Programme worksheets (www.casp-uk.net), copyright http://creativecommons.org/licenses/by-nc-sa/3.0/

---

between 'no evidence of effect' and 'evidence of no effect': the former may be derived from results that are either underpowered or non-significant, whereas the latter implies a sufficient sample size to show superiority, equivalence or noninferiority. Information about sample size calculations should therefore be provided in the published report of clinical trials.

Comparable standards can be applied to the critique of observational studies. A framework called Strengthening the Reporting of Observational Studies in Epidemiology (STROBE) can be used to explore the quality of the reporting of an observational study [6,7], with CASP checklists available to appraise the methodological quality of observational studies [5].

Reviews: Narrative and Systematic

Reviews have long been used to provide summary statements of the evidence for clinical practice. Reviews can be narrative or systematic. Often written by experts in the field, narrative reviews provide an overview of the relevant findings, as well as being educational and informative. However, the content and summary of the evidence base in a narrative review will ultimately be based on what the authors feel is important.

On the other hand, systematic review methodology sets out to gather the totality of the evidence on a subject and summarise it in an objective way using prespecified methods for study identification, selection, quality assessment and analysis. The aim is to be explicit and to limit biases at all stages of the systematic review process. The output is a synthesis of the results of primary studies – a synthesis that is accessible to clinicians, researchers and policymakers alike.

Systematic reviews also form the background for clinical trial design by establishing what is currently known, what methods were used to achieve that knowledge and what gaps remain. Systematic reviews are not substitutes for adequately powered clinical trials, but should be considered as complementary methods of clinical research.

There are generally accepted 'rules' about how to undertake a systematic review, which include:

- developing a team to undertake the systematic review, including clinicians who know the clinical area of the review and methodologists skilled in all aspects of the systematic review process;
- developing a focused review question: being clear on what is the intervention and comparator, who are the participants and what are the outcomes of relevance to the review (the PICO criteria);
- comprehensively searching for all material relevant to this question (Box 46.2 provides

---

Box 46.2   Selected sources that can be searched to identify reports of trials and clinical evidence.

Writing the question and selecting search terms

It is best to construct your question as simply as possible, ideally by combining any two of the four parts of the PICO formula (patient/condition; intervention; comparison; outcome), and then adding any relevant synonyms and/or alternative spellings. For example, the question 'Are red cell transfusions effective in the treatment of hip fracture?' is best searched for as patient/condition AND intervention, which for a quick search in PubMed could be constructed like this:

> ((hip OR hips OR intertrochanteric OR subtrochanteric OR trochanteric OR pertrochanteric OR peritrochanteric OR femur OR femoral OR acetabul*) AND fracture*) AND (blood OR erythrocyte* OR red cell* OR RBC* OR trigger* OR level* OR threshold* OR rule* OR restrict*) AND (transfus* OR hypertransfus* OR retransfus*)

Additional tips for searching in PubMed

- Use Boolean operators AND/OR to combine groups of search terms, but use NOT with care
- Use truncation to reduce the number of search terms used, e.g. bleed* OR haemorrhag*
- For a narrow, targeted search, try searching by title alone, e.g. tranexamic acid[TI]
- For quick therapy searches, try using PubMed Clinical Queries: www.ncbi.nlm.nih.gov/pubmed/clinical

Choosing the study design

Search for information from the highest level evidence, working down this list if there is little or no relevant evidence at higher levels:

1) Evidence from at least one **systematic review**
2) Evidence from at least one **randomised controlled trial**
3) Evidence from a well-designed **observational study** (e.g. **cohort or case–control studies**)
4) Evidence from well-designed nonexperimental studies (e.g. **case series** and **case reports**)
5) Expert opinion (e.g. overviews, editorials, narrative reviews).

Sources for searching for different study designs

Systematic reviews and randomised controlled trials

- Transfusion Evidence Library: www.transfusionevidencelibrary.com
- PubMed Clinical Queries: www.ncbi.nlm.nih.gov/pubmed/clinical – Category: Therapy; Scope: Narrow
- TRIP database: www.tripdatabase.com
- Cochrane Library (Wiley): onlinelibrary.wiley.com/cochranelibrary/search

Ongoing clinical trials

- WHO International Clinical Trials Registry Platform: http://apps.who.int/trialsearch/
- ClinicalTrials.gov: https://clinicaltrials.gov/

Observational studies

- PubMed Clinical Queries: www.ncbi.nlm.nih.gov/pubmed/clinical – Category: Therapy; Scope: Broad

Diagnostic and prognostic studies

- PubMed Clinical Queries: www.ncbi.nlm.nih.gov/pubmed/clinical – Category: Therapy; Scope: Broad/Narrow

(Continued)

Box 46.2   (Continued)

Cost-effectiveness studies

- NHS EED database in the Cochrane Library: www.cochranelibrary.com

Uncertainties about treatment effects

- DUETS database: www.library.nhs.uk/duets/

Further suggestions

- If time is at a premium, look first at sources that synthesise the evidence – for example, the Transfusion Evidence Library, TRIP Database, BMJ Clinical Evidence, UpToDate.
- Stay up to date by saving your searches and setting up regular alerts in PubMed, or by signing up for the monthly Transfusion Evidence Alert (www.transfusionevidencelibrary.com/newsletter).
- Manage your search results by downloading into bibliographic software – for example, EndNote or Reference Manager – and for research projects, always record the search terms used and the databases and dates searched.
- For further help, or for more comprehensive searching, make a friend of your hospital librarian!

---

some practical suggestions for use when developing a more comprehensive search strategy);

- using predefined, explicit criteria to assess eligibility and methodological aspects of identified studies;
- reporting and explaining why studies were excluded;
- using predefined, explicit methods for combining data from identified studies including, where appropriate, meta-analysis of the study data.

Meta-analysis, strictly speaking, means mathematically pooling data from primary studies. This method is acceptable for a systematic review when primary studies are sufficiently homogeneous in their design and quality to show any difference in treatment effect between the two treatment groups. Results from each study within a systematic review are typically presented in the form of a graphical display, called a 'forest plot'. A hypothetical example is shown in Figure 46.1.

The result for the outcome point estimate in each trial is represented by a square, together with a horizontal line that corresponds to the 95% confidence intervals (CIs). For summary statistics of binary or dichotomous data, effect measures are typically summarised as either a relative risk or an odds ratio (for definitions, see Figure 46.1). The 95% CI provides a very useful measure of effect, in that it represents the range of values that will contain the true size of treatment effect 95% of the time, should the study be repeated again and again. The solid vertical line corresponds to no effect of treatment (or a relative risk of 1.0 for the analysis of dichotomous data, see Figure 46.1). Forest plots, therefore, are a visual representation of the size of treatment effects between different trials and allow the reader to assess:

- the effect of treatment by examining whether the bounds of the confidence interval exceed or overlap the minimal clinically important benefit;
- the consistency of the direction of the treatment effects across multiple studies;
- outlying results from some studies relative to others.

Appraisal of Systematic Reviews

Figure 46.2 provides an overall guide for assessing the validity of evidence for treatment

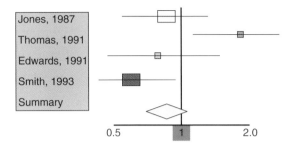

- The figure shows a forest plot display for four hypothetical studies.
- The point estimates for each trial have been presented as a relative risk for an outcome with discrete data. The blocks for the point estimates are different sizes, in proportion to the weight that each study takes in the analysis. Weighting is used in order to draw the reader's eye to the more precise studies.
- The relative risk (RR) is the ratio of risk in the intervention group to the risk in the control group. A RR of one (RR = 1.0) indicates no difference between comparison groups. For undesirable outcomes an RR that is less than 1 indicates that the intervention was effective in reducing the risk of that outcome.
- The diamond shape represents a summary point estimate for all trials. The vertical line corresponds to no effect of treatment. Thus if the 95% confidence interval crosses the vertical line, this indicates that the difference in effect of intervention therapy compared to control is not statistically significant at the level of $p > 0.05$ (please note there will be a 1 in 20 chance that the confidence interval does not include the true value). Such is the case in this example.
- Perhaps, the most important aspect of displaying the results graphically in this way is that it helps the reader look at the overall effects for each trial. Therefore, in this example, it should prompt the reader to ask why the results for one trial seem to be so different from the others (Thomas, 1991)?

Figure 46.1 A hypothetical forest plot.

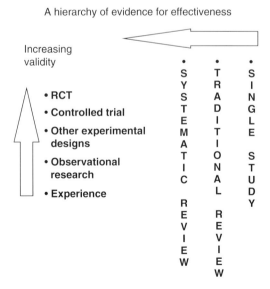

Figure 46.2 A guide for judging the validity of evidence for treatment decisions from different types of studies and reviews.

decisions for the different types of studies, trials and reviews mentioned in this section. Although sometimes criticised for their overemphasis on methodology at the expense of clinical relevance, and the inappropriate use of meta-analysis, systematic reviews have an important place in clinical practice as a means of transparently summarising evidence from multiple sources. As for RCTs, guidelines for the reporting of systematic reviews have been developed, including Preferred Reporting Items for Systematic reviews and Meta-Analyses (PRISMA) for the reporting of systematic reviews of RCTs and Meta-analysis of Observational Studies in Epidemiology (MOOSE) for the reporting of systematic reviews and meta-analyses of observational studies [8,9]. Quality assessment tools have also been developed for critical appraisal of systematic reviews (the Critical Appraisal Skills Programme, CASP) (Box 46.3).

Box 46.3   Key components of the critical appraisal process for systematic reviews.

Did the review ask a clearly focused question?

Do you think all the important, relevant studies were included?

Did the authors look for the right type of papers?

Did the review's authors do enough to assess the quality of the included studies?

If the results of the review have been combined, was it reasonable to do so?

What are the overall results of the review?

How precise are the results?

Were all the important outcomes for the review question considered?

Can the results be applied to the local population?

Are the benefits worth the harms and costs?

Source: Adapted from the Critical Appraisal Skills Programme worksheets (www.casp-uk.net), copyright http://creativecommons.org/licenses/by-nc-sa/3.0/.

Evaluating Systematic Reviews and Guidelines

The Grading of Recommendations Assessment, Development and Evaluation (GRADE) tool has been devised as a system for evaluating and rating the quality of evidence in systematic reviews and grading the strength of recommendations in guidelines. The system is designed for reviews and guidelines that examine alternative management strategies or interventions, which may include no intervention or current best management. An example relevant to transfusion medicine is the recent guidelines on immune thrombocytopenia from the American Society of Hematology, which utilised GRADE methodology to evaluate the strength of recommendations [10].

Comparative Effectiveness Research

Comparative effectiveness research (CER) is gaining support from both researchers and funding agencies, particularly in the USA and Canada. CER is defined as the conduct and synthesis of systematic research comparing different interventions and strategies to prevent, diagnose, treat and monitor health conditions. While experimental study designs like RCTs are highly valued methods of CER, they are costly and resource intensive and their results may not be easily generalisable to non-study patients. Nonexperimental approaches using observational data are also useful tools for CER but they are inherently limited by heterogeneous methodologies, diverse designs and susceptibility to bias. As methods of observational studies continue to be refined, the data they derive may become more widely applicable, such as advances in the design of clinical registries and the use of encounter-generated data from sources such as electronic medical records.

The informing fresh-versus-old red cell management (INFORM) pilot trial is an example of CER in transfusion medicine [11]. The design was pragmatic; patients were randomised to receive one of two treatments that are already routinely used, thus obviating the need for individual informed consent; data were collected in real time from existing electronic databases, thereby reducing costs; and study procedures were streamlined, enabling randomisation of more than 900 patients from a single centre in six months at very low cost. A larger pragmatic RCT with a similar design is planned to answer the question of the risk of mortality with fresh-versus-older blood [12]. These data will continue to address policy decisions around the maximum storage threshold that would optimise the balance between adequate supply and acceptable risk.

Evidence Base for Transfusion Medicine

So, how good is the evidence base for transfusion medicine? As a first step, identification of all relevant RCTs in transfusion medicine is essential. The UK Blood Services' Transfusion Evidence Library (www.transfusionevidencelibrary. com) is a comprehensive online database of systematic reviews and RCTs relevant to transfusion medicine (updated monthly). The Transfusion Evidence Library includes high-quality systematic reviews and RCTs from 1950 to the present, identified from comprehensive searches of MEDLINE and from extensive handsearching of transfusion-related conference proceedings. It also contains a growing number of clinical commentaries on recent important research articles in transfusion, in which the findings of the research are discussed within the context of other research, the difference the research could make to clinical practice is explained and any opportunities for further research are highlighted.

Another excellent resource is the Cochrane Collaboration's database of RCTs; the Cochrane Central Register of Controlled Trials (CENTRAL) (updated monthly) is a good starting point. This database uses sensitive literature search filters that aim to identify all RCTs that have been catalogued on MEDLINE from 1966 and on the European medical bibliographic database EMBASE from 1980. Other online resources containing collections of high-level evidence for clinicians include the TRIP Database, BMJ Clinical Evidence and PubMed's Clinical Queries. Box 46.2 presents a list of suggested sources that can be searched to identify relevant reports of clinical trials and systematic reviews.

Evidence Base for Transfusion Medicine: Individual Examples

In the following section, we provide two examples of developments in the evidence base for the practice of transfusion medicine following a systematic review. The first is an updated review on platelet transfusions, the second is a systematic review on an alternative to transfusion: activated recombinant factor VII (rFVIIa).

Platelets

An update of previous Cochrane systematic reviews on the use of platelet transfusions has been recently published [13]. The aim was to determine whether a therapeutic-only platelet transfusion policy (platelet transfusions given to treat bleeding) was as effective and safe as a prophylactic platelet transfusion policy (platelet transfusions given to prevent bleeding usually when the platelet count falls below a given trigger level) in patients with haematological disorders undergoing myelosuppressive chemotherapy or haemopoietic stem cell transplantation (HSCT). An important point illustrated by this review is that it represents an update of previous systematic reviews [14–16]. It therefore illustrates the iterative process for new reviews to incorporate new trial evidence. These earlier reviews also addressed the following questions.

- What is the appropriate threshold platelet count to trigger prophylactic platelet transfusions?
- What is the optimal dose for platelet transfusions?
- What is the evidence that a strategy of prophylactic platelet transfusions is superior to the use of platelet transfusions only in the event of bleeding (therapeutic-only use)?

In total seven RCTs met the predefined selection criteria (one of which is still ongoing), leaving a total of six trials eligible for the review and a total of 1195 participants. These trials were carried out over a 35-year period. For the systematic review's primary outcome (number of patients with at least one bleeding episode within 30 days), significant heterogeneity was noted ($I^2 = 88\%$). This heterogeneity may in part reflect the different methodology and grading systems used to analyse and categorise bleeding in the individual studies. Four studies in the review reported clinically significant bleeding events and all showed a similar effect: higher rates of bleeding in participants receiving a therapeutic-only platelet transfusion strategy. But major differences were noted between the four studies, including indications for platelet transfusion, red cell transfusion policy and study end points, as well as classification of bleeding events. A meta-analysis could not be performed with the data from these four studies.

The conclusions of the systematic review were that overall prophylactic platelet transfusions appeared to reduce the number of bleeding events and the number of days with clinically significant bleeding, therefore supporting the continued use of prophylactic platelet transfusions [13]. The studies in the review showed that major bleeding events did occur despite prophylactic platelet transfusions at platelet counts greater than 10×10^9/L. The limitation of the review to combine studies in a meaningful way raises important concerns about the reporting of bleeding outcomes, and the need for consistency in platelet transfusion trials. This was also a key message in a Cochrane review of platelet pathogen inactivation [17].

Alternatives to Transfusion

Many patients without haemophilia have now been treated, off-licence, with activated recombinant factor VII (rFVIIa). The patient settings are very diverse, including surgery (especially cardiac), gastrointestinal bleeding, liver dysfunction, intracranial haemorrhage and trauma, for example. Data from 25 RCTs enrolling around 3500 patients have now evaluated the use of rFVIIa as both prophylaxis to prevent bleeding (14 trials) or therapeutically to treat major bleeding (11 trials), in patients without

haemophilia [18]. This literature provides a more robust means of assessing the effectiveness and safety of rFVIIa, and formed the basis of a recent updated Cochrane review. When combined in meta-analysis, the trials showed modest reductions in total blood loss or red cell transfusion requirements (equivalent to less than one unit of red cell transfusion). However, the reductions were likely to be overestimated due to the limitations of the data. For other end points, including clinically relevant outcomes, there were no consistent indications of benefit and almost all the findings in support of and against the effectiveness of recombinant factor VIIa could be due to chance. The one, and important, exception was thromboembolic events. In both groups of trials, there was an overall trend to increased thromboembolic events in patients receiving rFVIIa. The forest plot for total arterial thromboembolic events is shown in Figure 46.3 and reaches statistical significance.

Common Practices of Transfusion and Interventions to Improve Transfusion Practice

Systematic reviews may also be applied to important questions about the evidence base for common or well-established practices in transfusion [19–21]. For example, reviews based on observational, nonrandomised studies have addressed the following question.

- What is the maximum time that one unit of red cells can be out of the fridge before it becomes unsafe? [19]
- How often should blood administration sets be changed while a patient is being transfused? [20]
- Which blood transfusion administration method – one-person or two-person checks – is safest? [21]

It is surprising and salutary to realise that some of these common recommendations appear to have little firm evidence base, yet are commonly reproduced in guidelines and protocols.

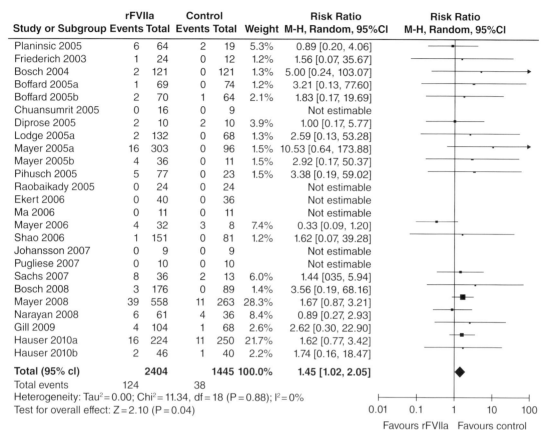

Study or Subgroup	rFVIIa Events	Total	Control Events	Total	Weight	Risk Ratio M-H, Random, 95%CI
Planinsic 2005	6	64	2	19	5.3%	0.89 [0.20, 4.06]
Friederich 2003	1	24	0	12	1.2%	1.56 [0.07, 35.67]
Bosch 2004	2	121	0	121	1.3%	5.00 [0.24, 103.07]
Boffard 2005a	1	69	0	74	1.2%	3.21 [0.13, 77.60]
Boffard 2005b	2	70	1	64	2.1%	1.83 [0.17, 19.69]
Chuansumrit 2005	0	16	0	9		Not estimable
Diprose 2005	2	10	2	10	3.9%	1.00 [0.17, 5.77]
Lodge 2005a	2	132	0	68	1.3%	2.59 [0.13, 53.28]
Mayer 2005a	16	303	0	96	1.5%	10.53 [0.64, 173.88]
Mayer 2005b	4	36	0	11	1.5%	2.92 [0.17, 50.37]
Pihusch 2005	5	77	0	23	1.5%	3.38 [0.19, 59.02]
Raobaikady 2005	0	24	0	24		Not estimable
Ekert 2006	0	40	0	36		Not estimable
Ma 2006	0	11	0	11		Not estimable
Mayer 2006	4	32	3	8	7.4%	0.33 [0.09, 1.20]
Shao 2006	1	151	0	81	1.2%	1.62 [0.07, 39.28]
Johansson 2007	0	9	0	9		Not estimable
Pugliese 2007	0	10	0	10		Not estimable
Sachs 2007	8	36	2	13	6.0%	1.44 [035, 5.94]
Bosch 2008	3	176	0	89	1.4%	3.56 [0.19, 68.16]
Mayer 2008	39	558	11	263	28.3%	1.67 [0.87, 3.21]
Narayan 2008	6	61	4	36	8.4%	0.89 [0.27, 2.93]
Gill 2009	4	104	1	68	2.6%	2.62 [0.30, 22.90]
Hauser 2010a	16	224	11	250	21.7%	1.62 [0.77, 3.42]
Hauser 2010b	2	46	1	40	2.2%	1.74 [0.16, 18.47]
Total (95% cl)		**2404**		**1445**	**100.0%**	**1.45 [1.02, 2.05]**
Total events	124		38			

Heterogeneity: Tau² = 0.00; Chi² = 11.34, df = 18 (P = 0.88); I² = 0%
Test for overall effect: Z = 2.10 (P = 0.04)

Favours rFVIIa   Favours control

Figure 46.3 The forest plot for total arterial thromboembolic events.

Are There Limitations to Evidence-Based Practice?

It is important to acknowledge some of the limitations of EBM that have been discussed by critics and supporters alike. EBM alone cannot provide a clinical decision; instead, the findings generated from EBM are one strand of input driving decision making in clinical practice. Each clinician will also need to consider the available resources and opportunities, the values and needs (physical, psychological and social) of the patient, the local clinical expertise and the costs of the intervention. Patients enrolled in clinical trials are not always the same as the individual patients requiring treatment, and generalising to different clinical settings may not be appropriate. It has also been said that, within EBM, there is an overemphasis

on methodology at the expense of clinical relevance, with the risks of generating conclusions that are either overly pessimistic or inappropriate for the clinical question. Perhaps we need to get away from the mentality that 'there is no good RCT evidence available to answer this clinical question' to thinking more about why this should be so, what can be learned from those studies that have already been completed and what design of trial would answer the main area of uncertainty in this transfusion setting.

Conclusion

This chapter has attempted to explain why it is essential to assess the quality of primary clinical research and consider the risks of evidence being misleading, for example in the case of few trials or a failure to identify appropriate clinical research questions. Systematic reviews and the statistical method of meta-analysis are useful tools to achieve this, but, like trials themselves, can become outdated and must be carefully scrutinised to ensure unbiased results. Transfusion medicine is no different from many other branches of medicine, and the evidence base that informs much of the practice has not developed to the point that it can be universally applied with confidence. There is a need to recognise these uncertainties and to identify those transfusion issues that require high priority for clinical research.

Appraising the evidence base for transfusion medicine is one part of improving practice; another is the effective dissemination of the evidence to clinicians. For example, clinicians may not have the time to search and evaluate the evidence themselves given the increasing numbers of publications and journals. As many of the sources are web based, access at any one moment may be easier but the skills of appraisal need to be regularly maintained.

There has been growing recognition that research, especially empirical research (based on observing what has happened), has been underutilised in making healthcare decisions at all levels. This appears to be as true for transfusion medicine as for other clinical areas. EBM is an approach to developing and improving skills to identify and apply research evidence to clinical decisions. Even the most ardent proponents of EBM have never claimed it is a panacea, and there is recognition that it should amplify rather than replace clinical skills and knowledge, and be a driver for keeping healthcare practices up to date.

Systematic reviews can help bring together relevant literature on a particular problem and assess its strengths, weaknesses and overall meaning. Such reviews can be used in different ways, including improving the precision of estimates of effect, generating hypotheses, providing background to new primary research or informing policy. Progress is being made to ensure that most areas in transfusion medicine are being systematically reviewed and some of these have encouraged plans for new RCTs.

KEY POINTS

- The process of EBM consists of question formulation, searching for literature, critically appraising studies (identifying strengths and weaknesses) and decisions around applicability to one's patients.
- It is essential to assess the quality of primary clinical research and consider the risks of evidence being misleading, for example in the case of few trials or a failure to identify appropriate clinical research questions.

- Systematic reviews of RCTs combine evidence most likely to provide valid (truthful) answers on particular questions of effectiveness, and form an important component to the evaluation of evidence-based practice in transfusion medicine.
- There is a common perception that much of transfusion medicine practice is based on limited evidence, but this is changing and systematic reviews are an important tool to collate, analyse and update the evidence base.

References

1 Sackett DL, Strauss SE, Richardson WS, Rosenberg W, Haynes RB. Evidence Based Medicine: How to Practice and Teach EBM, 2nd edn. Churchill Livingstone, Edinburgh, 2000.

2 The Streptomycin in Tuberculosis Trials Committee, Streptomycin treatment of pulmonary tuberculosis. BMJ 1948;**2**(4582):769–82.

3 Moher D, Hopewell S, Schulz KF et al. CONSORT 2010 explanation and elaboration:

updated guidelines for reporting parallel group randomised trials. BMJ 2010;**340**:c869.

4 Schulz KF, Altman DG, Moher D, CONSORT Group. CONSORT 2010 statement: updated guidelines for reporting parallel group randomised trials. BMJ 2010;**340**:c332.

5 www.casp-uk.net

6 Von Elm E, Altman DG, Egger M, Pocock SJ, Gøtzsche PC, Vandenbroucke JP, for the STROBE Initiative. The Strengthening the Reporting of Observational Studies in Epidemiology (STROBE) statement: guidelines for reporting observational studies. Ann Intern Med 2007;**147**(8):573–7.

7 Von Elm E, Altman DG, Egger M, Pocock SJ, Gøtzsche PC, Vandenbroucke JP, for the STROBE Initiative. The Strengthening the Reporting of Observational Studies in Epidemiology (STROBE) statement: guidelines for reporting observational studies. Lancet 2007;**370**(9596):1453–7.

8 Moher D, Liberati A, Tetzlaff J, Altman DG, PRISMA Group. Preferred Reporting Items for Systematic Reviews and Meta-Analyses: the PRISMA Statement. PLoS Med 2009;**6**(7):e1000097.

9 Stroup DF, Berlin JA, Morton SC et al, for the MOOSE (Meta-analysis of Observational Studies in Epidemiology) Group. Meta-analysis of observational studies in epidemiology: a proposal for reporting. JAMA 2000;**283**(15):2008–12.

10 Guyatt GH, Oxman AD, Schünemann HJ, Tugwell P, Knotterus A. GRADE guidelines: a new series of articles in the Journal of Clinical Epidemiology. J Clin Epidemiol 2011;**64**(4):380–2.

11 Heddle NM, Cook RJ, Arnold DM et al. The effect of blood storage duration on in-hospital mortality: a randomized controlled pilot feasibility trial. Transfusion 2012;**52**(6):1203–12.

12 Effect of Short-Term vs. Long-Term Blood Storage on Mortality after Transfusion. Heddle NM, Cook RJ, Arnold DM, Liu Y, Barty R, Crowther MA et al. N Engl J Med 2016;**375**:1937–45.

13 Estcourt LJ, Wood EM, Stanworth S, Trivella M, Doree C, Tinmouth A, Murphy MF. A therapeutic-only versus prophylactic platelet transfusion strategy for preventing bleeding in patients with haematological disorders after chemotherapy or stem cell transplantation. Cochrane Database Syst Rev 2015;**9**:CD010981.

14 Cid J, Lozano M. Lower or higher doses for prophylactic platelet transfusions: results of a meta-analysis of randomized controlled trials. Transfusion 2007:**47**(3):464–70.

15 Estcourt L, Stanworth SJ, Hopewell S, Heddle N, Tinmouth A, Murphy MF. Prophylactic platelet transfusion for haemorrhage after chemotherapy and stem cell transplantation. Cochrane Database Syst Rev 2012;**4**:CD004269.

16 Tinmouth AT, Freedman J. Prophylactic platelet transfusions: which dose is the best dose? A review of the literature. Transfus Med Rev 2003;**17**(3):181–93.

17 Butler C, Doree C, Estcourt LJ et al. Pathogen-reduced platelets for the prevention of bleeding. Cochrane Database Syst Rev 2013;**3**:CD009072.

18 Simpson E, Lin Y, Stanworth S, Birchall J, Doree C, Hyde C. Recombinant factor VIIa for the prevention and treatment of bleeding in patients without haemophilia. Cochrane Database Syst Rev 2012;**3**:CD005011.

19 Brunskill S, Thomas S, Whitmore E et al. What is the maximum time that a unit of red blood cells can be safely left out of controlled temperature storage? Transfus Med Rev 2012;**26**(3):209–23.

20 Blest A, Roberts M, Murdock J, Watson D, Brunskill S. How often should a red blood cell administration set be changed while a patient is being transfused? A commentary and review of the literature. Transfus Med Rev 2008;**18**(2):121–33.

21 Watson D, Murdock J, Doree C et al. Blood transfusion administration – 1 or 2 person checks, which is the safest method? Transfusion 2008;**48**(4):783–9.

Further Reading

Centre for Reviews and Dissemination. Systematic Reviews CRD's guidance for undertaking reviews in healthcare. CRD, University of York, 2009. Available at: www.york.ac.uk/crd/(accessed 21 November 2016).

Egger M, Davey Smith G, Altman DG. Systematic Reviews in Health Care. Meta-analysis in Context, 2nd edn. BMJ Publishing Group, London, 2001.

Greenhalgh T. How to Read a Paper: The Basics of Evidence Based Medicine, 5th edn. Wiley, Chichester, 2014.

Guyatt GH, Rennie D. Users' Guide to the Medical Literature: Essentials of Evidence-Based Clinical Practice. American Medical Association, Chicago, 2002.

Higgins JPT, Green S (eds). Cochrane Handbook for Systematic Reviews of Interventions, Version 5.1.0. Cochrane Collaboration, 2011. Available at: www.cochrane-handbook.org (accessed 21 November 2016).

Hyde CJ, Stanworth SJ & Murphy MF. Can you see the wood for the trees? Making sense of the forest plot. 1. Presentation of the data from the included studies. Transfusion 2008; **48**(2): 218–220.

Hyde CJ, Stanworth SJ, Murphy MF. Can you see the wood for the trees? Making sense of the forest plot. 2. Analysis of the combined results from the included studies. Transfusion 2008;**48**(4):580–3.

The Equator Network. Enhancing the Quality and Transparency of Health Research. Available at: www.equator-network.org/(accessed 21 November 2016).

47

A Primer on Biostatistics

Andrew W. Shih[1] and Nancy M. Heddle[2]

[1] Department of Pathology and Molecular Medicine, Transfusion Medicine Fellowship Program, McMaster University, Hamilton, Canada
[2] Department of Medicine, McMaster University and Canadian Blood Services, Hamilton, Ontario, Canada

Incidence and Prevalence

There are several measures of disease frequency that are used in epidemiological and medical literature. Two commonly used terms are *prevalence* and *incidence*. In general, statistics pertaining to *prevalence* are geared towards the question 'How many people have this disease at the moment or during a specific period?' and *incidence* is related to the question 'How many people newly acquire this disease?' Incidence can be calculated as an incidence proportion (typically referred to as risk) or as an incidence rate (typically calculated from cohort studies with long-term follow-up). Definitions of these terms and their calculations are summarised in Figure 47.1.

Statistics in Diagnostic Testing

A perfect diagnostic test would always identify patients as positive if they have the disease and would always be negative in patients without a disease. Unfortunately, the perfect diagnostic test rarely occurs in medical practice. There is typically variation in valid test results for both patients with and without a disease and, a certain degree of overlap between the two.

To help clinicians using diagnostic tests for clinical management, statistics are used to describe the accuracy characteristics of the test, derived from a 2×2 table with the test results generally on the y-axis (positive or negative) and disease/outcome (present or absent) generally on the x-axis (Table 47.1). Disease status is typically categorised by a test termed the 'gold standard'. Table 47.2 defines the characteristics that describe various aspects of a diagnostic test and their calculations. The terms most commonly used in the literature are sensitivity and specificity, where a test with a high sensitivity can be used to rule out disease if negative and a test with a high specificity can be used to rule in disease if positive. An example from the literature is demonstrated in Table 47.3.

Statistics used in diagnostic testing can assist clinicians in determining the probability of disease after the results of diagnostic testing are received. The pretest probability of having disease is often the prevalence of the disease in the population, if there are no other factors to adjust the pretest probability. With knowledge of the pretest probability, the result of the diagnostic test and the likelihood ratio of that test (defined in Table 47.4), the post-test

Practical Transfusion Medicine, Fifth Edition. Edited by Michael F. Murphy, David J. Roberts and Mark H. Yazer.
© 2017 John Wiley & Sons Ltd. Published 2017 by John Wiley & Sons Ltd.

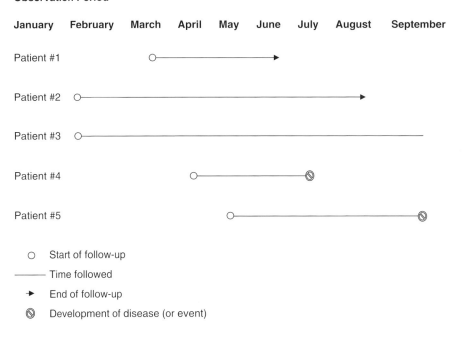

Observation Period

	January	February	March	April	May	June	July	August	September

Patient #1

Patient #2

Patient #3

Patient #4

Patient #5

○   Start of follow-up

──   Time followed

➔   End of follow-up

◎   Development of disease (or event)

Measure	Formula	Example
Point prevalence	New and existing cases/total population(at a <u>specific time point</u>)	Point prevalence in July: 1 case/5 patients = 20%
Period prevalence	New and existing cases/total population (in a <u>specific period of time</u>)	Period prevalence from January to September: 2 cases/5 patients = 40%
Incidence proportion	New cases within a time period/total population at risk <u>within a time period</u>	Incidence proportion from January to September: 2 case/5 patients = 40%
Incidence rate	New cases within a time period/<u>total person-time of observation of those at risk</u>	Incidence rate from January to September: 2 cases/(3 person-months + 7 + 8 + 3 + 4) = 2 cases/25 person-months

Figure 47.1   Measurements of disease/case frequency.

Table 47.1   Example of a 2 × 2 table for diagnostic tests.

		Disease (often categorised by a test result considered the gold standard)	
		Present	Absent
Test result	Positive	A: True positives	B: False positives
	Negative	C: False negatives	D: True negatives

Table 47.2 Statistical terms used for diagnostic testing.

Descriptive statistic	Definition	Method of calculation
Sensitivity	The proportion of positives identified of those who have the disease. Tests with high sensitivity are commonly used for ruling out disease if negative (if the test is negative, the rate of false negatives is low)	True positive/(true positive + false negative) A/(A + C)
Specificity	The proportion of negatives identified of those who do not have the disease. Tests with high specificity are commonly used for ruling in disease if positive (if the test is positive, the rate of false positives is low)	True negative/(true negative + false positive) D/(B + D)
Positive predictive value	The probability that a positive test correctly identifies an individual who has the disease. This value is affected by the prevalence of the disease in the population	True positive/(true positive + false positive) A/(A + B)
Negative predictive value	The probability that a negative test correctly identifies an individual who does not have the disease. This value is affected by the prevalence of the disease in the population	True negative/(true negative + false negative) D/(C + D)
Positive likelihood ratio	The probability that the patient with disease tests positive divided by the probability that the patient without disease tests positive. The higher the positive likelihood ratio, the better the test when positive to rule in disease. Excellent positive likelihood ratios are usually >10	Sensitivity/(1−specificity) True positives/false positives
Negative likelihood ratio	The probability that the patient with disease tests negative divided by the probability that the patient without disease tests negative. The lower the negative likelihood ratio, the better the test when negative to rule out disease. Excellent negative likelihood ratios are usually <0.10	(1−sensitivity)/specificity False negatives/true negatives

Table 47.3 Example of a 2×2 table and diagnostic test characteristics. Erez et al published a single-centre retrospective study to generate a pregnancy adjusted disseminated intravascular coagulation (DIC) score, compared to a chart diagnosis of DIC as a gold standard [15]. In 684 women with abruption, 43 had DIC. The investigators used a cut-off score of ≥26 to identify pregnant women with DIC and applied it to those with abruption as a sensitivity analysis.

		DIC diagnosis charted in pregnant woman (disease)	
		Present	Absent
Investigator DIC score ≥26 (test result)	Positive	A: 38	B: 26
	Negative	C: 5	D: 615

Descriptive statistic	Method of calculation	Calculation from example
Sensitivity	True positive/(true positive + false negative) A/(A + C)	38/(38 + 5) = 38/43 = 88.3%
Specificity	True negative/(true negative + false positive) D/(B + D)	615/(26 + 615) = 615/641 = 95.9%
Positive predictive value	True positive/(true positive + false positive) A/(A + B)	38/(38 + 26) = 38/64 = 59.3%
Negative predictive value	True negative/(true negative + false negative) D/(C + D)	615/(5 + 615) = 615/620 = 99.2%
Positive likelihood ratio	Sensitivity/(1−specificity) True positives/false positives	0.883/(1−0.959) = 0.883/0.041 = 21.5
Negative likelihood ratio	(1−Sensitivity)/specificity False negatives/true negatives	(1−0.883)/0.959 = 0.117/0.959 = 0.122

Table 47.4 Descriptive statistics. Definitions and example calculation.

Descriptive statistic	Definition	Value derived from example number set: 2, 3, 7, 8, 9, 5, 5, 4, 3, 2
Mean	The measure of the central tendency of a probability distribution. Calculated by taking the sum of a list of numbers divided by the number of numbers in that list	$(2 + 3 + 7 + 8 + 9 + 5 + 5 + 4 + 3 + 2)/10 = 48/10 = 4.8$
Median	The number separating the higher half of a data sample from the lower half. The median is more informative than the mean if the distribution is skewed	2, 2, 3, 3, **4**, **5**, 5, 7, 8, 9 Median = 4.5 (note that in an even set of numbers, it is the average of the middle two values)
Mode	The value that appears most often in a set of data. The mode is infrequently used in medical research	2, 3 and 5, appear twice. Those three numbers are the mode
Interquartile range (IQR)	A rank-ordered data set can be divided into four equal parts (quartiles). The values that divide each part are called the 1st, 2nd and 3rd quartiles, denoted by Q1, Q2 and Q3, respectively. The difference from Q1 to Q3 is called the IQR. It is often reported by providing the Q1 and Q3 values	Upper quartile = 7 Lower quartile = 3 IQR = 4 Often reported as IQR 3,7

probability of having the disease can be determined. An example of calculating the post-test probability using the Fagan nomogram is given in Figure 47.2 [1].

Descriptive Statistics

Descriptive statistics are used to summarise and describe distributions of data. They are also useful to guide more advanced analyses, which are used to make inferences from the data or to test for differences between groups.

Most statistical programmes compute statistics regarding the central tendency of the data as well as some measure of variability within the data [2]. The descriptive statistic that provides the most meaningful summary of the data will depend on whether the data are normally distributed or skewed; hence, it is useful to create a visual display of the data, such as a histogram or a Q–Q plot (quantile–quantile) [3]. When data are normally distributed, it is appropriate to report the mean and standard deviation. When

the data are skewed, the mean may not represent the central tendency of the data as it is easily affected by extreme observations or outliers [4]. Thus, the median is more appropriate to report along with at least one measure of variability (i.e. interquartile range, minimum/maximum) which provides the reader with more information about the distribution.

Table 47.4 provides a definition of these measures of central tendency, including an example of how they are calculated. Discussion regarding guidelines for summarising descriptive statistics is outside the scope of this chapter [5].

Differentiating Types of Data and Statistical Tests to be Used

Data analysis will always depend on the research question being addressed, the study hypothesis, the study design and the type of data collected during the study. Thought should always be given to the analysis approach during the design

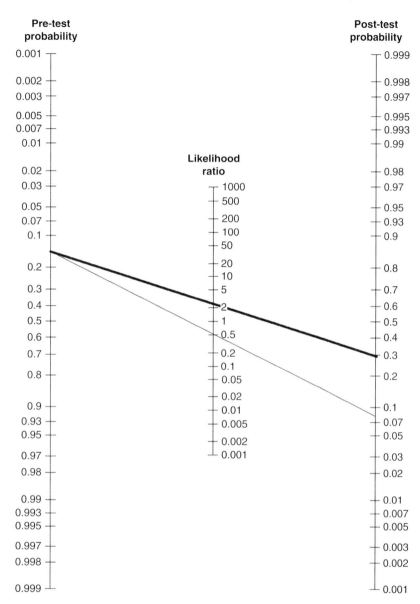

Pre-test probability

Post-test probability

Likelihood ratio

Figure 47.2 Example of the use of a Fagan nomogram. You wish to assess whether a young male seen in your clinic has splenomegaly as a potential reason for thrombocytopenia. Assuming the prevalence of splenomegaly is 3% in the general population, we would normally take the pretest probability as 0.03. However, on history, he has been complaining of early satiety and was referred to you with lymphadenopathy. You assume his pretest probability is higher at 0.15. Now you wish to use percussion of Traube's space (a physical examination manoeuvre) to try and investigate this further. If this test is positive, it has a positive likelihood ratio of 2.21. If this test is negative, it has a negative likelihood ratio of 0.53. The thick line on the nomogram demonstrates the post-test probability if the test were positive and the thin line demonstrates the post-test probability if the test were negative. This patient would have a post-test probability of 0.3 if positive and 0.085 if negative.

phase of the study. Ideally, each clinical study should have a biostatistician who is a member of the investigative team working with the principal investigator during the planning stages of the study. Bringing in a biostatistician at the end of the study just to do the analysis is typically problematic and developing a statistical analysis plan should be done as part of the study protocol. Although we identify some considerations for selecting the most appropriate statistical test to use, there are often issues of which most

investigators without advanced statistical experience will be unaware.

Considerations for selecting the most appropriate test for analysis are summarised in Table 47.5 and include the following.

- Identifying the dependent and independent variables in a study. The dependent variable(s) is/are the outcome(s) of interest in a study whereas the independent variable(s) is/are the exposure/intervention(s).

Table 47.5 Considerations for data analysis.

Independent variables			Dependent variables	
The output or outcome of interest (a variable that responds to an intervention or exposure)			The input or exposure/intervention (varied by and under the control of the investigator)	
Type of variable	Interval	Ratio	Ordinal	Nominal/ categorical
Definition	Numeric scale that has order and intervals between each value are evenly split	Numeric scale that has order and exact value between units but it also has a clear definition of zero	A set of ordered categories	Named categories
Examples	Systolic blood pressure	Weight, height Haemoglobin	Grades of agglutination +, ++, +++, ++++ WHO Bleeding Scale (measured from Grade 1 to 4, with 4 as the most severe)	Dead/alive

Data dependency*	Independent data/samples/observations	Dependent data/samples/observations[†]
Definition	When data, samples or observations are obtained from different subjects and/or samples are not dependent on each other, the data are said to be independent	When data, samples or observations are obtained by repeated measures from the same individual (i.e. before and after an intervention/exposure), the data are said to be dependent
Example	An observational study of acute reactions in 20 patients receiving their first platelet transfusions. Each patient is transfused platelets and followed for evidence of a reaction following only their first transfusions. Each observation (reaction yes/no) comes from an individual patient, thus the data are independent	An observational study of acute reactions in 20 patients receiving platelet transfusions. Ten patients are followed during two different transfusion episodes; the other 10 only receive one transfusion. Data are dependent, as there are 30 observations with 10 patients contributing two different measurements

* Not to be confused with the dependent/independent variables described above.
[†] Requires additional considerations during analysis to account for the fact that observations in some patients may be related or dependent on each other (i.e. bootstrapping).

- Categorisation of the dependent and independent variables by variable type (continuous, categorical, ratio or interval).
- Understanding the distribution of the data.
- Consideration of the study design (i.e. independent groups, before/after, repeated measures, etc.). For randomised controlled trials, the data should be analysed by the unit of randomisation (i.e. if patients are randomised then analyse by patient).

Examples of these considerations for data analysis are listed in Table 47.6. After these considerations, selecting an analysis approach that matches the hypothesis is paramount. For this chapter, statistical tests have been categorised as parametric, nonparametric and regression techniques.

Parametric methods of analysing data assume that the data follow a probability distribution such as a normal distribution (i.e. a bell curve). These methods are not used for data that are categorical (ordinal or nominal) and are typically not used for data that are skewed. Skewed data can sometimes be log transformed to create a normal distribution, an approach that should be done if possible [6]. If the data do not follow a parametric distribution (i.e. the data are skewed or there is no information about the data distribution), nonparametric approaches can be used. Kaplan–Meier estimates are nonparametric and are used for time-to-event analyses such as doing a survival analysis on the results of a randomised controlled trial. Regression analyses allow the investigator to assess the change in the dependent variable in relation to the change of an independent variable, making them a powerful tool for clinical research. A list and brief description of the more frequently used tests are provided in Table 47.7.

Table 47.6 Examples of considerations for data analysis.

Study	ABLE Study [16] Multicentre RCT comparing ICU patients receiving fresh blood (age <8 days) to patients receiving the oldest available blood, with 90-day mortality as the primary outcome	MIRACLE Study [17] Multicentre RCT comparing patients with chemotherapy-induced thrombocytopenia receiving pathogen-reduced platelets to patients receiving standard platelet products, with the 1-hour corrected count increment (CCI) as the primary outcome
Independent variables	The transfusion of fresh or older blood – categorical variable Age (days) is an interval variable but was used as a categorical variable for the intervention in this study	The transfusion of pathogen-reduced platelets or standard platelet products – categorical variable
Dependent variables	90-day mortality – categorical variable (dead or alive) Length of hospital stay (days; secondary outcome) – interval variable	1-hour CCI – interval variable Bleeding defined by WHO Bleeding Scale (secondary outcome) – ordinal variable
Data dependency	Independent – patients in either transfusion group (fresh or older blood) do not affect each other; each patient only contributes one outcome as well (assuming that patients are studied during just one hospital admission)	Dependent – because different patients had different (and multiple) episodes of platelet transfusions, each patient would contribute a different number of events; one patient contributing six events is not the same as three patients contributing two events, requiring a specialised analysis approach to deal with the dependency

ICU, intensive care unit; RCT, randomised controlled trial.

Table 47.7 Commonly used parametric, nonparametric and regression statistics.

	Application	Example
Parametric tests		
t-test	Compares continuous outcomes in two independent samples	A study comparing quantitative antibody levels after vaccination between immune thrombocytopenic purpura (ITP) patients receiving rituximab versus placebo [18]
Paired t-test	Compare continuous outcomes in two matched or paired samples	A study comparing platelet counts in ITP patients before romiplostim and after romiplostim was started (assuming that the values of the differences are a normal distribution) [19]
One-way ANOVA	Comparison of two or more groups where the independent variable is interval or continuous	A study assessing pulmonary hypertension in sickle cell disease patients chronically transfused, nontransfused sickle cell disease patients and age-matched controls (assuming the outcome is in a normal distribution) [20]
Repeated measures ANOVA	Used for analysis of repeated measure study designs. The test requires one categorical independent variable (either nominal or ordinal) and one dependent variable (continuous: interval or ratio)	A study assessing FiO_2 levels measured repeatedly in patients before and after transfusion who have transfusion-related acute lung injury (TRALI) or do not have TRALI [21]
Factorial ANOVA	Used to consider the effect of more than one factor on differences in the dependent variable	A study assessing nitric oxide levels in blood samples with different durations of storage of red cells and different pO_2 levels set by the investigators [22]
Nonparametric tests		
Mann–Whitney U test (Wilcoxon rank sum)	To compare a continuous outcome in two independent samples given the data is ordinal or in a nonparametric distribution	A study comparing the plasma to red cell ratio in massive haemorrhage patients who survived the protocol and those who did not survive the protocol (the distribution of plasma:red cell ratios is expected to be skewed) [23]
Sign test	To compare a continuous outcome in two matched or paired samples when the actual test value between pairs is expressed as <, > or equal to, rather than an actual numerical value	A study assessing whether there was either an increase or a decrease in transfusion requirements (but not assessing the actual difference in the number of units transfused) in chronic myelogenous leukaemia patients receiving splenectomy [24]
Wilcoxon sign rank test	To compare a continuous outcome from two related samples, matched samples or repeated measurements on a single sample to assess whether their population mean ranks differ	A study comparing IVIG utilisation in ITP patients before romiplostim and after romiplostim was started (assuming that the values of the differences do not meet a parametric distribution) [19]
Kruskal Wallis test	To compare a continuous outcome in more than two independent samples	A study assessing pulmonary hypertension in sickle cell disease patients chronically transfused, nontransfused sickle cell disease patients and age-matched controls (assuming the outcome is not in a normal distribution) [20]

(Continued)

Table 47.7 (Continued)

	Application	Example
Chi-square test	To test for significance using categorical frequency data	A study comparing successful immunity after vaccination between ITP patients receiving rituximab versus placebo (provided there are at least five events in each cell of a 2×2 table) [18]
Fisher exact test	To test for significance using categorical frequency data when the numbers in one or more of the cells in the 2×2 table are less than or equal to five	A study comparing successful immunity after vaccination between ITP patients receiving rituximab versus placebo (provided there are five or fewer events in each cell of a 2×2 table) [18]
McNemar test	Used with categorical frequency data when observations are paired/matched	A study comparing seroconversion rates for heparin-induced thrombocytopenia (HIT) antibodies in orthopaedic patients receiving fondaparinux and enoxaparin in separate episodes [25]
Survival analysis	Allows an analysis of how long people are in one state (i.e. alive) followed by a discrete outcome (death). People enter the study at different times and are followed for variable periods of time. Allows a comparison between two or more groups. A common method used is the Kaplan–Meier method, with the log-rank rest used to test the null hypothesis	A study following patients after receiving a massive haemorrhage protocol with a 1:1:1 ratio compared to a 1:1:2 ratio up to 24 hours and 30 days [26]
Regression		
Simple linear regression	Analysis of data with one independent variable and one or more dependent variables that are interval. This analysis assumes that the relationship between the dependent variables and the independent variable is linear	A study assessing in intensive care unit (ICU) patients after red cell transfusion the association between severity of illness at ICU admission (via the APACHE II score) and nadir haemoglobin on the day of red cell transfusion [27]
Multiple linear regression	Analysis data with one dependent variable and several independent variables (interval level data)	A study assessing how different variables (such as platelet age and patient body surface area) affect posttransfusion absolute count increments for platelet counts in ABO-compatible and ABO-incompatible platelet transfusions [28]
Logistic regression	Regression analysis is used when the dependent variable is binary. This analysis assumes that the relationship between the log odds of the dependent variable and the independent variable is linear. Multiple independent variables may also be included in a multiple logistic regression test	A study assessing 90-day all-cause mortality in ICU patients receiving fresh (<8 days) compared to those receiving the oldest available compatible blood, after adjusting for confounding variables such as age, sex, illness severity and coexisting illnesses [16]
ANCOVA	Combines ANOVA and regression (example: can be used to assess treatment effects while controlling for baseline characteristics)	A study comparing plasma volume used in patients receiving plasma prepared with pathogen inactivation and conventional plasma, while adjusting for co-variates such as patient demographics or model end-stage liver disease (MELD) score [29]

Determining Statistical Significance

P values and confidence intervals are often used to determine whether a test result is statistically significant. However, an understanding of all the following terms is important not only for interpretation of results but also for sample size calculation.

- Type 1 error (or α error) is the probability of a false positive conclusion by chance, and is usually set at 0.05. In other words, it is the probability of concluding an effect when the effect is not present.
- Type 2 error (or β error) is the probability of a false negative conclusion by chance – the probability of not detecting an effect when it is present. This value is typically set at 0.1–0.2.
- The power of the study to detect an effect if it does exist is defined as 1–β error. Hence, a β error of 0.1 will result in 90% power and 0.2 will have 80% power.
- The P value is a probability (between 0 and 1) of getting the observed value of the test statistic or a value with even greater evidence against the null hypothesis, if the null hypothesis is actually true. The smaller the P value, the greater the evidence against the null hypothesis. A relatively simple way to interpret a P value is to think of it as representing how likely a result would occur by chance. For a calculated P value of 0.001, we can say that the observed outcome would be expected to occur by chance only 1 in 1000 times in repeated tests on different samples of the population. A P value of less than 0.05 is typically used as the cut-point to reject a null hypothesis [7].

A confidence interval (CI) is a type of interval estimate of a population parameter. A 95% CI is a range of values that you can be 95% certain will contain the true effect in the population. Another way of expressing this is that if the study were repeated on multiple samples, the calculated CI (which would differ for each sample) would encompass the true population parameter 95% of the time. The CI provides more information than a P value.

Multiple Tests of Significance

A common mistake seen in some publications is the use of multiple tests of significance using the same data. As stated previously, if we took a set of data and performed a single test of significance with the type 1 error set at 0.05, the probability of obtaining a significant result by chance would be 5% or 1 in every 20 tests performed. If three tests of significance are done and each uses a P value of 0.05, now the probability of obtaining at least one statistically significant test result by chance would be 14%, calculated as $1 - (1 - 0.05)$ [3]. This reflects the higher probability of a false positive finding if more tests of significance are used on the same dataset.

This mistake is frequently seen in baseline characteristic data reported from a randomised controlled trial where many different variables are compared with individual tests of significance. In this example, randomisation should have provided balance between the two treatment groups and if the test on a variable is statistically significant, it would simply be due to chance.

To deal with multiple tests of significance, statistical approaches that adjust the P value based on the number of tests performed are used. The Bonferroni correction is one of the most commonly used methods where the desired level of significance of the group of tests is divided by the number of hypotheses being tested. This correction can be conservative and produce false negative results. Other methods include Tukey's Honestly Significant Difference and Scheffe's Test.

Trial Hypotheses and Common Pitfalls of Interpretation

A well-defined research question using the PICOT format is necessary for the proper design of a clinical study [8]. The question should clearly state or imply the hypothesis for the study. In clinical research, there are three possible hypotheses: superiority, noninferiority and equivalence. Each of these hypotheses requires different sample size calculations, different approaches to analyses and interpretation that is specific to the hypothesis being studied [9].

Superiority Trial

Superiority trials are usually designed to determine if a new treatment is better than an active control (such as current standard of care) or placebo. Thus, they attempt to prove the hypothesis that the intervention will have Δ_e (the true difference in effect) over the control group. This is the most common type of trial reported in the medical literature.

The analysis for the primary outcome for a superiority study should be an intention-to-treat analysis, where groups are analysed based on the initial treatment assignment and not on the treatment received (the latter termed a 'per-protocol' analysis). This type of analysis reflects what occurs in a 'real-world' setting where there are likely to be co-interventions, cross-overs and dropouts in trials. For example, the effect of a placebo-controlled trial of a new drug with many side effects would likely be overestimated with a per-protocol analysis compared to an intention-to-treat analysis.

When performing a superiority trial, the null hypothesis is that the effect of the treatment is not different from the control group. If the P value of the analysis is significant (≤ 0.05), the null hypothesis can be rejected and superiority claimed. One of the most common pitfalls when interpreting a negative superiority trial ($P > 0.05$) is a conclusion of equivalence or noninferiority that is not valid.

Equivalence Trial

Equivalence trials are designed to show that two treatments are equal within an acceptable defined boundary (referred to as the zone of equivalence). It is statistically impossible to demonstrate that two treatments have identical efficacy. Therefore, the design of an equivalence trial would demonstrate that the observed effect of an intervention, as indicated by the width of the confidence interval, should not be outside a boundary of $-\Delta_e$ and Δ_e (the true difference in a negative or positive direction respectively). The null hypothesis in an equivalence study is that the treatment effect is not similar, so a significant P (≤ 0.05) allows for rejection of the null hypothesis and a conclusion of equivalence.

Noninferiority Trial

Noninferiority trials are often used to demonstrate that the effect of an intervention is not inferior to the comparison treatment, usually with the assumption that the intervention has other ancillary benefits (such as fewer side effects, ease of administration or monitoring or decreased cost). The null hypothesis in a noninferiority trial is that the experimental treatment being compared is inferior to the control. If the P value of the analysis is ≤ 0.05, the null hypothesis can be rejected and noninferiority claimed.

In a noninferiority trial, the boundary for establishing noninferiority (zone of noninferiority) is a clinical decision as to what physicians are prepared to accept as a trade-off between risk and benefit [10]. The sample size for a noninferiority study should generally be calculated with a relative risk difference rather than an absolute risk difference, as this gives a more conservative sample size. A new intervention should ideally be compared to the current or most effective standard of care, or a phenomenon known as 'biocreep' can occur. When a slightly inferior treatment becomes the active control for future generations of trials, this may lead to the efficacy of the intervention getting worse with repeated cycles. This phenomenon has been described by Murphy in relation to platelet product efficacy [11].

Finally, both intention-to-treat and per-protocol analyses should be included in a noninferiority study. While intention-to-treat analyses in a poorly run superiority trial with unintended cross-over, loss to follow-up and nonadherence will produce a negative result, intention-to-treat analyses in a poorly run noninferiority trial will tend to favour a 'positive' result of noninferiority. Results in this situation require careful consideration.

Meta-analyses and Forest Plots

Meta-analyses

A systematic review is a focused literature review on a research question, where articles are identified and selected, and information synthesised together to provide the best summary of the literature available. The search strategy for the literature, the eligibility criteria for inclusion in the review and the methodology for data extraction and assessment of the articles are defined *a priori* before the search begins.

If studies are similar enough in nature in terms of clinical and methodological characteristics and the risk of publication bias is minimal, a statistical summary called a meta-analysis can estimate a pooled 'effect size' of several studies. Typically, it estimates a 'weighted' average across all the included studies. This can aid in summarising literature, resolving conflict in an area of medical therapy, increasing statistical power and identifying gaps in the literature.

The correct statistical model should be determined for the meta-analysis. A comparison of fixed and random effects models is shown in Table 47.8. If it is possible, both fixed and random effects models can be used and compared [12].

Forest Plots

Forest plots are graphs that summarise the individual study results in a systematic review and the pooled effect if the results are meta-analysed [13]. Generally, point estimates of each study are shown on the right of the forest plot around the vertical 'line of no difference'. Although the literature commonly formats point estimates to the left of the line of no difference as favouring the intervention, occasionally this is reversed. An example of a forest plot is given in Figure 47.3.

Often, below the numerical pooled estimate, the consistency between results of the included studies is reported. Heterogeneity can be assessed in different ways. If the chi-square statistic is greater than the number of studies minus one, then there is heterogeneity outside what would be expected by chance. Cochrane's Q Test or I^2 is generally considered a more robust test, given that the chi-square is not robust if studies have very small or large sample sizes. The higher the I^2 statistic, the more heterogeneity and if this is greater than 50%, it indicates that the validity of the overall estimate may be in question. An imaginary vertical line from the point pooled estimate intersecting all the 95%

Table 47.8 Comparison of fixed and random effects models in meta-analyses.

	Fixed effects models	Random effects models
Assumptions	Assumes the 'true' effect of the intervention is similar across studies	Assumes the 'true' effects of the intervention may be different across individual studies
Common example used	Mantel–Haenszel method	DerSimonian–Laird method Consider Knapp–Hartung correction or profile likelihood approach to adjust confidence intervals to avoid type 1 error
Type of model with the inverse variance method	When variance is within studies	When variance is between studies
Advantages	Produces a more accurate and precise result in studies without heterogeneity	Likely more applicable in medical literature given heterogeneity
Disadvantages	Not applicable in fields where there is heterogeneity between studies	Direction and magnitude of pooled estimates influenced more by smaller studies; produces wider confidence intervals

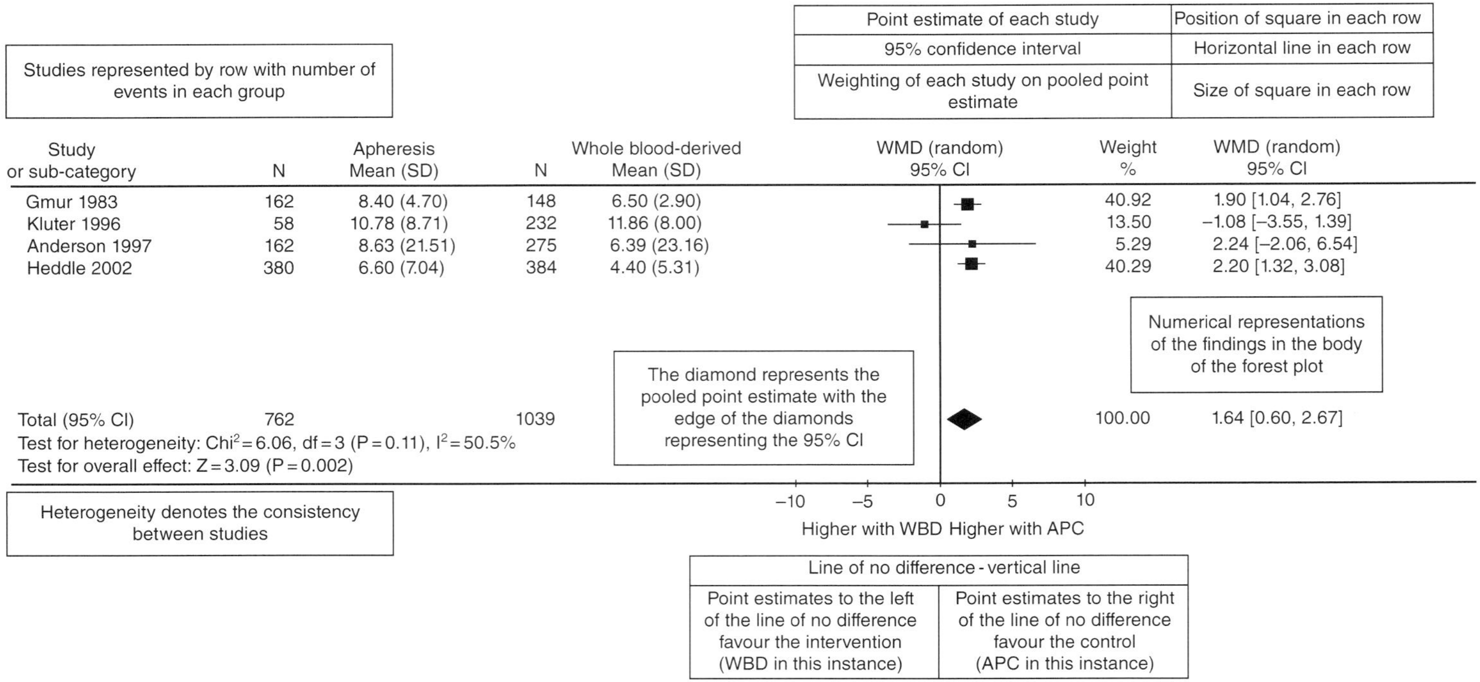
Studies represented by row with number of events in each group
Point estimate of each study
Position of square in each row
95% confidence interval
Horizontal line in each row
Weighting of each study on pooled point estimate
Size of square in each row
Study or sub-category
N
Apheresis Mean (SD)
N
Whole blood-derived Mean (SD)
WMD (random) 95% CI
Weight %
WMD (random) 95% CI
Gmur 1983 162 8.40 (4.70) 148 6.50 (2.90) 40.92 1.90 [1.04, 2.76]
Kluter 1996 58 10.78 (8.71) 232 11.86 (8.00) 13.50 −1.08 [−3.55, 1.39]
Anderson 1997 162 8.63 (21.51) 275 6.39 (23.16) 5.29 2.24 [−2.06, 6.54]
Heddle 2002 380 6.60 (7.04) 384 4.40 (5.31) 40.29 2.20 [1.32, 3.08]
Numerical representations of the findings in the body of the forest plot
The diamond represents the pooled point estimate with the edge of the diamonds representing the 95% CI
Total (95% CI) 762 1039 100.00 1.64 [0.60, 2.67]
Test for heterogeneity: Chi² = 6.06, df = 3 (P = 0.11), I² = 50.5%
Test for overall effect: Z = 3.09 (P = 0.002)
Heterogeneity denotes the consistency between studies
−10 −5 0 5 10
Higher with WBD Higher with APC
Line of no difference - vertical line
Point estimates to the left of the line of no difference favour the intervention (WBD in this instance)
Point estimates to the right of the line of no difference favour the control (APC in this instance)

Figure 47.3 Example of a forest plot. Meta-analysis of the weighted mean difference in the 1-hour corrected count increments of whole blood-derived (WBD) platelets compared to apheresis platelet concentrates (APC). *Source:* Adapted from Heddle NM et al. Transfusion 2008;**48**:1447–58.

confidence intervals can also be used as a rough estimate that the summary statistic is consistent with the results of the included studies [14].

Conclusion

While we have only scratched the surface of biostatistics with this chapter, the concepts discussed provide a framework for the interpretation of studies commonly seen in the medical literature. When performing research, consulting with a biostatistician is paramount to ensure that the study is designed in a way that facilitates proper analysis. However, having knowledge of the concepts in biostatistics ensures that the clinical goals of the study meet the study design and the analytical plan.

KEY POINTS

1) When using descriptive statistics, the mean is generally used when data follow a normal distribution. When data are skewed, the median and interquartile ranges are a better representation.
2) In diagnostic testing, a negative test that has a high sensitivity helps to rule out disease. A positive test that has a high specificity helps to rule in disease.
3) The higher the positive likelihood ratio, the better the test when positive to rule in disease. The lower the negative likelihood ratio, the better the test when negative to rule out disease.
4) The best statistical test to determine whether there is a relationship between independent and dependent variables depends on the variable type, independence of the data and the number of variables.
5) Type 1 error is the probability of a false positive result, which is best reduced by setting the P value to 0.05 or lower when calculating sample sizes. When reporting results, consider using 95% confidence intervals rather than the P value. Type 2 error is the probability of a false negative result, which is best reduced by setting the power of the study to 80% or higher when calculating sample size.
6) If multiple tests of significance are done, statistical approaches to adjust the P value are necessary.
7) A negative finding in a superiority study does not mean equivalence or noninferiority.
8) The following are optimal for the design of a noninferiority study: setting sample size based on relative risk difference, use of an active control which is the most effective standard of care and including a per-protocol analysis.
9) Studies should not be meta-analysed when the clinical diversity is too great, there is a significant risk of publication bias, or methodological diversity is too great.
10) Beware of meta-analyses that use fixed effects models and have heterogeneity. Random effects models may be more appropriate but will still be greatly affected by heterogeneity.

References

1 Grover SA, Barkun AN, Sackett DL. The rational clinical examination. Does this patient have splenomegaly? JAMA 1993;**270**:2218–21.
2 Kandane-Rathnayake RK, Enticott JC, Phillips LE. Data distribution: normal or abnormal? Why it matters. Transfusion 2013;**53**:480–1.
3 Ghasemi A, Zahediasl S. Normality tests for statistical analysis: a guide for non-statisticians. Int J Endocrinol Metab 2012;**10**:486–9.
4 Kandane-Rathnayake RK, Enticott JC, Phillips LE. Data distribution: normal or abnormal? Transfusion 2013;**53**:257–9.

5 Liu Y. Box plots: use and interpretation. Transfusion 2008;**48**:2279–80.

6 Kandane-Rathnayake RK, Enticott JC, Phillips LE. Data distribution: normal or abnormal? What to do about it. Transfusion 2013;**53**:701–2.

7 O'Brien SF, Osmond L, Yi QL. How do I interpret a p value? Transfusion 2015;**55**:2778–82.

8 Heddle NM. The research question. Transfusion 2007;**47**:15–17.

9 Lesaffre E. Superiority, equivalence, and non-inferiority trials. Bull NYU Host Joint Dis 2008;**66**:150–4.

10 Schumi J, Wittes JT. Through the looking glass: understanding non-inferiority. Trials 2011;**12**:106.

11 Murphy S. Radiolabeling of PLTs to assess viability: a proposal for a standard. Transfusion 2004;**44**:131–3.

12 Cornell JE, Mulrow CD, Localio R et al. Random-effects meta-analysis of inconsistent effects: a time for change. Ann Intern Med 2014;**160**:267–70.

13 Hyde CJ, Stanworth SJ, Murphy MF. Can you see the wood for the trees? Making sense of forest plots in systematic reviews. Transfusion 2008;**48**:218–20.

14 Hyde CJ, Stanworth SJ, Murphy MF. Can you see the wood for the trees? Making sense of forest plots in systematic reviews 2. Analysis of the combined results from the included studies. Transfusion 2008;**48**:580–3.

15 Erez O, Novack L, Beer-Weisel R et al. DIC score in pregnant women – a population based modification of the International Society on Thrombosis and Hemostasis score. PloS One 2014;**9**:e93240.

16 Lacroix J, Hebert PC, Fergusson DA et al. Age of transfused blood in critically ill adults. N Engl J Med 2015;**372**:1410–18.

17 Mirasol Clinical Evaluation Study Group. A randomized controlled clinical trial evaluating the performance and safety of platelets treated with MIRASOL pathogen reduction technology. Transfusion 2010;**50**:2362–75.

18 Nazi I, Kelton JG, Larche M et al. The effect of rituximab on vaccine responses in patients with immune thrombocytopenia. Blood 2013;**122**:1946–53.

19 Zeller MP, Heddle NM, Kelton JG et al. Effect of a thrombopoietin receptor agonist on use of intravenous immune globulin in patients with immune thrombocytopenia. Transfusion 2016;**56**:73–9.

20 Detterich JA, Kato RM, Rabai M, Meiselman HJ, Coates TD, Wood JC. Chronic transfusion therapy improves but does not normalize systemic and pulmonary vasculopathy in sickle cell disease. Blood 2015;**126**:703–10.

21 Rashid N, Al-Sufayan F, Seshia MM, Baier RJ. Post transfusion lung injury in the neonatal population. J Perinatol 2013;**33**:292–6.

22 Stapley R, Owusu BY, Brandon A et al. Erythrocyte storage increases rates of NO and nitrite scavenging: implications for transfusion-related toxicity. Biochem J 2012;**446**:499–508.

23 Borgman MA, Spinella PC, Perkins JG et al. The ratio of blood products transfused affects mortality in patients receiving massive transfusions at a combat support hospital. J Trauma 2007;**63**:805–13.

24 Bouvet M, Babiera GV, Termuhlen PM, Hester JP, Kantarjian HM, Pollock RE. Splenectomy in the accelerated or blastic phase of chronic myelogenous leukemia: a single-institution, 25-year experience. Surgery 1997;**122**:20–5.

25 Warkentin TE, Cook RJ, Marder VJ et al. Anti-platelet factor 4/heparin antibodies in orthopedic surgery patients receiving antithrombotic prophylaxis with fondaparinux or enoxaparin. Blood 2005;**106**:3791–6.

26 Holcomb JB, Tilley BC, Baraniuk S et al. Transfusion of plasma, platelets, and red blood cells in a 1:1:1 vs a 1:1:2 ratio and mortality in patients with severe trauma: the PROPPR randomized clinical trial. JAMA 2015;**313**:471–82.

27 Murphy DJ, Howard D, Muriithi A et al. Red blood cell transfusion practices in acute lung injury: what do patient factors contribute? Crit Care Med 2009;**37**:1935–40.

28 Pavenski K, Warkentin TE, Shen H, Liu Y, Heddle NM. Posttransfusion platelet count increments after ABO-compatible versus ABO-incompatible platelet transfusions in noncancer patients: an observational study. Transfusion 2010;**50**:1552–60.

29 Cinqualbre J, Kientz D, Remy E, Huang N, Corash L, Cazenave JP. Comparative effectiveness of plasma prepared with amotosalen-UVA pathogen inactivation and conventional plasma for support of liver transplantation. Transfusion 2015;**55**:1710–20.

Further Reading

Kleinbaum DG, Kupper LL, Nizam A, Rosenberg ES. Applied Regression Analysis and Other Multivariable Methods. Cengage Learning, Boston, 2014.

Mann CJ. Observational research methods. Research design II: cohort, cross sectional and case-control studies. Emerg Med J 2003;**20**:54–60.

Pagano M, Gauvreau K. Principles of Biostatistics. Duxbury, Australia, 2000.

Schulz KF, Grimes DA. Sample size calculations in randomised trials: mandatory and mystical. Lancet 2005;**365**:1348–53.

48

A Primer on Health Economics

Seema Kacker and Aaron A. R. Tobian

The Johns Hopkins University School of Medicine and Bloomberg School of Public Health, Baltimore, USA

Introduction

Healthcare costs within the United States as well as globally are rising, and has also impacted the field of transfusion medicine. In the United States, national health spending is expected to grow by an average of 5.8% per year between 2014 and 2024, with healthcare costs as a portion of gross domestic product expected to rise to 19.6% by 2024 [1,2]. Similarly, blood transfusion costs have grown over the past two decades [3–5], due in part to increased demand for transfusion services, increased utilisation of risk reduction methods to improve blood supply safety and the implementation of new technologies in donation and transfusion [6].

Blood transfusion costs may seem negligible when considering the overall cost of healthcare – transfusion represents just 1% or less of total costs for most conditions [7]. However, the proportion of total hospital costs attributable to blood transfusion varies greatly by disease and procedure. For some treatments, including liver and bone marrow transplantation, transfusion plays a more substantial financial role; the cost of blood products alone for these treatments can exceed $3800 (equivalent to £2300) or 5–9% of total hospital costs [7]. Transfusion-associated complications can also result in costly hospital stays and treatments [8,9].

As our population ages and we increasingly use procedures and treatments that require transfusion, the demand for blood products will likely be sustained. These trends and the associated expenditures raise concerns about sustainability and value in our healthcare system, and have prompted increased attention to the field of health economics. Health economics is concerned with effectiveness, efficiency and behaviour as they relate to the allocation of health and healthcare, and uses rigorous analytical methods to understand the behaviour of the many players within the healthcare system – patients, providers, public and private payers, communities, etc. It addresses questions such as: is technique A or B more cost effective? Or, how have various donor policies or donation campaigns affected the supply of blood and blood products? Or, in a context of a limited blood supply, what resource allocation strategies would help to maximise total welfare? Or even, what is the overall economic impact of transfusion-transmitted HIV infection? Using an economic lens to understand issues in transfusion medicine can have important implications for policy design and, ultimately, for patient care.

How Economists Think about Transfusions

Economists think about how to allocate a limited set of resources given some consumer demand. Health economists can view health as a stock variable – individuals have some initial endowment

Practical Transfusion Medicine, Fifth Edition. Edited by Michael F. Murphy, David J. Roberts and Mark H. Yazer.
© 2017 John Wiley & Sons Ltd. Published 2017 by John Wiley & Sons Ltd.

of 'health', and in the absence of investments, like nutrition and physical activity and medical care, the stock of 'health' declines over time. In this set-up, 'health' leads to some level of happiness, or utility, and individuals choose to 'purchase' some amount of medical care to improve their overall utility, given a set of preferences and trade-offs [10]. Of course, in the actual healthcare market, it's difficult to simply 'purchase' an amount of healthcare to keep up stocks of health and happiness. Health and healthcare are complex, because the market for healthcare is not one where individuals receiving care are fully responsible for paying for it. Furthermore, individuals receiving care often do not know exactly what they are getting, and another agent – a physician, for example – is often largely responsible for determining the kind and quantity of care provided. Still, the framework of understanding health as being produced by a number of factors, including healthcare, can be useful.

To further illustrate an economic perspective when it comes to transfusion medicine, let us consider the blood supply. The blood supply is primarily reliant on voluntary donation – donors may be given small gifts (e.g. T-shirts, pens, cookies) for their donation, but are usually not financially compensated. This leads to a blood supply that becomes a common resource, or a 'common good'. Furthermore, it can result in the problem of 'free-riding': anyone can benefit from use of the blood supply but only some individuals choose to contribute to it. In the United States, although roughly 38% of the population is eligible to donate at any given time, less than 10% donate annually [11]. The NHS Blood and Transplant (NHSBT) in England estimates that only 4% of the eligible population donates blood [12]. Alternatively, if the blood supply were set up as a free market system, individuals would purchase an amount of blood consistent with their value for blood, subject to their own financial constraints.

Although blood is usually donated for free by altruistic individuals, there are significant costs associated with collection, testing, component preparation and labelling, storage, shipping and transfusion. These 'processing fees' vary substantially across different blood products, as well as across different geographic regions and facilities [5]. A costing analysis of four hospitals transfusing surgical patients found a range of red cell unit costs from $522 to $1183 (£344 to £766). This variation can be partly explained by differences in the efficiency and scale of processing and other overhead charges. Additional processing and laboratory testing, as well as a decrease in the donor pool, have also led to an overall increase in the cost of blood and blood products [9,13].

Although the supply of blood remains limited, the demand for blood products in the United States has declined; an AABB study found an 8.2% decrease in the collection of red cell units between 2008 and 2011 [14]. This decrease may be attributable to increased use of patient blood management programs to reduce unnecessary transfusion and associated risks [15], as well as an increased use of surgical techniques and methods that minimise blood loss. A blood management program at Stanford Hospital using real-time electronic best practices alerts resulted in a 24% reduction in total red cell transfusions and a reduction in the number of patients transfused outside haemoglobin trigger guidelines by nearly 50%. This led to savings of $1.6 million (£1 million) in purchase costs per year [16]. Similar results have been reported elsewhere [17,18]. Decreased transfusion could, of course, also be beneficial by reducing the risk of transfusion-transmitted infections and other associated complications.

Economic Evaluation in Transfusion Medicine

Design

The field of transfusion medicine has increasingly relied on economic evaluation in the past several years to help clinicians and policymakers maximise efficiency and patient benefit while minimising cost [19]. These analyses are particularly relevant for evaluating risk reduction methods in blood collection and processing as well as in transfusion, but also for evaluating the patient, hospital and social impact of new policies and management strategies.

Multiple forms of economic evaluation exist, including cost analyses, cost minimisation analyses, cost-effectiveness analyses, cost-utility analyses and cost-benefit analyses. Each of these will be described briefly, including relevant examples, to provide a general understanding of how to understand and interpret these types of analyses. A summary is provided in Table 48.1. Further guidance on how to perform these economic evaluations is detailed elsewhere [19–23].

Cost analyses assess the resources being used for a given program or policy. For example, a blood supplier might be interested in evaluating the overall costs associated with a donation campaign and a subsequent blood drive held in a community centre. This type of analysis might consider costs associated with designing and producing advertisements, training, salaries or compensation for individuals involved in the campaign, rental fees for the community centre space, equipment and supplies necessary for the drive and for donors, salaries for nurses and technicians, waste management, product testing and processing.

While many studies focus on direct medical expenses only, others incorporate a broader set of costs, also including direct nonmedical expenses and intangible and productivity-related costs. Direct medical expenses include the costs of goods, services or other resources consumed for the provision of healthcare. These costs could be associated with the diagnosis, treatment or management of disease (physician time, laboratory testing, hospital services, medication, etc.). Direct nonmedical expenses are costs that are not inherently medical but still associated with the provision of healthcare, including costs of transportation, patient and caregiver time, training of technicians and medical professionals and hospital facilities and equipment. Intangible costs monetise other forms of burden, such as pain and suffering, and

Table 48.1 Summary of economic evaluation designs.

Type of economic evaluation	Outcomes	Example	Notes
Cost analysis	Costs ($)	Lifetime cost of chronic transfusion for patient with sickle cell disease	Cost discounting may be important for long-term analyses
Cost minimisation	Costs ($)	Comparison of cost for hospital to store emergency blood in operating rooms or in blood transfusion laboratory	Similar to cost analysis
Cost effectiveness	Costs ($) Effectiveness (natural units – infections averted, lives saved, cases identified, etc.)	Financial and health impact of incorporating HIV nucleic acid testing in the blood supply	Estimate cost-effectiveness ratio (average or incremental) Effectiveness discounting
Cost-utility	Costs ($) Utility (QALYs, DALYs)	Cost-utility analysis of an electronic medical record check to confirm that a transfusion is appropriate for a particular patient	Similar to cost-effectiveness but using a standard effectiveness measure
Cost-benefit	Costs ($) Benefits ($)	Cost-benefit analysis of alternative blood donation campaigns	Monetises health outcomes

DALY, disability-adjusted life-year; HIV, human immunodeficiency virus; QALY, quality-adjusted life-year.

costs associated with lost productivity account for missed opportunities (in the workplace, in school, at home, etc.) attributable to disease. It should also be noted that different costs are often associated with different individuals within the healthcare system: the blood supplier, the hospital, the patient or the caregiver, for example.

In our blood collection example above, we focused on direct medical and non-medical expenses from the perspective of the blood supplier. If we had been thinking about costs from the donor perspective, or if we were using a broader societal approach, we would factor in indirect costs of lost productivity/wages and any pain or suffering associated with donation.

When thinking about the context of transfusion, it can be useful to organise costs into three categories: 'pre-transfusion', 'transfusion' and 'post-transfusion' (Figure 48.1) [20]. Each of these stages consists of several distinct processes, all associated with costs, and the costs within each stage can be further classified into the categories described above: 'direct medical', 'direct non-medical' and 'intangible/productivity'. Furthermore, each cost can be associated with specific individuals or groups involved in transfusion.

In addition, when conducting cost analyses (or any economic evaluation) over a period of years, outcomes may need to be discounted. Discounting incorporates the understanding

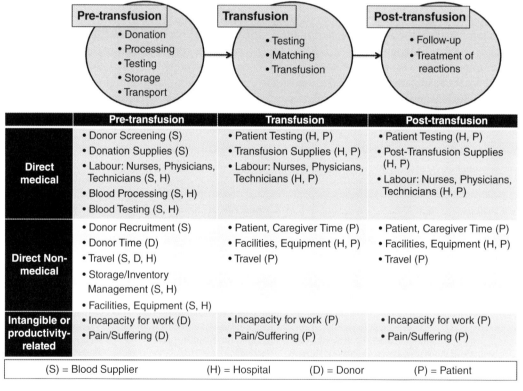

Figure 48.1 Representative costs associated with transfusion. Costs associated with transfusion can be categorised by the order in which they are experienced: pre-transfusion, transfusion and post-transfusion. Within each of these categories, direct medical, direct nonmedical and intangible costs are borne by donors (D), blood suppliers (S), hospitals (H) and patients (P). For hospitals that both collect and transfuse blood products, both the supplier and hospital costs would be incorporated. An economic evaluation may choose to focus on one of these perspectives and some or all of these cost categories. *Source:* Kacker et al. 2013 [20]. Reproduced with permission of John Wiley and Sons.

that costs experienced in the future are worth less than those experienced today. This is because, given a choice, humans prefer to have an increase in money or health now, rather than later. While there is some debate over the value of discounting health effects (effectiveness, utility), it is generally accepted that future costs should generally be discounted at a rate of 3% per year [24]. Monetary outcomes also need to be expressed using a common base year (i.e. 2017 US dollars), and this may require conversion of financial input parameters to a base year. Conversion between costs of different years often utilises the medical care component of the Consumer Price Index [25]. Depreciation of capital (equipment, facilities) may also need to be considered in some evaluations.

Cost minimisation analyses are very similar to cost analyses but compare multiple programs or policies to select the least costly option. While the interpretation of these studies is generally straightforward, their exclusive focus on financial impact may not be appropriate or optimal for clinicians or policymakers also concerned with health impact. Building on our blood collection example, a blood supplier might be interested in holding a blood drive, but with minimal costs, and could use a cost minimisation analysis to compare costs associated with alternative donation campaigns or venues.

Cost-effectiveness analyses account for financial impact as well as 'effectiveness', a natural measure of a health-related outcome of interest. Effectiveness is defined by the research team, and can vary from infections averted to adverse reactions prevented to lives saved to cases identified. Including a measure of effectiveness provides an additional dimension for the analyses, but because different analyses may use different measures of effectiveness, it is not always straightforward to compare alternatives. Continuing with our blood drive example, a blood supplier might want to minimise costs associated with their donation campaign, while also attracting the greatest number of donations. In this framework, they might be most interested in a cost per red cell unit collected, cost per donor, cost per new donor or some other measure incorporating effectiveness.

Cost-utility analyses resolve the issue of difficult comparisons by standardising the measurement of health outcomes in terms of quality-adjusted life-years (QALYs) or disability-adjusted life-years (DALYs). Health utility, in the form of QALYs or DALYs, is not a particularly concrete concept, but is a method used to compare various health outcomes using a single index [26]. The QALY is a measure of life-years discounted by a disability weight, such that one QALY is a year of life in perfect health. The DALY is a measure of the gap between life expectancy in perfect health and actual lifetimes, and is defined by: $DALY = YLL + YLD$, where YLL is years of life lost due to premature death and YLD is years of life lived with disability. Further explanation of these measures and their definitions has been provided elsewhere [26]. Cost-utility analysis is especially common in transfusion medicine literature related to interventions to reduce transfusion-transmitted infections or other potential transfusion risks. For example, transfusion services might be interested in methods of pathogen reduction to decrease transmission of HIV, HCV, HTLV, etc., and might use a measure of cost ($) per QALY to compare alternative interventions.

Finally, cost-benefit analyses go a step further by monetising the effects of a program or policy, making the costs and benefits directly comparable in monetary terms. While this can be very helpful in decision making, the best method of monetising benefits may not be entirely clear.

Model Analysis

Since policymakers, payers, providers and patients frequently use economic evaluation to select between alternative investment decisions, these analyses are often set up as comparisons between proposed strategies (or technologies, interventions, programs, policies, etc.) and baseline strategies, which could describe current methods, or another (generally less effective) option. In a simple decision analysis, only two strategies are compared, but more complicated analyses may involve multiple options.

In the case that only two strategies are being compared (proposed versus baseline), net cost and net effectiveness are calculated for the proposed strategy, using the baseline strategy as comparison. For a given pair of compared strategies, four scenarios are possible, as illustrated in Figure 48.2 [16]:

1) the proposed strategy can be less costly and more effective than the baseline
2) the proposed strategy can be more costly and more effective than the baseline
3) the proposed strategy can be more costly and less effective than the baseline

4) the proposed strategy can be less costly and less effective than the baseline.

In the first scenario, the proposed strategy is clearly preferable to the baseline strategy; it is optimal in terms of cost and effectiveness. In the third scenario, the baseline strategy is clearly preferable. However, in scenarios 2 and 4, the preferred strategy is less clear since the proposed strategy is preferable in one dimension (health or financial), but not preferable in the other dimension.

When a decision involves multiple mutually exclusive proposals, the method of analysis is similar. Typically, the proposed strategies could be arranged in order of increasing effectiveness,

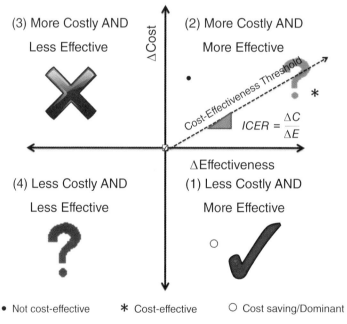

Figure 48.2 Illustration of cost-effectiveness outcomes. Each quadrant of this graph represents one of four potential scenarios resulting from a cost-effectiveness analysis comparing one proposed strategy to a baseline strategy. The lower right quadrant (1) represents a scenario where the change in costs (ΔC) is negative (the cost of the proposed is less than the cost of the baseline), and the change in effectiveness (ΔE) is positive (the effectiveness of the proposal is greater than the effectiveness of the baseline). Any scenario falling in this quadrant will be cost saving and considered dominant over the baseline. The upper right quadrant (2) represents the situation where both ΔC and ΔE are positive. If the incremental cost-effectiveness ratio (ICER), calculated as shown, falls below a given threshold (e.g. $50 000/QALY), the proposed strategy is considered cost effective. However, if the ICER is greater than the threshold, the proposed strategy would not be considered cost effective. The upper left quadrant (3) represents the scenario where ΔC is positive and ΔE is negative. Any scenario falling in this quadrant would be excluded, since neither of the dimensions (cost or effectiveness) is enhanced under the proposed strategy. Finally, in the lower left quadrant (4), ΔC and ΔE are both negative. This is not a commonly considered scenario, since the proposed strategy being evaluated is generally either more costly or less effective than a baseline. *Source:* Kacker et al. 2013 [23]. Reproduced with permission of John Wiley and Sons.

and an incremental cost-effectiveness ratio (ICER) is calculated. The ICER is defined as:

$$ICER = \frac{(C_1 - C_0)}{(E_1 - E_0)}$$

where C_1 and C_0 are the costs associated with a proposed strategy and a comparison strategy, respectively, and E_1 and E_0 are the effectiveness measures associated with each. The strategy used for comparison is generally the strategy with the next lowest effectiveness. No ICER would be calculated for the strategy with the lowest effectiveness. The ICERs associated with each strategy are then compared to determine if particular strategies can be eliminated, as demonstrated in Figure 48.3 [13].

Strategy	Costs ($)	Effectiveness (QALY)	ACER ($/QALY)	ICER ($/QALY)
Strategy 1 (Baseline)	0	0	---	---
Strategy 2	80	2	(80–0)/(2–0) = 40	(80–0)/(2–0) = 40
Strategy 3	160	4	(160–0)/(4–0) = 40	(160–80)/(4–2) = 40
Strategy 4	150	5	(150–0)/(5–0) = 30	(150–160)/(5–4) = –10

Strategy 3 is "strongly dominated": more costly and less effective than an alternative (Strategy 4)

Strategy	Costs ($)	Effectiveness (QALY)	ACER ($/QALY)	ICER ($/QALY)
Strategy 1 (Baseline)	0	0	---	---
Strategy 2	80	2	(80–0)/(2–0) = 40	(80–0)/(2–0) = 40
Strategy 3	160	4	(160–0)/(4–0) = 40	(160–80)/(4–2) = 40
Strategy 4	150	5	(150–0)/(5–0) = 30	(150–160)/(5–4) = –10

Strategy	Costs ($)	Effectiveness (QALY)	ACER ($/QALY)	ICER ($/QALY)
Strategy 1 (Baseline)	0	0	---	---
Strategy 2	80	2	(80–0)/(2–0) = 40	(80–0)/(2–0) = 40
Strategy 4	150	5	(150–0)/(5–0) = 30	(150–80)/(5–2) = 23.33

Strategy 2 is "weakly dominated": higher ICER than next most effective strategy (Strategy 4)

Strategy	Costs ($)	Effectiveness (QALY)	ACER ($/QALY)	ICER ($/QALY)
Strategy 1 (Baseline)	0	0	---	---
Strategy 2	80	2	(80–0)/(2–0) = 40	(80–0)/(2–0) = 40
Strategy 4	150	5	(150–0)/(5–0) = 30	(150–80)/(5–2) = 23.33

ACER = average cost–effectiveness ratio (Calculated using Strategy 1 as comparison group)

ICER = incremental cost–effectiveness ratio (Calculated using strategy with next lowest effectiveness as comparison group)

Figure 48.3 Illustration of example calculations and comparisons for cost-effectiveness ratios. In this example, the decision involves four mutually exclusive strategies, where Strategy 1 represents a baseline, and Strategies 2–4 represent alternative proposals. Costs and effectiveness are shown for each of these strategies, and the proposed strategies are arranged in order of increasing effectiveness. The average cost-effectiveness ratio (ACER) for Strategies 2–4 is calculated using Strategy 1 as comparison group, while the incremental cost-effectiveness ratio (ICER) is calculated using the next lowest effectiveness strategy as the comparison (Strategy 4 uses Strategy 3 as comparison, Strategy 3 uses Strategy 2 as comparison and Strategy 2 uses Strategy 1 as comparison). The ICER values are then compared to determine if particular strategies can be eliminated. The top table shows that Strategy 3 is 'strongly dominated' by Strategy 4: Strategy 3 is less effective and more costly than Strategy 4. Thus, Strategy 4 is clearly preferable to Strategy 3, and we eliminate Strategy 3 from our list of potential strategies (second table). The ICERs are then recalculated, using Strategy 2 as the comparison group (next lower effectiveness) for Strategy 4. These results show that Strategy 2 is 'weakly dominated' by Strategy 4: the ICER for Strategy 4 is less than the ICER for Strategy 2 (third table). This indicates that the marginal cost of obtaining the effectiveness associated with Strategy 2 is greater than the marginal cost of an alternative. Strategy 2 is thus eliminated (fourth table). *Source:* Kacker et al. 2013 [20]. Reproduced with permission of John Wiley and Sons.

A generally accepted threshold for 'cost effectiveness' is somewhere between $50 000 (£32 000) and $100 000 (£64 000)/QALY. The World Health Organization also supports using an income-dependent measure of three times the per capita gross domestic product [27]. The role of these threshold values in transfusion medicine policy remains somewhat unclear; expanded donor blood screening for HIV-1 using p24 antigen testing or nucleic acid testing has been shown to not be cost effective in the context of most other medical interventions [28], but is still widely implemented. One study suggested that in the United States, nucleic acid testing for HIV, HCV and HBV in whole-blood donations is expected to cost between $4.7 million (£3 million) and $11.2 million (£7.2 million) per QALY saved [29,30].

Economic evaluations can also be incorporated into more complex models. Markov models, for example, are frequently used in scenarios where a process is recurrent or involves multiple stages or phases, such as chronic transfusion therapy or screening for infection at fixed intervals. Markov models are state transition models defined by a set of mutually exclusive states – each can be associated with certain costs and effectiveness – and a set of transition probabilities between those states. Further description on these models is provided elsewhere [24].

Unrealistic assumptions in an economic evaluation can frequently lead to unreliable results, making it particularly important to keep in mind general guidelines for economic evaluations and to clearly report assumptions and methods, in addition to uncertainty. Nearly every parameter incorporated in a model – costs, probabilities, effectiveness measures – comes with some uncertainty or may vary over the time period analysed, and this uncertainty may affect the robustness of outcomes. Thus, any economic evaluation should address the impact of uncertainty in parameter estimates on reported outcomes. One-way sensitivity analysis is a method of varying only one input parameter (holding all other parameters fixed at 'base-case values') and reporting the resulting range in the outcome variable. A tornado diagram can be generated from a series of one-way sensitivity analyses, each varying a different parameter [23]. Two-way sensitivity analysis is also possible to modify two variables simultaneously. The extent of variation in the input parameters should reflect a range of generally realistic values.

Probabilistic sensitivity analysis is an additional method to vary multiple input parameters at one time. Each input parameter to be varied is described by a distribution (uniform, triangular, Beta, normal, etc.), depending on its characteristics, and a value for each parameter is randomly selected from the appropriate distributions. The distribution underlying any input parameter is often unknown, and must be assumed by the research team based on expectations about the relative likelihood of different values for any particular variable.

Conclusion

Health economics, and especially economic evaluation, is becoming increasingly relevant in transfusion medicine. While it has previously been suggested that transfusion medicine is somehow different from other areas of healthcare in that, as a society, we are willing to spend more for a given health improvement related to blood safety than we are willing to spend for a similar health improvement in other areas [31], costs are rising, demand is persisting despite implementation of patient blood management measures and budgets are increasingly proving to be restrictive. Applying the tools of health economics to transfusion medicine can and will be increasingly valuable.

KEY POINTS

1) Healthcare costs worldwide are rising, and the field of transfusion medicine is not isolated from these changes.

2) Health economics is concerned with effectiveness, efficiency and behaviour as they relate to the allocation of health and healthcare, and uses rigorous analytical methods to understand the behaviour of the many players within the healthcare system – patients, providers, public and private payers, communities, etc.

3) The field of transfusion medicine is increasingly relying on economic evaluation to help clinicians and policymakers maximise efficiency and patient benefit while minimising cost.

4) Multiple forms of economic evaluation exist, including cost analyses, cost minimisation

analyses, cost-effectiveness analyses, cost-utility analyses and cost-benefit analyses.

5) In the context of transfusion, it can be useful to organise costs into three categories ('pre-transfusion', 'transfusion' and 'post-transfusion') and important to pay careful attention to which individuals or groups are affected by each cost.

6) Policymakers, payers, providers and patients may use economic evaluation to decide between alternative investments, and may incorporate this evaluation into different models to structure these comparisons.

7) Health economics, and especially economic evaluation, is becoming increasingly relevant in transfusion medicine. Applying the tools of health economics to transfusion medicine can and will be increasingly valuable.

References

1 Keehan SP, Cuckler GA, Sisko AM et al. National Health Expenditure Projections, 2014–24: spending growth faster than recent trends. Health Affairs 2015;**34**:1407–17.

2 McCarthy M. US healthcare spending will reach 20% of GDP by 2024, says report. BMJ 2015;**351**:h4204.

3 Varney SJ, Guest JF. The annual cost of blood transfusions in the UK. Transfus Med 2003;**13**:205–18.

4 Amin M, Fergusson D, Aziz A, Wilson K, Coyle D, Hebert P. The cost of allogeneic red blood cells – a systematic review. Transfus Med 2003;**13**:275–85.

5 Shander A, Hofmann A, Ozawa S, Theusinger OM, Gombotz H, Spahn DR. Activity-based costs of blood transfusions in surgical patients at four hospitals. Transfusion 2010;**50**:753–65.

6 Custer B, Hoch JS. Cost-effectiveness analysis: what it really means for transfusion medicine decision making. Transfus Med Rev 2009;**23**:1–12.

7 Jefferies LC, Sachais BS, Young DS. Blood transfusion costs by diagnosis-related groups in 60 university hospitals in 1995. Transfusion 2001;**41**:522–9.

8 Blumberg N. Allogeneic transfusion and infection: economic and clinical implications. Semin Hematol 1997;**34**:34–40.

9 Shander A, Hofmann A, Gombotz H, Theusinger OM, Spahn DR. Estimating the cost of blood: past, present, and future directions. Best Pract Res Clin Anaesthesiol 2007;**21**:271–89.

10 Mankiw NG. Principles of Economics, 7th edn. Cengage Learning, Stamford, 2015.

11 American Red Cross. Blood facts and statistics. Available at: wwwredcrossbloodorg/learn-about-blood/blood-facts-and-statistics (accessed 22 November 2016).

12 NHS Blood and Transplant. New NHSBT research reveals 20% drop in young donors in the last decade. Available at: www.nhsbt.nhs.uk/news-and-media/news-archive/news_2011_06_14.asp (accessed 22 November 2016).

13 Toner RW, Pizzi L, Leas B, Ballas SK, Quigley A, Goldfarb NI. Costs to hospitals of acquiring and processing blood in the US: a survey of hospital-based blood banks and transfusion services. Appl Health Economics Health Policy 2011;**9**:29–37.

14 Department of Health and Human Services. The 2011 National Blood Collection and Utilization Survey Report. Available at: www.aabb.org/research/hemovigilance/bloodsurvey/Documents/11-nbcus-report.pdf (accessed 22 November 2016).

15 Anthes E. Evidence-based medicine: save blood, save lives. Nature 2015;**520**:24–6.

16 Goodnough LT, Shieh L, Hadhazy E, Cheng N, Khari P, Maggio P. Improved blood utilization using real-time clinical decision support. Transfusion 2014;**54**:1358–65.

17 Mehra T, Seifert B, Bravo-Reiter S et al. Implementation of a patient blood management monitoring and feedback program significantly reduces transfusions and costs. Transfusion 2015;**55**:2807–15.

18 Frank SM, Oleyar MJ, Ness PM, Tobian AA. Reducing unnecessary preoperative blood orders and costs by implementing an updated institution-specific maximum surgical blood order schedule and a remote electronic blood release system. Anesthesiology 2014;**121**:501–9.

19 Custer B, Janssen MP, Alliance of Blood Operators Risk-Based Decision-Making I. Health economics and outcomes methods in risk-based decision-making for blood safety. Transfusion 2015;**55**:2039–47.

20 Kacker S, Frick KD, Tobian AA. The costs of transfusion: economic evaluations in transfusion medicine, Part 1. Transfusion 2013;**53**:1383–5.

21 Kacker S, Frick KD, Tobian AA. Establishing a framework: economic evaluations in transfusion medicine, part 2. Transfusion 2013;**53**:1634–6.

22 Kacker S, Frick KD, Tobian AA. Constructing a model: economic evaluations in transfusion medicine, Part 3. Transfusion 2013;**53**:1885–7.

23 Kacker S, Frick KD, Tobian AA. Data and interpretation: economic evaluations in transfusion medicine, Part 4. Transfusion 2013;**53**:2130–3.

24 Drummond M, Drummond M. Methods for the Economic Evaluation of Health Care Programmes, 3rd edn. Oxford University Press, Oxford, 2005.

25 United States Department of Labor. Consumer Price Index. Available at: www.bls.gov/cpi/ (accessed 22 November 2016).

26 World Health Organization. Global Burden of Disease. Available at: http://www.who.int/topics/global_burden_of_disease/en/ (accessed 22 November 2016).

27 World Health Organization. Cost Effectiveness and Strategic Planning. Available at: http://www.who.int/choice/en/ (accessed 22 November 2016).

28 AuBuchon JP, Birkmeyer JD, Busch MP. Cost-effectiveness of expanded human immunodeficiency virus-testing protocols for donated blood. Transfusion 1997;**37**:45–51.

29 Custer BS. Good evidence begets good policy: or so it should be. Transfusion 2012;**52**:463–5.

30 Brooks JP. Using basic ethical principles to evaluate safety efforts in transfusion medicine. J Blood Transfus 2012;**2012**:407326.

31 Custer B. Economic analyses of blood safety and transfusion medicine interventions: a systematic review. Transfus Med Rev 2004;**18**:127–43.

Further Reading

Amin M, Fergusson D, Aziz A, Wilson K, Coyle D, Hebert P. The cost of allogeneic red blood cells – a systematic review. Transfus Med 2003;**13**:275–85.

Custer B, Hoch JS. Cost-effectiveness analysis: what it really means for transfusion medicine decision making. Transfus Med Rev 2009;**23**:1–12.

Custer B, Janssen MP, Alliance of Blood Operators Risk-Based Decision-Making I. Health economics and outcomes methods in risk-based decision-making for blood safety. Transfusion 2015;**55**:2039–47.

Drummond M, Drummond M. Methods for the Economic Evaluation of Health Care Programmes, 3rd edn. Oxford University Press, Oxford, 2005.

Kacker S, Frick KD, Tobian AA. The costs of transfusion: economic evaluations in transfusion medicine, Part 1. Transfusion 2013;**53**:1383–5.

Kacker S, Frick KD, Tobian AA. Data and interpretation: economic evaluations in transfusion medicine, Part 4. Transfusion 2013;**53**:2130–3.

Mankiw NG. Principles of Economics, 7th edn. Cengage Learning, Stamford, 2015.

Shander A, Hofmann A, Gombotz H, Theusinger OM, Spahn DR. Estimating the cost of blood: past, present, and future directions. Best Pract Res Clin Anaesthesiol 2007;**21**:271–89.

49 Scanning the Future of Transfusion Medicine

Jay E. Menitove[1], Paul M. Ness[2] and Edward L. Snyder[3]

[1] Greater Kansas City Blood Center, Kansas City, USA (Retired)
[2] Transfusion Medicine Division: Professor, Pathology and Medicine, Johns Hopkins Medical Institutions, Baltimore, USA
[3] Transfusion Medicine Service, Cellular Therapy Center, Yale-New Haven Medical Center, Yale University, New Haven, USA

Introduction

Transfusion medicine is a technology-based discipline undergoing continuous change. This chapter summarises recent significant changes and likely future changes to blood collection and component processing, hospital-based transfusion medicine and cellular therapies. Automation, standardisation and a focus on quality and safety will continue to characterise blood component production. Although pathogen reduction technology remains an area of key interest, blood product safety initiatives will require a perspective grounded in cost-effectiveness and informed by risk-based decision making. Patient blood management initiatives have reduced blood utilisation in developed countries, but the costs of improved components with reduced patient risk may be difficult to sustain and place community blood centres and national health service programmes in jeopardy. Increased data on clinical transfusion decisions will allow haemovigilance to improve patient outcomes. Evidence-based guidelines are being implemented and potentially better formulations of blood components, including whole blood and refrigerated platelets, will undergo investigation and implementation if proven beneficial. Haematopoietic stem cell transplantation will need to minimise the toxicities of graft-versus-host disease. Other cellular therapies are exploring immunotherapy against cancer and non-malignant disorders and, in some cases, will justify the extreme cost of these treatments.

Blood Donor and Blood Supply Issues

Blood collection agencies serve society as the link between altruistically motivated blood donors and fellow citizens facing medical, surgical, obstetric and traumatic events. These agencies require organisational structure, mission and vision alignment, skilled managers, compliance with professional and governmental regulations, financial strength for future growth, risk tolerability and strategic planning.

'Saving and Improving Lives: Strategic Plan 2015–20' from the UK National Health Service Blood and Transplant (NHSBT) illustrates near-term opportunities for UK blood services [1]. The plan builds on accomplishments achieved by combining blood and transplantation services into one organisation 10 years previously and the more recent merging of three separate regional blood donor databases into a single national system. An overall £70 million in savings resulted through consolidation and lean

Practical Transfusion Medicine, Fifth Edition. Edited by Michael F. Murphy, David J. Roberts and Mark H. Yazer.
© 2017 John Wiley & Sons Ltd. Published 2017 by John Wiley & Sons Ltd.

process improvements. Economy of scale dominates the narrative that includes enhancing digital communication and connection with blood and potential organ donors, increasing income from diagnostic and therapeutic services, providing expert support for next-generation cellular and molecular therapy and investing in information technology (IT) infrastructure. Importantly, the plan contains key performance indicators for monitoring future initiatives.

These topics are not unique to the NHSBT. Currently, blood services in developed nations face systemic change and financial constraints requiring modern organisational structures. Will they sustain resources to implement new technological advances? Will the donor base remain adequate? Will quality and safety policy continue to reflect the 1980s post-HIV demand for absolute safety or moderate to reflect optimal safety consistent with prudent fiscal management? Will efficiency initiatives dampen 'surge capacity' for events requiring immediate, large increases in the blood supply? We will learn the answers to these provocative questions in the near future.

New Technologies Applied to Blood Donations

The new technologies, discussed below, represent next-generation advances. Implementing them requires fiscal constraint. 'New' must be 'improved' and offset existing costs.

Pathogen reduction (PR) technology, photochemically treated plasma and platelets, carries CE marking and received US Food and Drug Administration approval in December 2014. Previously, in response to concerns about vCJD transmission, the NHSBT provided methylene blue-treated plasma; a pharmaceutical pathogen-reduced plasma product is also available. PR technology inactivates viruses, bacteria and lymphocytes in platelet and plasma products, mitigating the hazard imposed by bacteria contaminating one in 3000 platelet transfusions and the need for x-ray or gamma irradiation to prevent transfusion-associated graft-versus-host disease in susceptible patients. Emerging and new infectious agents, such as chikungunya, dengue and *Anaplasma phagocytophilum*, will be likely inactivated prior to test detection development and implementation, an important benefit considering the thousands of HIV transmissions that occurred prior to virus identification and testing [2].

Cost represents the greatest barrier to implementation. Many see the additional charges as noncost-effective, since transfusion-associated infectious risks are extremely low, surveillance for emerging pathogens is robust and processes for red cell pathogen reduction (needed for *Babesia* inactivation) await clinical trial results and regulatory approval. Proponents suggest PR would result in reduction of infectious disease tests eliminating cost, longer platelet shelf-life reducing outdating and waste and eliminating costs associated with current and proposed newer platelet bacterial detection methods.

Red cell genomic testing appears at the threshold of transitioning immunohaematology from a serology-based discipline to one based on DNA testing. Mounting evidence demonstrates satisfactory concurrence rates between serological test results and those obtained by molecular techniques. Limited examples show feasibility of genomic blood donor–recipient matching for patients with sickle cell disease at the community hospital or regional level [3]. Nationally, barriers include expenses for testing millions of blood donors and patients, appropriate IT systems for storing and pairing patient and donor information and public understanding, approval and consent for the use of genetic information in this scenario. Potential transfusion recipients currently undergo genetic testing for antithrombotic medication effectiveness and chemotherapy treatment. As such, extending molecular testing to include blood group genotyping for these patients focuses and potentially lowers alloimmunisation incidence and immunohaematology reference laboratory costs.

Advances associated with metabolomics research present opportunities for improving stored blood quality. At present, uncertainty exists about currently used criteria and predictability of red cell functional activity. Metabolomics provides the tools for investigating peptide, lipid membrane and red cell metabolite changes under various storage conditions and anticoagulant/preservative solutions. Presumably, this will identify markers that more accurately reflect storage lesions impacting oxygen delivery and patient outcomes or potentially foster matching blood donors with red cell preservative preparations most compatible with their red cell physiology [4].

None of the above will achieve success without robust analytic capacity. All require sophisticated IT systems that link blood donors and patients, blood centres and hospitals, red cell metabolites and functional results and interventions and outcomes. Consistent with the NHSBT strategic plan, next-generation customer intimacy relationships (previously considered long-term, close, personal relationship seeking to understand and fulfil customer needs) will be based on digitally derived analytics that discern customer needs and expectations.

However, the ultimate barrier involves linkage between the centralised system and the 'last mile', i.e. transport of specimens from the field to reference laboratories. Drone transport potentially provides a mechanism for speeding delivery of vital samples.

All of these advances require highly skilled personnel and fiscal investments that favour large-scale enterprise over niche providers, furthering the trend towards consolidation and centralisation.

Maintaining an Adequate Donation Base

In contrast to the above, blood collection will remain a local and regional undertaking for the foreseeable future (possibly to be superseded by synthetic, bioengineered or 'bio-pharmed' cells). Technology will improve the product (and, in the long term, possibly the need for individual blood donation), but cannot replace the current interaction between phlebotomists and blood donors. Will the donor base remain adequate despite the reduced need?

Blood supply adequacy equates to a balance between supply and demand. In 2008–9, demand was 35.1 red cell units per 1000 population in the UK, 32.8 in Canada and 48.9 in the US, decreasing to 30.0, 28.7 and 37.6 in 2014–15, respectively. Forecasts project further declines as the tenets of patient blood management programmes become fully integrated into practice guidelines. These utilisation trends suggest overall blood inventory shortfalls will not occur, as the blood donating 'greatest' and baby boomer generations transition from donors to recipients. The theory of planned behaviour plays a pivotal role in decisions about donating blood [5]. Millennials, born between the early 1980s and 2000s, represent the next generation of blood donors. They appear community oriented and passionate, with values, attitudes and subjective norms favourable to maintaining blood donation adequacy.

Evidence correlating frequent blood donation and iron deficiency coupled with the variable relationship between iron stores and haemoglobin levels foreshadows a requirement to measure blood donor iron status as an acceptability criterion for blood donation in addition to haemoglobin levels. This assumes that low iron stores present a risk to blood donors that requires corrective action, for example performing ferritin measurements at the current donation or repeating them based on results obtained at prior donations, conducting health assessments and targeting iron supplementation based on these results and haemoglobin determinations [6]. Determining the extent to which iron deficiency represents a health issue opens a broader discussion of risk tolerability as a factor in triggering interventions.

Process for Decision Making in Times of Rapid Change and Uncertainty

Risk tolerability, public perception of fairness and related issues reflect upon blood donor eligibility requirements and all aspects of transfusion safety. For example, the revised men who have sex with men (MSM) regulations for donor eligibility by multiple national regulatory agencies, including the US FDA, exemplify changes brought about by scientific advances, changes in public attitudes and acceptance of some, albeit minimal, additional risk. The discussions leading to these modifications identified a need for an orderly public policy decision-making process for deciding 'how safe is safe enough?' [7].

Risk-based decision making (RBDM) offers an option for informing these conversations. The RBDM framework involves stakeholders, includes risk tolerability and evaluates health risks and economic and broad societal factors. It uses an integrated approach that identifies, assesses, evaluates, decides and communicates the decision-making process. In these times of rapid change and high-complexity technology advances, further dialogue seems certain and will likely benefit from a structured process.

Fiscal Sustainability of the Blood Supply

In the UK, despite a 9.5% decline in blood use between 2011–12 and 2014–15, the NHSBT maintained revenues in excess of expenses as a result of excess capacity reductions and efficiency improvements. In 2017, local testing and processing laboratory consolidation that started in 2006 will continue with work transfer from supercentres at Sheffield and Newcastle to Manchester. Samples from up to 12 designated genomic sites are slated for a central biodepository at Milton Keynes. Hospital charges for red cells, set annually through a national commission process, fell from £140 per red cell unit in 2007–8 to £120 in 2015–16. In contrast, in the US, hospitals view their relationship with blood collection agencies as 'customer–vendor'; blood products are just another commodity. The customer intimacy relationship that tied US blood centres and transfusion service professional staff faded into history, replaced by hospital procurement department staff conducting supply chain contract negotiations. Concurrent with the decline in blood utilisation, hospital buying power increased as local hospitals formed alliances, hospital systems grew through regional or national mergers and acquisitions

and group purchasing organisations gained dominance.

In response to this, independent, regional US blood centres consolidated through mergers, acquisitions or other alliances (including group purchasing alliances) to eliminate duplication, waste and excess capacity. America's Blood Centers, a trade organisation of independent US blood centres collecting approximately 50% of the US blood supply, shrank to 63 members from 77 secondary to industry consolidation. To optimise management levels, streamline processes and reduce expenses, the American Red Cross Biomedical Services reduced to 19 from 36 blood regions, consolidating collections, finance, human resources, information technology and manufacturing at the national level (Tony DiPasquale, Senior Director, American Red Cross, personal communication). Unlike the UK, with its single-payer NHS public system, most hospitals and all blood centres in the US reside in the private sector. Cost savings achieved through process improvements and consolidation now translate into lower prices in an intense bidding process for hospital blood supplier contracts to achieve a larger slice of a smaller market. The impact of these efficiency-driven changes on surge capacity, i.e. the ability to increase blood collections in the face of urgent situations, remains uncertain.

Currently, price competition for market share affects US blood centre margins (profitability). During 2014, 28.1% of independent blood centres had negative margins; 23.5% had negative margins in 2013 (Louis M. Katz, Chief Medical Officer, America's Blood Centers, personal communication). Most likely, there will be further reductions in excess capacity, more blood centre consolidation and a revised reimbursement relationship between US blood centres and payers, possibly similar to the UK NHS, in which hospitals and blood collection agencies receive payments from a single payer. In the US, this corresponds to the Centers for Medicare and Medicaid Services or insurance companies. Additionally, patient outcome metrics will drive payment instead of the current fee-for-product or volume-based system. Regardless, international differences are likely to converge and transfusion medicine services will join with healthcare in receiving payment related to patient outcomes (value) rather than volume.

Hospital Transfusion Service and Patient Care Perspectives

Immunohaematological Progress

Future therapies will take advantage of the explosion of development in molecular testing of blood groups on red cells and other cellular components that are now applied to pretransfusion testing. Although the serological tests used to identify blood donor antigens and recipient blood groups and antibodies will probably not disappear from hospital and donor centre settings, the capability of these standard testing systems will be enhanced by automated methodology that reduces human testing errors and enhances turnaround time in transfusion services.

Many blood centres and transfusion services will use molecular red cell antigen detection methods to screen blood donor inventories and to resolve difficult patient problems where recent transfusions, autoantibodies or complicated transfusion histories make these testing systems a valuable adjunct to routine methods [8]. With these methodologies, blood centres are performing routine red cell genotype analysis that permits more specific donor–patient matching and will help hospitals to find blood for difficult-to-match recipients. Hospitals will also use molecular methods to better identify women who need Rh immune globulin, avoiding the unnecessary treatment of many women with current testing protocols. Similar systems may enhance platelet transfusion therapy as well. Although prospective matching has not been shown to reduce alloimmunisation for red cells or platelets in the past, even for high-risk patient groups, future studies are likely to continue to explore the utility of prospective

matching; if shown to have value for patients, it will then be determined if the clinical advantages justify the costs of these developments. Enhanced antigen screening capability for cellular antigen systems, such as HLA, may prove to be particularly important for cellular therapies that are expected to grow rapidly in the future.

It is encouraging that a number of investigators are applying immunological methods in animal systems to determine how the process of alloimmunisation occurs and whether there are therapies that could be applied to prevent alloimmunisation or reverse clinically significant alloantibodies in affected patients. Our future transfusion therapies will be enhanced by learning which patients are at risk for alloimmunisation and the pathophysiological underpinnings of alloimmunisation as they apply to transfusion therapy. Prevention or reversal of alloimmunisation to HLA would enhance solid organ transplant programmes where previously immunised recipients are currently denied transplant options or required to undergo dangerous and expensive treatments to permit an incompatible solid organ or haematopoietic cell transplant.

Our increased understanding of immunohaematological principles has improved our capability to reduce adverse transfusion complications. Persistent transfusion problems, such as delayed haemolytic transfusion reactions, TRALI not caused by donor antibodies and allergic transfusion reactions should be amenable to detection and prevention by better use of our evolving knowledge of immunohaematology. It may also be possible to gain better understanding of the pathophysiological mechanism and adverse effects due to immunomodulation, such that we can reduce this transfusion complication for patients.

Complications of Transfusion

As we take pride in this collective record of accomplishment and recent track record in mitigating transfusion-transmitted infections, complacency is not an option; diligence in reducing and eliminating transfusion risks must remain a primary transfusion medicine objective. In the US, there is growing evidence that *Babesia* transmission, chikungunya and dengue infection should remain high on the surveillance list of emerging concerns [9, 10]. A number of blood safety issues will be reduced by adoption of pathogen reduction systems, now available for platelets and plasma and hopefully available for red cells in the future. Even if licensure is achieved, adoption may be stymied by cost considerations if pathogen reduction is advantageous for disease transmission issues alone. If these systems can be shown to reduce or eliminate some donor loss through travel history exclusions or elimination of unnecessary tests, or demonstrate other advantages for patients such as reduction of alloimmunisation or prevention of graft-versus-host disease, the case for adoption by transfusion services will be enhanced and reimbursement strategies will become more cogent.

We are also gaining perspective on the controversial debate of whether older blood has deleterious effects on transfused patients that could potentially be reduced by using fresher red cells [11] Recent publication of the RECESS study in cardiac surgery patients and the ABLE study from ICUs demonstrated no advantage to fresher units compared to blood in the middle of the acceptable storage range. On the other hand, it remains difficult to perform randomised studies of blood near outdate and the studies of older red cells in animals demonstrating worse outcomes remain a large concern. Ongoing research will determine whether the suggested culprits of nitric oxide, microparticles, non-transferrin-bound iron or other biological modifiers can be manipulated by storage systems to reduce adverse effects for patients. Commercial development of new anticoagulants, washing systems or anaerobic blood storage may be proved valuable and implemented.

Clinical Transfusion Practice

One of the positive outcomes from blood safety initiatives has been our response to regulatory pressures to standardise blood collection and preparation processes. Although there are clear benefits in terms of blood safety from standardised procedures, we have become increasingly aware that modifications in the components we transfuse are required to meet the unique needs of different patient populations. These modifications have created an opportunity to test new transfusion medicine concepts and practices with evidence-based methodology [12]. Neonatal and paediatric transfusions have required hospital transfusion services to modify their practices to administer effective therapies in reduced volumes to these patients. Fresher blood components may be required for subsets of these patients, and blood components with reduced potassium loads for massively transfused children will be needed, perhaps prepared with potassium-reducing filters or better systems of cell washing. The availability of recombinant coagulation factors has revolutionised the care of haemophilia, and recently developed formulations with longer half-life should enhance care. In a similar manner, new factors such as recombinant factor VIIa will continue to be introduced for broader patient groups with acute haemorrhage, but concerns about efficacy, toxicity and costs for these agents make the availability of yet to be released newer recombinant proteins subject to prospective analysis and discussion.

We now recognise that our approaches to patients with massive blood loss require rethinking. Data from the military suggested that early resuscitation using large volumes of plasma can save lives, leading to the development of massive transfusion protocols in hospitals with red cells, plasma and platelets being administered in a 1:1:1 ratio [13]. These practices are now being extended to other patients with major haemorrhage who clearly require red cell support. It may be time to go back to the future and reinstitute the use of whole blood for these indications. Most of us incorrectly learned that whole blood does not provide platelet support, but recent data demonstrate that whole blood stored in the cold maintains adequate functional platelets for 10–14 days. Whole blood provided from donors with low anti-A titres or filtered to remove isohaemagglutinins may make a better universal trauma component in the future.

At the same time as frozen plasma use is increasing dramatically in trauma, we recognise that frozen plasma is our most inappropriately ordered blood component, commonly used to correct trivial elevations of coagulation tests or prevent bleeding in procedures where evolving evidence has shown no medical value from this risky transfusion intervention. Complicating these issues are the many problems with plasma administration: ABO antibodies that make products unavailable as a universal therapy, large volumes that put patients at risk when acute care is needed, slow processing times due to thawing requirements and inadequate potency for acute haemorrhage or reversal of anticoagulation. Plasma formulations that are concentrated, pathogen reduced and with low isohaemagglutinin titres should enhance therapy for acutely bleeding patients or those who are volume overloaded due to liver or cardiac disease.

Another plasma issue that is now recognised but perhaps inadequately addressed is the role of plasma therapy to correct the endotheliopathy of trauma [14]. In addition to providing coagulation support, it is now recognised that plasma has a corrective role for this important clinical entity and the corrective factor may not be maintained in some plasma formulations such as thawed plasma. Studies are under way to determine what plasma factor plays a therapeutic role and how best to deliver it in transfusion therapy.

Platelet therapy has been enhanced by recent developments such that platelets are widely available, alloimmunisation has been reduced by leukoreduction and managed by platelet matching, bacterial sepsis and other reactions have been reduced and platelet triggers and dosage are evidence based, at least for patients with haematological malignancies. Unfortunately, the advantages of platelet therapy have not been maximised for patients bleeding from trauma or surgery. Recent evidence suggests that the decision to provide all platelets with room-temperature storage may underserve bleeding patients since 4° storage

of platelets enhances haemostasis more promptly [15]. If clinical studies verify these evolving reports, cold storage platelets will enhance transfusion support for acute bleeding and may enable us to store platelets well beyond the current five-day period. Platelet particles or frozen platelets may also become available and provide better haemostatic support.

These evolving medical transfusion issues suggest that the transfusion service will become more important as a source of product modifications, becoming more of a wet pharmacy for blood components. As a parallel development, transfusion services and their leadership will need to emphasise their critical role as transfusion consultants for clinicians, who will be faced with a growing menu of product modifications and new offerings from donor blood or the recombinant engineers. Many transfusion medicine specialists are now actively involved in the patient blood management movement; in addition to its focus on reducing unnecessary transfusions, the clinical interactions that will result should provide better opportunities for transfusion specialists to help clinicians target the unique needs of their patients. As we embrace the growing heterogeneity of products we offer from donor blood, recombinant proteins, cellular engineering and bone and tissue banking, and continue to offer these services with emphasis upon our critical consultative role, the transfusion medicine discipline will continue to grow and flourish with benefits to patients and their supporting clinicians.

Alternatives to Transfusion

The transfusion community will continue to learn from patients who refuse blood therapy, and treatment modifications that provide care to these patients that results in outcomes that are similar if not better than patients accepting blood transfusions will continue to be recognised. Bloodless medicine programmes have emphasised the development of impeccable surgical technique, the recruitment of physicians willing to care for these patients understanding this therapeutic limitation, the use of transfusion alternatives, the restriction of transfusions to lower triggers based upon evolving clinical evidence and the need for presurgical assessments and informed consent discussions with patients well in advance of surgical procedures.

Our enthusiasm for transfusion alternatives will hopefully be rewarded with new therapies in the future. Tranexamic acid use will continue to grow and potentially fill the gap created by the withdrawal of aprotinin from clinical use. The long search for a haemoglobin-based oxygen carrier (HBOC) to replace blood in trauma was impaired by clinical evidence from a major trial in trauma showing limited efficacy and a meta-analysis demonstrating that the HBOC class has adverse effects of increased myocardial infarctions and mortality compared to controls as a result of nitric oxide effects. The continuing clinical need for patients with severe anaemia who cannot be transfused due to autoantibodies, alloantibodies or religious objection will hopefully be fulfilled as increased knowledge of haemoglobin function and nitric oxide effects are applied to modifications of old products or development of new formulations [16].

Cellular Therapy – A View to the Future

The roots of cellular therapy in transfusion medicine began in the nineteenth century with transfusion of whole blood and continues today with the transplantation of haematopoietic stem cells, progenitor cells and whole organs [17]. The development and growth of regenerative medicine as a subdiscipline of cellular therapy has also increased exponentially in the last decade. The use of mononuclear cell-impregnated biodegradable scaffolds to repair and replace tissues and organs, and to restore organ function, has shown great potential in the treatment of a variety of clinical disorders. Some other major areas for future cell therapy research include studies involving chimeric antigen

receptor (CAR) T-cells, CD34+ cell *in vitro* expansion, mesenchymal stem cells (MSC), immunotherapeutic dendritic cell therapies and adipose tissue-associated stem cells. Overarching all of these studies is an ongoing need to deal with the increasing regulatory hurdles associated with initiation and conduct of phase I/II clinical trials.

Mesenchymal stem cells are multipotent, nonhaematopoietic stromal cells present in the bone marrow and other tissues, including adipose, peripheral blood and placental. MSC can differentiate into various other cells, including osteoblasts, myocytes, adipocytes and chondrocytes. Although there are many unanswered questions regarding MSCs when injected intravenously, they are believed to home in to sites of inflammation, post tissue injury; differentiate into various cell types, secrete various biological response modifiers, stimulate recovery of injured cells and inhibit inflammation [18]. There are over 400 clinical trials using mesenchymal stem cells currently being conducted around the world.

As with many new technologies, the initial hopes of success have not always been confirmed with further study. While initial studies suggested that after these various types of cells carried out their repair function in patients, they would persist *in situ*, further research suggested that they do not always persist in the host. Current evidence, however, suggests that some subsets of transplanted T-cells may persist in the patient for long periods of time. Cellular therapies, such as the use of T-regulatory (Tregs), natural killer (NK) and dendritic cells to treat tumours or graft-versus-host disease, currently show much future therapeutic promise.

Chimeric Antigen Receptors/T-Cells

In the past few years, there has been substantial research into the use of chimeric antigen receptors (CARs), as well as research into the use of another form of gene-modified cancer therapy involving T-cell receptors (TCRs). CARs are used to redirect T-cell specificity to antibody-recognised target antigens on cell surfaces and TCRs are used to direct HLA-presented peptide epitopes intracellularly. Unlike TCR-mediated antigen recognition, CARs are able to recognise antigen and function independently of HLA and are therefore able to work in any genetic background [19].

The potential for gene-modified T-cell-based therapy to be an effective method to target and kill cancer cells is now being appreciated. While a few initial phase trials using CARs/T-cells have been completed, more than 100 trials are in progress worldwide. In paediatrics, the use of CARs/T-cells to treat relapsing acute lymphoblastic leukaemia was associated with an approximately 90% remission rate in children who had exhausted all other treatment options [20].

Immunotherapies

The costs and time necessary for developing new cellular therapy products are substantial and are often the limiting factors for continuing clinical trials. Failure of cell therapy companies occurs for a variety of reasons, and some clinical trials have not made it past phase II or phase III clinical studies, often due to the inadequacy of the cells being used, inadequate trial design, poor patient selection, slow enrolment or loss of commercial funding. While it was thought that cellular therapies would save money for the healthcare system, this advantage has not yet been proven, as most novel therapies are not FDA approved and are not yet eligible for reimbursement by third-party payers [21]. Once on the market, struggles continue as the initial costs of development and delivery are so high that the price of treatment may be prohibitive.

The rise and fall of the autologous cellular immunotherapy therapeutic Sipuleucel-T (Provenge®) is an example of the challenges faced by cellular therapy manufacturers. Provenge is a cell-based cancer immunotherapy, a form of therapeutic cancer vaccine, used for the treatment of hormone-refractory metastatic prostate cancer [22]. Patient dendritic cells are extracted by leucapheresis and incubated with a fusion protein consisting of prostatic acid phosphatase (PAP), a prostate antigen and granulocyte-macrophage colony-stimulating factor which acts as an immune cell activator. These stimulated antigen-presenting cells then act as a cancer vaccine and when reinfused into the (autologous) patient, induce a response against the PAP antigen, resulting in tumour cell destruction. The development of this cancer immunotherapy was the first example of complete navigation from a phase I clinical trial to approval, availability on the market and associated reimbursement from insurance companies. The phase III trial data, however, showed that its use extended a patient's life only by about four months at a cost of $94 000 per treatment. Due to the expensive cost of development, production, competition from other treatment modalities and the relatively limited benefit achieved, demand for the technology waned, the company was unable to remain solvent and the venture failed.

Nevertheless, this protocol has much therapeutic potential and several other diseases have been targeted using a similar approach. Clinical trials involving patients with melanoma, lymphoma or myeloma are being conducted.

CD34 Cell Expansion

The use of cord blood for haematological transplantation has been increasing. The limited number of haematopoietic stem and progenitor cells obtainable in one unit of cord blood, however, has been one factor limiting the widespread adoption of cord blood transplantation. At the moment, there is no standard cord blood enhancement technology approved or used in clinical practice except for the use of very expensive double unit cord blood transplantation. Multiple methods have been tried to increase engraftment of haematopoietic stem cells. During *ex vivo* expansion, however, stem cells rapidly lose their 'stemness' and their capability for long-term engraftment. Recent clinical trials have demonstrated that cord blood haematopoietic progenitors, rather than the actual stem cells, do expand *ex vivo* and may provide clinical benefit by significant acceleration of platelet and neutrophil recovery [23].

The field of cord blood enhancement/expansion is still in a state of flux. Clinical trials have not shown the long-term therapeutic benefit as determined by stem cell engraftment or whether these *ex vivo* expansion techniques have any influence on stem cells. Whether *ex vivo* cord blood expansion is a viable option in cord blood transplantation, and whether such techniques will become medically and commercially viable, are among the unanswered questions that will influence the future development of this field.

Stem Cell Tourism

Many researchers have expressed concerns that the administrative burden imposed by the FDA regulation of existing cellular therapies may be slowing down the process of bringing these biological products to the thousands of patients who might benefit from them. Others have opined that these regulatory requirements are so burdensome that patients seeking these types of medical care are increasingly turning to 'stem cell tourism'. Stem cell tourism refers to the situation in which physicians and private medical practices outside the US offer patients access to cellular therapies in countries where these techniques can be used, unfettered by US FDA regulation. The efficacy of many of these experimental therapies, however, is unproven and, worse than providing no benefit to the patient, may actually result in harm or even patient death.

The majority of cellular therapies approved by the FDA use haematopoietic stem cells to treat disease. Stem cell clinics across the United States, however, are marketing an aspirated-adipose tissue product derived from a stem cell-stromal vascular fraction (SVF) [24]. The stem cells obtained from this procedure are multipotent and may have the potential to regenerate injured tissue. Although the use of this product has become very popular, the risks are not known and in addition to the risk of harming patients, any medical serious adverse events arising from such treatment in unlicensed

clinics may result in a considerable setback for the future licensure of these stem cell products.

As clinical trials continue and substantial improvements in outcomes are achieved, the utility of these therapies to treat tumours and conditions other than those evaluated in the original studies is being explored. Would more effective use of these cells require that they be targeted to each different tumour type is a question remaining to be answered. Many more clinical trials will be needed to determine if these various types of therapies will be useful as a tool in personalised medical care.

Manufacturing Issues in Cellular Therapeutics

Cellular products from autologous and allogeneic donors are biological materials that are subjected to varying degrees of federal regulations which, however burdensome, are designed to ensure appropriate collection and processing and the safe and informed use of these products in patients. The FDA requires that novel products or products that are greater than minimally manipulated, including cells in culture that may undergo differentiation, cell expansion and gene modification, must be closely regulated [9]. These novel biological cell therapy products are viewed by the FDA as a drug, requiring a similar regulatory pathway to that required for chemical drug compounds or other biologicals. Requirements for use of special facilities such as clean rooms, use of good manufacturing practices (GMPs) and maintenance of high levels of quality control are mandatory in order to obtain licensure permission to release and market these products to patients. Cellular products that are collected for homologous use and that undergo minimal manipulation, such as red cell depletion of haematopoietic grafts or cryopreservation without combination with, or use with, other drugs or medical devices, are less highly regulated [25].

Another limiting factor besides the production cost of these cells is the availability of the specialised clean laboratory environments required to manufacture them for use in clinical trials. Other major challenges for cellular transplantation and regenerative medicine therapies also remain to be addressed. Obtaining adequate numbers of the cells needed for these various clinical trials including procurement by apheresis and/or expansion of the specific cells needed for a specific disease treatment remains a major problem. Complying with FDA regulation for the use of these biological products in patients and establishment and completion of clinical trials with subsequent approval of regulatory groups and third-party payers are required before these technologies can become a standard of care in medical practice.

The participation of transfusion medicine specialists in overseeing and directing these highly regulated areas will be critical for the foreseeable future. The quality controlled cell-processing procedures ensure that the participation of our specialty in these developing programmes still requires guidance from transfusion medicine clinicians. As cell therapy continues to be a major part of our specialty, we can look forward to forming stronger relationships with our clinical colleagues in many other specialties. Despite the challenges, future clinical trials are sure to provide exciting information that will help develop new technologies for the treatment of cancer and other diseases afflicting tens of thousands of patients around the world.

Afterthoughts

We appreciate the editor's invitation to provide this prospective view of transfusion medicine and cellular therapies. We came into the field at a time when transfusion practices were rarely questioned, cost pressures were minimal and the overriding concern was the development of a sufficient donor base to meet the growing demands for red cells and platelets. HIV and viral hepatitis brought this quiet era to an abrupt end, generating a revolution to embrace blood safety as a preeminent cause and generating incisive questions from patients and physicians about whether they really need the blood we could provide and what they might do to avoid the risks. Our track record in enhancing blood safety has been remarkable, but new infections, haemovigilance systems that demonstrate persistent non-infectious problems for patients and conflicting clinical data that suggest that blood transfusions are a two-edged sword continue to perplex us. We are addressing these concerns with clinical trials, innovations in blood component design and expansion of transfusion services beyond our traditional boundaries. As a primary example, the long-sought but difficult-to-achieve accomplishments in cellular therapy are just beginning to be realised and their eventual role cannot be overestimated. There is no question that patients are receiving better components and therapies based upon more accurate testing and getting therapy targeted to their specific needs. *Practical Transfusion Medicine* has reviewed much of the recent history, provides an update of where we are in this expanding field and reminds us of the continuing challenges that we must address. This concluding chapter can only speculate on where we will go in the coming years.

References

1 NHS Blood and Transplant. Saving and Improving Lives: Strategic Plan 2015–20. Watford: National Health Service Blood and Transplant, 2015.

2 Kleinman S, Stassinopoulos A. Risks associated with red cell transfusions: potential benefits from application of pathogen inactivation. Transfusion 2015;**55**:2983–3000.

3 Tormey CA, Hendrickson JE. Routine non-ABO blood group antigen genotyping in sickle cell disease: the new frontier in pretransfusion testing? Transfusion 2015;**55**:1374–7.

4 Zimring JC. Widening our gaze of red blood storage haze: a role for metabolomics. Transfusion 2015:**55**:1139–42.

5 France JL, Kowalsky JM, France CR et al. Development of common metrics for donation attitude, subjective norm, perceived behavioral control, and intention for the blood donation context. Transfusion 2014;**54**: 839–47.

6 Magnussen K, Ladelund S. Handling low hemoglobin and iron deficiency in a blood donor population: 2 years' experience. Transfusion 2015;**55**:2473–8.

7 Menitove JE, Leach Bennett J, Tomasulo P, Katz LM. How safe is safe enough, who decides and how? From a zero-risk paradigm to risk-based decision making. Transfusion 2014;**54**:753–7.

8 Moulds JM, Ness PM, Sloan SR (eds). Bead Chip Molecular Immunohematology. New York: Springer, 2011.

9 Perkins HA, Busch MP. Transfusion-associated infections: 50 years of relentless challenges and remarkable progress. Transfusion 2010;**50**:2080–9.

10 Vamvakas EC, Blajchman MA. Blood still kills: six strategies to further reduce allogeneic blood transfusion-related mortality. Trans Med Rev 2010;**24**:257.

11 Glynn SA. The red blood cell storage lesion: a method to the madness. Transfusion 2010;**50**:1164–9.

12 Josephson CD, Glynn SA, Kleinman ST, Blajchman MA, for the State of the Science Symposium Transfusion Medicine Committee. A multidisciplinary "think tank": the top 10 clinical trial opportunities in transfusion medicine from the National Heart, Lung, and Blood Institute-sponsored 2009 State of the Science Symposium. Transfusion 2011;**51**:828–41.

13 Young PP, Colton BA, Goodnough LT. Massive transfusion protocols for patients with substantial hemorrhage. Trans Med Rev 2011;**25**:293.

14 Kozar RA, Peng Z, Zhang G et al. Plasma restoration of endothelial glycocalyx in a rodent model of hemorrhagic shock. Anesth Analg 2011;**112**:1289–95.

15 Reddoch KM, Pidcoke HF, Montgomery RA et al. Hemostatic function of apheresis platelets stored at 4C and 22C. Shock 2014;**41**:54–61.

16 Weiskopf RB, Silverman TA. Balancing potential risks and benefits of hemoglobin based oxygen carriers. Transfusion 2013;**53**:2327–33.

17 Seifried E, Mueller M. The present and future of transfusion medicine. Blood Transfus 2011;**9**: 371–6.

18 Wang S, Qu X, Zhao RC. Clinical application of mesenchymal stem cells. J Hematol Oncol 2012;**5**;19.

19 Strauss H, Morris E, Abken H. Cancer gene therapy with T cell receptors and chimeric antigen receptors. Curr Opin Pharm 2015;**24**:113–18.

20 Maude SL, Frey N, Shaw PA et al. Chimeric antigen receptor T cells for sustained remissions in leukemia. N Engl J Med 2014;**371**(16):1507–17.

21 McAllister T, Audley D, L'Heureux N. Autologous cell therapies: challenges in the US FDA regulation. Regen Med 2012;**7**(Suppl. 6): 94–7.

22 Goldman B, DeFrancesco L. The cancer vaccine roller coaster. Nat Biotechnol 2009;**27**:129–39.

23 http://celltrials.info/2013/02/18/trends-cord-blood-expansion-enhancement/ (accessed 3 November 2016).

24 Taylor-Weiner H, Zivin JG. Medicine's Wild West – unlicensed stem-cell clinics in the United States. N Engl J Med 2015;**373**(11):985–7.

25 FDA 21CFR, Part 127.

Index

Practical Transfusion Medicine, Fifth Edition. Edited by Michael F. Murphy, David J. Roberts and Mark H. Yazer.
© 2017 John Wiley & Sons Ltd. Published 2017 by John Wiley & Sons Ltd.